FUNDAMENTALS FOR

Ophthalmic Technical Personnel

FUNDAMENTALS FOR

Ophthalmic Technical Personnel

Barbara Cassin, MEd, CO, COMT
Former Program Director
Ophthalmic Technology Training Program
Department of Ophthalmology
College of Medicine
University of Florida
Gainesville, Florida

Content Editor
Latif M. Hamed, MD, FACS
Associate Professor
Departments of Ophthalmology and Pediatrics
Chief, Pediatric Ophthalmology and Strabismus Service
Medical Director, Orthoptic Training Program
Department of Ophthalmology
College of Medicine
University of Florida
Gainesville, Florida

SAUNDERS

An Imprint of Elsevier

SAUNDERS

An Imprint of Elsevier

The Curtis Center
Independence Square West
Philadelphia, Pennsylvania 19106

Library of Congress Cataloging-in-Publication Data

Cassin, Barbara
    Fundamentals for ophthalmic technical personnel / Barbara Cassin ;
content editor, Latif M. Hamed.
       p.   cm.
    ISBN-13: 978-0-7216-4931-3   ISBN-10: 0-7216-4931-9
    1. Ophthalmic assistants.   2. Ophthalmology.   I. Title.

RE72.5.C37   1995
617.7—dc20   94–13135

Fundamentals for Ophthalmic Technical Personnel

Permissions may be sought directly from Elsevier's Health Sciences Rights Department in Philadelphia, PA, USA: phone: (+1) 215 239 3804, fax: (+1) 215 239 3805, e-mail: healthpermissions@elsevier.com. You may also complete your request on-line via the Elsevier homepage (http://www.elsevier.com), by selecting 'Customer Support' and then 'Obtaining Permissions'.

ISBN-13: 978-0-7216-4931-3
ISBN-10: 0-7216-4931-9

Printed and bound by CPI Group (UK) Ltd, Croydon, CR0 4YY

Transferred to digital print 2012

Contributors

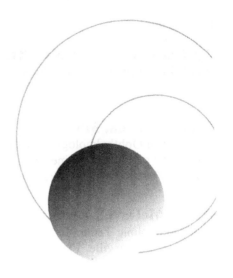

Sidney Cassin, MA, PhD
Professor of Physiology and Joint Appointment, Pediatrics, University of Florida,
College of Medicine, Gainesville, Florida
Autonomic Nervous System

Lindreth DuBois, MEd, MMSc (CO, COMT)
Associate in Ophthalmology, Department of Ophthalmology, Emory University,
Atlanta, Georgia
Peripheral Nervous System

Donald Enkerud, CRA, MBA
Assistant in Ophthalmology, University of Florida Eye Center, Gainesville, Florida
Ophthalmic Photography

Alison Guber, CO, COMT
Orthoptist, Ophthalmic Medical Technologist, Guber Eye Center, Orlando, Florida
Examination Strategy

Eileen Harrell, BS
Staff Ophthalmic Technologist, University of Florida Eye Center; Chief Contact
Lens Technologist, University of Florida Eye Center, College of Medicine,
Gainesville, Florida
Contact Lenses

Charisse Barcelo Hines, CO, COMT, CST
Houston, Texas
Surgical Assisting

David Hodgetts
Technologist/Orthoptist, University of Florida Eye Center; Instructor, University of
Florida Eye Center, College of Medicine, Gainesville, Florida
Biometry

Patricia T. Lamell, MEd, CO, COMT
Ophthalmic Technologist/Orthoptist, Baptist Eye Institute, Jacksonville, Florida
Surgical Assisting

Tom M. Maida, MS
Assistant in Ophthalmology, Ocular Echography, and Visual Electrophysiology,
University of Florida, Gainesville, Florida
Clinical Visual Psychophysics

Donna McDavid, Associate of Arts
Staff Ophthalmic Technologist, University of Florida Eye Center, College of
Medicine, Gainesville, Florida
Biomicroscopy, Eye Disorders

Diana J. Shamis, MHSE, CO, COMT
Assistant in Ophthalmology, Department of Ophthalmology, University of Florida,
Gainesville, Florida
Pharmacology, Automated Perimetry, Eye Disorders

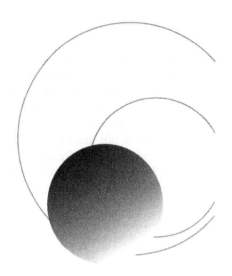

Preface

The need for skilled technical personnel in ophthalmology continues to grow along with technological advances. In the last 25 years, almost 20 formal training programs, mostly at the technician and technologist level, have emerged. Most programs have evolved independently, as program directors discarded lecture and workshop topics that were not successful or necessary for what was required by the job market. What resulted in competent, efficient personnel able to facilitate eye care remained. To a large extent, program directors have had to decide how much of what topics was covered. Over the years, much more has been added than subtracted.

Almost anyone can punch buttons that spit out answers from computerized equipment. Technical personnel, however, can gather better information on patients when they understand what they are doing and know why they are doing it, and if that information is valid. Learning terminology and testing techniques by rote, without understanding the basic principles underlying the data collecting tasks, may result in invalid data. Reading alone, without supervised practice, will not result in reliable testing either. There has to be a combination of all of these factors.

Students always seem to want more lectures and tests, yet their instructors realize the importance of supervised clinical skills development. Monitoring such skills, however, is labor intensive.

The emphasis in *Fundamentals for Ophthalmic Technical Personnel* is on how to perform the various tasks and avoid the pitfalls so that the necessary information is provided to the ophthalmologist. Other tests that may be substituted when the most desirable tests cannot be performed for various reasons are provided. Most ophthalmic texts use terminology appropriate for residents and ophthalmologists, stress diagnosis and treatment, and assume that everyone reading these texts has completed medical school and understands most of the complexities of the human body. About a decade ago, my contributors and I began to formalize material that we had developed as classroom handouts for our own students. As instructors, we had to decide what was appropriate for technical personnel, translate this material into layperson's language, and add basic science information that was required of nonphysicians. *Fundamentals for Ophthalmic Technical Personnel* is the culmination of those processes.

Since many technologist students have bachelor's degrees in nonscientific fields, we have always taught the basic sciences as though students have had no science courses beyond the high school level. Chapters 1 to 14 are especially valuable, therefore, as a reference source for ophthalmic assistants and technicians who are on-the-job trained. This text will also meet the needs of many applicants trained on the job for skills evaluation who wish to better understand the reasons for testing, but who are unable to enroll in a formal training program because of location or finances or both.

We also recommend weekend in-office or weekend JCAHPO–approved continuing education courses, especially if they can be supplemented by assigned reading and discussion. Although ophthalmic technical personnel are not responsible for diagnosis or treatment, with experience they are often able to understand why ophthalmologists make their decisions.

This text is not meant to be totally comprehensive, but it does include enough of the basics to provide a framework for further professional development. It is hoped that this initiation into pertinent basic ophthalmic information will provide a solid foundation for improved quality of data collecting by eye care professionals.

Acknowledgments

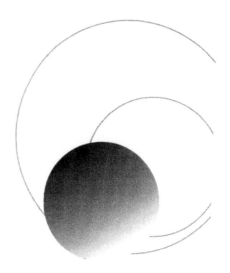

My gratitude to Dr. Melvin Rubin, chairman of the Department of Ophthalmology at the University of Florida College of Medicine, for his continued support of the training programs for ancillary personnel. In the 18 years that I was privileged to be the program director for the orthoptic/ophthalmic technology training programs at the University of Florida, I worked with and helped train over 100 ophthalmology residents, 40 orthoptists, and 70 technologists. I worked with over 20 staff ophthalmologists, especially with eight pediatric ophthalmologists. From most I learned more than I taught.

Some of my best ideas came from students. Many contributed study methods, mnemonics, and descriptions found in many chapters of *Fundamentals for Ophthalmic Technical Personnel*. It is impossible for me to recognize each one individually; however, Barbara Brown Castleman was most helpful in critiquing many of the earliest chapters. She assisted immeasurably in bringing order out of chaos. Her comments brought cohesiveness and relevance to what is included and in what order. Dr. Latif M. Hamed warrants special acknowledgment for his helpful suggestions and medical content editing of this text.

Over the years a succession of ophthalmic photographers—Jerry Hoover, Don Enkerud, Dale Pennell, and Harry Rosa—have made our department's photography collection what it is today: an excellent resource for teaching and lecturing materials. This book too has benefited in no small measure from this invaluable resource. Harry Rosa in particular has provided endless solutions to tricky problems. Kay Barker, our department's assistant photographer, warrants a special thank you for furnishing photographs and working like a detective to find appropriate slides in departmental files.

Most of all, a special note of appreciation to my husband Sidney, who helped sharpen my computer skills in addition to supplying me with love, understanding, and support.

Contents

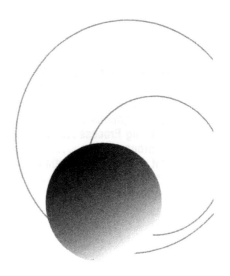

FUNDAMENTALS FOR

Ophthalmic Technical Personnel

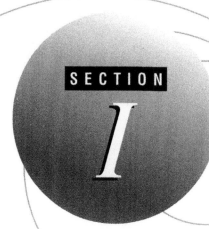

Basic Ophthalmic Sciences

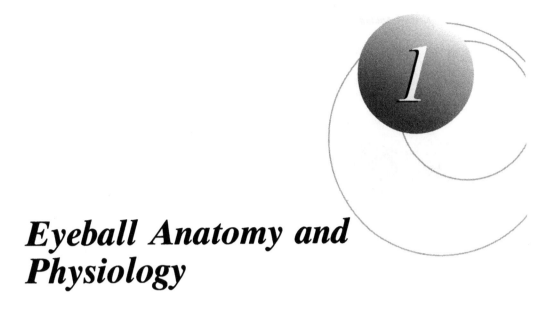

Eyeball Anatomy and Physiology

LEARNING OBJECTIVES

- List the three coats of the eye
- List the three spaces found within the eye
- List the three layers of the tear film from the layer closest to the cornea outward
- List the five layers of the cornea

- Describe the flow of aqueous from its formation to its outflow from the eye
- List those structures found in the anterior segment of the eye
- List those structures found in the posterior segment of the eye
- List the ten layers of the retina

● EXTERNAL EYE

The surface of the external eye needs no introduction, but some of the terminology used to describe it does. The black circle, the pupil, is actually a hole in the middle of the iris, which is the structure that colors the eye. The cornea is a transparent, rigid cover over the iris (Fig. 1–1).

The external eye can be apportioned differently to make different observations. We can describe directions by cylinder axis notations, by likening the directions to a clock, or by referring to other anatomical planes of reference (Fig. 1–2).

● ADNEXA

The orbit contains, besides the eyeball itself, the eyelids, lacrimal apparatus, nerves, blood vessels, extraocular muscles, fat, and connective tissues.

Eyelids

The eyelids, which cover, protect, and lubricate the eyeball, are modified, movable folds of skin and muscle composed of four layers: the skin, orbicularis oculi muscle, tarsus, and conjunctiva. The outer layer of very thin skin extends across the top of the lid margin and connects the inner conjunctival layer near the posterior edge of the lid margin at a junction called the gray line. The skin portion of the margin contains the eyelashes embedded in hair shaft follicles and openings for oily Zeiss's glands. Meibomian gland openings are found just behind the gray line. Sensation from the upper eyelid comes from the ophthalmic division (V_1) of the 5th (trigeminal) cranial nerve (CN V), but sensation from the lower eyelid comes from the maxillary division (V_2) of the same nerve. Near the medial (inner) canthus in both upper and lower eyelids are the puncta, holes marking the beginning of the nasolacrimal drainage system.

The palpebral fissure is the almond-shaped opening from the upper to the lower lid margin. The orbicularis oculi muscle lies just beneath the skin layer, encircling the palpebral fissure in a sphincter-like fashion. Innervated by the 7th (facial) cranial nerve (CN VII), it closes the eyelids. The palpebral portion of the orbicularis causes blinking. The outer orbital portion functions for forcible lid closure (Fig. 1–3).

When the eye is open, the upper eyelid creases and forms a lid fold for the excess tissue. The crease is created by attachments from the levator muscle to the front of the orbicularis muscle. The crease approximates the upper border of the tarsus. The levator

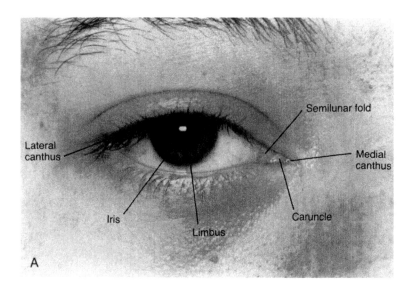

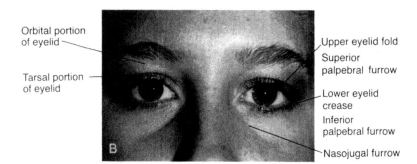

FIGURE 1–1. External topography. *A,* Eyeball. *B,* Eyelids. *C,* Medial canthal area.

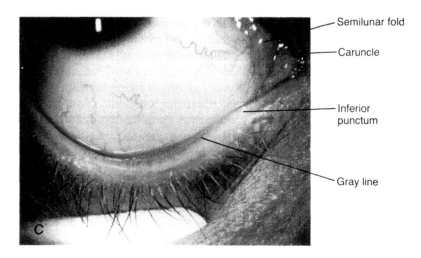

moves the eyelid about 15 mm as the eye moves from looking straight down to straight up. Lack of an upper eyelid fold indicates poor levator function. Lack of an upper eyelid crease indicates no levator function. The levator is controlled by the superior division of the 3rd (oculomotor) cranial nerve (CN III).

The tarsus is a rigid plate of fibrous tissue underneath the orbicularis, giving the eyelid its form and firmness at the lid margin. The orbital septum provides the front barrier against spread of superficial infection or hemorrhage into the orbit and attaches to the tarsal plate that also contains the oily meibomian glands. The tarsus is the primary site of insertion of the levator muscle (levator palpebrae superioris) that opens the upper eyelid. Müller's muscle is innervated by sympathetic fibers and acts as an accessory lid elevator. It inserts into the upper edge of the tarsal plate in the upper eyelid just above the conjunctiva of the eyelid (Fig. 1–4).

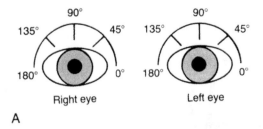

A

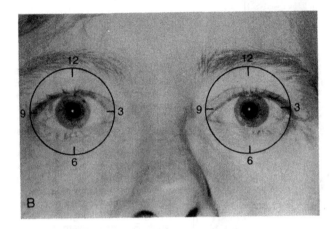

B

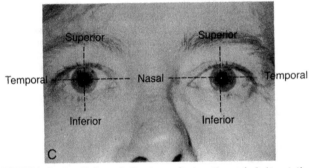

C

FIGURE 1–2. *A* to *C*, Descriptive terms for locations. *A*, Axis notation as used for cylindrical refractive errors. *B*, Defining location in terms of clock hours. *C*, Defining location in terms of quadrants.

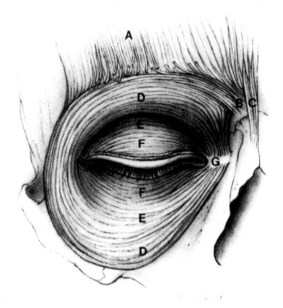

FIGURE 1–3. Orbicularis oculi muscle. D = orbital portion of the orbicularis, E = pre-septal, F = pretarsal, G = medial canthal tendon. E and F together form the palpebral portion of the orbicularis. The following muscles surround the orbicularis: A = frontalis muscle, B = corrugator superciliaris muscle, C = procerus muscle. (Courtesy of Crowell Beard, M.D.)

Lacrimal Apparatus

Tears are secreted by the lacrimal gland, which lies against the lacrimal fossa in the upper outer aspect of the orbit near the front margin. Tears empty into the superior fornix through 10 to 12 fine ducts, flowing across the eye by the blinking action of the eyelids. The drainage system begins at the superior and inferior punctal openings at the head of the superior and inferior canaliculi. The two canaliculi join as the common canaliculus, then drain through the Rosenmüller's valve into the lacrimal sac next to the nose. This opens into the lacrimal duct before it opens into the nose underneath the inferior turbinate by way of Hasner's valve.

Blinking creates a negative pressure by shortening the canaliculus and expanding the lacrimal sac, thus drawing tears into it. Opening the eye produces positive pressure as the sac collapses and forces fluid into the nose. The blink also serves to sweep "old" tears into the nasolacrimal pump system (Fig. 1–5).

Innervations responsible for tear secretion are complex. Reflex tearing from strong odors, bright light, or eye irritation originates from afferent stimulation of the ophthalmic division (V_1) of the 5th (trigeminal) cranial nerve (CN V). Schirmer's test measures reflex tearing.

Efferent innervation of the lacrimal gland is both parasympathetic and sympathetic. The efferent parasympathetic is more important, occurring as the greater superficial petrosal branch, part of the 7th (facial) cranial nerve (CN VII), which merges with sympathetic fibers traveling with the maxillary division (V_2) of CN V, before joining the lacrimal nerve. Parasympathetic innervation to the lacrimal gland may be responsible

The conjunctiva is a thin mucous membrane that lines the inner surface of the eyelid (palpebral portion) and overlies the anterior sclera of the eyeball (bulbar portion). The junction of these two portions is the fornix (cul-de-sac). The very thin, transparent bulbar portion moves freely except at its juncture with the cornea at the limbus. When blinking, the conjunctiva acts to reduce friction on the eyeball.

The crescent-shaped semilunar fold, or plica, and a reddish fleshy mound, or caruncle, adjacent to the inner canthus, are composed of modified tissue. The former is a fold of the conjunctiva containing goblet cells and the latter modified skin containing sebaceous and sweat glands.

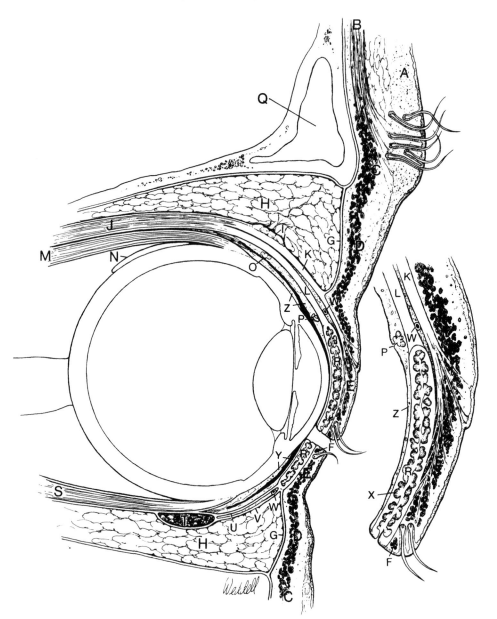

FIGURE 1–4. Schematic cross section of the eyelids. A = skin, B = frontalis muscle, C = orbital orbicularis, D = pre-tarsal orbicularis, E = superior tarsus, F = muscle of Riolan, G = orbital septum, H = orbital fat pad, I = superior transverse ligament (Whitnall's), J = levator muscle, K = levator aponeurosis, L = Mueller's muscle, M = superior rectus muscle, N = superior oblique tendon, P = gland of Wolfring, Q = frontal sinus, R = meibomiam glands, S = inferior rectus muscle, T = inferior oblique muscle, U = superior ligament of Lockwood, V = capsulopalpebral fascia, W = peripheral arterial arcade, X = inferior tarsus, Y = Tenon's capsule, Z = conjunctiva. (Courtesy of Crowell Beard, M.D.)

for the gross production of tears for reflex tearing that results from foreign body sensations or crying. Sympathetic innervation to the lacrimal gland occurs by other routes. One route travels from the carotid plexus to the ophthalmic division (V_1) of CN V, then to the lacrimal nerve. Another starts from the cavernous plexus and travels with the ophthalmic and lacrimal arteries, before hopping to the lacrimal gland. Sympathetic fibers are thought to have some minor, indefinite regulatory role for secretion.

• EYEBALL

The adult eyeball is an imperfect sphere. Approximately 24 mm (little more than 1 inch) in diameter and 7 mL in volume, the eyeball is encased and pro-

tected by the bony orbit. It is suspended within the socket—where it is cushioned with fat and connective tissue and covered with two protective eyelids.

The divisions of the eyeball are not exactly geometric. The equator is an imaginary circle just in front of the vortex veins. The anatomical equator is about 14 mm from the limbus. The vortex veins are found a few millimeters behind the equator. Although the equator is near the middle, the division into anterior and posterior segments breaks behind the lens. The cornea, the front quarter of the sclera, the anterior chamber, the iris, the posterior chamber, and the lens constitute the anterior segment or the front third of the eye. The posterior segment consists of the vitreous, the retina, the choroid, most of the sclera, and the optic disc. The ciliary body bridges the two segments (Fig. 1–6).

The surface of the retina is divided differently for

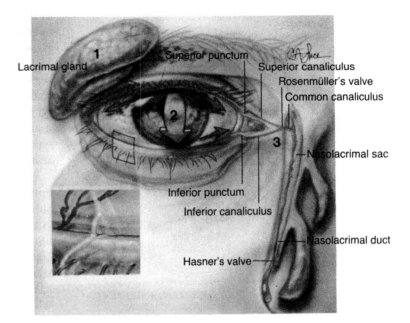

FIGURE 1–5. Secretion, distribution, and drainage of the lacrimal system. As the eye closes with a blink negative pressure is created in the nasolacrimal sac, drawing tears into it. Opening the eye creates positive pressure and forces the tears out into the nose through the nasolacrimal duct. (From Zide BM, Jelks GW: Surgical Anatomy of the Orbit. New York, Raven Press, 1985.)

various purposes. For example, theoretical vertical and horizontal lines divide the retina at the center of the optic disc for consideration of the blood supply, because the superior and inferior nasal arteries and veins supply the upper and lower nasal quadrants of the retina, respectively, and the superior and inferior temporal arcades supply the upper and lower temporal quadrants, respectively. For the purpose of fixation, spatial localization, binocular function, and perimetry, the retina is divided into nasal and temporal halves, and upper and lower halves, by lines drawn vertically and horizontally through the fovea. The horizontal line will strike the lowest third of the optic disc (Fig. 1–7).

The eye has three distinct layers—*sclera, choroid,* and *retina*—enclosing the lens. There are three fluid-filled spaces—*anterior chamber, posterior chamber,* and *vitreous* (Fig. 1–8).

The outer layer is the semirigid, tough sclera (''white of the eye''), with tissue similar to the cornea but not transparent. The outer surface of the sclera is covered with thin, elastic episclera that contains blood vessels. The sclera's rigidity gives the eyeball its form and serves as a framework to support and protect the eyeball's contents. Scleral thickness varies from its thinnest (less than 0.3 mm) beneath the rectus muscle insertions to its thickest (1.0 mm) at the posterior pole. The opaque sclera acts, along with the pigment epithelium layer, to provide a light-tight box preventing stray light rays from degrading the retinal image. At the optic disc the sclera thins at the lamina cribrosa, allowing retinal nerve fibers to penetrate and form the optic nerve. The posterior sclera is also penetrated by short and long posterior ciliary arteries and nerves surrounding the optic nerve (Fig. 1–9).

Clear cornea meets opaque, white sclera at a transition zone, the limbus. The 12-mm-diameter cornea is the clear front window of the eye, providing both transparency through which light may pass and two thirds (45 diopters) of the focusing power of the eye. Without a clear cornea, the retina cannot produce a clear image. The cornea, which has no blood supply, receives its nutrients from the underlying aqueous fluid and its oxygen from the air. Because of its steep curvature, 7 mm radius compared to 12 mm for the entire eyeball, the cornea protrudes like a dome. The central third is nearly spherical. It flattens and thickens near the peripheral limbal edge. A cornea measuring less than 10 mm in diameter is a microcornea, and a cornea measuring more than 13 mm in diameter is a macrocornea.

A thin precorneal tear film covers the conjunctiva and cornea and lubricates them. This produces a smooth optical surface and provides immunoglobulins for protection against infections and allergies. Tears prevent the front part of the eyeball from drying out and wash away foreign and harmful materials.

The tear film itself is constructed of three distinct layers. The oily lipid layer is secreted by the meibomian glands and Zeiss's glands. Being fatty, this outermost layer retards evaporation from the aqueous layer. It provides a smooth anterior refracting surface and prevents tears from overflowing onto the face. The thick middle aqueous layer secreted by the main lacrimal gland and Krause's and Wolfring's accessory lacrimal glands is sandwiched between the oily and mucin layers. The aqueous layer contains water-soluble nutrients such as salt, glucose, oxygen, and proteins necessary to sustain corneal health and to keep the cornea and conjunctiva hydrated. Krause's and Wolfring's glands

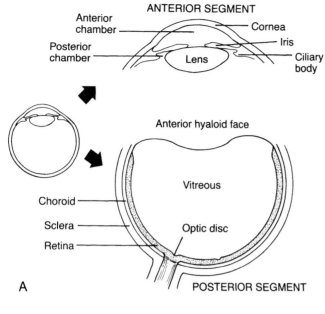

ANTERIOR SEGMENT

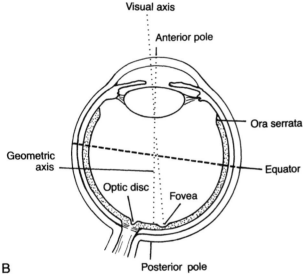

A

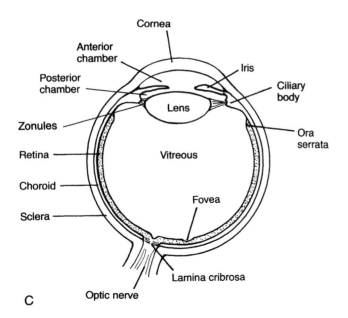

B

C

in the conjunctiva provide the basic secretion of tears, as opposed to reflex tears provided by the main lacrimal gland. This secretion wets the filter paper the first 8 to 15 minutes of a Schirmer's test. The secretion usually decreases with the patient's age. The innermost hydrophilic mucin layer, the one secreted by the conjunctiva's goblet cells, lies against the cornea. It helps to maintain uniform spread of the tear film and acts as a wetting agent to stabilize the tear film by keeping it from sticking to the hydrophobic corneal epithelium.

The cornea has five layers of tissue. The outermost epithelium is composed of cells that are continually sloughed and replaced, allowing minor injuries to the cornea to heal in 24 to 48 hours. Just beneath the epithelium is the cornea's thin basement membrane, the basal lamina, and then Bowman's membrane. Once destroyed, Bowman's membrane cannot regenerate. It scars as it heals. The middle layer, the stroma, contains 90% of the cornea's thickness. Desçemet's membrane, the dense basement membrane of the endothelium, separates the stroma from the innermost endothelial layer, and provides both rigidity and a barrier to water from the anterior chamber.

Any increase in the cornea's water content decreases its transparency. The endothelium keeps the cornea clear by actively pumping water out of the stroma. Damage to the endothelium often results in cloudiness and swelling of the cornea (Fig. 1–10).

At birth the eyeball is only about 16 mm in diameter (axial length). This short distance from the front of the cornea to the retina produces farsightedness. As the eyeball grows during development, it may grow too long. If its diameter becomes greater than 24 mm, the eyeball may become nearsighted (Fig. 1–11).

Uvea

The middle layer of the eye, the uvea, consists of the iris anteriorly, the ciliary body, and the choroid posteriorly. The uvea contains blood vessels that supply the eye's tissues with nutrients and pigment. The spongy iris regulates the amount of light entering the eye by acting like a camera's diaphragm with the pupil as its central hole. Iris stroma contains pigment, the amount of which determines the color of the eye, i.e., less pigment results in a blue or gray eye color, more in brown or black. Beneath the iris stroma lie the iris muscles, which regulate the size of the pupil. The radially oriented muscle fibers of the iris dilator muscle (dilator pupillae) pull the pupil open. A second muscle,

FIGURE 1–6. Divisions of the eyeball. *A,* A coronal cut divides the globe into anterior and posterior segments. *B,* The geometric axis divides the eye into right and left halves. *C,* A transverse cut divides the globe into upper and lower halves.

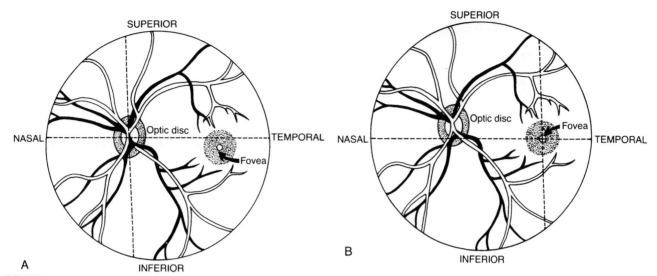

FIGURE 1–7. Division of the retina into quadrants at the posterior pole. *A,* Schema for retinal blood vessels. *B,* Schema for fixation, visual axis, and visual fields.

delineated on the anterior iris by the jagged concentric collarette, is the iris sphincter (sphincter pupillae). Its smooth fibers are arranged circularly near the pupil margin. When light intensity is high, as in bright sunlight, the sphincter contracts and the dilator relaxes. When light intensity is low, as in a movie theatre, the

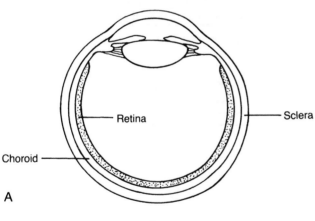

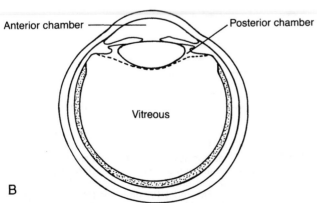

FIGURE 1–8. Layers and spaces of the eyeball. *A,* Three layers. *B,* Three spaces.

dilator contracts and the sphincter relaxes. A dilated pupil can reach 8 mm in size. A constricted pupil can decrease to 1 mm (Fig. 1–12).

The pupillary margin of the iris rests on the lens, where it acts like a one-way valve, allowing aqueous to pass from the posterior to the anterior chamber. The posterior epithelial layer, which may curve around the pupillary margin, is highly pigmented. The iris root inserts at the ciliary body. When it disinserts, it is an iridodialysis. The ciliary muscle, the iris dilator, and the iris sphincter are the intrinsic eye muscles within the eyeball just as the extraocular muscles are the extrinsic eye muscles attached to the outside of the eyeball.

The ciliary body, located in the posterior chamber circumferential to the lens, bridges the anterior and posterior segments of the eye, extending backward from the root of the iris to the anterior border of the choroid. It has two sections, one flat and one folded. The front folded section, the pars plicata, has a corrugated appearance from its more than 60 folds (processes), which contain outer pigmented epithelial cells and inner nonpigmented epithelial cells. Many zonules run from the ciliary processes to suspend the crystalline lens. The relatively smooth and flat posterior section is the pars plana. This transition zone between the mobile ciliary processes and the delicate, stationary retina abruptly ends as a jagged, scalloped edge at the ora serrata (Fig. 1–13).

The ciliary body has two functions, accommodation and aqueous production. Nonpigmented epithelial cells secrete the fluid containing aqueous humor and hyaluronic acid that flows into the posterior chamber between the lens and the iris, then through the pupil into the anterior chamber in front of the iris. The ciliary body has three types of fibers: mostly longitudinal, some

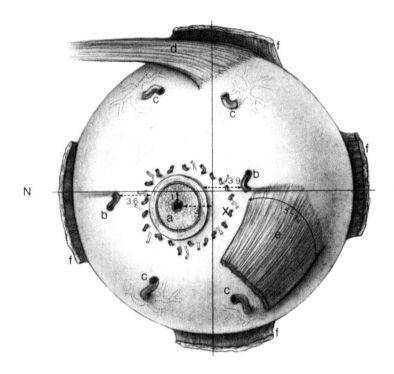

FIGURE 1–9. Posterior view of the left eyeball. N = nasal, T = temporal, a = optic nerve, b = long ciliary artery, c = vortex vein, d = superior oblique muscle, e = inferior oblique muscle, and f = rectus muscle. (From Hogan M, Alvarado J, Weddell J: Histology of the Human Eye. Philadelphia, WB Saunders, 1971.)

circular, and some radial. They tend to work together as a unit. Some muscle fibers contract to relax tension on the zonules, thus increasing the optical power of the lens by accommodation. Other muscle fibers connect to the trabecular meshwork, increasing the facility of outflow by pulling on the scleral spur. This opens the meshwork and increases its pore size.

The choroid portion of the uvea, mostly composed of large blood vessels, provides nutrients to the outer third of the retina. Sandwiched between the sclera and the retina, its extends backward from the ora serrata. Its blood supply is from the long and short posterior ciliary arteries. Bruch's membrane, the innermost layer, separates the choroid from the underlying retinal pigment epithelium (RPE). The outer surface of Bruch's membrane interlocks with a layer of small sinuses and large capillaries called the choriocapillaris. The inner surface of Bruch's membrane constitutes the basement membrane of the pigment epithelium. Cuboidal pigment epithelial cells interdigitate with the rods and cones of the retina. Breaks in Bruch's membrane lead to subretinal neovascularization.

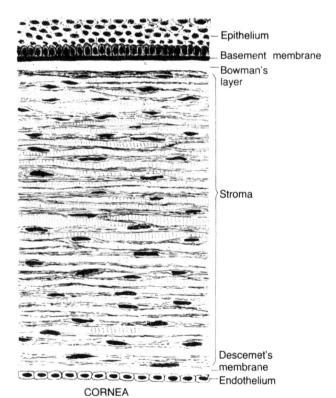

CORNEA

FIGURE 1–10. Cornea consists mostly of stroma and is lined on both sides with a membrane and a cellular layer. (From Hamming NA, Apple D: Anatomy and embryology of the eye. In Peyman GA, Sander DR, Goldberg MF (eds): Principles and Practice of Ophthalmology, vol. I. Philadelphia, WB Saunders, 1980.)

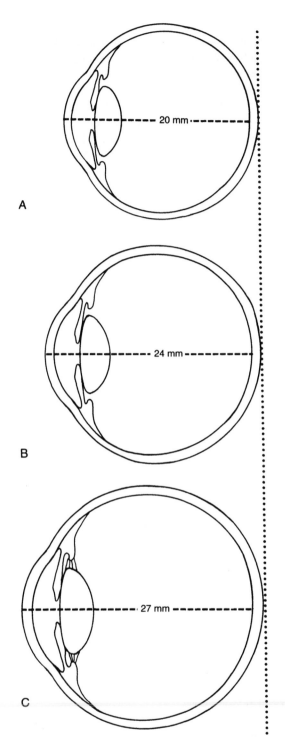

FIGURE 1–11. Size of the eye determines its axial length. *A,* Short eye has axial hyperopia. *B,* Normally sized eye has minimal, or no, refractive error. *C,* Long eye has axial myopia.

Retina

This innermost layer is responsible for the primary function of the eyeball as a photosensitive surface similar to photographic film. Rods and cones are the two types of light-sensitive photoreceptors. The retina

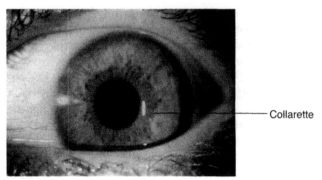

FIGURE 1–12. External view of the iris.

adapts very well to varying light intensities by a dual system: photopic and scotopic. The photopic system functions in bright daylight and employs cone photoreceptors, whereas the scotopic system functions under dim light and employs rod photoreceptors. Cones are comparable to fine-grain camera film, less sensitive to light but with excellent image resolution. Rods are comparable to coarse-grain camera film, more sensitive to light but poorer in image quality. Light rays enter the eye through the cornea, are refracted through the clear optical media (anterior chamber, lens, posterior chamber, vitreous, and retinal inner layers), and form an image on the photoreceptors in the outer layer. This image is converted into electrical impulses for transmission to the brain for processing. All surrounding tissues support this retinal function.

The retina is transparent but appears to be pink, from the blood in the underlying choroid. The outer third of the retina receives its blood supply from the choroid. The inner two thirds of the retina receives blood from branches of the central retinal artery. The dual blood vessel systems, one from the choroid, the other from the central retinal artery, do not connect.

Retinal landmarks include the optic disc (nerve head), macula, fovea, and foveola. (See Color Plate 36.) Nerve fibers that become the optic nerve pass through the sieve-like lamina cribrosa within the disc. The macula is the posterior focal point for the eye's

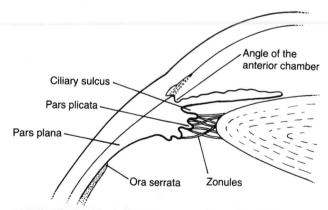

FIGURE 1–13. Structures found in and near the ciliary body.

optical system. At its center is the fovea, a retinal depression formed by sideways displacement of some internal retinal layers, exposing cones. The fovea contains only cones. The central pit within the fovea is the foveola. The fovea has no blood supply in the central 0.3 to 0.45 mm, an area called the foveal avascular zone (FAZ). Its nutrients are supplied only by the choriocapillaris.

The fovea and the optic disc have 1.5-mm diameters, and the macula 3 mm. The size of the optic disc can be used as a measure of retinal distances. For example, the fovea lies the equivalent of two disc diameters temporal to the optic disc.

The central posterior fundus runs forward to the equator. From the equator forward to the ora serrata is the periperal fundus. The ora serrata is the serrated anterior limit of the retina, demarcating its junction with the pars plana.

The sequence of retinal layers appears inverted because light has to penetrate the full thickness of the retina before reaching the photoreceptors. The outermost retinal layer next to the choroid consists of delicate, transparent, sensory nerve tissue (photoreceptors). The retina contains three layers of neuron cell bodies—photoreceptors, bipolar cells, and ganglion cells. In addition are two plexiform layers containing synapses from one neuron type to another, two nuclear layers containing cell bodies of one of the neuron types, and two limiting membranes. In all, we find 10 approximately separate layers (Fig. 1–14):

1. The outermost layer, i.e., closest to the choroid, is the *retinal pigment epithelium* (RPE). This is a single layer of hexagonal cells just inside Bruch's membrane continuous with the pigment epithelium of the ciliary body. Its cells serve as a base for the vertically arranged

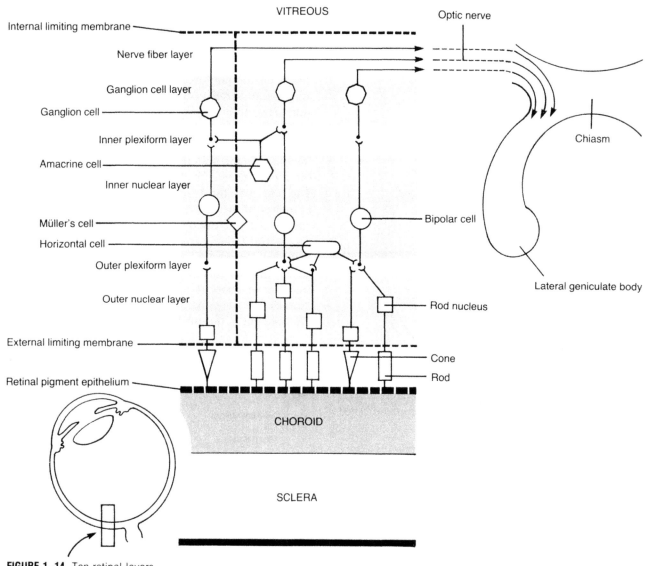

FIGURE 1–14. Ten retinal layers.

visual cells. Among the many functions of the RPE are maintenance of the blood-retinal barrier and metabolism of vitamin A needed by the visual pigments. The potential space between the pigment epithelium and the sensory retina enlarges when the retina detaches.

2. The *photoreceptors* (rods and cones) are imbedded in the RPE. Cone cells are most densely packed in the macula, the central part of the retina responsible for providing sharp central vision and color discrimination. Best visual acuity is achieved by the one-to-one coupling between cone and bipolar cells in the fovea. Rod cells are evenly distributed except for the fovea, which has none. The extreme peripheral retina has about 10 rods per cone. Visual resolution decreases in the far periphery, where rods are associated in multiples with each bipolar cell.

3. The sieve-like *external limiting membrane*, more a zone than a membrane, interdigitates around the rods and cones and forms the limit of the outer nuclear layer. It is composed of the outermost ends of Müller's cells, which stretch vertically from the external to the internal limiting membrane and lend structural and nutritional support to the retina.

4. The *outer nuclear layer* contains the cell bodies (with their nuclei) of the rods and cones.

5. The rod and cone axons synapse with adjacent bipolar horizontal and amacrine dendrites in the *outer plexiform layer*. Within this layer, at the fovea, photoreceptor axons travel obliquely to meet bipolar cells.

6. The bipolar cell, or *inner nuclear*, layer contains not only the nuclei of the bipolar cells, but also nuclei of horizontal, amacrine, and Müller's cells, which transmit information within the retina. Bipolar cells of this middle cell layer are the first order neurons for vision. Horizontal and amacrine cells distribute information sideways, almost like cross wiring, to other areas of the retina. Horizontal cells, found in the outermost zone, send processes to specialized contact points at each synaptic junction to provide an alternate side pathway, bringing information from more distant rods and cones to the bipolar cells. Amacrine cells, found in the innermost zone, have processes that store glycogen and other enzymes needed for energy. Amacrine cells sidewise connect bipolar cells to ganglion cells.

7. Bipolar cells axons and ganglion cell dendrites synapse in the *inner plexiform layer*, the second and final intraocular synapse.

8. The *ganglion cell layer*, the third cell layer, contains the second order neurons for vision. This continuous single layer of cells is thicker in the macula, because of the one-to-one coupling in this area of bipolar to ganglion cells, than in the periphery.

9. The *nerve fiber layer* (NFL), a roughly concentric arrangement of the one million ganglion cell axons, begins in the peripheral retina, turns almost 90° to run horizontally, and progresses toward the optic disc. The heaviest concentration of nerve fibers is found in the papillomacular bundle. The surrounding fibers form upper and lower arches radiating toward the optic disc. The horizontal raphe demarcation along the horizontal meridian appears only on the temporal side.

10. The *internal limiting membrane* is the basement membrane, which lies against the vitreous, probably secreted by vertically oriented Müller's cells. It covers the entire surface of the retina from ora serrata up to, but not over, the optic disc.

Electrodiagnostic procedures are useful in retinal diseases. These tests are, however, rarely performed in a private practice setting.

Electroretinogram (ERG)

When light strikes the retina an electrical potential is generated. The ERG measures the change in this action potential as the retina is stimulated with diffuse light or patterns. The ERG is recorded by placing electrodes on the cornea, as a contact lens or filament, and on the forehead or temple.

The photopic ERG produced by light flash stimulation has three wave components (A, B, and C) generated by different portions of the retina. The A wave is a negative deflection generated by the photoreceptor cells. The rod and cone portions are generated separately and are electrically additive. They can be separated by appropriate changes in light adaptation, intensity, or color of the stimulus. The A wave decreases with dark adaptation. It is followed by the positive deflection of the B wave generated by Müller's and bipolar cells. The amplitude of the B wave deflection should be at least 1.5 times that of the A wave. The C wave, which has little clinical use, is a slow positive deflection generated by the retinal pigment epithelium. The lag time between stimulation and response is called the latency period. The ganglion cell and nerve fiber layers do not contribute to the ERG (Fig. 1–15).

The ERG is a mass response of the entire retina. A large portion of the retina must be damaged in order to cause a change. Small retinal lesions or opacities of

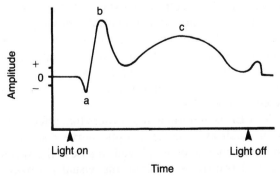

FIGURE 1–15. ERG wave.

the ocular media do not affect the ERG, but media opacities that scatter light may increase it.

Electro-oculogram (EOG)

The electro-oculogram (EOG) evaluates the condition of the RPE. Like the ERG, the EOG is a mass response and is not affected by localized retinal lesions. The EOG measures the resting potential between the cornea and the retina. The cornea is more positive than the retina. An electrode is placed at the medial and lateral canthus of each eye. Potential changes are measured as the patient moves the eyes rhythmically from side to side between two fixation points. The electrode closest to the cornea becomes positive and causes a deflection in the recording system. A baseline is established in a light adapted state. Next the recording is continued first through 15 minutes of dark adaption and then 15 minutes of light.

The EOG is expressed using Arden's ratio, which is the ratio of the maximum amplitude deflection in the light-adapted state (light peak) compared with the minimum amplitude deflection in the dark-adapted state (dark trough). In diseases of the RPE, such as retinitis pigmentosa, the Arden's ratio decreases.

Visual Evoked Response (VER)

The VER or visual evoked potential (VEP) is the electrical response of the visual cortex to visual stimulation, measured with electrodes placed on the scalp over the occipital cortex. Repeated visual stimulation, such as flashing lights or moving checkerboards, is presented to the patient who must be reasonably attentive to obtain an accurate assessment. It cannot be used in patients with opaque media. The repeated, synchronized electrical response to the visual stimulus can be filtered out of the remainder of the electrical activity produced by the occipital lobe. The binocular VER is greater than the monocular VER caused by binocular summation.

The VER represents the visual system as a whole. Damage to any portion of the sensory visual pathway may alter the VER. Because a large proportion of the visual cortex represents the small area of central retina, the VER is the electrodiagnostic test that correlates best for macular function and visual acuity evaluation. Although not sufficiently precise to place an exact value on visual acuity, it can establish an approximate range. For this reason it is useful to assess visual potential in nonresponsive infants and in patients with suspected functional visual loss.

The VER is abnormal in disorders that affect central vision, such as macular or optic nerve disease. The response can also be employed to assess the speed of electrical transmission along the visual pathway. In demyelinating diseases, which slow transmission, such

as multiple sclerosis, there is a prolonged latency period.

Optic Disc

Nerve fiber layer axons become myelinated at the lamina cribrosa, a sieve-like portion of the sclera sitting in the optic disc. Once through the lamina cribrosa, these myelinated axons become the optic nerve. No further synapse occurs until the optic nerve fibers reach the lateral geniculate body.

These holes (lamina cribrosa) weaken the sclera, allowing outward bowing of the disc into the optic nerve when intraocular pressure remains abnormally elevated over time. The disc is then *cupped*. Pressure-induced death of axons contributes to the cupping. This happens with increased intraocular pressure, as in glaucoma. Increased pressure external to the eyeball within the orbit or around the optic nerve bows the disc inward and elevates it, causing papilledema. (See Color Plate 37.)

Because no rods or cones are on the retina at the optic disc, this area cannot perceive light. The result is a normal physiological blind spot within the visual field. Visual field defects involving the retina and optic nerve often affect nerve fiber bundles.

Spaces

The space between the cornea and the iris is called the anterior chamber. Its clear watery fluid, the aqueous humor, contains most of the same soluble components as blood, but in different concentrations. Aqueous bathes the cornea with needed nutrients. Aqueous is secreted by the nonpigmented (inner layer of) epithelium of the ciliary processes into the posterior chamber, the space between the iris and the lens. Aqueous flows toward the center of the posterior chamber, lifting the iris off the lens, then flows through the pupil into the anterior chamber. Here it circulates partly by convection currents, as warmer aqueous strikes cooler cornea (Fig. 1–16).

Aqueous oozes through the trabecular meshwork (TM) into Schlemm's canal, a large venous channel that circles inside the trabecular meshwork circle. Aqueous next flows into collector channels that form the deep scleral plexus. This plexus drains into anterior ciliary and episcleral veins, entering the eye's venous system and terminating in conjunctival veins near the limbus. Secretion of aqueous fluid is balanced by its drainage at the angle, maintaining an intraocular pressure between 10 and 20 mm Hg. When the balance is upset by resistance to percolation through the trabeculum, abnormally high intraocular pressure results. If this

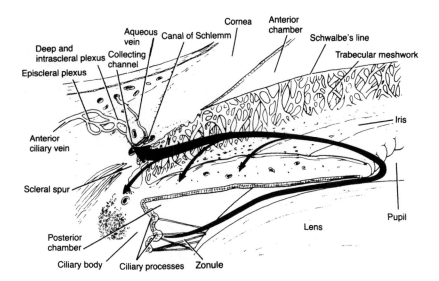

FIGURE 1–16. Flow of aqueous humor. (From Snell RS, Lemp MA: Clinical Anatomy of the Eye. Boston, Blackwell Scientific Publishing, 1989. Reprinted by permission of Blackwell Scientific Publications, Inc.)

persists, optic nerve damage occurs with subsequent loss of vision. This is called glaucoma.

The angle of the anterior chamber includes Schwalbe's line (end of Desçemet's membrane), Schlemm's canal, the trabecular meshwork, the scleral spur, the anterior border of the ciliary body, and the iris (Fig. 1–17).

Adhesions between iris and lens are called posterior synechiae. Anterior synechiae are adhesions from the cornea to the iris. Those in the anterior chamber near the angle are peripheral anterior synechiae (PAS). When PAS become numerous, they close the angle. The area of closure is referred to colloquially as a *zipped up* angle (Fig. 1–18).

The posterior chamber contains the ciliary sulcus and is bounded on the front of the iris and behind by the zonules. After cataract removal, posterior chamber intraocular lenses (PC IOL) may be inserted into the remains of the capsular bag, or positioned in the sulcus.

Lens

The crystalline lens is a flexible, transparent, biconvex structure located just in front of the vitreous in the posterior chamber, lying against the back of the iris and the front of the vitreous face. The lens is suspended behind the iris and is held in place by a double ring of transparent, filamentary, elastic zonules, which run from the lens equator to the pars plana and the pars plicata of the ciliary body. An elastic capsule encloses the lens fibers, thus preventing cell movement in or out and serving as a thick basement membrane. It permits the lens its own metabolism with diffusion from nutrients in the surrounding aqueous. This isolates the lens from nerve and blood supply because it is not continuous with other intraocular tissues. The anterior capsule is twice as thick as the posterior. The pupillary

margin of the iris rests on the lens and acts as a valve, allowing aqueous to pass in only one direction from the posterior to the anterior chamber.

Embryonic development produces two Y-shaped sutures in the nucleus that are visible with the slit lamp (the anterior Y is upright, the posterior Y inverted). The lens, arranged concentrically (onion-like) constantly adds layers throughout life. The more superficial layers are the youngest (subcapsular). With age, the lens increases in size and density but decreases in elasticity, often becoming opaque (cataractous) and requiring surgical removal.

The lens provides about a third of the eye's optical power (20 D). Lens power varies with the distance of a viewed object. In the unaccommodated state, the ciliary muscle is at rest, putting the zonular fibers "on the stretch," keeping the lens thinner and as flat as possible. The ciliary muscle's contraction causes accommodation. It bunches up toward the lens, which relaxes the zonular fibers and allows the lens to expand so that it becomes more nearly spherical, mostly by increasing the convexity of the anterior lens surface, which moves forward with the iris to make the anterior chamber shallower. The refractive power of the lens increases and its focal length decreases, permitting the eye to keep near objects in focus. As an object comes closer to the eye, the lens accommodates only enough to keep the image of the object in focus on the retina. Equal impulses are sent to each eye through parasympathetic fibers from CN III for increasing the power of the lens (Fig. 1–19).

Vitreous

The clear, gelatinous vitreous body occupies 80% of the inside of the globe and fills the large sphere behind the lens. The vitreous is supported by a filamentary

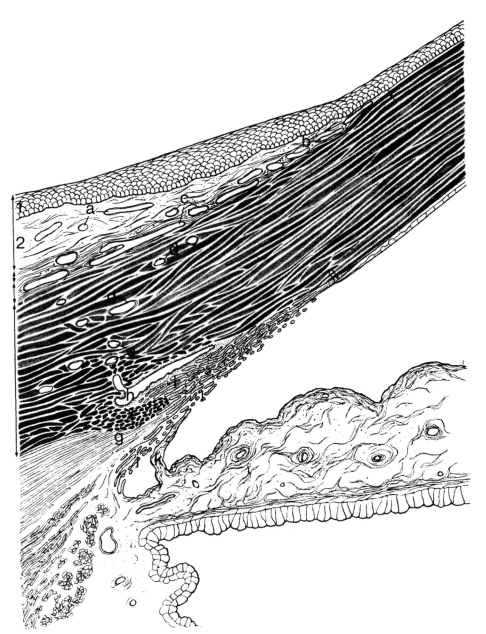

FIGURE 1–17. Cross section of the angle of the anterior chamber. a = conjunctival stromal vessels, b = peripheral corneal arcade, c = episcleral vessels, d = intrascleral plexus, e = deep scleral plexus, f = scleral spur, g = ciliary muscle, h = Schlemm's canal, i = trabecular meshwork, j = uveal meshwork, k = iris process. (From Hogan M, Alvarado J, Weddell J: Histology of the Human Eye. Philadelphia, WB Saunders, 1971.)

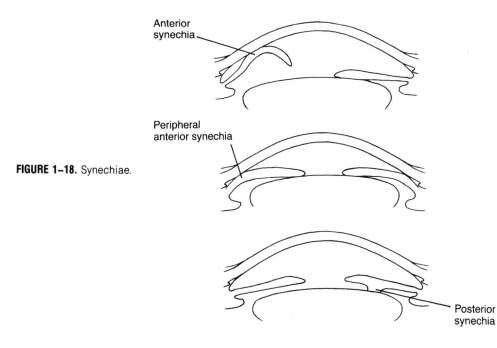

FIGURE 1–18. Synechiae.

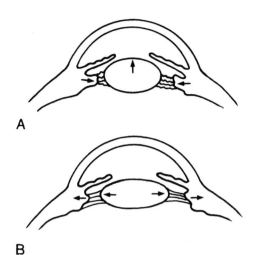

FIGURE 1–19. Change in the shape of the lens with accommodation. *A,* Accommodation. With added lens power, the ciliary muscle tightens and the zonules are loose. *B,* No accommodation. With lens at rest, the ciliary muscle relaxes and the zonules are stretched.

connective tissue matrix and water-attracting polysaccharides, especially hyaluronic acid, which accounts for its near total (more than 99%) water content. Collagenous filaments connect the vitreous to the retina and are strongest at the vitreous base around the ora serrata and at the margin of the optic disc. Anterior condensation of vitreous tissue forms the hyaloid face, which acts as a barrier between the anterior and posterior segments of the eye. Light rays refracted by the cornea and lens must travel through the vitreous to produce an image on the retina. For the image to be clear, the vitreous must be clear. The vitreous liquefies with age, often separating from the retina.

Bibliography

Cogan DG: Neurology of the Visual System. Springfield, IL, Charles C Thomas, 1976.

Doxanas MT, Anderson DL: Clinical Orbital Anatomy. Baltimore, Williams & Wilkins, 1984.

Warwick R: Eugene Wolff's Anatomy of the Eye, 7th ed. Philadelphia, WB Saunders, 1976.

• CHAPTER 1 EYEBALL ANATOMY AND PHYSIOLOGY

1. The eyeball divides into front and back portions
   a. at the equator
   b. at the geometric axis
   c. behind the lens
   d. at the visual axis
   e. behind the ora serrata.

2. The average axial length in millimeters of an adult's eyeball is
   a. 8
   b. 12
   c. 16
   d. 24
   e. 29.

3. The space between the lens and the iris is the
   a. anterior chamber
   b. pupil
   c. angle
   d. posterior chamber
   e. vitreous.

4. Which freely moving, thin mucous membrane reduces friction on the eyeball?
   a. conjunctiva
   b. eyelid
   c. fornix
   d. Tenon's capsule
   e. tear film.

5. The part of the eye that provides the clearest visual image, such as occurs with fine grain film in a camera, is the
   a. lens
   b. rods
   c. cornea
   d. nerve fiber layer
   e. cones.

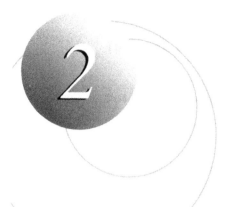

Anatomy of the Skull and Orbit

LEARNING OBJECTIVES

- Describe the floor of the cranial vault, including the three fossae
- Identify the seven bones of the orbit
- Identify the three openings into the orbit from the cranial vault
- List those vessels and nerves that course through each of the three openings
- List those structures that travel through the muscle cone
- List and locate the four sinuses that surround the orbit
- Describe the nerve fibers that flow through the ciliary ganglion

BONES OF THE SKULL

The brain is completely enclosed by the bony skull except for the foramen magnum at the base where the brain stem and spinal cord connect. The cranial wall varies in thickness in different regions of the skull, e.g., the ethmoid bone is extremely thin, whereas the sphenoid can be a quarter of an inch thick (Fig. 2–1).

The top surface of the mushroom-shaped brain has the precise contour of the inner surface of the skullcap. However, it is difficult to imagine the shape of the *base* (undersurface) of the brain. The undersurface rests on a three-tiered skull base with progressively lower levels. The highest and most forward tier, the anterior cranial fossa, forms the roof above the orbits and supports the frontal lobes. Each sphenoid ridge is the edge of the cliff at the back of each anterior cranial fossa. Just under each sphenoid ridge is an optic foramen, a superior orbital fissure, and an orbit's back wall.

The optic foramen and the superior orbital fissure connect the back of the orbit with the middle cranial fossa, providing a pathway to the orbit for nerves and blood vessels passing through the cavernous sinus. The temporal lobes rest in the middle cranial fossa, which resembles a butterfly's wings.

A portion of the sphenoid bone (clivus) serves as a slide in the middle as it slopes down toward the posterior cranial fossa. This lowest, largest, and hindmost tier contains the cerebellum, with the pons and medulla

almost resting on the clivus. In the foramen magnum, a large hole at the bottom of the clivus, the spinal cord widens to become the brain stem (Fig. 2–2).

The sella turcica (a Latin phrase meaning Turkish saddle) is in the midline of the middle cranial fossa at the top of the slide. The optic nerves exit the orbit through the optic foramina and pass over the sella. At the front of the sella are two anterior clinoid processes. The back of the saddle, the dorsum sellae, is formed into two posterior clinoid processes. Housed in the sella is the pituitary body with the optic chiasm crossing just above it. On either side of the sella turcica, just behind each orbit, lies a cavernous sinus, a pool of venous blood that contains nerves and blood vessels to supply the orbit and the eye. If the sella turcica resembles a Turkish saddle, then the two cavernous sinuses resemble two saddlebags attached to either side (Fig. 2–3).

The spinal vertebrae are divided into five sections, starting just below the skull:

1. Seven *cervical* segments in the back of the neck, labeled C1–C7
2. Twelve *thoracic* segments behind the chest, labeled T1–T12
3. Five *lumbar* segments in the lower back, labeled L1–L5
4. Five *sacral* segments, labeled S1–S6
5. One *coccygeal* segment at the bottom (Fig. 2–4).

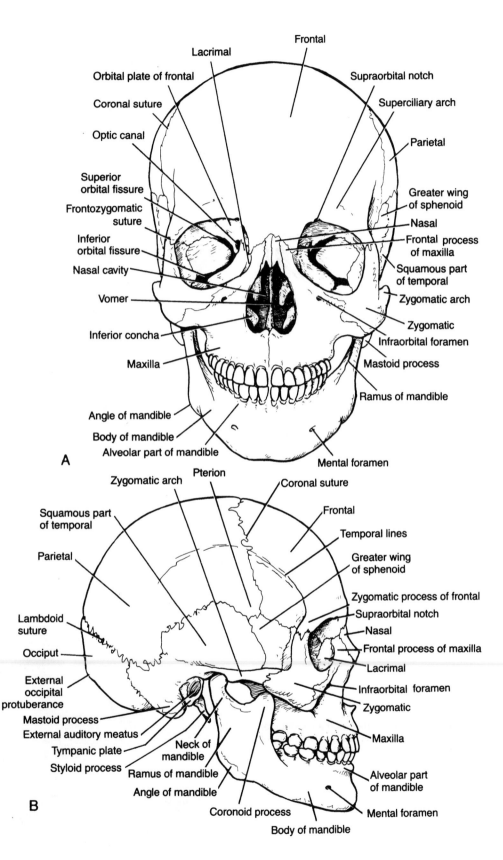

FIGURE 2–1. *A,* Anterior view of the skull. *B,* Lateral view of the skull. (From Snell RS, Lemp MA: Clinical Anatomy of the Eye. Boston, Blackwell Scientific Publications, 1989. Reprinted by permission of Blackwell Scientific Publications, Inc.)

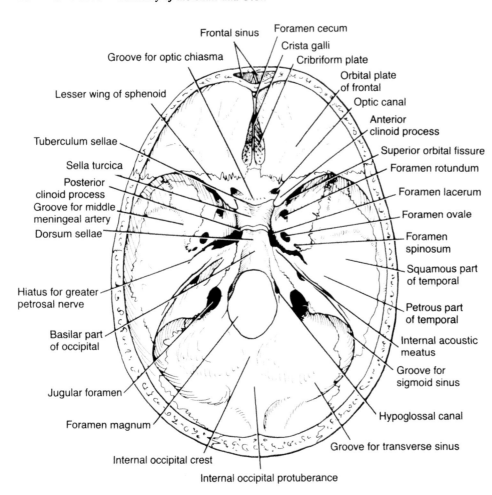

Frontal sinus
Foramen cecum
Crista galli
Groove for optic chiasma
Cribriform plate
Orbital plate of frontal
Lesser wing of sphenoid
Optic canal
Anterior clinoid process
Tuberculum sellae
Superior orbital fissure
Sella turcica
Foramen rotundum
Posterior clinoid process
Foramen lacerum
Groove for middle meningeal artery
Foramen ovale
Dorsum sellae
Foramen spinosum
Squamous part of temporal
Hiatus for greater petrosal nerve
Petrous part of temporal
Internal acoustic meatus
Basilar part of occipital
Groove for sigmoid sinus
Jugular foramen
Hypoglossal canal
Foramen magnum
Groove for transverse sinus
Internal occipital crest
Internal occipital protuberance

FIGURE 2–2. Floor of the skull. (From Snell RS, Lemp MA: Clinical Anatomy of the Eye. Boston, Blackwell Scientific Publications, 1989. Reprinted by permission of Blackwell Scientific Publications, Inc.)

FIGURE 2–3. Middle portion of the middle cranial fossa. (From Zide BM, Jelks GW: Surgical Anatomy of the Orbit. New York, Raven Press, 1985.)

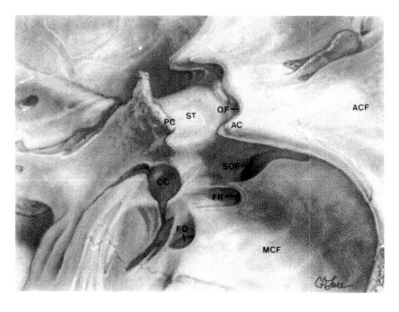

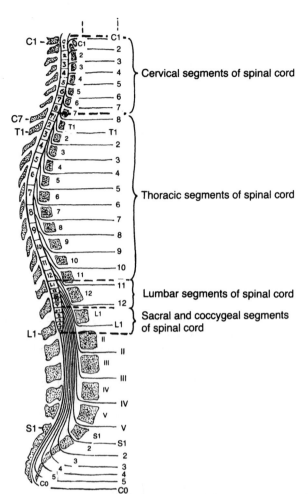

FIGURE 2–4. Spinal vertebrae number designations. C = cervical, T = thoracic, L = lumbar, S = sacral. (From Ranson S, Clark S: Anatomy of the Nervous System, 10th ed. Philadelphia, WB Saunders, 1959.)

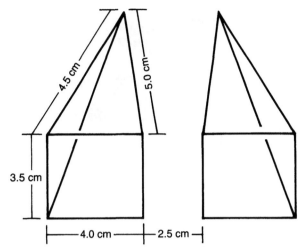

FIGURE 2–5. Schematic diagram of the shape of the orbit.

Many sympathetic nerve fibers destined for the eye and orbit leave the central nervous system from vertebrae in the cervical and upper thoracic segments.

● BONES OF THE ORBIT

The eye and the tissues around it (periorbita) are housed in a bony socket, the orbit, that envelops and protects the eye. Each orbit is shaped like a pyramid tipped over backward 90°, up and toward the midline of the skull, so that the apex of the pyramid is the back of the orbit, next to the nasal bones. The squarish base of the pyramid is upended as the four sides of the front rims of the orbit. The apex contains the optic canal and the superior orbital fissure (SOF). The 7-mL volume of the eye easily fits within the 30-mL volume of the orbit. Seven bones compose the roof, floor, and medial and lateral walls of the orbit. The roof, floor, and lateral wall are triangular, whereas the medial wall is approximately oblong (Fig. 2–5).

The roof is formed almost entirely by the thick frontal

bone. At the superonasal margin of the frontal bone is the supraorbital notch to which the trochlea, the pulley for the superior oblique, attaches. The back end of the roof is formed by the lesser wings of the sphenoid bone.

The medial (nasal) wall is formed mostly by the paper-thin ethmoid bone (lamina papyracea). The remaining frontal portion of the medial wall is formed by the maxillary and lacrimal bones.

The floor is formed by the maxilla medially, the zygoma laterally, and the tiny palatine bone at the back of the orbit. Thin orbital floor bones and the maxillozygomatic suture make this area especially susceptible to traumatic blow-out fracture. The zygomatic and frontal bones also form part of the lateral (temporal) wall, the strongest wall of the orbit. The rear two thirds are formed by the greater wing of the sphenoid (Fig. 2–6).

● OPENINGS IN THE ORBIT

The inferior orbital groove and canal on the floor of the orbit form a gap between the greater wing of the sphenoid and the maxilla. Branches of the maxillary division (V_2) of the trigeminal nerve (CN V) and blood vessels to the anterior portion of the face travel through here to supply the skin below the orbit.

Inferior Orbital Fissure

Infraorbital nerve (V_2)

Zygomatic nerve (V_2)

Infraorbital artery (branch from maxillary artery)

Inferior ophthalmic vein (possibly)

The apex separates the other two openings, the SOF and the optic foramen. The optic foramen transmits the optic nerve and the ophthalmic artery. Most sympathetic fibers from the plexus surrounding the internal carotid artery enter the optic foramen, traveling near

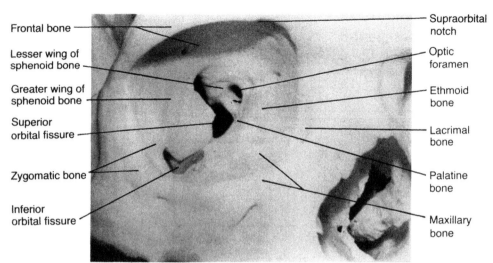

Frontal bone

Lesser wing of
sphenoid bone

Greater wing of
sphenoid bone

Superior
orbital fissure

Zygomatic bone

Inferior
orbital fissure

Supraorbital
notch

Optic
foramen

Ethmoid
bone

Lacrimal
bone

Palatine
bone

Maxillary
bone

FIGURE 2–6. Topography of the right orbit.

the ophthalmic artery. Some of these fibers innervate the iris dilator. Some probably innervate Müller's muscle.

Optic Foramen

Optic nerve

Ophthalmic artery

Sympathetic nerve fibers

All the other nerves and veins for the eye and extraocular muscles enter or leave the orbit through the *superior orbital fissure,* the principal opening from the cranial vault to the orbit for nerve passage. The superior orbital fissure is formed by a gap between the greater and lesser wings of the large sphenoid bone. The origin of most of the extraocular muscles is a tendinous ring, Zinn's annulus, that spans the superior orbital fissure and the optic foramen. The first three nerves that enter the orbit do so through the fissure *above* the annulus, remaining outside the muscle cone, whereas the next four enter *through* the annulus near the lateral rectus origin, traveling into the orbit within the muscle cone space.

Those nerves, starting at the top, that pass through the fissure are listed in Table 2–1. Not included in the table are the veins, the inferior ophthalmic, which passes through below the annulus, and the superior ophthalmic, which passes through above the annulus (Fig. 2–7).

Because the 3rd, 4th, and 6th cranial nerves (CN III, IV, and VI), and branches from the ophthalmic division (V_1) of the 5th trigeminal cranial nerve (CN V) pass through the superior orbital fissure to enter the orbit from the cavernous sinus, decreased extraocular muscle function (ophthalmoplegia) associated with pain or lack of sensation is called the superior orbital fissure syndrome. The same findings result from disorders in the cavernous sinus itself, although the terms cavern-

ous sinus syndrome and parasellar syndrome are also used. When there is involvement of the optic nerve, however, indicating that the problem extends into the orbit, it becomes an orbital apex syndrome. If the condition is painful and inflammatory, it becomes the Tolosa-Hunt syndrome. Tolosa-Hunt resembles a pseudotumor in the orbit, but localizes farther back. Inflammation, trauma, tumors, or aneurysms may also produce these symptoms.

● SINUSES AROUND THE ORBIT

The orbit is surrounded on three sides by sinuses. The frontal sinus is in the frontal bone, just above the supraorbital notch. The ethmoid sinus is in the nose, separated from the orbit only by the very thin nasal wall of the ethmoid bone. The maxillary sinus lies under the floor of the orbit behind the maxilla (cheekbone). Infections and inflammations in the sinuses may expand into the orbit, and vice versa. A 4th sinus, the sphenoid, is found under the sella turcica within the body of the sphenoid bone (Fig. 2–8).

TABLE 2–1.

Nerves that Pass Through the Superior Orbital Fissure

Nerve	Letter	Enters
Lacrimal	L	
Frontal	F	Above
Trochlea	T	
Superior div. III	S	
Nasociliary	N	Through
Inferior div. III	I	
Abducens	A	

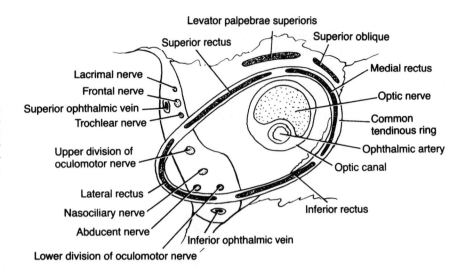

FIGURE 2–7. Relationship of Zinn's annulus to the superior orbital fissure and optic foramen. (From Snell RS, Lemp MA: Clinical Anatomy of the Eye. Boston, Blackwell Scientific Publications, 1989. Reprinted by permission of Blackwell Scientific Publications, Inc.)

● DIAGNOSTIC IMAGING

X-rays are a form of radiation that can affect a sensitized plate to produce a shadow-photograph of objects located within an opaque substance, such as the body. Details of structures can be shown in a predetermined plane of the body. X-ray films show transmitted radiation from bone, water, and air, but are not good for studying soft tissue, and so have been largely supplanted by computed tomography (CT scans) and magnetic resonance imaging (MRI).

CT scanners also use radiation. As tissues absorb the radiation, thin beams are detected as thousands of points in lines. A computer changes the lines to intersecting points to construct the picture, thus measuring the amount of x-ray absorbed. The CT image consists of a grid of small squares. The resolution increases with the number of small squares used to create the image. A contrast medium is sometimes given to enhance absorption of radiation. Because different tissues have different electron densities, absorption of radiation varies, making tissue definition possible. Bone absorbs the best, water the least, but brain, blood, and soft tissues enough to allow them to be examined in a noninvasive manner. Areas appearing light have greater absorption, darker areas less. Orbital

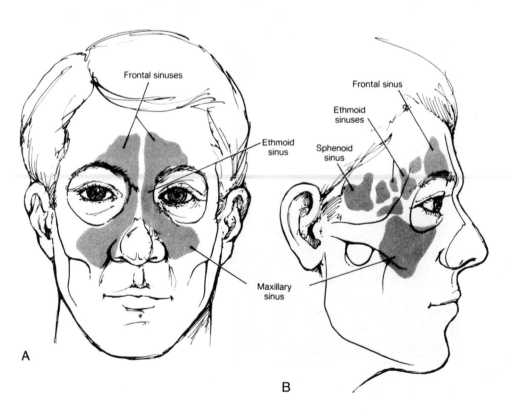

FIGURE 2–8. Sinuses that surround the orbit. *A,* Frontal view. *B,* Lateral view. (From Doxanas MT, Anderson RL: Clinical Orbital Anatomy. Baltimore, Williams and Wilkins, 1984.)

anatomy can be delineated. Because the patient goes "through a big white doughnut" on a stretcher, axial (transverse) cuts are obtained.

By its other name, nuclear magnetic resonance (NMR), MRI has been performed for years in chemistry laboratories for compound identification. No radiation is involved. Hazards are minimal. MRI uses a computer and a giant cylindrical magnet to produce detailed images of the body's layers of skin, fat, mus-

cle, and blood vessels provided by the response of hydrogen protons within the body to the magnetic field. The molecular structure of tissues depends on the number of protons ($+$), neutrons, and electrons ($-$). The MRI's strong magnetic field aligns some of the body's hydrogen ions into upright, parallel rows. The machine then sends out radiofrequency signals causing the nuclei to spin off course. The magnetic field is turned off. As the nuclei return to their previous positions they

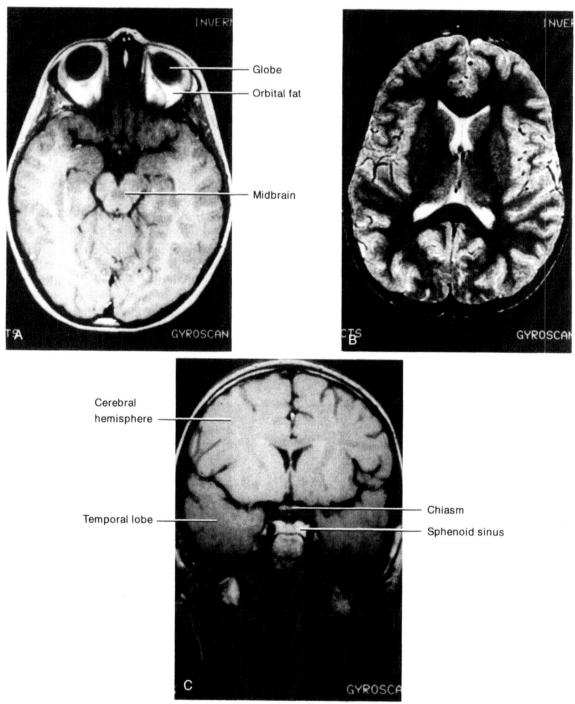

FIGURE 2–9. Examples of normal MRI pictures *A*, T_1-weighted transverse cut at the level of the mid-brain. *B*, T_2-weighted transverse cut above the floor of the anterior cranial fossa. *C*, T_1-weighted coronal cut through the chiasm and sphenoid sinus. (Courtesy of L. Hamed.)

give off their own particular signals, which are fed into a computer that translates the data from each tissue's different signal intensity and duration into "slices" imaged for our viewing. The time for the energized nuclei to relax is described by two time constants, T_1 and T_2, specific for different tissues. Lesions in tissues are shown by changes in the T_1 and T_2 images.

MRI breaks down specific densities of brain, blood, water, and fat, thus providing higher image resolution. Solids such as bone produce low intensity signals, whereas liquids are higher in intensity. Nerve, muscle, and brain give distinct intermediate intensity signals. White matter is distinguished from gray matter. Soft tissues such as brain and spinal cord can be studied in previously impossible detail. T_1-weighted images are especially good for visualizing the soft tissues of the orbit. Intracranial identification of optic nerves, chiasm, and optic tracts is more effective than that by CT. MRIs are considerably more expensive, however. Figure 2–9 is useful for orientation.

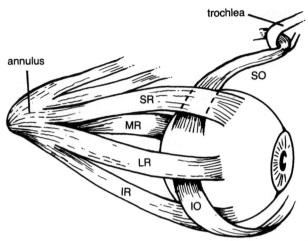

FIGURE 2–10. Muscle cone begins at Zinn's annulus with origins of the four rectus muscles and ends with muscle insertions onto the eyeball.

● CONNECTIVE TISSUE

Each extraocular muscle is encased in its own sheath of connective tissue condensed from Tenon's capsule. The blending of the sheaths of the inferior oblique and the inferior rectus muscle and its extension upward to the sheaths of the medial and lateral rectus muscles forms a sling under the eyeball called Lockwood's suspensory ligament. Condensation of tissue, Whitnall's ligament, blends the sheaths of the superior oblique and the superior rectus in a similar manner above the eyeball. Many extensions (check ligaments) from the muscle sheaths form a complex system of fibrous attachments interconnecting the muscles, attaching them to the orbit, supporting the globe, and limiting extraocular muscle movement. An expansion of connective tissue, the intermuscular septum, interconnects the four rectus muscles near the equator of the globe, thus

contributing to the muscle cone. This fascial tissue reduces retraction of the eyeball into the orbit and enhances smooth eye movements by reducing vibration of the contents of the orbit when the eye suddenly stops or changes direction.

Orbital fat pads act as cushions, supporting the eyeball, optic nerve, and extraocular muscles, and are present both inside and outside the muscle cone.

The eyeball itself is enveloped in a thin, fibroelastic connective tissue socket, Tenon's capsule, that covers the eye from the limbus to the optic nerve, fusing with the intermuscular septum as it approaches the limbus, where it merges with the conjunctiva 3 mm from the limbus. The inner surface of Tenon's capsule is smooth, allowing the sclera, muscles, and intermuscular septum to glide back and forth within it. Tenon's capsule keeps the sclera free of fat behind the equator and the muscles free of fat in front of the equator. If Tenon's capsule is perforated, however, fat may bulge through the hole, fuse to the eyeball, and so restrict its normal movements.

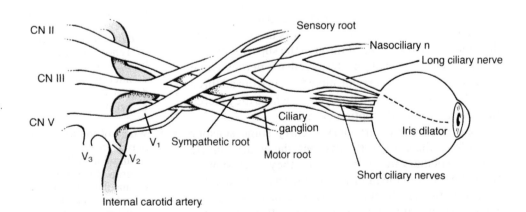

FIGURE 2–11. Ciliary ganglion.

• MUSCLE CONE

The superior oblique muscle and the levator superioris muscle originate just outside and above Zinn's annulus. The four rectus muscles originating at Zinn's annulus form the tip of the cone. The muscles separate from one another as they run forward toward the eyeball. The bottom of the muscle cone is near the back of the eye. The optic nerve, the ophthalmic artery and veins, the ciliary ganglion, the inferior and superior divisions of CN III, CN VI, and the nasociliary nerve also travel inside the muscle cone. (Fig. 2–10).

• OPTIC NERVE

The optic nerve consists of ganglion cell axons of the retinal nerve fiber layer that form the optic nerve as they exit through the lamina cribrosa. The optic nerve fibers are covered by myelin. The nerve is surrounded by the same sheaths as the brain. Blood supply to the optic nerve comes from the ophthalmic, ciliary, and central retinal arteries.

From its origin at the optic disc, the optic nerve runs through the muscle cone to exit the orbit through the optic canal at the apex, then ends at the chiasm. The optic nerve is about 50 mm long, with 30 mm in the orbit pressed into an S shape to provide for slack.

• CILIARY GANGLION

The ciliary ganglion is a collection of nerve fibers, roughly crab-shaped, located within the muscle cone near the orbital apex. It receives three roots from the back of the orbit. One short motor root has preganglionic parasympathetic fibers from the inferior division of CN III (oculomotor). These are the only fibers that synapse here. The nasociliary nerve (branch of the ophthalmic division (V_1) of CN V) gives off another, the long sensory sympathetic root that carries sensory information from the cornea, iris, and ciliary body. The 3rd root has motor sympathetic fibers from the cavernous sinus plexus that travel through the ciliary ganglion without synapsing, carrying constrictor fibers to uveal blood vessels. All three roots are from fibers that enter or leave the orbit through the superior orbital fissure. Six to 10 short posterior ciliary nerves leave the ciliary ganglion, carrying mixed fibers from all three roots to travel forward to the eyeball, where they pierce the sclera around the optic nerve.

Long posterior ciliary nerves carry some sensory fibers from the cornea, the iris, and the ciliary muscle to the nasociliary nerve, but mostly they carry sympathetic fibers from the internal carotid artery plexus that innervate the iris dilator. The iris dilator fibers bypass the ciliary ganglion but often merge with some of the short ciliary nerves. Parasympathetic postganglionic fibers from the ciliary ganglion to the iris sphincter and ciliary body, along with the iris dilator fibers from the long posterior ciliary nerves, run between the sclera and choroid in the suprachoroidal space to the ciliary muscle, where they form the ciliary plexus (Fig. 2–11).

Bibliography

Beard C, Quickert M: Anatomy of the Orbit. Birmingham, Aesculapius, 1977.
Doxanas MT, Anderson DL: Clinical Orbital Anatomy. Baltimore, Williams & Wilkins, 1984.
Garrity JA, Forbes GS: Computed tomography of the orbit. In Duane TD, Jaeger EA (eds): Biomedical Foundations of Ophthalmology, vol 2. Philadelphia, Harper & Row, 1990.
Kronish JW, Dortzbach RK: Magnetic resonance imaging. In Duane TD, Jaeger EA (eds): Biomedical Foundations of Ophthalmology, vol. 2, Philadelphia, Harper & Row, 1990.
Rootman J: Diseases of the Orbit. Philadelphia, JB Lippincott, 1988.
Warwick R: Eugene Wolff's Anatomy of the Eye and Orbit, 7th ed. Philadephia, WB Saunders, 1976.
Zide BM, Jelks GW: Surgical Anatomy of the Orbit. New York, Raven Press, 1985.

• CHAPTER 2 SKULL AND ORBIT

1. Which of the following is *not* an orbital bone?
   a. palatine
   b. lacrimal
   c. frontal
   d. maxilla
   e. clivus

2. The ophthalmic division of the fifth (trigeminal) cranial nerve (CN V) enters the orbit through the
   a. optic canal
   b. ethmoid sinus
   c. superior orbital fissure
   d. sphenoid sinus
   e. inferior orbital fissure.

3. Under which part of the base of the skull does the eyeball rest?
   a. sella turcica
   b. sphenoid ridge
   c. middle cranial fossa
   d. anterior cranial fossa
   e. anterior clinoid processes

4. The first layer covering the eyeball is the
   a. Tenon capsule
   b. conjunctiva
   c. intermuscular septum
   d. tear film
   e. periorbita.

5. Which of the following structures pierces the fat in the muscle cone?
   a. annulus of Zinn
   b. cranial nerve IV
   c. maxillary nerve
   d. ophthalmic artery
   e. inferior ophthalmic vein

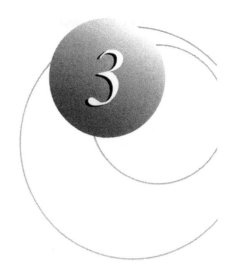

Blood Supply

LEARNING OBJECTIVES

- Trace the blood supply to the brain from the heart
- Explain the relationship between the vertebrobasilar artery system and the internal carotid artery system
- Explain the importance of the circle of Willis

- Identify the various portions of the circle of Willis
- Trace the blood supply to the eye and orbit from the internal carotid artery in the cavernous sinus
- Trace venous drainage from the eye and its orbit back to the heart

● BLOOD SUPPLY TO THE HEAD

The aorta is the main artery arising from the heart. Its branches eventually supply blood to the entire body. The first three blood vessels to branch off from the aorta emerge at the aortic arch: the brachiocephalic, the left common carotid, and the left subclavian arteries. The brachiocephalic almost immediately throws off two branches, the right common carotid and the right vertebral arteries. The rest of the brachiocephalic artery changes name to the right subclavian artery.

The left and right common carotid arteries travel up the neck to the jaw line, where each splits into an external and an internal carotid artery. The external carotid arteries supply the outside of the head and neck. The internal carotid arteries supply the front and midportions of the brain, including the eyes and orbit, with terminal branches exiting the orbit to the forehead and nose.

The left vertebral artery is the first branch of the left subclavian artery. The right vertebral is the second branch of the brachiocephalic artery. The vertebral arteries and their branches supply the back of the brain, the cervical spinal cord, the brain stem, and the cerebellum. As the branches of the two internal carotid and two vertebral arteries travel upward, all areas of the brain and related structures are supplied. We concentrate on the branches of the internal carotid and vertebral that supply areas related to the eye and vision (Fig. 3–1).

Basilar System

The two vertebral arteries pass upward through side holes in the upper six cervical vertebrae, entering the base of the skull through the foramen magnum. The vertebrals unite to form the basilar artery on the underside of the brain stem at the level of the pons. Branches from the basilar supply the medulla oblongata, the cerebellum, and the spinal cord.

The basilar travels upward on the ventral surface of the brain stem, finally splitting into two posterior cerebral arteries at the top border of the pons. Each posterior cerebral artery sends a posterior communicating artery branch to meet each middle cerebral artery branch from the internal carotid system. The posterior cerebrals then travel around to the topside of the midbrain, where branches supply the temporal and occipital lobes (Fig. 3–2).

Internal Carotid System

In the neck, the internal carotid artery (ICA) runs from the common carotid fork to the base of the skull, which it enters through the carotid canal in the temporal bone, then turns sharply upward to penetrate into the cavernous sinus. As it travels forward through the sinus, it assumes a characteristic S-shape, bending up, then backward, then up again, giving off three smaller arteries before or just after leaving the sinus. The oph-

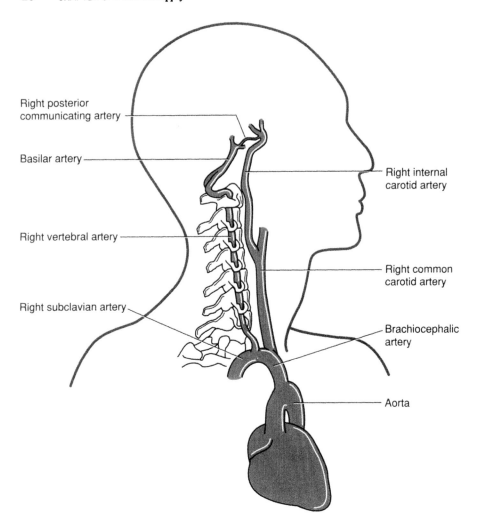

Right posterior communicating artery

Basilar artery

Right vertebral artery

Right subclavian artery

Right internal carotid artery

Right common carotid artery

Brachiocephalic artery

Aorta

FIGURE 3–1. Schematic drawing of the arterial blood supply from the heart to the head.

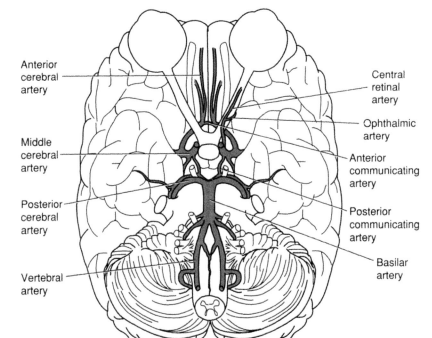

FIGURE 3–2. Schematic drawing of the major arterial blood vessels on the ventral surface of the brain and brain stem.

Anterior cerebral artery

Middle cerebral artery

Posterior cerebral artery

Vertebral artery

Central retinal artery

Ophthalmic artery

Anterior communicating artery

Posterior communicating artery

Basilar artery

thalmic artery is the first branch coming off the front bend of the S just under the optic nerve, traveling with the optic nerve to the orbit through the optic canal. The ophthalmic artery provides all the blood supply to the globe, extraocular muscles, and other orbital structures. As the ICA bends up through the top of the cavernous sinus, the small posterior communicating artery emerges as its second branch, traveling back to anastomose with the posterior cerebral artery, the large terminal branch of the basilar system. The posterior communicating artery runs just above and parallel to the third (oculomotor) cranial nerve (CN III), connecting the internal carotid and basilar systems as part of the circle of Willis.

Traveling back between the optic and oculomotor nerves, the internal carotid now divides into its terminal branches, the anterior cerebral and middle cerebral arteries. The middle cerebral is the larger, supplying a large midportion of the brain. The middle is the cerebral artery most commonly involved in blood vessel disease. The anterior cerebral loops over the chiasm, forming most of the front of the circle of Willis, then supplies the front of the brain (Fig. 3–3).

Circle of Willis

The circle of Willis is a cerebral arterial circle, linking the internal carotid artery and the basilar system, interconnecting the anterior, middle, and posterior cerebral arteries. This unique formation is found at the base of the brain on the ventral surface of the brain stem just under the optic chiasm in the interpeduncular fossa (Fig. 3–4). The brain structures lying within the circle of Willis include the optic chiasm and the stalk from the pituitary body. The fore and midportions of the circle are supplied by the internal carotid system, the back portion by the basilar system.

At the front of the circle lie the two anterior cerebral arteries joined by one short anterior communicating artery, the front bridge of the circle of Willis. The two middle cerebral arteries form the midportion of the circle. The posterior portion is formed by the two posterior cerebral arteries that connect with the two middle cerebral arteries by way of the two posterior communicating arteries. Blood supplies from the internal carotid and vertebral arteries meet but do not mix at that point in each posterior communicating artery where the blood pressure from the two arteries is equal. Blood passes forward or back across that point, however, to keep the blood pressure equalized to the brain from both systems. It also provides alternate routes for blood supply if any arteries are damaged.

• BLOOD SUPPLY OF THE VISUAL PATHWAY

Retina. The retinal circulation is from two sources. The central retinal artery supplies the layers close to the vitreous, and the long posterior ciliary arteries from the choroidal circulation supply the layers close to the choroid.

Optic Nerve. This nerve varies from one segment to another. Branches from the posterior ciliaries, the central retinal artery, and the cilioretinal arteries supply the optic nerve head. Within the orbit, the ophthalmic artery nourishes the optic nerve. Closer to the chiasm, the nerve is still partially supplied by the ophthalmic artery but also by the anterior cerebral and anterior communicating arteries.

Optic Chiasm. Blood supply is from the internal carotid, anterior communicating, and anterior cerebral arteries from above and from the posterior communicating, posterior cerebral, and basilar arteries from below.

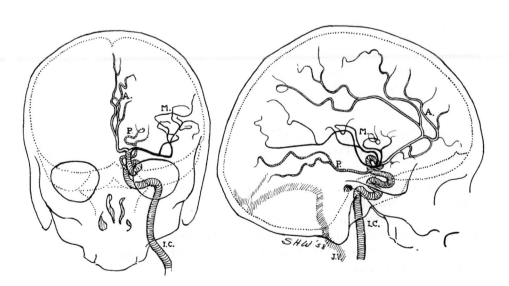

FIGURE 3–3. Schematic drawing of the internal carotid artery system. A = anterior cerebral artery, IC = internal carotid artery, MC = middle cerebral artery, P = posterior cerebral artery. (From Ranson SW, Clark SL: The Anatomy of the Nervous System, 10th ed. Philadelphia, WB Saunders, 1959.)

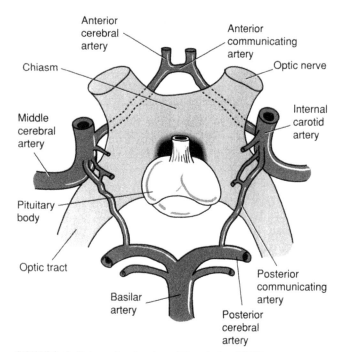

FIGURE 3–4. Schematic drawing of the circle of Willis.

Optic Tract. The major supply is from the anterior choroidal artery branch of the internal carotid.

Lateral Geniculate Body. The major contributors are the posterior choroidal artery branch from the posterior cerebral and the anterior choroidal artery branch from the internal carotid artery.

Optic Radiations. The upper portion of the radiations is supplied by the deep optic branch of the middle cerebral artery. The lower portion is mainly supplied from branches of the posterior cerebral arteries.

Visual Cortex. The visual cortex is nourished by terminal branches of the posterior cerebral artery. Some blood supply also comes from terminal branches of the middle cerebral artery. There are many interconnections between the posterior and middle cerebral arteries.

Frontal Gaze Centers. These centers are nourished by the middle cerebral artery branch of the internal carotid.

Pons, Midbrain, Cerebellum. These structures are nourished by branches of the basilar artery.

• BLOOD SUPPLY TO THE ORBIT: OPHTHALMIC ARTERY

The blood supply to the orbit comes from the ophthalmic artery branch of the internal carotid (Fig. 3–5). The ophthalmic artery enters the orbit through the optic foramen in the sheath of the optic nerve at the apex of the orbit, running forward near the medial orbital wall below the medial rectus muscle. Its terminal di-

visions are the supraorbital, nasal, and palpebral branches.

The branches of the ophthalmic artery can be divided into two groups. One group supplies the orbit and surrounding structures, and the other supplies the eye and its muscles. The ophthalmic artery's main branches are:

Orbital	Ocular
Lacrimal	Central retinal
Supraorbital	Posterior ciliaries
Ethmoidal	10 to 15 short
Posterior	2 long
Anterior	
Muscular	7 Anterior
Lateral (LR, SR, SO, LEV)	
Medial (MR, IR, IO)	
Supratrochlear	
Dorsal nasal	

Orbit (Fig. 3–6)

The ophthalmic artery next gives off the posterior ciliary arteries. These subdivide into 10 to 20 short posterior ciliary arteries (SPCA), which enter the posterior portion of the globe near the optic nerve to supply the choroid and optic disc. The two long posterior ciliary arteries (LPCA) pierce the sclera, then travel forward between the sclera and the choroid to supply the ciliary body, iris, and front part of the choroid. They branch and reanastomose to create the major and minor arterial circles of the iris.

Circulation to the extraocular muscles is supplied by lateral and medial muscular branches of the ophthalmic artery. Many variations exist in the number and location of the muscular branches. Commonly, the lateral branch supplies the lateral rectus, superior rectus, and superior oblique muscles. The medial muscular branch

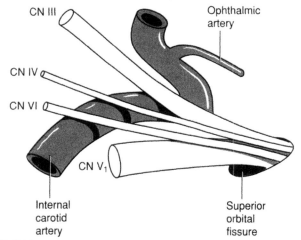

FIGURE 3–5. Schematic drawing of the portion of the internal carotid artery found within the cavernous sinus.

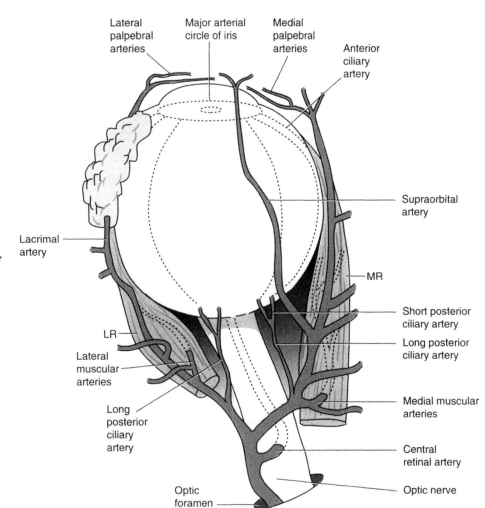

Lateral palpebral arteries

Major arterial circle of iris

Medial palpebral arteries

Anterior ciliary artery

Supraorbital artery

MR

Short posterior ciliary artery

Long posterior ciliary artery

Medial muscular arteries

Central retinal artery

Optic nerve

Lacrimal artery

LR

Lateral muscular arteries

Long posterior ciliary artery

Optic foramen

FIGURE 3–6. Pattern of the major branches of the ophthalmic artery.

is larger than the lateral, supplying the medial rectus, inferior rectus, and inferior oblique muscles. The inferior rectus and inferior oblique also receive a branch from the infraorbital artery. Two arteries emerge from each muscle tendon, except the lateral rectus, which only has one.

The seven arteries that leave the four rectus muscles become the anterior ciliary arteries (ACAs). The ACAs penetrate the sclera near the muscle's insertions to supply the iris and ciliary body, joining with the two LPCAs to form the major arterial circle of the iris. The major arterial circle nourishes the front third of the eye.

The lacrimal artery branches off the ophthalmic artery as it runs over the optic nerve. It travels toward the temporal side of the orbit with the lacrimal nerve, running between the superior and lateral recti to supply the lacrimal gland. The artery then sends a twig to the lateral rectus and further splits into terminal vessels, the superior and inferior palpebral arteries. These supply the conjunctiva and the upper eyelid. Other lacrimal artery branches freely anastomose with branches from

the external carotid system to form the arterial arcades of the eyelids.

Two ethmoidal arteries arise from the ophthalmic as it travels forward along the medial wall to supply the ethmoidal air cells, frontal sinus, and mucous membranes of the ethmoid and nose. The supraorbital artery branch from the ophthalmic artery travels along the skull through the supraorbital notch, supplying the upper eyelid, forehead, and scalp. Medial and lateral palpebral branches anastomose with lacrimal artery branches to help form the arterial arcades of the eyelids. At the front of the orbit, the ophthalmic artery splits into its terminal branches, the supratrochlear, and the dorsal nasal.

Eyeball

The central retinal artery, the first division of the ophthalmic artery, pierces the optic nerve 12 mm behind the globe and penetrates the lamina cribrosa with the central retinal vein. The retinal arteries and veins travel through the nerve head, but split immediately

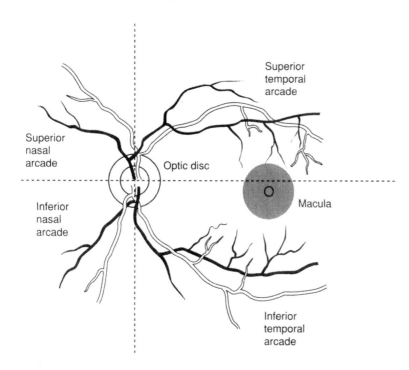

FIGURE 3–7. Schematic drawing of the main branches of the central retinal artery.

once within the eye, dividing the retina into four quadrants, two supplied by the superior and inferior temporal arcades and two supplied by superior and inferior nasal vessels.

The blood supply to the retina comes from two systems. Blood is supplied to the five inner layers of the retina closer to the vitreous by the central retinal artery (Fig. 3–7). The outer five layers of the retina closer to the choroid are supplied by the choroidal system. The macula is nourished by branches of the inferior and

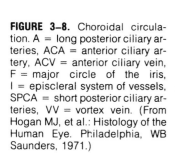

FIGURE 3–8. Choroidal circulation. A = long posterior ciliary arteries, ACA = anterior ciliary artery, ACV = anterior ciliary vein, F = major circle of the iris, I = episcleral system of vessels, SPCA = short posterior ciliary arteries, VV = vortex vein. (From Hogan MJ, et al.: Histology of the Human Eye. Philadelphia, WB Saunders, 1971.)

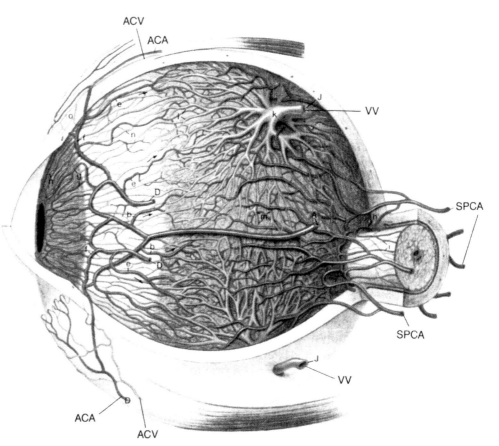

superior temporal arcades. The fovea is nourished from the choriocapillaris below it. The transparent retina allows easy visualization to the level of the pigmented epithelium, where some of the color and detail of the choroid are screened out (Fig. 3–8).

The choroidal vessels are usually only noted as an orange background on fundus examination. The arterial supply to the choroid comes partly from the short ciliary arteries entering about the optic nerve and partly from anterior ciliary arteries entering the eye from the extraocular muscles.

The central retinal artery and vein system does not connect to the choroidal circulation (Fig. 3–9).

● VENOUS RETURN FROM THE HEAD

From the Orbit

As in other parts of the body, ocular arterial blood flow is transferred to veins through a fine capillary network that progresses into sequentially larger vessels that carry venous blood out of the orbit. Blood that arrived by way of the central retinal artery is carried out of the globe by the central retinal vein. The blood drains out of the choroid by four vortex veins, one in each posterior quadrant. The upper pair collects into the superior ophthalmic vein, as do the lacrimal and

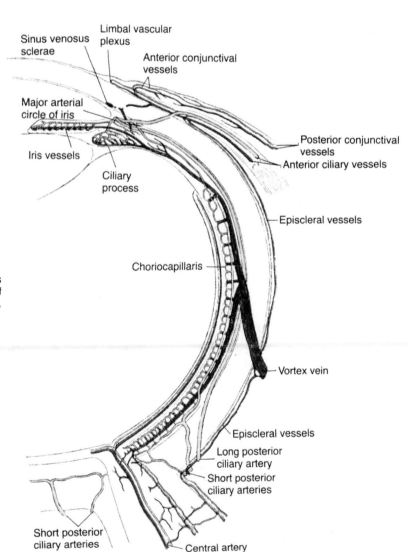

FIGURE 3–9. Blood supply to the eye as shown in cross section. (From Warwick R: Eugene Wolff's Anatomy of the Eye and Orbit, 7th ed. Philadelphia, WB Saunders, 1976.)

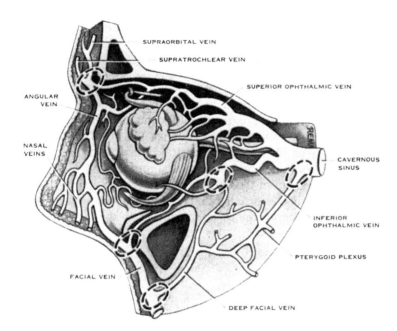

FIGURE 3-10. Venous drainage from the orbit. (From Warwick R: Eugene Wolff's Anatomy of the Eye and Orbit, 7th ed. Philadelphia, WB Saunders, 1976.)

FIGURE 3-11. Venous drainage from the head. (From Carpenter MB: Human Neuroanatomy, 7th ed. Baltimore, Williams & Wilkins, 1976.)

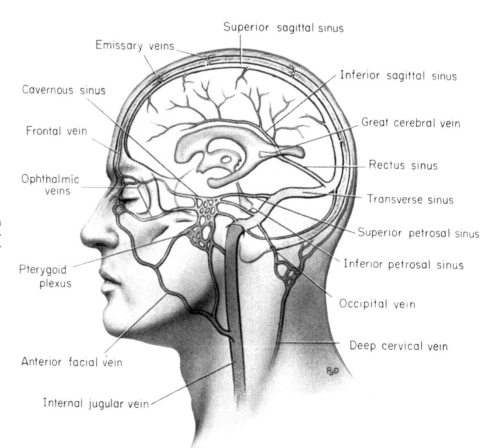

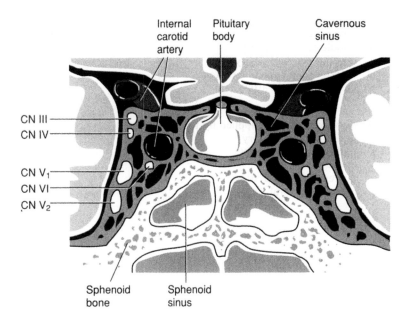

FIGURE 3–12. Coronal section through the cavernous sinus.

ethmoidal veins. The lower pair drains into the inferior ophthalmic vein. To a lesser extent, blood drains from the ciliary body into anterior ciliary veins. These drain into muscular veins from the extraocular muscles, which empty into the superior and inferior ophthalmic veins (Fig. 3–10). The larger, superior ophthalmic vein and the smaller, inferior ophthalmic vein carry blood away from the globe and orbit backward, the superior through the superior orbital fissure into the cavernous sinus. The inferior sometimes joins the superior but can exit through the inferior orbital fissure into the pterygoid plexus under the orbit floor. The central retinal vein can join the superior ophthalmic vein before both enter the cavernous sinus, usually above the annulus. Some drainage also occurs out of the orbit over the lacrimal sac from the supraorbital and palpebral veins connecting to the facial blood vessel system.

From the Brain

The blood drainage system from the brain is divided into two large interrelated categories, the cerebral veins and the dural sinuses.

Superficial cerebral veins, named according to their location, collect blood from the surface of the brain. Deep cerebral veins return blood from the area around the midbrain.

Fourteen dural sinuses provide most of the venous drainage from the brain. Each sinus is an area of "pooling," receiving deoxygenated blood that is eventually carried out of the skull through the internal jugular veins. Each internal jugular vein travels down the side of the neck, merging with its respective subclavian vein to form respective brachiocephalic veins. The right and left brachiocephalic veins unite to form the superior

vena cava, which empties into the right atrium of the heart (Fig. 3–11).

We are mainly interested in the two cavernous sinuses that lie on either side of the sella turcica in the middle cranial fossa. The front end of the cavernous sinus abuts the superior orbital fissure. The superior ophthalmic vein drains blood from the eye and orbit through the superior orbital fissure into the cavernous sinus. On the inner wall of the sinus lies the internal carotid artery (Fig. 3–12). In or near the outer wall are the third (oculomotor), fourth (trochlear), ophthalmic divisions (V_1) of the fifth (trigeminal), sixth (abducens), and maxillary division (V_2) of the fifth (trigeminal) cranial nerves. These nerves enter the orbit through the superior orbital fissure. The two cavernous sinuses communicate with each other around the pituitary body.

Bibliography

Doxanas MT, Anderson RL: Clinical Orbital Anatomy. Baltimore, Williams & Wilkins, 1984.

Miller NR: Vascular supply of the visual pathways. In Miller NR (ed): Walsh & Hoyt's Clinical Neuro-ophthalmology, 4th ed, Vol. I. Baltimore, Williams & Wilkins, 1985.

Warwick R: Eugene Wolff's Anatomy of the Eye and Orbit, 7th ed. Philadelphia, WB Saunders, 1976.

● CHAPTER 3 BLOOD SUPPLY

1. The internal carotid artery interconnects with the basilar system at the
   a. cavernous sinus
   b. ophthalmic artery
   c. vertebral artery
   d. circle of Willis
   e. pituitary body.

2. The ophthalmic artery branches off the
   a. internal carotid artery
   b. middle cerebral artery
   c. anterior cerebral artery
   d. anterior communicating artery
   e. common carotid artery.

3. The occipital lobe is supplied by the
   a. internal carotid artery
   b. middle cerebral artery
   c. circle of Willis
   d. posterior cerebral artery
   e. anterior cerebral artery.

4. The superior and inferior ophthalmic veins drain into the
   a. vortex veins
   b. supraorbital vein
   c. cavernous sinus
   d. ethmoid sinus
   e. muscular veins.

5. The blood supply to the outer retina is partly from the
   a. central retinal artery
   b. short ciliary arteries
   c. anterior cerebral artery
   d. ethmoidal artery
   e. supraorbital artery.

Barbara Cassin
Diana J. Shamis

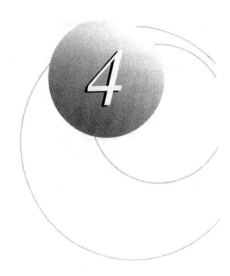

Pharmacology

LEARNING OBJECTIVES

- Describe proper technique for instillation of topical ophthalmic drops and ointment
- List the advantages and disadvantages of four methods of drug delivery
- Explain the technique and rationale of punctal occlusion
- Differentiate between mydriatic and cycloplegic medications

- Describe four different types of glaucoma medications with an example of each type
- List three antibiotics, three antiviral agents, three antifungal medications, three corticosteroids, and three anesthetic agents used for the care of eyes

Although ophthalmic technical personnel are not responsible for prescribing drugs, they must understand what drugs are commonly prescribed and why. Because they are often the first personnel to hear patient complaints about symptoms subsequent to taking such medications, it is especially important to be aware of side effects from drugs taken for ocular disorders, as well as ocular side effects from drugs taken for systemic diseases. New drugs appear every year, often supplanting those in use for decades. As you become more familiar with your ophthalmologist's drug preferences, you may use this information to explain to the patient how and why a drug is taken.

Drugs are substances that affect body functions. They may be described in three ways:

1. Chemical formula (e.g., 5-iodo-2-deoxyuridine, acetylsalicylic acid, 2,6-dichloro-N'-2-imidazolidinylidene-1,4-benzenediaminemine monohydrochloride)
2. Approved generic name (e.g., idoxuridine, aspirin, apraclonidine)
3. Brand name (e.g., Bufferin or Ecotrin, Iopidine).

An important part of any history taking is trying to discover any sensitivity to drugs the patient knows he or she has. Any chemical or drug in sufficiently high doses can become toxic to the patient. Even the appropriate therapeutic dose may cause a toxic reaction in the susceptible patient. Ophthalmologists continually evaluate the risk-benefit ratio, i.e., the chances the toxic effect will exceed the benefit to the patient. Drugs are generally prescribed with the lowest concentration needed to be effective. To take an accurate drug history, ophthalmic technical personnel should become familiar with the usual doses of common ophthalmic medications.

Often the patient may not be able to tell you what medications he or she is taking or the dosage. Patients should be encouraged to bring medications with them. You should try to assess how the patient actually does take them, rather than how he or she is supposed to take them.

● ROUTES OF ADMINISTRATION

Drugs may be administered to the eye by various methods. Topical medications are applied locally to the surface of the eye, either as drops or ointment. This route is the simplest and the most common, and it can be self-administered.

Drops may also be solutions or suspensions. Solutions have the drug completely dissolved in them. Suspensions contain very small, undissolved, drug particles. With time, the particles settle to the bottom of the bottle. Suspensions must be shaken thoroughly just before use. Ocular steroids are commonly in suspension form.

Topical drugs have the advantage of being absorbed directly by the eye, with little being absorbed by the body as a whole, thus avoiding undesirable systemic side effects. The disadvantages are that an insufficient dose may penetrate the cornea and the beneficial effects will not extend beyond the anterior segment. Corneal penetration increases when the corneal epithelium is disrupted. This may occur following applanation tonometry, corneal abrasion, or topical anesthetic drug application. A higher concentration may also be achieved by increasing the length of time a topical medication remains on the eye. The patient should be instructed to block the punctum after drops are instilled to avoid the drug exiting into the nasolacrimal duct, so more medication will stay on the eye. This not only increases the corneal penetration, but also decreases the amount of drug entering the bloodstream through blood vessels in the nasal mucosa, and so reduces systemic side effects. Ointments and suspensions persist longer than drops.

Ophthalmic technical personnel frequently apply topical medications as ordered by the ophthalmologist and instruct the patient on proper procedure (Fig. 4–1). Teach the patient to pull down the lower eyelid for instillation into the lower conjunctival cul-de-sac. The tip of the dropper bottle or the ointment tube must never touch the eye or eyelid. If it does, the contents are considered contaminated and must be discarded. Replace the cap immediately after use to prevent contamination. One or two drops or a bead of ointment is all that is needed. Have the patient close the eye for about 30 seconds to contain the drop, or open and shut the eye to spread the ointment. Ointment remains in contact with the eye longer, but it blurs vision and tends to be more difficult to apply. It is often used in children because it is more difficult to "cry out" than drops.

Drugs administered systemically to the whole body reach therapeutic levels more quickly in highly vascular tissues such as the eyelids, optic nerve, retina, and uvea, but not in the anterior segment or the aqueous. A large amount of drug is absorbed by the body to supply the relatively smaller amount that reaches the eye. The increased risk of possible systemic side effects is weighed against the benefit to be gained when an eye has a severe problem.

Systemic administration may be taken orally, i.e., by mouth, (per os, p.o.). Because this method is easiest for the patient, it is the most common systemic route. When taken by mouth, a drug enters the intestines, then passes from the gut into blood vessels, and finally from the blood vessels into eye tissues. Its disadvantage is the uneven distribution of the drug to the target organ.

Systemic administration may be parenteral (outside the intestinal tract) by injection. The organ is affected more quickly, and the dose is more accurate. Injections are given intravenously (IV or into a vein) or intramuscularly (IM or into the muscle), when even higher levels of drug must reach the eye, as for more severe infections and inflammations. Intramuscular injection is used for large doses needing slower absorption. Intravenous injection is absorbed more rapidly than an oral administration.

When steroids and antibiotics are injected into tissues around the eye (periocular) there is better and longer delivery to the anterior segment of the eye when compared with topical administration, with less systemic absorption than with oral medications and IM or IV injections. Drugs may be injected subcutaneously (subq, s.c.)—under the skin—retrobulbar—behind the eye within the muscle cone (primarily for local anesthesia)—or subconjunctivally (subconj)—under the conjunctiva. Intracameral injection into the anterior chamber is used for thick elastic gel (viscoelastic substances) before cataract extraction. Intravitreous injection into the vitreous substance may be used in a heroic effort to save an eye with severe endophthalmitis.

• AUTONOMIC DRUGS FOR OPHTHALMOLOGY
(Table 4–1)

Cholinergic Agents (Parasympathomimetics)

These direct-acting drugs simulate the effect of acetylcholine. Among the ocular effects are constriction of the pupil, by contraction of the iris sphincter, and contraction of the ciliary body, causing accommodative spasm and increased myopia. Mechanical traction on the scleral spur opens the trabecular meshwork and increases the aqueous outflow. Dropper bottles containing parasympathetic agonists have green tops.

Glaucoma Treatment

Pilocarpine HCl. This drug, in drops, 0.5 to 6%, qid, will last 6 hours. This safe, low cost, common

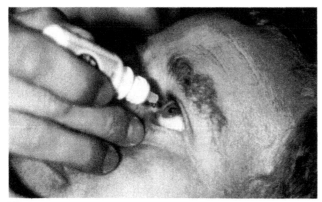

FIGURE 4–1. Technique for application of topical eye drops. Middle and fourth finger pull out lower eyelid, exposing lower cul-de-sac as thumb and forefinger squeeze dropper bottle.

TABLE 4–1

Common Ocular Medications

Medication	Common Dosage	Bottle Cap Color	Frequency	Common Side Effects
Glaucoma Medications				
Pilocarpine	0.5–6%	Green	QID	Miosis, induced myopia, blurring, brow ache
Timolol (Timoptic)	0.25%	Lt. blue	BID	Bradycardia, hypotension, bronchial constriction, shortness of breath
	0.50%	Yellow	BID	
Timolol (Timoptic XE)	0.25%	Lt. blue	QID	(Same as Timoptic)
	0.50%	Yellow	QID	
Betaxolol (Betoptic)	0.25%		BID	(Same as Timoptic)
	0.50%	Dk. blue	BID	
Levobunolol (Betagan)	0.25%	Lt. blue	BID	(Same as Timoptic)
	0.50%	Yellow	BID	
Dipivefrin (Propine)	0.10%	Purple	BID	Conjunctival injection, topical irritation, mydriasis
Acetazolamide (Diamox)	125 mg, 250 mg	(tablets)	BID or QID	Nausea, diarrhea, loss of appetite, lethargy, tingling in extremities
	500 mg	(sequels)	BID or QID	
Methazolamide (Neptazane)	25 mg, 50 mg	(tablets)	BID or QID	

	Common Dosage	Bottle Cap Color	Effective Period	Common Side Effects
Cycloplegics				Uncommon
Tropicamide (Mydriacyl)	1%	Red	5–6 hours	Dry mouth, excitation, facial flushing, tachycardia
Cyclopentolate (Cyclogyl)	0.5–1.0%	''	24 hours	Angle closure due to dilation
Homatropine		''	36 hours	
Scopolamine		''	48–72 hrs	
Atropine	1%	''	2 weeks	
Mydriatics				
Phenylephrine (Neo-Synephrine)	2.5–10.0%	Red	4–6 hours	Uncommon, irregular heart beat, hypertension, angle closure due to dilation

antiglaucoma agent has been used since 1876. Ocular side effects occur frequently. Not only do these drops sting, but younger people may experience ciliary spasm, which produces pain, brow ache, and accommodative spasm, all of which do subside. Myopia induced by the accommodative spasm causes visual acuity to decrease initially, only returning to normal 6 hours later. Patients have decreased vision in dim illumination because pharmacologically miotic pupils cannot dilate. With mild cataracts, the miosis often blocks the visual axis significantly and decreases vision. This drug may cause conjunctival and anterior uveal blood vessel congestion, allergic conjunctivitis and dermatitis, and cataracts.

Patients taking long-term miotics may develop posterior synechiae (scars binding the back of the iris to the lens) from the chronically small, immobile pupil. Pilocarpine should be discontinued before ophthalmic surgery because it has inflammatory properties.

Pilocarpine's systemic side effects include slow heart rate, sweating, tearing, nausea, vomiting, salivation, diarrhea, gastrointestinal cramps, and bronchial muscle constriction. The antidote of choice is atropine.

Pilocarpine Ocuserts. Formulations are P-20 and P-40 (20 μg/hr; 40 μg/hr). These are membrane wafers, impregnated with pilocarpine and designed to give slow release. The wafer is worn under the upper or lower eyelid and is replaced weekly. This delivery system eliminates many of the side effects of pilocarpine drops. Because patients may still develop accomodative spasm during the first 12 to 24 hours after placement of a fresh membrane, they should be advised to replace it before going to sleep.

Pilopine Gel. Pilocarpine gel (4%) may be used at bedtime for prolonged therapeutic effect while the patient sleeps.

Carbachol. This miotic, 0.75 to 3%, tid, is no longer widely used, unless intolerance to pilocarpine occurs. Its actions and side effects are similar to those of pilocarpine.

Nonglaucoma Applications. A rapid acting, direct parasympathetic agonist is given as an intraocular injection for immediate miosis following cataract extraction. Constricting the pupil allows the iris to act as a barrier, assuring that the implanted posterior chamber intraocular lens remains in the posterior chamber. Examples include Miochol (acetylcholine chloride 1 : 100) as an intraocular injection and Miostat (carbachol).

Indirect Cholinergic Agents

Anticholinesterase inhibitors stimulate the parasympathetic system by inactivating the enzyme cholinesterase. Cholinesterase chemically breaks down acetylcholine. Decreased cholinesterase activity allows naturally released acetylcholine to stay longer in the synaptic space and continue parasympathetic action.

Ocular effects include ciliary muscle and iris sphincter spasm resulting in brow ache, accommodative spasm with its induced myopia, and miosis. Physical opening of the trabecular meshwork increases aqueous outflow.

Glaucoma Treatment

Echothiophate Iodide (Phospholine Iodide). This drug, 0.03 to 0.25%, bid, may be used for open angle glaucoma when patients are not compliant with pilocarpine. It tends to be badly tolerated.

Its ocular side effects are similar to those produced by pilocarpine. It slows the heart rate and causes nausea, vomiting, increased inflammation, and diarrhea. Phospholine iodide is also cataractogenic in older patients and should be avoided in phakic patients. Chronically miotic pupils may cause posterior synechiae. To prevent formation of iris cysts in children Neo-Synephrine (which contracts the iris dilator, counteracting the chronic miosis) should be given concurrently. Because of the additional side effects, direct-acting cholinergic agents are preferred.

The patient should be warned that anticholinesterase inhibitors may interact with commonly taken muscle relaxants (such as succinylcholine), enhancing and prolonging the apnea (lack of breathing) produced. If general anesthesia is necessary, phospholine iodide should be discontinued for at least 2 weeks. Organophosphate pesticides present in garden chemicals and dog dips should also be avoided as these produce compounding effect and may quickly reach toxic levels. These compounds can be absorbed through the skin and result in illness or respiratory arrest. Ocular side effects are more common with cholinesterase inhibitors than with direct-acting parasympathomimetics. The antidote is atropine.

Other Agents. The following drugs are similar to phospholine iodide, but are now rarely used:

Demecarium bromide (Humorsol): 0.12% to 0.25%, bid

Isofluorophate (Floropryl): 0.25%, bid

Physostigmine salicylate (Eserine): 0.25%

Nonglaucoma Applications

Edrophonium Chloride (Tensilon Chloride, Reversol). This drug, IM or IV, is a short-lived, rapid-acting, anticholinesterase inhibitor, given IV for the diagnosis of myasthenia gravis, a nerve-muscle junction weakness. Side effects include bradycardia (slow heart rate) and hypotension (low blood pressure). Atropine is the usual antidote.

Pyridostigmine Bromide (Mestinon). This long-acting, oral medication is used for the long-term treatment of myasthenia gravis.

Phospholine Iodide. This topical eye drop is used as an alternative method to glasses for controlling accommodative esotropia.

Parasympatholytic Agents

These parasympathetic blockers prevent acetylcholine action at the nerve endings in the muscle. The ocular effects are paralysis of iris sphincter and ciliary muscle causing pupil dilatation (mydriasis) and loss of accommodation (cycloplegia). With more heavily pigmented irides, and darker eye color, more medication is needed to achieve complete dilation and cycloplegia.

Parasympatholytics are used to provide improved dilation for retina examination and to suspend accommodation to allow accurate retinoscopy and refraction. In addition, these drugs treat ocular inflammatory processes such as uveitis, and in postoperative patients. Cycloplegia relieves the pain caused by ciliary spasm associated with iritis and corneal abrasion. With chronic uveitis, the pupil is miotic and does not move much, allowing posterior synechiae to form. Dilation with atropine can often bounce the pupil, thus breaking the synechiae. If the eye is inflamed, the dosage of atropine is often increased. In sensitive individuals, parasympatholytics can cause facial flushing, excitation, tachycardia (increased heart rate), dry mouth, fever, hallucination, convulsion, uncoordinated body movement, speech impairment, and disorientation. In case of overdose, discontinue the next dose, then resume. When overdose is severe, physostigmine, Tensilon (edrophonium chloride), or phospholine iodide is to be given as an antidote. Dropper bottles containing cycloplegic drugs have red tops.

The following parasympatholytics are commonly used.

Tropicamide (Mydriacyl). This drug, 0.50 to 2%, is weak, but lasts 5 to 6 hours, with one drop every 5 min × 2. Its effect is seen in 20 min. This is the most common cycloplegic for adults because of its short duration.

Cyclopentolate (Cyclogyl). This agent, 0.50 to 2%, lasts 24 hours. Instill one drop every 5 min × 2 with effect in 45 min. This is the most common cycloplegic given to children.

Homatropine. This drug, 2 to 5%, lasts 36 hours but is *rarely used.*

Scopolamine. This agent, 0.25%, lasts 48 to 72 hours and is *rarely used.*

Atropine Sulfate. This drug is available as 0.5 to 1% ointment, 0.5 to 1% drops, given at one bead bid × 2, or one drop tid × 3. Effects may last for 10 to 14 days. Atropine ointment is preferred over drops for children because it remains in the eye longer and is, therefore, less likely to be absorbed into the systemic circulation through the naso-lacrimal mucosa. A small dot of ointment is easier for the parents to administer to a child. No ointment is applied the day of the appointment because it is difficult to refract through the sticky film. Atropine is the most powerful cycloplegic.

Adrenergic Drugs (Sympathomimetics)

Direct-acting sympathomimetics dilate the eye by contraction of the iris dilator, but they have no cycloplegic effect because they do not act on the ciliary muscle involved with accommodation. Sympathetic agonists are also used to decrease the intraocular pressure. Alpha agonists mildly decrease aqueous production. Beta agonists increase aqueous production. Both increase uveal-scleral and trabecular aqueous outflow.

Glaucoma Treatment

Epinephrine HCl (Epifrin, Glaucon) or Epinephrine Borate (Eppy/N, Epinal). This agent, 0.50 to 2%, is given bid. Epinephrine has significant topical ocular side effects including local rebound vasodilation after vasoconstriction, chronic irritation, itching, tearing, blepharitis, and allergic conjunctivitis. Mild pupillary dilation may close an already narrow angle. Chronic use may cause adenochrome (black pigment) deposition in the lower conjunctival cul-de-sac. Epinephrine should not be given to aphakic patients because of the potential for macular edema. Systemic side effects are less common, but epinephrine may cause increased blood pressure, increased heart rate, palpitations, and vasoconstriction.

Dipivefrin HCl (Propine). This drug, 0.1% bid, is an inactive form (prodrug) of epinephrine. Propine has no therapeutic effect in its initial form until it is converted to epinephrine inside the eye. Once converted, it has the same effect of decreasing intraocular pressure (IOP) as epinephrine with fewer side effects. Enhanced absorption allows application of lower concentrations. The side effects are the same as those of epinephrine but milder.

Apraclonidine HCl (Iopidine). This agent, 0.50 to 1%, tid, is highly effective at lowering IOP, probably by decreasing aqueous production. It is given 1 hour before and immediately after anterior segment laser procedures to prevent postlaser IOP spike. It is also given to glaucoma patients on maximum medical therapy who need about a month's additional therapy to delay surgery. Side effects include ocular injection, irregular heart rate, and mydriasis.

Mydriatric Agents

Phenylephrine HCl (AK-Dilate, Mydfrin, Neo-Synephrine). Phenylephrine, 2.5%, 10%, with an effect that lasts 2 to 6 hours, enhances pupil dilation for retinal examinations. This agent is often used with cycloplegics to effect faster dilation, but it transiently elevates blood pressure and produces heart arrhythmias. Susceptible patients may be supersensitive.

Decongestants

Eye "whiteners" are not strong enough to dilate the pupil, but are weak topical ocular vasoconstrictors, enough to blanch the sclera in minutes, acting as a decongestant. Agents in current use include the following:

Naphazoline HCl (Naphcon, Albalon, Vasocon, Degest-2): 0.012 to 0.1%

Tetrahydrozoline (Murine Plus, Visine): 0.05%

Oxymetazoline (OcuClear): 0.025%

Phenylephrine (AK-Nefrin, Isopto Frin): 0.12%

Ephedrine

Adrenergic Drugs (Sympathomimetics)

Indirect acting adrenergic drugs are of limited clinical application in ophthalmology.

Cocaine

Topical *cocaine* stimulates the iris dilator by preventing the reuptake of norepinephrine. An intact sympathetic pathway is necessary for norepinephrine to be made available. Cocaine can be used to diagnose Horner's syndrome but does not enable one to differentiate preganglionic from postganglionic lesions.

Hydroxyamphetamine (Paredrine)

This topical sympathomimetic drug stimulates the iris dilator to contract by the release of norepinephrine from nerve terminals. An intact postganglionic sympathetic pathway is necessary for norepinephrine to be released. The Paredrine test can be used to differentiate a preganglionic from a postganglionic lesion in Horner's syndrome. This drug will not dilate the pupil if there is a postganglionic defect but will dilate one with a preganglionic defect. The drug is no longer available (Table 4–1).

Adrenergic Blocking Agents

Nonselective beta blockers, having both $beta_1$ and $beta_2$ receptor antagonist, are the current first choice for glaucoma control. They are generally well tolerated and without significant ocular side effects. Beta blockers decrease intraocular pressure by decreasing aqueous production. The dropper bottle has a yellow or blue top.

These medications can have very serious systemic side effects. $Beta_1$ blocker effects include bradycardia (decreased heart rate), hypotension (decreased blood pressure), and syncope (fainting). Check the patient's pulse periodically. $Beta_1$ blockers should not be given to any patient with a history of heart problems. $Beta_2$ blocker side effects include bronchial constriction and increased airway resistance. $Beta_2$ blockers should not be given to a patient with a history of asthma or COPD (chronic obstructive pulmonary disease).

Some typical drugs of this class are

Timolol maleate (Timoptic): 0.25%, 0.50%, bid

Levobunolol HCl (Betagan): 0.25%, 0.50%, bid

Metipranolol HCl (Optipranolol): 0.3%, bid

Betaxolol HCl (Betoptic): 0.25% suspension, 0.50% solution, qd or bid.

Betaxolol, a $beta_1$ cardiac blocker only, is similar to timolol and levobunolol but safer to give to patients with a history of lung problems.

Carbonic Anhydrase Inhibitors

These sulfa derivatives are powerful oral medications for control of glaucoma. Inhibition of the enzyme carbonic anhydrase slows aqueous production and decreases intraocular pressure.

Carbonic anhydrase inhibitors have many systemic side effects. Patients often complain about paresthesia (tingling in hands and feet), gastrointestinal upset, nausea, vomiting, diarrhea, increased urination, decreased appetite, weight loss, lethargy, kidney stones, mental changes, depression, and impotence. Because of their common and intolerable side effects, carbonic anhydrase inhibitors are used only if topical medications fail to provide adequate intraocular pressure control. Carbonic anhydrase inhibitors in glaucoma treatment include the following:

Acetazolamide (Diamox): 125- and 250-mg tabs, 500-mg sequels, bid, qid

Methazolamide (Neptazane): 25- and 50-mg tabs, bid, qid

Dichlorphenamide (Daranide): 50-mg tabs, bid

Hyperosmotic Agents

Osmotic agents are administered to obtain rapid, short-term decrease in intraocular pressure. The effect occurs within an hour and lasts about 4 hours. The eye is hypo-osmotic compared with the hyperosmotic agent. The increased osmotic gradient draws fluid out of the eye into the bloodstream. The fluid is filtered through the kidneys but not reabsorbed in the usual percentage because of the hyperosmotic agent's molecules. It is excreted as additional urine instead.

Because this fluid may overload the circulation, these drugs are not advised for heart patients; such drugs may trigger acute congestive heart failure.

Oral Agents

Oral agents have the advantage of easy administration. Unfortunately, they commonly cause nausea and vomiting. This side effect can be reduced by diluting the hyperosmotic with Gatorade, lime juice, or orange juice. Other side effects of osmotics include increased urine volume, headache, and mental confusion.

Glycerin (Glyrol, Osmoglyn): 50%. This should not be given to diabetics because it increases blood glucose levels.

Isosorbide (Ismotic). This drug, 45% solution, may be given to diabetics because it does not increase blood glucose levels as glycerin does.

Intravenous Osmotic Agents

Mannitol (Osmitrol): 20%. This drug has several side effects, e.g., increased plasma volume and marked increase in urine output, but remains the drug of choice because of its lack of other side effects, except in patients with renal disease.

Urea: 30%. This older drug is rarely given.

Anesthetics

All medications ending in -aine or -caine are anesthetics. These drugs produce a transient loss of feeling and pain by prevention of transmission of sensory nerve impulses.

Topical Ocular Anesthetics

These drugs are used for painless, comfortable measurement of intraocular pressure, examination of otherwise painful eye conditions such as corneal abrasions, and removal of superficial foreign bodies. The drops may cause momentary corneal irritation, conjunctival redness, and punctate epithelial erosion. Topical anes-

thesia occurs within one minute of instillation and lasts 15 to 20 minutes.

Topical anesthetics should never be prescribed to ease pain from corneal injury or disease. Continued application leads to softening of the corneal epithelium, retards corneal healing, and possibly results in perforation of the cornea. Topical anesthetics are never prescribed for home use. Some topical ocular anesthetics are as follows.

Cocaine. Severe side effects, including addiction, have resulted in a decline in the use of this excellent anesthetic.

Proparacaine HCl. (AK-Taine, Alcaine, Ophthaine, Ophthetic). This is the most commonly chosen anesthetic for applanation tonometry and other minor clinical procedures.

Tetracaine. (Pontocaine): 0.5%. This drug is more irritating, but longer lasting, than proparacaine, and it is given for minor surgical procedures in the operating room.

Periocular Local Anesthetics

Because of the risks of general anesthesia, much ocular surgery is done with injectable periocular anesthetics.

Retrobulbar injection of anesthetic agents into the muscle cone is used for much intraocular surgery, thus preventing neural transmission from CN II through CN VI. The patient cannot see (CN II), cannot feel (CN V), and cannot move (CN III, IV, and VI) the eye. A tranquilizer is often added to help the patient relax during the procedure. Although rare, adverse reactions are possible, including decreased blood pressure, tremors, convulsions, and respiratory or cardiac arrest. Surgical rooms should be equipped with devices for monitoring vital signs and suction apparatus for clearing airways. Physicians and allied health personnel must always be prepared to perform cardiopulmonary resuscitation when anesthetics are injected.

Lidocaine HCl (Dalcaine, Xylocaine). Lidocaine diffuses more readily through tissue than procaine and lasts longer, permitting up to 2 hours of operating time from one injection.

Procaine HCl (Novocain) and Choloroprocaine HCl (Nesacaine). Although these anesthetics have the advantage of rapid onset of effect, they are rarely used in ophthalmic procedures because of short duration (30 minutes to 1 hour).

Mepivacaine HCl (Carbocaine). Mepivacaine is absorbed more slowly than lidocaine, with an effective period of 2 to 3 hours.

Bupivacaine HCl (Marcaine). Bupivacaine is absorbed more slowly than lidocaine, slowing the onset of effect, but has the advantage of a long effective period (4 to 6 hours). It is frequently used in combination with lidocaine to achieve rapid onset of effect and a long effective period.

Additives to Retrobulbar Anesthetics

Epinephrine. Causes vasoconstriction that slows the absorption of local anesthetic injections, prolonging duration of action.

Hyaluronidase. Improves the spread of anesthetic through orbital tissues.

Antibiotics

Derived from living organisms or synthesized commercially, these antibacterial drugs are used to destroy disease-causing micro-organisms. Drugs that kill bacteria ("bugs") are bactericidal, whereas bacteriostatic drugs only stop bacterial reproduction and proliferation. Sulfonamides such as sulfacetamide sodium (AK-Sulf, Bleph 10, Cetamide, Sulamyd, Vasosulf) and sulfisoxazole (Gantrisin), are bacteriostatic drugs often administered for bacterial conjunctivitis.

Most currently used antibiotics are bactericidal. In order to effectively fight bacteria, the physician has to know what antibiotics they are sensitive to. Cultures of the infecting micro-organisms should be taken before treatment is begun because the antibiotics may prevent growth of the micro-organisms in culture media and prevent an accurate diagnosis. Once cultures are taken, a broad-spectrum antibiotic is tried in a *shotgun* approach. If this approach does not work, sensitivity testing of the bacterial culture will indicate which antibiotic will be most effective against the infection. In intraocular infections, cultures from the vitreous yield better cultures than those from the aqueous. Overuse and unnecessary use of antibiotics may lead to increased adverse side effects and development of antibiotic-resistant microorganisms.

Different types of infection require different modes of antibiotic administration. Topical medications are effective for superficial infections such as conjunctivitis or corneal ulcers. An important consideration in topical antibiotic therapy is how well the medication penetrates the cornea. Penicillin and tetracycline, two common systemic antibiotics, penetrate the cornea so poorly that they are rarely applied topically. Periocular or subconjunctival injections are given for more severe corneal ulcers, and intravitreal injections are given for severe intraocular infections.

The commonest gram-negative rod is *Pseudomonas*. Sources of *Pseudomonas* include contaminated mascara or contact lens solutions. Because of its virulence, ulcers from contact lens wear are treated for *Pseudomonas* until proved otherwise. Effective antibiotics include neomycin, gentamycin, tobramycin, cephazolin, and carbenicillin.

Two unwanted effects that may be produced by antibiotics in the treatment of eye infections are hypersensitivity and destruction of micro-organisms normally found in eye tissue. Hypersensitivity causes a local allergic reaction but on occasion will produce serious anaphylaxis, an extreme allergic reaction that is potentially fatal. Once this occurs the involved drug cannot be given to that patient again. Destroying normal micro-organisms allows other bacteria, normally inhibited, to grow rampantly.

A discussion of commonly used antibiotics follows:

Aminoglycosides

As a group, these drugs are especially effective against gram-negative organisms but have possible side effects involving the kidneys and hearing.

Amikacin. Often used when organisms are resistant to gentamycin.

Gentamycin (Garamycin, Genoptic). This broad-spectrum antibiotic is especially effective against gram-negative organisms such as *Pseudomonas*. Used topically it may cause nausea, vomiting, and headache. When the drug is injected, it may cause hearing or kidney problems.

Neomycin. This drug is being phased out of common usage because of increased allergic reactions.

Tobramycin (Tobrex). This drug is used in treating corneal abrasions, as is neomycin. It is the usual first choice for serious gram-negative infections.

Bacitracin (Baciguent)

This drug is often selected to treat blepharoconjunctivitis caused most commonly by *Staphylococcus aureus*. Pneumococcus and hemophilus also commonly cause conjunctivitis.

Cephalosporins

Cefaclor (Ceclor)

Cefotaxime (Claforan)

Cefoxitin (Cephamycin, Mefoxin)

Cephalexin (Keflex)

Cephalothin (Keflin)

Cephazolin (Ancef, Kefzol)

Chloramphenicol (Chloromycetin, Chloroptic, Econochlor, Ophthochlor)

Chloramphenicol has serious side effects, e.g., bone marrow suppression, renal disease, and anemia. It has less toxicity than penicillin, however, and is effective against a wide variety of microorganisms. It is exceptionally well suited in the treatment of intraocular infections, such as Haemophilus influenzae, following penetrating trauma or surgery.

Other Single-Agent Antibiotics

Ciloxin

Clindamycin: often used to treat ocular toxoplasmosis

Colistin (Coly-Mycin S)

Erythromycin (Ilotycin)

Gramacidin

Lincomycin

Penicillins

   Ampicillin

   Carbenicillin

   Methicillin

   Penicillin G

   Penicillin V

Polymixin B

Streptomycin

Tetracycline (Achromycin, Aureomycin): effective for treating chlamydia

Vancomycin: one of the most effective antibiotics for resistant staphylococcus infections; kidney or hearing toxicity possible

Antibiotic Mixtures

Sometimes medications are mixed to facilitate administration.

Neosporin (Neomycin, polymyxin B, and bacitracin)

Polysporin (Polymyxin B and bacitracin)

Statrol (Neomycin and polymyxin B)

Antifungals

Fungi are plants that reproduce by spores and spread by hyphae. Microscopic fungi, such as molds, mildews, and yeasts, are found in every environment. Corneal trauma involving plant material, such as walking into a tree branch, is a common source of fungal infection. Fungi thrive in moist, warm environments, and consequently, are most common in the southern United States.

Once a fungal infection is under control, patients frequently need a corneal graft. The following ocular antifungal medications are commonly administered:

Amphotericin B (Fungizone)

Natamycin (Natacyn, Pimaricin): current agent of choice

Miconazole (Monistat)

Antivirals

Antiviral drugs for the treatment of ocular herpes simplex infections were the first antiviral medications developed. Antiviral agents may cause an allergic contact dermatitis. The following drugs are common ocular antiviral medications:

Idoxuridine (Herplex, IDU, Stoxil). Side effects include punctate keratitis, follicular conjunctivitis, punctal stenosis, and atopic dermatitis.

Trifluorothymidine (Viroptic, TFT). This most effective drug is most commonly used.

Vidarabine (Vira-A). This agent is less toxic than IDU.

Acyclovir (Zovirax). Used in genital herpes and herpes zoster ophthalmicus.

Artificial Tears and Lubricants

Solutions containing wetting agents such as polyvinyl alcohol or methylcellulose can be used for long-term tear replacement in patients with dry eyes. Tear supplements extend tear film breakup, reducing the gritty, burning sensation typical of dry eyes. Many varieties are available without prescriptions. Patients usually try several brands to find the most suitable. Preservatives in a particular solution may be irritating to the eye. If patients use artificial tears more than six times a day, it is recommended that they use a nonpreserved form.

Solutions

Absorbotear

Dry Eye Therapy

Lacril

Liquifilm

Murine

Refresh

Tears Naturale

Ointments

Hypotears

Refresh

Lacri-Lube

Anti-inflammatory Agents

Corticosteroids

Natural corticosteroids are produced in the adrenal cortex. Synthetic corticosteroids are administered for their excellent anti-inflammatory properties. They reduce the swelling, redness, exudation, and scarring which accompany ocular surgery, trauma, allergy, or inflammatory processes, such as uveitis. Delicate ocular tissues are particularly susceptible to damage from inflammation and scarring.

The serious drawback of corticosteroids is that they are immunosuppressive and decrease the body's natural resistance to invading or opportunistic microorganisms. The ocular side effects of corticosteroids include proliferation of viral, fungal, or bacterial infections; retarded wound healing; corneal perforation; increased intraocular pressure; and posterior subcapsular cataract formation.

One serious side effect of systemic steroids is a fluid imbalance that leads to water retention with tissue swelling and puffiness and causes a typical "moonfaced" appearance. Patients may become hypertensive and may experience muscle wasting and weakness, bone demineralization (producing stress fractures), retarded growth, diabetes from increased blood glucose levels, hirsutism, and decreased ability to deal with other illness. Steroid dosages need to be tapered because sudden termination can cause recurrent inflammation, systemic adrenal shut-down, and even death.

After organ transplantation, steroid therapy in children for immunosuppression may retard growth. As with most medications, corticosteroids are effective longer when injected, but topical drops have markedly fewer side effects.

The following is a list of common corticosteroids:

Prednisolone (AK-Pred, Predforte, Econopred, Inflamase)

Fluorometholone (FML Liquifilm, Fluor-Op)

Dexamethasone (Decadron, Maxidex, AK-Dex)

Medrysone (HMS Liquifilm)

Mixture of Corticosteroid and Antibiotic

This mixture often eases the administration of the medication.

Blephamide (prednisolone and sulfacetamide)

Cortisporin (hydrocortisone, neomycin, bacitracin, and polymixin B)

Maxitrol (dexamethasone, neomycin, and polymixin B)

TobraDex (dexamethasone, tobramycin)

Nonsteroidal Anti-inflammatory Drugs (NSAIDs)

These substances are clinically valuable because they can often achieve the required anti-inflammatory effect without the undesirable side effects produced by corticosteroids. These medications block the synthesis of prostaglandins.

A list of common NSAIDs follows:

Acetylsalicyclic acid (Aspirin, Anacin, Bufferin, Empirin, Excedrin)

Diflunisal (Dolobid)

Fenoprofen (Nalfon)

Flurbiprofen (Ocufen)

Ibuprofen (Motrin, Advil)

Indomethacin (Indocin)

Naproxen (Naprosyn)

Sulindac (Clinoril)

Tolmetin (Tolectin)

Systemic Medications

During the history taking part of the ocular examination, technical personnel must record current medications the patient may be taking. The following lists common systemic medications eye patients may be using:

Antianxiety Agents

Chlorediazepoxide (Librium)

Diazepam (Valium)

Lorazepam (Ativan)

Anticonvulsant Agents

These are taken to prevent seizures.

Diazepam (Valium)

Phenobarbital (Luminal)

Phenytoin (Dilantin)

Valproic acid (Depakene)

Antidepressants

These mood elevators are often called "nerve pills." Common side effects are drowsiness and dizziness. Common agents are

Amitryptyline (Elavil)

Chlordiazepoxide (Librium)

Desipramine (Norpramin)

Doxepin (Adapin, Sinequan)

Imipramine (Tofranil)

Perphenazine (Triavil)

Analgesics (Pain Relief)

Acetaminophen (Tylenol)

NSAIDs:

Acetylsalicylic acid (Aspirin, Anacin, Bufferin, Empirin, Excedrin)

Diflunisal (Dolobid)

Fenoprofen (Nalfon)

Ibuprofen (Motrin, Advil)

Indomethacin (Indocin)

Naproxen (Naprosyn)

Sulindac (Clinoril)

Opiate-Related Analgesics

Codeine (Tylenol 3)

Meperidine (Demerol)

Oxycodone (Percocet, Percodan)

Pentazocine (Talwin)

Propoxyphene (Darvon, Darvocet)

Cardiac Drugs

What the patient describes as "heart pills" may be for congestive heart failure (CHF), such as

Digitalis (Digoxin, Lanoxin)

Propranolol (Inderal)

Diuretics are prescribed to increase urination and reduce excess fluid. Some examples are

Acetazolamide (Diamox)

Chlorothiazide (Diuril)

Furosemide (Lasix)

Hydrochlorothiazide (HCTZ)

Little pink or white pills (vasodilators) given for chest pain (angina) include

Nitroglycerin

Isosorbide (Isordil)

Verapamil (Calan)

Nifedipine (Procardia)

Irregular heart beat (arrhythmia) is controlled by

Propranolol (Inderal)

Quinine (Quinidine, Quinidex)

Procainamide (Procan, Pronestyl)

Hypertension (high blood pressure) is frequently treated by beta blockers such as

Atenolol (Tenormin)

Metoprolol (Lopressor)

Nadolol (Corgard)

Propranolol (Inderal)

Timolol (Blocadren)

Other physicians use calcium channel blockers, such as

Diltiazem HCl (Cardizem)

Nifedipine (Procardia)

Verapamil HCl (Calan, Isoptin)

Anticoagulants prescribed to decrease blood clotting include

Bishydroxycoumarin (Dicumarol)

Heparin

Warfarin (Athrombin-K, Coumadin)

The high cholesterol that complicates heart disease is moderated by drugs such as

Cholestyramine (Cuemid, Questran)

Clofibrate (Atromid S)

Lovastatin (Mevacor)

Diabetes Medications or "Sugar Pills"

Insulin injections

Chlorpropamide (Diabinese)

Glipizide (Glucotrol)

Glyburide (DiaBeta, Micronase)

Tolazamide (Tolinase)

Tolbutamide (Orinase)

Asthma or Chronic Obstructive Pulmonary Disease (COPD) Medications (Bronchodilators)

Albuterol (Proventil, Ventolin)

Aminophylline

Isoproterenol (Isuprel)

Metaproterenol (Alupent)

Oxtriphylline (Choledyl)

Terbutaline (Brethaire, Brethine)

Theophylline (Theo-Dur)

Immunosuppressants

These drugs decrease the effectiveness of the body's natural immune system. All have serious side effects. They are used to decrease organ rejection after organ transplants and in anticancer therapy. They interfere with DNA and RNA synthesis and stop the immuno-response by preventing antibody synthesis.

Azathioprine (Imuran)

Cyclophosphamide (Cytoxan)

Cyclosporine (Sandimmune)

Fluorouracil (5-fluorouracil): used in ophthalmology to prevent bleb closure after glaucoma filtering procedures

Methotrexate (Folex, Mexate)

Tranquilizers

Chlorpromazine (Thorazine)

Haloperidol (Haldol)

Prochlorperazine (Compazine)

Thioridazine (Mellaril)

• OCULAR REACTIONS TO SYSTEMIC MEDICATIONS

Aspirin: retinal hemorrhages

Hydroxy-chloroquine (Plaquenil): central scotomas, macular degeneration, severe bilateral irreversible retinal damage

Quinidine: toxic amblyopia

Ethambutol: severe, optic neuritis, optic atrophy

Digitalis: yellow color vision, central scotomas, decreased vision

Hydrochlorthiazide (HCTZ): transient changes in refractive error, retinal hemorrhages

Birth control pills: retinal changes, retinal vein occlusion

Rifampin: increased tearing, conjunctival redness

Antibiotics: optic neuritis

Phenothiazine tranquilizers: blurred vision from paralysis of accommodation, dilated pupils, and pigment deposits on the cornea, lens, and retina

Antidepressants: blurred vision from paralysis of accommodation, dilated pupils

Warfarin (Coumadin): blurred vision from paralysis of accommodation, dilated pupils, retinal hemorrhages

Antihistamines: blurred vision from paralysis of accommodation, dilated pupils, transient changes in refractive error

Corticosteroids: optic neuritis, papilledema, cataracts, open angle glaucoma, transient myopia

Bibliography

Albert DM, Jakobiec FA: Principles and Practice of Ophthalmology: Basic Sciences, Sect VII, Pharmacology, Sect VIII, Toxicology. Philadelphia, WB Saunders, 1994.

Ellis PP: Ocular Therapeutics and Pharmacology, 7th edition. St Louis, CV Mosby, 1985.

Gilman AG, Goodman LS, Rall TW, et al.: Goodman and Gilman's The Pharmacological Basis of Therapeutics, 8th ed. New York, Macmillan Publishing Company, 1990.

Havener WH: Ocular Pharmacology, 5th edition. St Louis, CV Mosby, 1983.

Ophthalmic Drug Facts. St Louis, JB Lippincott (Facts and Comparisons Div), 1989.

Pavan-Langston D (ed): Manual of Ocular Diagnosis and Therapy. Boston, Little Brown, 1984.

Thomas P: Pharmacology of the Eye. Chicago, Year Book, 1978.

• CHAPTER 4 PHARMACOLOGY

1. Which of the following methods of drug delivery is the most common systemic route?
   a. topical
   b. oral
   c. subconjunctival
   d. intramuscular
   e. intracameral

2. Which of the following drugs is *not* useful in controlling glaucoma?
   a. Neptazane
   b. Propine
   c. Mydfrin
   d. Timoptic
   e. Pilocar

3. Which of the following drugs dilates the pupil (by paralyzing the iris sphincter) and blocks the accommodation (by paralyzing the ciliary body)?
   a. Cyclogyl
   b. Propine
   c. Mydfrin
   d. Timoptic
   e. Pilocar

4. Which one of the following antibiotics is in common topical use for superficial eye infections?
   a. bacitracin
   b. penicillin
   c. idoxuridine
   d. methazolamide
   e. lidocaine

5. Which one of the following drugs reduces inflammation but slows wound healing?
   a. Naprosyn
   b. vancomycin
   c. Maxidex
   d. natamycin
   e. Betoptic

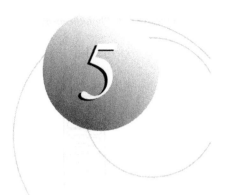

Photochemistry of Vision

LEARNING OBJECTIVES

- List four photosensitive pigments
- Compare differences between rods and cones
- Explain the bleaching process of visual pigments in the retina
- Explain the reformation of visual pigments in the retina
- Discuss light and dark adaptation

- List the primary colors
- Explain hue, saturation, and intensity
- Discuss the various types of color vision deficiencies
- Know how to test for color vision deficiencies

Just as a plant converts light energy into nourishment by photosynthesis, the retina converts light energy into an electric action potential by photochemistry for propagation as a nerve impulse. The rod and cone photoreceptors are the light-sensitive elements. They have separate functions in relaying information. More sensitive rods activate in low light levels with black and white vision. Less sensitive cones cannot respond at such low light levels. They activate at higher light levels with color vision. In high light levels the rods are maximally bleached.

● ANATOMY

Both rods and cones have two major segments, outer and inner, connected by thin microtubules of modified cilia. The outer segment imbeds into retinal pigment epithelium (RPE) tentacles. Approximately 700 dense membranous discs in the outer segment of cones, formed by infoldings of the cell membrane, serve as shelves to support attached visual pigments. Rod outer segments contain freely floating discs, similar to a stack of coins, with more visual pigment than cones have. The inner segment contains mitochondria, the "power packs" that provide most of the enormous amount of energy needed for the photoreceptors to function. As a result, the retina consumes more oxygen per unit weight than any other body tissue because of its relatively high metabolic rate (Fig. 5–1 and Table 5–1).

New visual pigment is continuously synthesized in the outer segment, using vitamin A from the RPE that has been converted to 11-*cis* retinal. New discs are also formed to balance the degeneration of old discs at the tip of the outer segment that are digested by the RPE.

Through two mechanisms the RPE controls the enormous metabolic needs of the photoreceptors. First, it stores large quantities of vitamin A in its alcohol form as retinol or as retinyl ester, which it exchanges with the overlying photoreceptors during the photochemical reaction. Second, the RPE acts as a barrier in the opposite direction, helping to conserve vitamin A and lipids within the eye. As these stores are depleted, vitamin A is replaced from supplies in the blood and liver.

Vitamin A (retinol) is essential for the formation of visual pigments and epithelial tissues in the body, especially the cornea and conjunctiva. Vitamin A is obtained from food, absorbed from the gastrointestinal tract, stored in the liver, and released to the blood stream until specific binding sites on the retinal pigment epithelium capture it. Most of the vitamin A in the retina is stored in the RPE except in prolonged darkness when most of it is converted to rhodopsin in the rods.

Light passes through the various media of the eye before being absorbed by the visual pigments on the outer segments. The absorbed high energy light causes complex chemical changes that decompose the visual pigments into products that excite the photoreceptors to discharge electrical signals our nervous system identifies. How absorption of light by visual pigments is

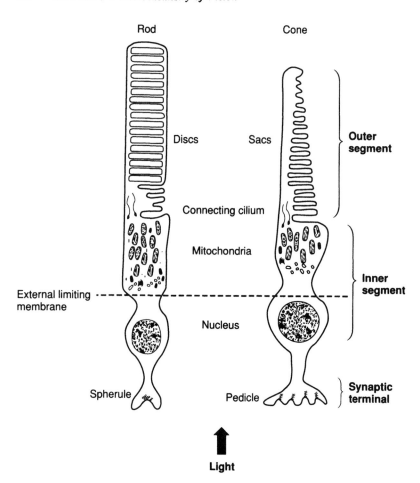

FIGURE 5–1. Schematic drawing of the functional parts of a rod and a cone.

linked to the change in electropolarization of the photoreceptors is not fully understood. The current theory is that a change in sodium conduction occurs across the surface membrane of the outer segment of the photoreceptor and alters its polarization. This amplifies the signal that stimulates the nerve impulse.

TABLE 5–1.

Comparison between Rods and Cones

Rods	Cones
Long and narrow	Short and conical
One visual pigment—rhodopsin	Three visual pigments—chlorolabe, erythrolabe, and cyanolabe
No color vision	Color vision
Spherical synapse terminal	Pedicle synapse terminal
120 million in number	6.5 million in number
Groups connecting to one nerve fiber	One to one cone to nerve fiber in fovea
Poor visual resolution	Excellent visual resolution
Better signal amplification	Poorer signal amplification
Lower threshold to light	Higher threshold to light
Best in dim light (scotopic)	Best in bright light (photopic)

● VISUAL PIGMENTS

The human eye contains at least four photosensitive pigments. Although they react chemically the same way, they are sensitive to different wavelengths of light. The cones contain three pigments: blue sensitive (cyanolabe), green sensitive (chlorolabe) and red sensitive (erythrolabe). Rhodopsin, the only visual pigment in the rods, has its peak absorption at 500 nm (deep green). The collective peak sensitivity for cones is at 565 nm. Three separate peaks have been measured, one for each pigment: 440 nm for cyanolabe, 540 nm for chlorolabe, and 570 nm for erythrolabe.

Each pigment has two parts: a colorless protein called opsin and a pigment called retinal, an aldehyde of vitamin A in the 11-*cis* configuration. The various forms of opsin are different in each of the four known pigments. The 11-*cis* retinal is the same in all pigments, but changes to different molecular shapes, or isomers, which are important in the chemical breakdown and reformation of all pigments.

● BLEACHING PROCESS

Retinol is the natural form of vitamin A found as an alcohol derivative. Retinal is an aldehyde derivative of vitamin A and is usually found in the all-*trans* configuration. It can only combine with opsin in the 11-*cis* configuration, however.

Vitamin A in the RPE changes to its all-*trans* configuration so that it can become the photosensitive form as a visual pigment, opsin, and the 11-*cis* retinal isomer in the discs. It is not known how all-*trans* retinol in the pigment epithelium converts to 11-*cis* retinal in the outer segment, although it is known that the 11-*cis* retinal configuration binds tightly to opsin.

On exposure to light, the pigment molecule (11-*cis* retinal) absorbs photons of energy and isomerizes to the all-*trans* retinal configuration. All-*trans* retinal is the most stable isomer but has the wrong shape for continued attachment to opsin. The uncoupling of retinal and opsin triggers the electrical charge. Retinal reduces to retinol as visual pigment bleaches (Fig. 5–2).

Bleaching depletes the supply of visual pigment. Once bleached, the pigments must regenerate to maintain retinal sensitivity. Bleaching is similar to running down a car battery by leaving the lights on when the motor is not running. Regenerating is similar to driving the car to recharge the battery. Regeneration allows us to see in bright light constantly without being dazzled by it.

● PHOTOREGENERATION

The liberated all-*trans* retinal reconstitutes visual pigment through two enzyme pathways. In low levels of light, the potentially toxic all-*trans* retinal does not accumulate but rapidly metabolizes to 11-*cis* retinal by one pathway. The opsin present locks with the 11-*cis* isomer to reform visual pigment. The production of pigment keeps pace with the slow breakdown rate (Fig. 5–3).

In prolonged daylight, most vitamin A is in the RPE and most of the rhodopsin is bleached. Rhodopsin breaks down faster than it is produced. The cones are better adapted for bright light because they break down less rapidly and reform more quickly. With these high levels of illumination, however, too much all-*trans* retinal is produced. More slowly, the second enzyme pathway converts the excess all-*trans* retinal to retinol, which diffuses from the outer segment back to the RPE for storage in an ester form of vitamin A. Bleaching and regeneration depend on enzymes found in the inner segment and the retinal pigment epithelium.

The rate of visual pigment bleaching and the rate of visual pigment regeneration establish a steady state, or equilibrium, depending on the amount of illumination. When the amount of illumination remains constant, the rates of bleaching and regeneration take place at an approximately constant rate. When the illumination increases, the steady state of the photochemical cycle shifts in the direction of an increased rate of bleaching with increased production of all-*trans* retinal. When the illumination decreases, the steady state shifts toward an increased rate of resynthesis.

● LIGHT AND DARK ADAPTATION

Light and dark adaptation is the retina's method of coping with the enormous range of light intensities from extremely high to extremely low. The retina automatically alters its sensitivity by changing the amount of light-sensitive pigments present in the photoreceptors. In darkness, the sensitivity of retina is at its maximum,

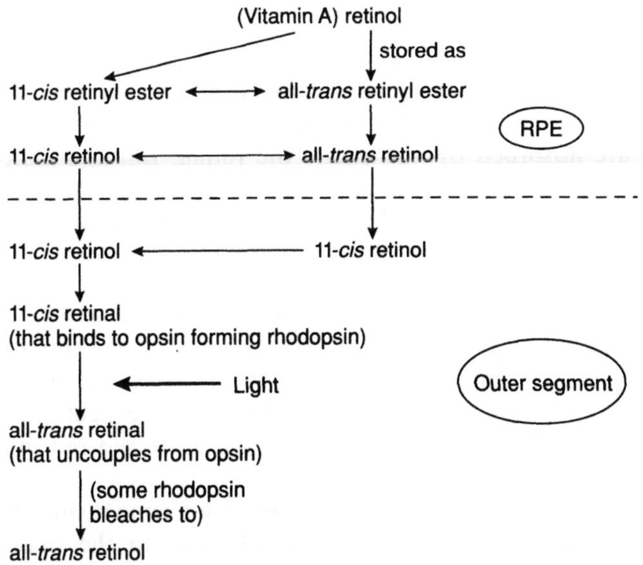

FIGURE 5–2. Bleaching pathway.

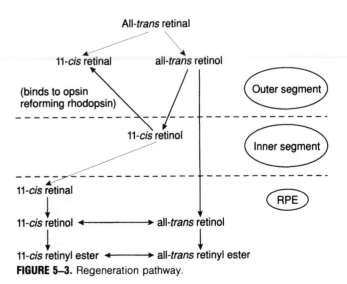

FIGURE 5–3. Regeneration pathway.

as is the amount of visual pigment. Change in the rod system leads to changes in the final threshold of the adaptation curve. Change in the cone system is seen as a change in the early phase (1 to 5 minutes) of the curve. Transretinal disease involving both rod and cone systems may affect both portions of the curve (Fig. 5–4).

Dark adaptation occurs when going from higher to lower light intensity. Retinal sensitivity is very low when first exposed to darkness, but within 1 minute the sensitivity increases 10-fold. By the end of the 7-minute initial phase of dark adaptation, there is a 100-fold increase in sensitivity caused by the regeneration of the cone pigments. The rod-cone break signals a very rapid increase in rod sensitivity. After 10 minutes, rod vision is more sensitive than cone vision. When fully dark-adapted the retina is 10,000 times more sensitive to light than when bleached.

Rods function best for this scotopic vision. Pupils dilate to allow as much light as possible to enter. Production of rhodopsin proceeds faster than its breakdown. When the retina is exposed to prolonged darkness, essentially all the retinal and opsins in both rods and cones combine to produce light-sensitive pigments. As the amount of visual pigment increases, retinal sensitivity increases. This decreases the visual threshold and allows rods to detect the minutest amount of light. In dark adaptation, the central part of the visual field becomes "blind" because cones are less sensitive than rods and cannot respond. We can see only shapes in the darkness. The cone pigments recover faster but are less sensitive. Rods adapt slowly but have much more sensitivity. The entire course of dark adaptation takes approximately 40 minutes.

When going from dark surroundings to a lighter one, light adaptation takes about 10 minutes. Vision under these daylight conditions is called photopic. Pupils constrict to prevent flooding the eye with an overload of light. Rhodopsin bleaches in a minute, thus breaking down faster than it regenerates. Cone pigments, being less sensitive, require bright light to increase the visual threshold for their breakdown and quick regeneration.

Both rods and cones are active in photopic vision, but the cones function better because they resolve fine detail, especially in the central foveal area. Large portions of the photochemicals in both rods and cones decompose into all-*trans* retinal and opsin. Most of the retinal converts to vitamin A. As these two reactions increase, the amount of light-sensitive pigments decreases, along with retinal sensitivity, whereas visual acuity increases.

The decrease in retinal sensitivity during light adaptation is only partially explained by regeneration of visual pigments. Rapid neural adjustments, such as feedback mechanisms to different light intensities, also occur through the horizontal cells and the cones themselves.

In summary, the vitamin A (retinol) stored in the retinal pigment epithelium is necessary to trigger the cascade of events that takes place in the outer segment of rods and cones for transmission of light signals. Rods have one visual pigment called rhodopsin. Cones have three. The bleaching and subsequent regenerating of visual pigments occur much more rapidly than esterifying the excess retinol for storage in the RPE as a retinyl ester. As the eye adapts to total darkness, rhodopsin builds up to high levels, and retinal sensitivity increases. The rods react to minute amounts of light. When this dark-adapted retina is exposed to light, rhodopsin bleaches. As more light is admitted, rhodopsin further decomposes. The farther the shift in this direction, the more light adapted the eye becomes. With these low levels of visual pigment, retinal sensitivity decreases. The cones react best under these conditions.

• COLOR VISION

Electromagnetic wavelengths of radiant energy from the sun consist of visible and invisible light. Only those wavelengths from 400 to 700 nm are visible, i.e., they are absorbed by and excite the retina. Infrared light has a longer wavelength than 700 nm and passes through the retina. Ultraviolet light's wavelength is shorter than 400 nm and is absorbed by the cornea and lens (Fig. 5–5).

White light is a combination of all visible wavelengths. When passed through a prism, it fans out into a series of separate hues, each with its own wavelength. The shorter the wavelength, the more the light rays bend. Violet wavelengths bend the most and red the least.

Absorption of light by a pigment in a cone results in transmission of electrical signals sent to the optic nerves. Coded messages of light that strike the retina

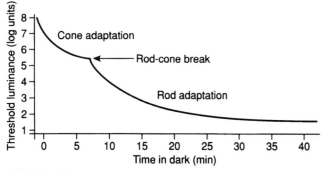

FIGURE 5–4. During dark adaptation, the rods become increasingly sensitive to low light levels. Cones cannot produce the same increase in their sensitivity.

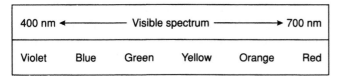

FIGURE 5–5. Visible spectrum.

are sent to a "hue center" in the brain. This hue center compiles the information and determines what color we see.

Most objects absorb at specific wavelengths of light and transmit or reflect not just one wavelength but a complex assortment of them. White objects *reflect* most of the light rays striking them. Black objects *absorb* most of the light rays striking them. Cones are not equally sensitive to all wavelengths. The color perception depends on how each of the three types of cones respond. Wavelengths around 450 nm initiate the perception of blue, around 540 nm initiate the perception of green, around 570 nm inititate yellow, and around 650 initiate red (Fig. 5–6).

The Young-Helmholtz trichromacy theory of color vision assumes three types of cones, each with one of three pigments that absorb specific wavelengths with peak sensitivities in the red, green, and blue regions of the spectrum. Any other color can be produced by mixing appropriate amounts of these three colors.

Red, green, and blue are primary colors. Light mixtures are additive and add different reflectances. Color acts differently for the pigments on an artist's palette because pigments and inks are subtractive. Here the resulting color from mixing comes from what is absorbed rather than what is reflected.

Colors are distinguished by hue, saturation, and intensity or brightness. *Hue* is the color we ascribe to

an object from its predominant reflected wavelength. People with normal color vision can discriminate 150 to 200 hues, from reds to oranges, yellows, greens, blues, and violets. *Saturation* is the amount of white in a given hue. A highly saturated color has very little white. Pink is a less saturated red. Light of a single wavelength, monochromatic, is the most highly saturated. If mixed with white light (a combination of all wavelengths), the light becomes washed out, or less saturated. *Intensity* is the brightness of a color. Brightness varies with wavelength. The range of visual intensities is thought of as a continuum, with black at one end and white at the other. Increased brightness occurs at the white end and decreased brightness at the black. Saturation and illumination produce variations in hue. As intensity changes, hues change, i.e., increased brightness makes reds appear more red, whereas decreased brightness makes them yellower.

Color Vision Deficiencies

Because we have three different cone pigments, humans with normal color vision are called trichromats. Those who are unable to distinguish hues correctly are best described as color deficient. They have a color weakness in one or more of the three types of cones. Many of those with a color vision defect learn to give color names to familiar objects in terms of their characteristic brightness. A true red to one type of red-green color-defective individual may appear to be dark gray. Both the true red and a dark gray object are "red" to such individuals.

Anomalous trichromats (6% of population) suffer from a less than optimal function of one of the three cone pigments. A deficiency of red-sensitive cones (protanomaly) results in poor red-green discrimination and so the red end of the spectrum appears dimmer than normal. A deficiency of green-sensitive cones (deuteranomaly) also results in poor red-green discrimination, although red appears normally bright. A deficiency of blue-sensitive cones (tritanomaly) results in blue-green and blue-yellow insensitivities. Anomalous trichromats have the least severe color vision defect.

Dichromats (2% of population) have only two functioning pigments. Depending on which pigment they lack, they are protanopes (lack red), deuteranopes (lack green), or tritanopes (lack blue). Tritanopia is extremely rare.

Cone monochromats have only one functioning pigment and are truly color blind. Their appreciation of color is limited to very dull tones or gray. Visual acuity is usually good, and electroretinograms are normal. Rod monochromats (achromats) have no pigment at all and are fortunately quite rare. Not only do they lack any color appreciation, but also they have nystagmus,

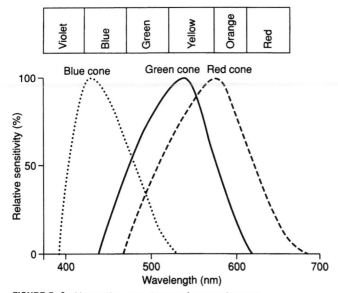

FIGURE 5–6. Absorption spectrums of cone pigments.

photophobia, and vision in the 20/200 range. Their color vision defect is the most severe.

Rare autosomal dominant color deficiencies can affect males or females and are usually characterized by difficulty with low saturation (pastels) or low intensity (dark) colors. Congenital defects do not change, affect both eyes in specific areas (both eyes can be tested at once), and are found with all target sizes and illumination. These individuals have characteristic test results and usually can name colors correctly. There are no other visual complaints. At present, congenital color defects cannot be cured.

Eight percent of white males have congenital, sex-linked, genetic defects in color vision: 5% are deuter-

---

Technique for Use of Farnsworth-Munsell D-15

1. Remove all caps from box, leaving the fixed blue-violet reference cap at one end.

2. Randomize the arrangement of the caps, color side up.

3. Instruct the patient to place the cap closest in color to the fixed reference cap next to it.

4. Instruct the patient to place the remaining caps, in order of color resemblance, into the box.

5. Flip the box over and record on the score sheet the order of the caps by the number on the underside.

6. Connect the numbers on the score sheet by the order in which the patient placed them.

7. Patients with normal color vision will arrange the caps from 1 to 15 in sequence.

8. Protans will arrange in the following order 15–1–14–2–13–12–3–4–11–10–5–9–6–8–7 (Fig. 5–7A).

9. Deutans will arrange in the following order 1–15–2–3–14–13–4–12–5–11–6–7–10–9–8 (Fig. 5–7B).

Farnsworth's Dichotomous Test for Color Blindness—Panel D-15

Name_____ Age_____ Date_____ File No._____

Department _____ Tester_____

Dichotomous Analysis				
Type	Axis of Confusion			
Protan	(RED-bluegreen)	☐	Pass ☐	
Deutan	(GREEN-redpurple)	☐		
Tritan	(VIOLET-greenishyellow)	☐	Fail ☐	

Test
Subject's Order ___ ___ ___ ___ ___ ___ ___ ___ ___ ___ ___ ___ ___ ___ ___

Retest   1   2   3   4   5   6   7   8   9   10 11 12 13 14 15
Subject's Order ___ ___ ___ ___ ___ ___ ___ ___ ___ ___ ___ ___ ___ ___ ___

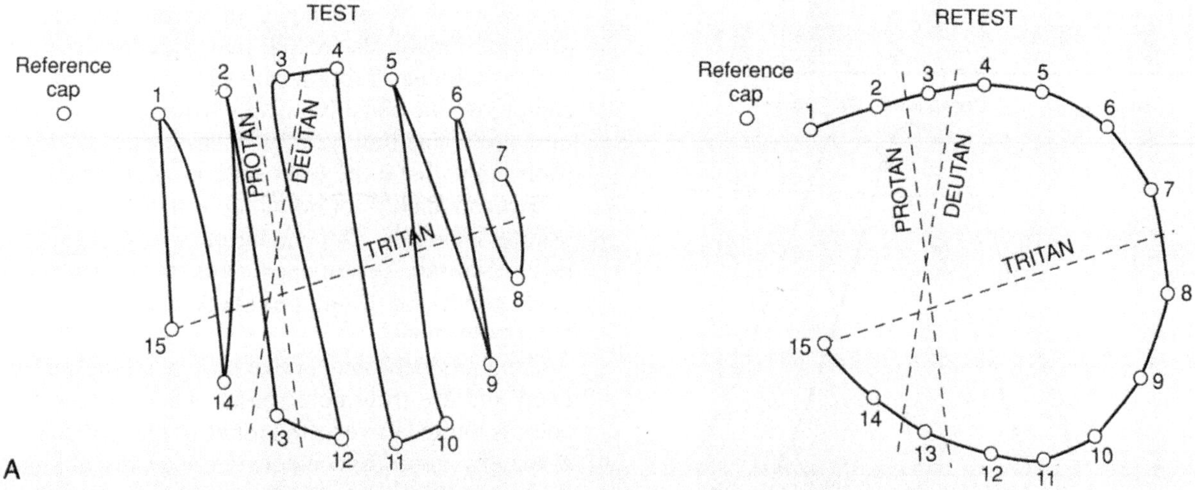

FIGURE 5–7. *A*, Chart for Farnsworth D-15 test illustrating the arrangement of discs for a protan defect on the left and for normal color vision on the right. *B* (*facing page*), Chart for Farnsworth D-15 test illustrating the arrangement of discs for a deutan defect.

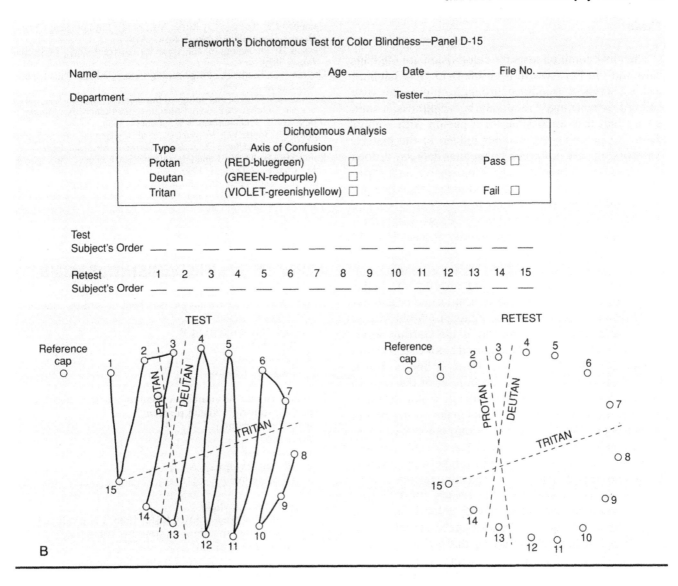

Farnsworth's Dichotomous Test for Color Blindness—Panel D-15

anomalous, 1% are protanomalous, 1% protanopic, and 1% deuteranopic. Females have two X chromosomes; males have one X and one Y. An X chromosome carries the defect. A defective recessive X chromosome is inherited by a female from her color-deficient father. The female has normal color vision from her normal, dominant X chromosome. Any of her sons who inherit the defective X chromosome will also be color deficient. The female is the carrier. The grandfather passes the defective gene through his daughter to some of his grandsons.

Acquired defects secondary to disease or trauma can be cured if the disease or trauma improves. Macular and optic nerve diseases (e.g., optic neuritis and thyroid ophthalmopathy) are most common. Other diseases that cause color vision defects include choroidal/retinal detachment, rod/cone dystrophies, and retinitis pigmentosa. Trauma is usually caused by an eye injury

or a chemical poisoning. Acquired defects give conflicting and variable test results and progress or regress with the disease or trauma. They are not classified as precisely as congenital defects, but they instead have a more general lower color discrimination ability. Classifying them as protan, deutan, and tritan is inappropriate. Each eye is affected differently and must be tested separately. The defect depends on target size and illumination.

Color vision testing should be done on all children before they start school, on all patients with undiagnosed low visual acuity, on all patients suspected of neuro-ophthalmologic disease (optic nerve, optic tract, optic radiations), and on all patients who report recent changes in color discrimination. Normal color vision with decreased visual acuity suggests no organic disease. Deficient color vision suggests retinal or optic nerve disease.

Tests

The most common tests for color vision are the Ishihara and the Farnsworth-Munsell D-15. The Ishihara test is a series of pseudoisochromatic color plates with colored dots arranged randomly by brightness in such a way that it is impossible for a person with a color defect to perceive the number hidden in the matrix. Designed to test red-green congenital defects, it does not classify acquired defects. Inexpensive and portable, this testing can be completed in less than five minutes. Clinically, the Ishihara test is used to see the number correctly identified, e.g., people with intact color vision should correctly identify at least 11 of 14 plates. (See Color Plate 16.)

The Farnsworth-Munsell D-15 test uses rainbow colored caps that must be arranged in order of similar hues. The caps have the same saturation and brightness but different hues. (See Color Plate 25.) A blue-violet cap fixed at one end of the tray is the starting point. It is often selected to study acquired color defects from retinal disease. On the score sheet, a line is drawn connecting the numbers on the bottom of the caps in the sequence chosen by the subject. Color-deficient patients show characteristic errors in the arrangements of the caps. Mild anomalous trichromats may pass. The Farnsworth 100 hue actually has 85 caps. Divided into four trays, there is no confusion between red and green or blue and yellow. Very sensitive testing is time-consuming, as is analyzing the results. Both Farnsworth tests more accurately classify color defects than the Ishihara. A Nagel's anomaloscope tests for congenital red-green defects by having the patient match a mixture of red and green wavelengths to a yellow screen. It is not as cheap and portable as the other tests, however, and is not common in clinical practice.

When testing color vision, the color depends on the ambient light. The Illuminant C Lamp (MacBeth) provides the same quantities of all wavelengths. It is best for testing. When not available, the next best lighting is daylight or fluorescent lighting.

Bibliography

Benson WE: An Introduction to Color Vision. In Duane T (ed): Clinical Ophthalmology, vol 3. Harper Medical, Philadelphia, 1978.
Berne RM, Levy MN: Physiology, 3rd ed. St Louis, CV Mosby, 1993.
Campbell CJ, Koester CJ, Rittler MC, et al.: Physiological Optics. Hagerstown, MD, Harper & Row, 1974.
Davson H: Physiology of the Eye, 5th ed. New York, Pergamon Press, 1990.
Guyton AC: Textbook of Medical Physiology, 8th ed. Philadelphia, WB Saunders, 1991.
Marmor MF: Clinical physiology of the retina. In Peyman GA, Sanders DR, Goldberg MF (eds): Principles and Practice of Ophthalmology, vol II. Philadelphia, WB Saunders, 1980.
Pokorny J, Smith VC, Verriest G, et al.: Congenital and Acquired Color Vision Defects. New York, Grune & Stratton, 1979.
Rubin ML, Walls GL: Fundamentals of Visual Science. Springfield, IL, Charles C Thomas, 1969.
Saari JC: Metabolism and photochemistry in the retina. In Moses RA, Hart WM (eds): Adler's Physiology of the Eye, 8th ed. St Louis, CV Mosby, 1987.

• CHAPTER 5 PHOTOCHEMISTRY OF VISION

1. Which of the following phrases best describes cones?
   a. scotopic vision
   b. high threshold to light
   c. no color
   d. 120 million
   e. long and narrow

2. Which isomer of vitamin A combines with a colorless protein to form a visual pigment?
   a. all-*trans* retinal
   b. retinol
   c. retinyl ester
   d. all-trans retinol
   e. 11-*cis* retinal

3. In prolonged daylight
   a. rhodopsin breaks down faster than it is produced
   b. most of the vitamin A is stored in the retinal pigment epithelium
   c. rate of visual pigment regeneration increases
   d. low levels of all-*trans* retinal are produced
   e. visual pigment bleaching decreases.

4. White light is a mixture of approximately equal amounts of
   a. red and green light
   b. red, blue, and yellow light
   c. red, green, and blue light
   d. red, yellow, and green light
   e. red and blue light.

5. The least severe color deficiency is
   a. monochromatism
   b. tritanopia
   c. deuteranopia
   d. anomalous trichromatism
   e. dichromatism.

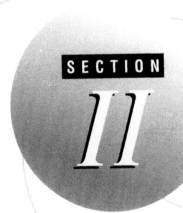

Neuroanatomy

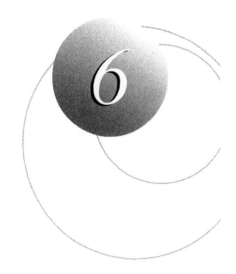

Nervous System

The basic unit of the nervous system is the *neuron* (nerve cell). Each neuron has a *cell body* and at least one more, usually many, processes called nerve fibers. A nerve fiber is either a *dendrite,* a short, branching fiber that receives information to send *to* the cell body, or an *axon,* a single long fiber that delivers information *from* the cell body for transmission to another nerve cell or to an effector organ, such as an eyelid. Neurons are stimulated at one set of terminals and conduct impulses in one direction only, as if on one-way streets. Billions of neurons are organized interdependently through innumerable interconnections and subsystems.

Nerve cell bodies are usually found in clusters. In the peripheral nervous system such a cluster is a *ganglion.* Such a cluster in the central nervous system is a *nucleus.* Gray matter, the central core of the brain and spinal cord, contains clumps of these nerve cell bodies. Gray matter is primarily surrounded by white matter, axons of those cell bodies found in the gray matter. These axons are covered with a white fatty sheath called myelin. An extra coating of gray matter is found on the outside of the cerebellar and cerebral cortices.

A pathway is a chain of communicating axons with a common origin and a common destination, giving it its name. For example, the occipitomesencephalic tract starts in the occipital cortex and ends in the midbrain (mesencephalon). In the central nervous system, a bundle of pathway axons can be called a tract, fasciculus (bundle), peduncle, or lemniscus. In the peripheral nervous system, these axon bundles are called nerves.

● ACTION POTENTIAL

The membrane surrounding each nerve fiber is polarized; i.e., it has opposing electrical charges on opposite sides. An electrical stimulus makes the nerve cell *excitable,* changing its polarity to allow ions to pass from one side of the membrane to the other. When a stimulus sufficiently excites an axon membrane, an explosive, temporary, two-phase sequential change in sodium conduction occurs called an *action potential.*

The action potential creates a minute voltage change. The tiny electrical current generated is just enough to push the impulse farther along the nerve fiber by exciting adjacent portions of the membrane, resulting in propagation of the action potential, which moves along by a series of these electrical nudges. These electric currents transmit undistorted signals from one region of the neuron to another. Once the impulse passes, the cell membrane reverts to its original polarity, ready for conduction of another impulse (Fig. 6–1).

● SYNAPSE

An impulse begins in an axon, travels the length of the axon, and meets a dendrite of another neuron. The contact point between the two neurons is a specialized junction, called a *synapse.* Neurons conducting information to synapses are presynaptic. Those conducting information away are postsynaptic. A narrow fluid-filled gap separates the pre- and postsynaptic neurons.

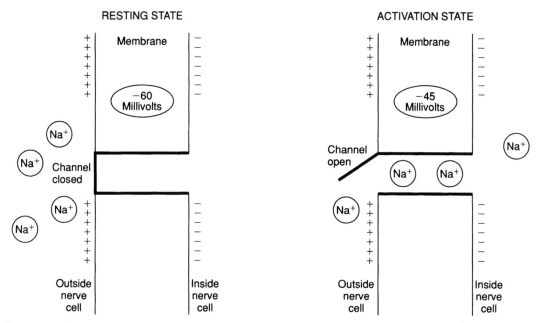

FIGURE 6-1. The nerve cell membrane has a positive charge outside and a negative charge inside. In its resting state, the negative charge inside is greater than the positive charge outside. In this example, a voltage change in membrane potential activates sodium (Na^+) channels to open. Sodium ions flow into the nerve cell. The sodium's positive charge decreases the negative charge on the inside surface of the membrane. Similar channels exist for potassium (K^+) ions.

This gap cannot be bridged electrically, thus preventing direct propagation of the action potential. At the synapse the electrical activity from the axon of the first neuron has to excite the dendrite of the second neuron. It does so chemically.

The presynaptic axon terminal ends in a slight swelling. When an action potential in the presynaptic neuron reaches the swelling, small quantities of an excitatory chemical neurotransmitter stored in the axon terminal are released into the gap. Acetylcholine is the most common chemical transmitter in the nervous system (Fig. 6-2).

The neurotransmitter diffuses through the gap between the nerve terminal and the next neuron, changes the membrane's polarity of the postsynaptic neuron, and thus allows ions to combine reversibly with receptors located on the postsynaptic neuron. The impulse jumps from the axon of the first excited nerve cell to the dendrite of the next excited nerve cell. The result is propagation of the action potential, which passes along the nerve impulse in the postsynaptic neuron.

The released transmitter does not remain in the gap indefinitely. If it did, the synapse would continue firing indefinitely, as long as acetylcholine remained in the extracellular fluid. For example, acetylcholine is inactivated by the enzyme cholinesterase, which is found in both pre- and postsynaptic neurons. As acetylcholine is destroyed, or returned to the presynaptic terminal, the membrane of the postsynaptic neuron returns to its normal resting state.

The amount and type of transmitter determine how much and in which direction the polarity of the next neuron will change. The transmitter substance may be

1. *Excitatory*—causing fewer negative changes in polarity in the postsynaptic neuron's membrane, opening receptor sites, and stimulating the postsynaptic neuron for continued transmission of the nerve impulse.

2. *Inhibitory*—causing more negative changes in polarity in the postsynaptic neuron's membrane, making it more difficult for the postsynaptic neuron to fire and preventing further transmission of the nerve impulse (Fig. 6-3).

• NERVOUS SYSTEM ORGANIZATION

The body's nervous system receives thousands of bits of information from the world around us through

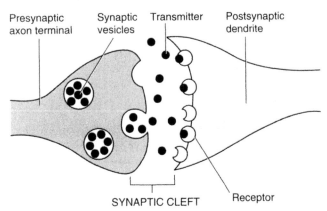

FIGURE 6-2. Schematic drawing of a synapse.

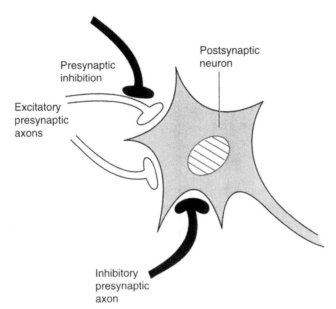

FIGURE 6–3. Presynaptic changes in polarization.

our sensory nerve fibers. Receptors in the skin for pain, touch, pressure, and temperature, and specialized receptors for taste, vision, smell, and hearing, send information to be analyzed by the thought processes of the nervous system. New sensory experiences are compared with stored memories, and important new data are selected and channeled into motor regions of the brain so that desired responses can be planned and carried out. The remainder is stored as memory, mostly in the cerebral cortex, for future control of motor activities and for use in thinking processes.

Three classes of neurons exist: sensory neurons, motor neurons, and interneurons. Afferent sensory neurons start the chain, relaying information through as-

cending pathways from all parts of the body *into* the central nervous system (CNS). Think of sensory information as being sent upstream. The CNS contains huge numbers of interneurons. Interneurons connect sensory and motor neurons, acting as intermediaries and analyzing incoming information and integrating responses. Efferent motor neurons transmit instructions *from* the central nervous system out through descending pathways to muscles or glands as the final, peripheral neurons in the chain. Think of motor responses as going downstream. All the decisions of the nervous system are harmoniously interdependent (Fig. 6–4).

That part of the nervous system which relates the body to the surrounding world is the somatic system. Its cell bodies are located in the central nervous system. The motor system carries signals to the body from directions given by various brain centers. Motor axons travel from the CNS to the skeletal muscles, which act on these signals, moving a body part or another object, or talking, for example. Skeletal muscle is striated (striped) by myofibrils, the functional contracting units of muscles (Fig. 6–5). This type of voluntary muscle remains in a resting state when unstimulated, in contrast to smooth and cardiac muscles, which are innervated by the autonomic nervous system. Smooth muscle, of which the body's internal organs are composed, is built of smaller fibers than skeletal muscle, and without striations. Though myofibrils are present, they are much smaller. Smooth or involuntary muscle receives dual antagonistic innervation from both sympathetic and parasympathetic divisions of the autonomic nervous system (ANS). The eye has innervation from both CNS and ANS.

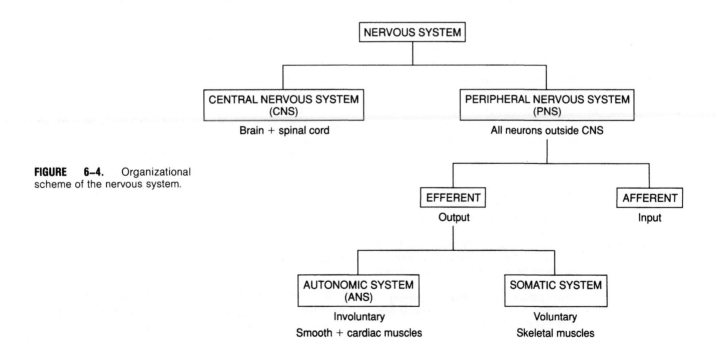

FIGURE 6–4. Organizational scheme of the nervous system.

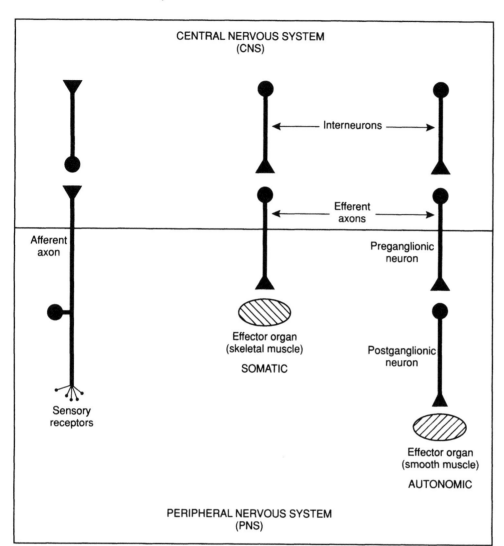

FIGURE 6–5. Differences between the autonomic system and the somatic system.

Nervous System as a Computer

Think of the nervous system as a computer. The input signal is fed to a programming unit, which determines the sequence of operations. The computer may store the information or send out commands by an output signal. This is similar to the thought processes in our brains that allow us to direct our attention first to one thought, then to another, until a complex sequence takes place. Our brain has these necessary computer components:

Input system (what is typed in)	= *afferent pathways*, sensory pathways bringing information from sense organs, receptors in the skin and viscera to the central mechanism.
Data processing (what is done with the data)	= *central mechanism*, analysis, interpretation, monitoring, fine-tuning information received from the afferent pathways, sending out instructions to the efferent pathways. Includes supranuclear and internuclear systems.
Output system (what is output)	= *efferent pathways*, motor pathways conveying instructions from the central mechanism to body parts. Includes infranuclear system.

The visual system has afferent mechanisms (optic nerve, optic tract, optic radiations), central mechanisms (frontal cortex, occipital cortex, brain stem), and efferent mechanisms (oculomotor, trochlear, abducens nerves). The vision data processing occurs at both cortical (cerebrum) and subcortical (brain stem) levels.

The *input system* for vision begins with sensory neurons found in the retina and ends in the occipital lobe around the calcarine fissure in the striate cortex (Brodman area 17). Secondary sensory input comes from the labyrinth in the inner ear. If defective signals are transmitted by the sensory visual pathway, the processing will deliver defective motor responses. This is similar to the computer phrase "garbage in, garbage out."

Levels of Control for Vision

Supranuclear and *cortical* refer to the highest brain centers in the cerebral hemispheres. Refer to these *highest* cortical centers as levels *above*. All interneuron pathways for computing, analysis, coding, decoding, integrating, storing, and executing are *supranuclear*.

For vision, the development of the CNS led to levels of control, descending from the dominant mental level in the frontal cortex, to a lower level around the occipital-parietal junction. Supranuclear cortical centers in the frontal and the occipital lobes are most important, controlling fast and slow eye movements, respectively.

Cortical commands are sent by supranuclear pathways from cortical centers downstream to *lower* subordinate levels of control in the brain stem. These subcortical gaze centers are considered as *lower levels* of control. Brain stem control centers are still supranuclear, *above* the level of cranial nerve nuclei. Brain stem centers are more primitive. They can operate subconsciously. They frequently receive information from the vestibular system or the higher centers in the cerebrum, however, overriding and modifying the messages to be sent to the oculomotor nerve nuclei. Commands are also sent to brain stem centers from the cerebellum for coordination and from the vestibular apparatus to keep the desired image on the fovea.

The brain stem contains vertical and horizontal gaze centers. The centers for vertical gaze are within the midbrain. The centers for horizontal gaze are within the pons. Internuclear pathways from brain stem centers enter the medial longitudinal fasciculus to send commands to even *lower* subordinate levels of control in the cranial nerve nuclei in the brain stem. Think of the medial longitudinal fasciculus as a highway interconnecting the cranial nerve nuclei.

The output or *infranuclear* system for vision begins with motor neurons in the nuclei of the 3rd, 4th, and 6th nerves in the brain stem, with some assistance from CNs VII and VIII. Infranuclear signals are sent through nerves that leave these nuclei, exit the brain stem, travel forward through the cavernous sinuses on either side of the chiasm, and then enter the orbits through the superior orbital fissures to innervate the eyes. The infranuclear system is even more primitive than the internuclear, requiring commands from control centers before it can send messages. The infranuclear system is a *lower,* more peripheral level than the brain stem. This system is below the cortical level. In fact, it is below the level of the brain stem gaze centers, the vestibular system, and the medial longitudinal fasciculus. The position of the eye at a given time is a synchronous integration of the various levels of control.

● DISRUPTION OF NERVOUS SYSTEM FUNCTION

Interruptions at different levels of control influence eye movements in different ways. The lower in the hierarchy the defect is found, the fewer more specific functions are lost. The reverse is also true. The higher the level of control where the defect is found, the more global the loss of function(s). If one of the supranuclear centers fails, none of the lower levels of command, the brain stem centers or nuclei, receive their orders. The messengers (oculomotor nerves) can transmit messages, but they need to get the command.

Supranuclear defects affect gazes, not specific nerves. They produce neither eye misalignment nor diplopia (except for skew deviations). The eyes remain parallel, although, e.g., they may be unable to move past the midline to the right.

Defects in the medial longitudinal fasciculus (MLF) connections are *internuclear*. Brain stem defects after instructions leave the gaze centers produce misalignments peculiar to this area; e.g., skew deviations and internuclear ophthalmoplegias (INO). They are not gaze palsies, but also do not obey the usual rules for extraocular muscle function pertinent to infranuclear misalignments. Infranuclear defects produce incomitant deviations with diplopia. An infranuclear ocular motor defect affects the *nerve* before it can innervate its extraocular muscle.

● DESCRIPTIVE TERMINOLOGY

Anatomic directional terminology originally developed for describing vertebrate animals. These specific directional terms refer to the relative locations of parts of the body. The directions are in common usage for the extremely complex nervous system structures. Without knowledge of these terms, too much time will be spent determining the orientation of diagrams and structures instead of integrating the desired information (Fig. 6–6).

● Directions

Caudal (inferior)	toward or at the tail or bottom
Central	located in the brain
Cephalic (superior)	toward or at the head or top
Contralateral	on the opposite side of the body
Cranial	toward or at the skull or top
Distal	farther from the trunk or point of origin
Dorsal (posterior)	toward or at the back of the body
Ipsilateral	on the same side of the body
Medial	toward or at the middle of the body
Peripheral	away from the brain, toward the extremities

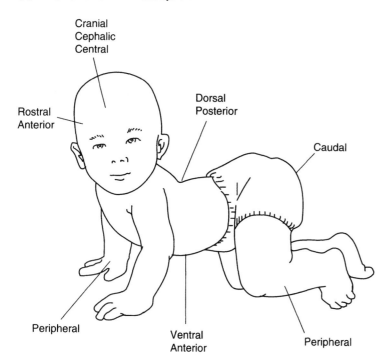

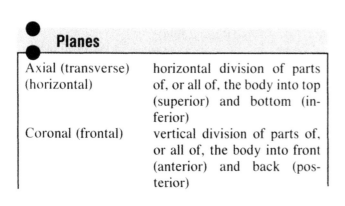

FIGURE 6–6. Relative directions of different parts of the body.

Proximal	nearer or at the trunk or point of origin
Rostral	toward the beak or head
Ventral (anterior)	toward or at the front of the body

Planes, on the other hand, are divisions of the body that are at right angles to one another. Computerized tomographic (CT) scans and magnetic resonance imaging (MRI) studies make liberal use of these planes. You will have difficulty identifying the slices of the body parts you are viewing without this knowledge.

● **Planes**

| Axial (transverse) (horizontal) | horizontal division of parts of, or all of, the body into top (superior) and bottom (inferior) |
| Coronal (frontal) | vertical division of parts of, or all of, the body into front (anterior) and back (posterior) |

| Sagittal | vertical division of parts of, or all of, the body into right and left (Fig. 6–7). |

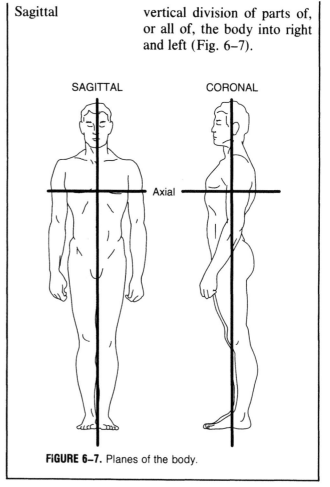

FIGURE 6–7. Planes of the body.

Bibliography

Angevine JB, Cotman CW: Principles of Neuroanatomy. Oxford, Oxford University Press, 1981.

Atwood HL, MacKay WA: Essentials of Neurophysiology. Toronto, BC Decker, 1989.

Berne RN, Levy MN: Physiology, 3rd ed. St. Louis, Mosby Year Book, 1993.

Cassin B, Solomon SAB: Dictionary of Eye Terminology, 2nd ed. Gainesville, FL, Triad, 1990.

Rhodes R, Pflanzer R: Human Physiology. Philadelphia, Saunders College, 1989.

Tortora GJ, Grabowski SR: Principles of Anatomy and Physiology, 7th ed. Hagerstown, MD, Harper & Row, 1992.

● CHAPTER 6 NERVOUS SYSTEM

1. Information from the retina is transmitted by
   a. efferent fibers
   b. ganglia
   c. interneurons
   d. afferent fibers
   e. gaze centers.

2. The highest level of commands begins in the
   a. parietal-occipital centers
   b. frontal centers
   c. brain stem centers
   d. cranial nerve nuclei
   e. cerebellum.

3. The temporary, two-phase sequential change in sodium conduction of a nerve membrane that allows transmission of an impulse is
   a. a synapse
   b. an axon
   c. an action potential
   d. a neurotransmitter
   e. a presynaptic terminal.

4. When describing the relative location of the hands, the following direction is appropriate.
   a. central
   b. proximal
   c. peripheral
   d. rostral
   e. dorsal

5. If an MRI of the head is performed so that the slices cut off from front to back similar to cutting tree rings, the plane is called
   a. axial
   b. coronal
   c. sagittal
   d. frontal
   e. distal.

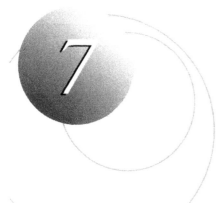

Sensory Visual Pathway

LEARNING OBJECTIVES

- Describe the characteristic patterns of the three basic areas constituting the nerve fiber layer of the retina
- Describe the anatomy of the sensory visual pathway
- Differentiate the composition of the origin of nerve fibers in the prechiasmal and postchiasmal portions of the pathway
- Describe the relationship between areas of the visual field and the origin of nerve fibers that represent that area
- Locate nerve fibers in the calcarine fissure in relation to their location in the nerve fiber layer of the retina (Fig. 7–1).

The eye's functions are controlled by both sensory and motor nerves. Sensory (afferent) nerves are those that receive environmental stimuli, e.g., light. Incoming visual information from space around us is transmitted through sensory nerves, following a characteristic pattern, to the visual area at the back of the occipital lobe for interpretation by the brain.

● ORGANIZATION OF THE SENSORY VISUAL PATHWAY

Reflected light from an object is refracted by the cornea and lens, travels through the aqueous and vitreous, then through the inner retina until the object's image falls on rod and cone *photoreceptors*. The image is sharp if the eye's optical system is normal. The photoreceptors are stimulated by the light to generate an electrical nerve impulse (Fig. 7–2). This electrical impulse starts the information on its way through the sensory visual pathway from the rods and cones through the bipolar cells to the ganglion cells. Each cone in the *macular* area connects to one bipolar cell, which in turn connects to one ganglion cell. Multiple numbers of *peripheral* rods and cones synapse with each bipolar cell, and multiple bipolar cells synapse with each ganglion cell, so that representation in the optic nerve from these other retinal areas is much less dense.

Ganglion cell axons form the nerve fiber layer, containing mostly central fibers from the macula, organized in a characteristic pattern with three distinct areas (Fig. 7–3).

1. A central concentric configuration, the papillomacular bundle, connects the macula with the optic nerve head. Defects here produce central or centrocecal scotomas.

2. Temporal to the macula, the superior and inferior nerve fibers are separate along an anatomical horizontal meridian, the raphe, which effectively serves as a boundary between the superior and inferior visual fields. Because the optic nerve head is nasal to the fovea, temporal fibers have to arc around the fovea to reach the nerve head.

3. Radial fibers nasal to the disc fan out toward the periphery without respecting the horizontal nasal meridian.

An optic neuropathy often creates a defect in one of the three characteristic nerve fiber bundle patterns, as does glaucoma.

As the nerve fiber layer bundles funnel through the optic disc to exit the eye together, they compose the *optic nerve*. Here the bundles become myelinated. Each optic nerve contains both nasal and temporal fibers from the same eye. Injury to one optic nerve, a prechiasmal defect, affects only fibers to the eye on that side, having no effect on any fibers from the opposite eye (Fig. 7–4).

Leaving the orbits through the optic foramina (canals), the optic nerves from each eye recede where they converge to meet at the *optic chiasm* where all

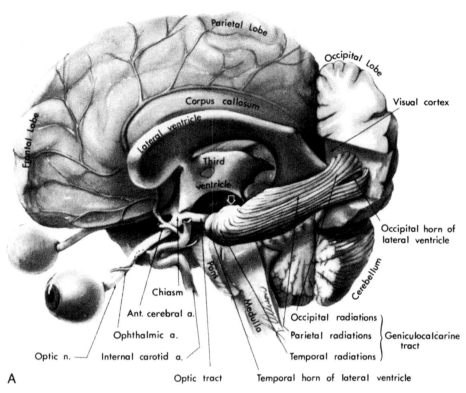

FIGURE 7-1. Sensory visual pathway from the eyeball through the optic nerve, chiasm, optic tract, and optic radiations to the visual cortex in the occipital lobe. *A,* Sagittal view. (From Glaser JS: Neuro-ophthalmology, 2nd ed. Hagerstown, MD, Harper & Row, 1990.) *B,* Axial view.

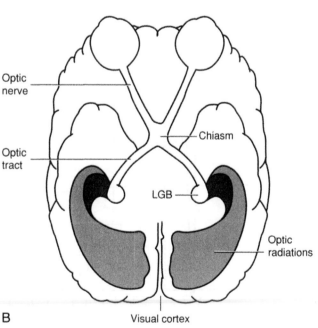

the nasal retinal fibers from both eyes cross over to the opposite side. The chiasm itself lies directly over the sella turcica, a bony depression in the floor of the skull that also houses the pituitary body. As each internal carotid artery exits the top of each cavernous sinus, which lies alongside the sella turcica, its branches surround the chiasm and the optic nerves.

Some of the inferior nasal fibers as they finish crossing near the bottom of the chiasm loop briefly up into the opposite optic nerve, forming von Willebrandt's

knee, before looping down into the opposite optic tract. This "knee" is the junction of one optic nerve (both nasal and temporal fibers) and inferior nasal fibers of the opposite eye.

Behind the chiasm, the crossed nasal fibers from the opposite (contralateral) eye join with the temporal fibers from the same (ipsilateral) eye to travel together as the *optic tracts*. Therefore, the right optic tract contains all the temporal fibers from the right eye and all the nasal fibers from the left eye. These fibers come

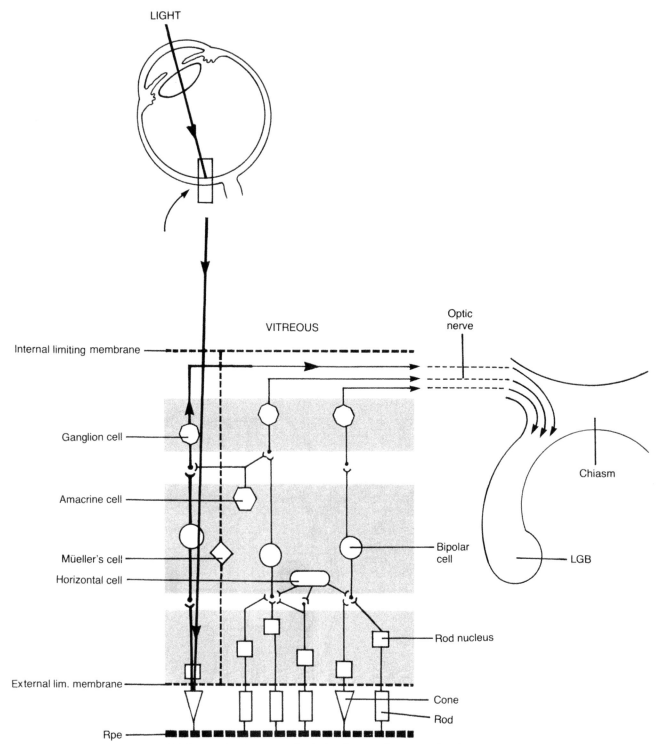

FIGURE 7–2. Schematic diagram of light entering the eye, refracted to form an image on the photoreceptors after traveling through the retina, then transmitted back out to the nerve fiber layer and exiting the eye at the optic disc.

from the right half of each eye's retina but contain information from the left half of each eye's visual field. The left optic tract has all of the left eye temporal fibers and all of the right eye nasal fibers. These fibers come from the left half of each eye's retina but contain information from the right half of each eye's visual field. Each side of the brain gets half its visual information

from each eye. These paired halves of each visual field are *homonymous* because they contain information from the same side of each eye (Fig. 7–5).

Each optic tract continues traveling backward around the outside of the midbrain portion of the brain stem to end in the lateral geniculate body (LGB). Nerve fibers from the ganglion cells synapse here, giving rise

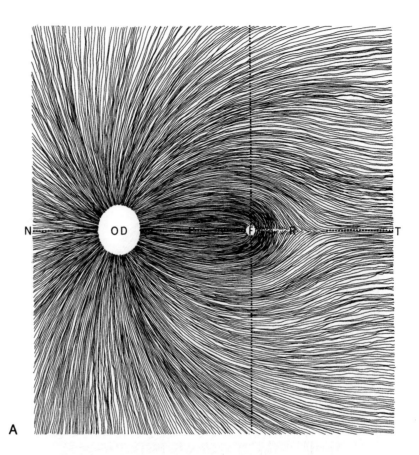

FIGURE 7–3. *A,* Characteristic pattern of the nerve fiber layer of the retina. Notice that the division into temporal and nasal retina occurs at the fovea rather than at the optic disc. (From Hogan MJ, Alvarado JA, Weddell JE: Histology of the Human Eye. Philadelphia, WB Saunders, 1971.) *B,* Central papillomacular bundle includes enormous numbers of macular fibers that travel nasally to enter the temporal border of the optic disc.

Figure continued on following page

A

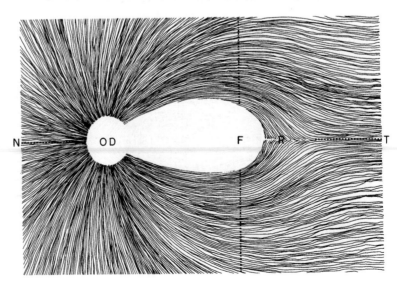

B

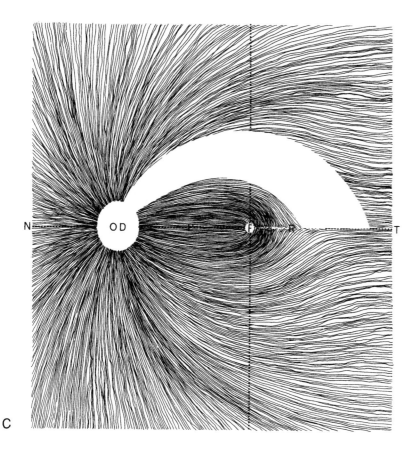

C

FIGURE 7–3. *Continued C*, Arcuate bundles run from the horizontal raphe in the temporal retina in the paracentral area above and below the papillomacular bundle to converge and enter the optic disc at its upper and lower temporal borders. *D*, Fibers nasal to the optic disc converge in straight lines in a fan pattern to the nasal border of the optic disc.

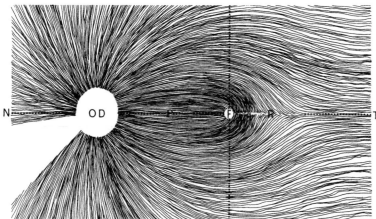

D

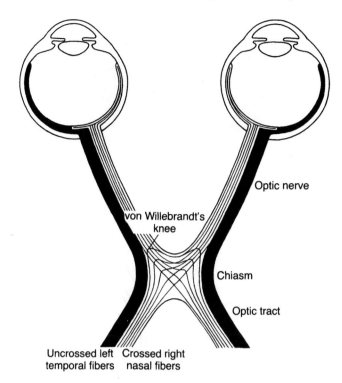

FIGURE 7–4. Crossing of nasal fibers from both optic nerves occurs at the chiasm. At the junction of each optic nerve and the chiasm, some inferior nasal fibers that have just crossed backtrack up into the opposite optic nerve for a short distance before resuming their course into the opposite optic tract. The fibers that backtrack form von Willebrandt's knee. Left temporal and right nasal fibers are illustrated. (From Hogan MJ, Alvarado JA, Weddell JE: Histology of the Human Eye. Philadelphia, WB Saunders, 1971.)

to the afferent neurons that travel together as the *optic radiations*.

As the nerve fibers forming this final portion of the visual system leave the lateral geniculate body, they fan out. Some swing forward and laterally around the lateral ventricle down into the temporal lobe of the brain (Meyer's loop), whereas others pass superiorly through the parietal lobe (Fig. 7–6).

Finally, the nerve fibers in the optic radiations terminate around the calcarine fissure, a cleft in the occipital lobe. The area responsible for vision at the termination of the afferent visual pathway is Brodmann area 17, also known as the striate, or visual, cortex. A large portion of the posterior tip of the occipital cortex contains macular fibers. Each area in the retina is represented in a corresponding area of the visual cortex (Fig. 7–7). The left visual cortex perceives objects situated in the right visual field of each eye, imaged on the left halves (left temporal, right nasal) of each retina. Superior fibers responsible for the inferior visual field terminate along the upper lip of the calcarine fissure, and inferior fibers responsible for the superior visual field terminate along the lower lip. For example, lower fibers

in the left occipital lobe contain information about upper fields to the right of visual space.

● SUMMARY

The retinal photoreceptors generate an electrical nerve impulse in the retinal bipolar cells, which travels to the retinal ganglion cells. Ganglion cell axons form a characteristic pattern of nasal and temporal nerve fiber bundles in the retina that leave through the optic disc to form the optic nerve. The optic nerves travel to the optic chiasm, where all the nasal fibers from both eyes cross. Behind the chiasm, each optic tract contains temporal fibers from the eye on that side and nasal fibers from the opposite eye. The fibers synapse in each lateral geniculate body, continuing backward as the optic radiations, which end in the visual cortex at the tail end of the occipital lobe.

Understanding the precise architecture of the sensory visual pathway is of paramount importance when looking for visual field defects.

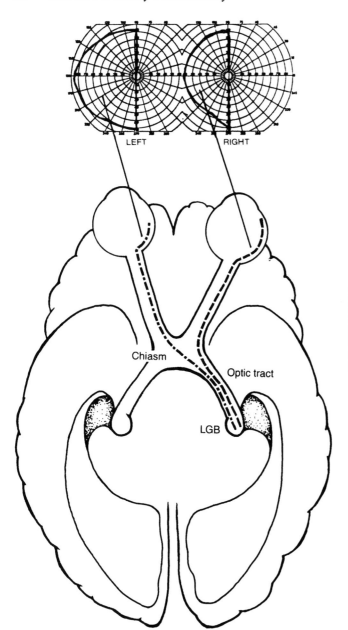

LEFT   RIGHT

Chiasm

Optic tract

LGB

FIGURE 7–5. The optic tracts travel from the chiasm to the lateral geniculate body. Each optic tract has temporal fibers from the eye on the same side and nasal fibers from the eye on the opposite side. In this example, the right optic tract contains all the temporal fibers of the right eye and all the nasal fibers of the left eye. This represents all the visual information from the right halves of both eyes about the left halves of both visual fields.

FIGURE 7–6. The optic radiations travel from the lateral geniculate body (LGB) to the visual cortex in the occipital lobe. Some inferior fibers in the temporal lobe have to circle down and around the lateral ventricles. Those fibers form Meyer's loop.(Modified from Warwick R: Wolff's Anatomy of the Eye and Orbit, 7th ed. Chapman & Hall, Hampshire, England.)

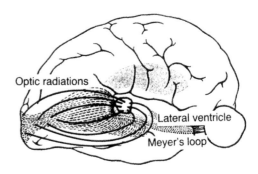

Optic radiations

Lateral ventricle

Meyer's loop

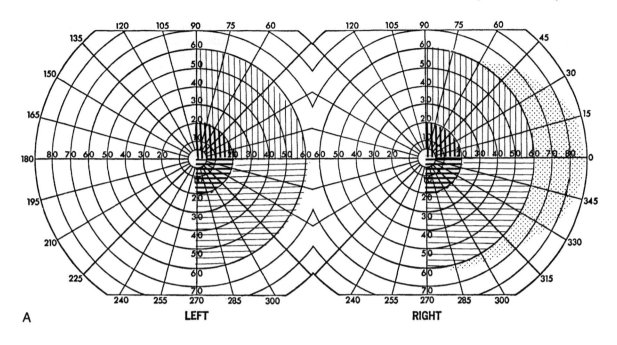

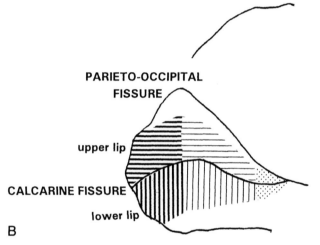

PARIETO-OCCIPITAL
FISSURE

upper lip

CALCARINE FISSURE

lower lip

B

FIGURE 7–7. Areas of visual field and retina represented by corresponding areas around the calcarine fissure of the visual cortex. Optic radiation fibers representing the inferior macula on the lower lip of the calcarine fissure project onto the upper visual field. *A,* Right half of visual fields from both eyes. *B,* Midsagittal view of left occipital lobe.

Bibliography

Cogan DG: Neurology of the Visual System. Springfield, IL, Charles C Thomas, 1976.

Glaser JS: Anatomy of the visual system. In Neuro-ophthalmology, 2nd ed. Hagerstown, MD, Harper & Row, 1990.

Miller NR: Walsh and Hoyt's Clinical Neuro-ophthalmology, 4th ed. Volume One, Section I: The Visual Sensory System. Baltimore, Williams & Wilkins, 1982.

Polyak S: The Vertebrate Visual System. Chicago, University of Chicago Press, 1957.

● CHAPTER 7 SENSORY VISUAL PATHWAY

1. Which choice represents the first synapse in the sensory visual pathway?
   a. bipolar cell to ganglion cell
   b. photoreceptor to ganglion cell
   c. optic nerve to optic tract
   d. photoreceptor to bipolar cell
   e. ganglion cell to lateral geniculate body

2. Identify the last synapse.
   a. bipolar cell to ganglion cell
   b. photoreceptor to ganglion cell
   c. optic nerve to optic tract
   d. photoreceptor to bipolar cell
   e. ganglion cell to optic radiations

3. After crossing at the chiasm, which inferior nasal fibers loop forward temporarily into the optic nerve before traveling back into the optic tract?
   a. Meyer's loop
   b. papillomacular bundle
   c. horizontal raphe
   d. lateral geniculate body
   e. von Willebrandt's knee

4. Incoming information to the brain for vision terminates
   in the
   a. calcarine fissure
   b. lateral geniculate body
   c. optic radiations
   d. Meyer's loop
   e. von Willebrandt knee.

5. Information from the left half of the visual field of the
   right eye is transmitted to the
   a. right visual cortex
   b. left optic radiations
   c. chiasm
   d. right frontal lobe
   e. left optic nerve.

Central Nervous System

LEARNING OBJECTIVES

- Locate and identify the lobes of the brain
- Locate and identify the structures on the undersurface of the brain
- Identify the structures viewed on a midsagittal view of the brain stem
- Relate the structure and function of the pons and midbrain to the eye and orbit
- Explain the relationship of specific areas of the brain to visual function
- Describe the formation and circulation of cerebrospinal fluid

The central nervous system (CNS) is composed of the brain and the spinal cord (Fig. 8–1). It has three distinct parts (cerebrum, brain stem, and cerebellum) encased within the bony skull and spine. A triple layer of membranes (meninges) protect and support the brain. The tough, dense dura mater lies just inside the skull and spine, the web-like arachnoid mater lies in the middle, and the thin pia mater sticks to the outer surface of the brain and spinal cord.

The subarachnoid space between the arachnoid and pia mater contains cerebrospinal fluid (CSF). CSF also fills four interconnected pools (ventricles) within the brain, providing additional protection as a liquid cushion (Fig. 8–2).

The brain is roughly mushroom-shaped. The cerebrum sits like the cap on top of the brain stem, the stalk. The top of the stalk contains the thalamus and hypothalamus. The main control area is the thalamus. It controls everything the CNS, peripheral nervous system (PNS), and autonomic nervous system (ANS) do. The cerebellum and brain stem are more primitive than the cerebrum. They are responsible for the *automatic* (involuntary) processes of the body (respiration, heartbeat, and so forth). The cerebellum regulates such subconscious activities as muscle coordination, perception of movement and position of body parts, and vestibular equilibrium. The brain stem is vital to the visual system in that it contains the horizontal and vertical gaze centers and the nuclei of the nerves that govern both internal and external ocular muscles, as well as the nerve tracts that coordinate their actions.

● CEREBRUM

The largest structure of the mammalian brain is the cerebrum, consisting of two cerebral hemispheres that are partially separated by a central, deep medial longitudinal fissure. At the bottom of this fissure are bands of fibers, the corpus callosum, whose axons transfer information between the two hemispheres (Fig. 8–3).

The cerebral hemispheres have an interior central core of gray matter surrounded by white matter with an added superficial covering of gray matter called the cerebral cortex. The cortex serves largely as an information storage center, responsible for the nonautomatic portion of our behavioral and thought processes. Cortical function is relatively advanced on the developmental ladder, allowing conscious, voluntary integration of both stored (memory) and new information.

The surface of the cerebral hemisphere is wrinkled by bulges (gyri) and indentations (sulci and deeper fissures). This infolding provides a large cortical surface area for enormous numbers of interneurons (Fig. 8–4). The cerebrum separates into four lobes:

1. Frontal
2. Parietal
3. Temporal
4. Occipital

The central sulcus (fissure of Rolando) separates the frontal and parietal lobes. The lateral sulcus (fissure of Sylvius) separates the temporal lobe from the frontal. The parietal occipital fissure separates the parietal and

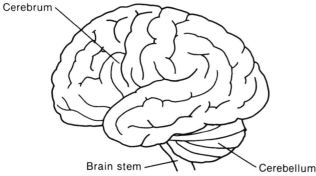

FIGURE 8–1. Parts of the brain.

occipital lobes. The calcarine fissure meets the parieto-occipital fissure.

The frontal lobe is the most advanced part of the brain. It is located at the front, above the bony orbits. Voluntary movements are initiated here, including fast eye movements (saccades) that position targets of interest on the fovea. Behavior is influenced here also. The parietal lobe, located in the upper midpart of the brain, is responsible for body sensations. The temporal lobe, located on the side next to the ear, contains the major portion of the optic radiations. Processing of sounds, sights, smells, and vestibular messages, including memory and retrieval, occurs here. The occipital lobe at the back of the brain contains the terminal end of the sensory visual pathway, where retinal images are transmitted.

One method of representing areas of the cerebrum is to map it with numbers according to function. The most widely used system was devised by Korbinian Brodmann. Areas of special interest for vision and eye movements are areas 8 in the frontal lobe and 17, 18, and 19 in the parietal and occipital lobes. We not only "see" here, we also interpret what we see, and relate it to past visual experiences. Area 17 is the primary sensory-visual one. Visual neural impulses transmitted from the retina are perceived here. Located at the occipital pole, it is responsible for recognition of incoming visual data brought to this end station by the sensory-visual pathway. Areas 18 and 19 translate visual data from area 17, beginning the recognition, interpretation, and decision-making that initiate signals to other parts of the cerebrum or the brain stem through supranuclear pathways for slow eye movements and accommodation. Brodmann area 8, often called the frontal eye field, originates conjugate fast eye movements (saccades). It exerts voluntary, intentional control over eye movements, as well as involuntary control. Decisions on what we prefer to look at any specified time occur here (Fig. 8–5).

A ventral view of the brain shows the undersurface that rests against the bottom of the skull. The bottom of the frontal lobe sits in the anterior cranial fossa of the skull, the temporal lobes sit in the middle, the

cerebellum rests in the posterior cranial fossa, and the medulla is just above the foramen magnum, the large hole in the bottom of the skull. The brain stem rests against the bony slide, the clivus (Fig. 8–6).

The cerebrum, the great command center, receives impulses from appropriate receptors, integrates them, then sends messages to the brain stem and to motor units of the spinal cord. Specific areas of the cerebral cortex are concerned with specific functions of the body. The cortex can be likened to the Pentagon in that it integrates and organizes the services of a number of substations housed in the brain stem. These substations regulate body functions such as breathing and digestion, maintaining them even in an emergency. But the planning and execution are decided by the cerebrum.

The cerebral cortex is the *highest* brain level and the origin for supranuclear pathways. Most of the memories of past experiences are stored here, including patterns of motor responses. Each time a portion of the cerebral cortex is destroyed, a vast amount of information is lost to the thinking process, and some of the mechanism for processing this information is also lost.

Diencephalon

The diencephalon, often called the *between brain*, is the upper end of the brain stem, but is more often considered as part of the cerebrum. The diencephalon sits above the midbrain, containing the thalamus and hypothalamus. The third ventricle separates its two hemispheres (Fig. 8–7).

The thalamus relays sensory information to the cerebral cortex. It gives us an awareness of quality, pleasant or unpleasant. The hypothalamus is the chief subcortical center for regulation of bodily functions. It controls both divisions of the autonomic nervous system as well as hormones secreted by the pituitary body, which dangles below the ventral surface of the hypothalamus. The optic chiasm lies over the pituitary body.

The hypothalamus maintains optimal internal body functions (temperature, digestion, excretion, water balance, and arterial blood flow). Except for the nerve fiber tracts for visual function that pass through it, the hypothalamus is unimportant for visual function.

• BRAIN STEM—SUBCORTICAL CONTROL CENTER

The brain stem controls the subconscious activities of the body. Large areas of the cerebral cortex can be removed without affecting these subconscious activities. This *subcortical* area (*lower* brain level) connects the spinal cord to the cerebrum.

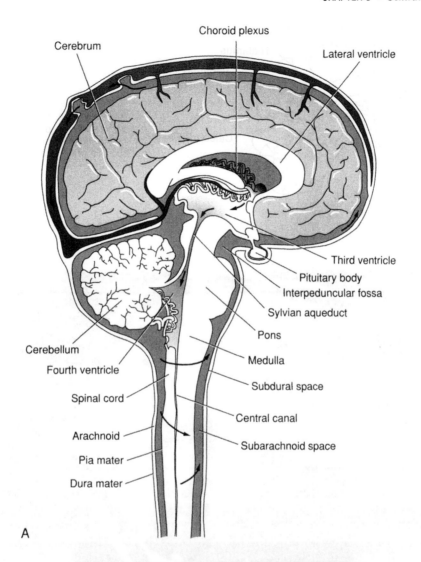

Cerebrum

Choroid plexus

Lateral ventricle

Third ventricle

Pituitary body

Interpeduncular fossa

Sylvian aqueduct

Pons

Medulla

Subdural space

Central canal

Subarachnoid space

Cerebellum

Fourth ventricle

Spinal cord

Arachnoid

Pia mater

Dura mater

A

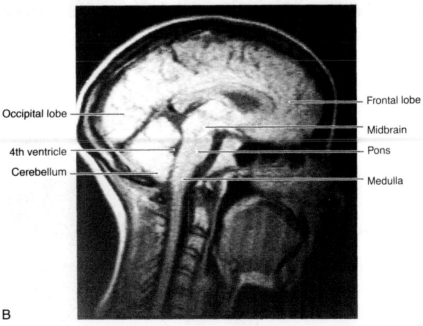

Occipital lobe

4th ventricle

Cerebellum

Frontal lobe

Midbrain

Pons

Medulla

B

FIGURE 8–2. Midsagittal section of the brain, spinal cord, meninges, and cerebrospinal fluid. (Adapted from Macmillan Publishing Company from The Principal Nervous Pathways, 3rd ed. Rasmussen T. Copyright 1945 Macmillan Publishing Company; copyright renewed © 1973. Roberts C, Rasmussen T.)

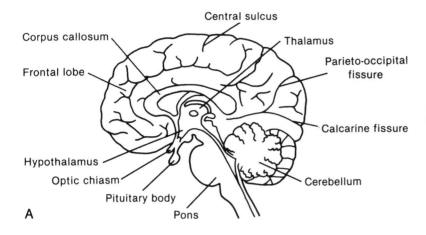

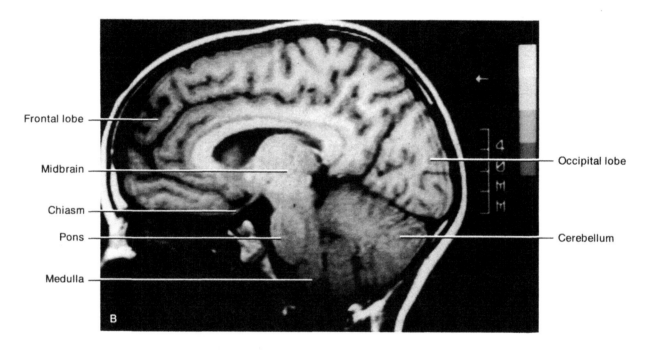

FIGURE 8–3. *A*, Midsagittal view of structure and landmarks of the right half of the brain. *B*, Magnetic resonance imaging (MRI) of the left half of the brain.

FIGURE 8–4. Location of the four lobes of the brain and the two deepest sulci.

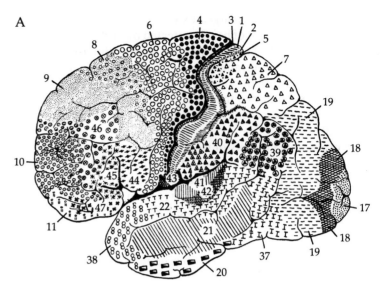

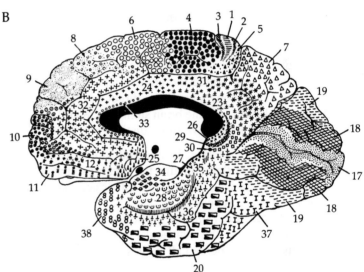

FIGURE 8–5. Inside and outside view of the brain divided into Brodmann's areas. (From Angevine JB, Cotman CW: Principles of Neuroanatomy. New York, Oxford University Press, 1981. Originally from Brodmann K: Vergleichende Lokalisationslehre der Grosshirrinde (Barth, Leipzig, 1909.)

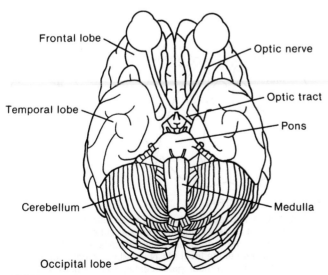

FIGURE 8–6. Ventral view of the undersurface of the brain.

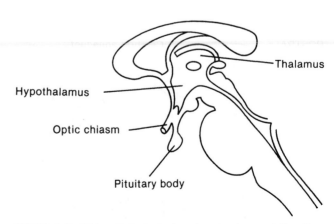

FIGURE 8–7. Midsagittal view of major structures of the diencephalon.

The brain stem is an enlarged extension at the top of the spinal cord. Instead of being protected by vertebrae like the spinal cord, the brain stem is found within the skull just above the foramen magnum. It consists of the medulla, pons, midbrain (mesencephalon), and diencephalon, each above the other. Compare it to the stalk of a mushroom with the cap being the cerebrum (Fig. 8–8).

The brain stem consists of white matter outside and islands of gray matter (e.g., the red nucleus and cranial nerve nuclei) inside. Ascending and descending tracts run throughout, bringing in information from the external environment and producing skeletal muscle movement from reflex signals. The reticular formation is a diffuse group of cells and fibers running from the spinal cord through the brain stem to the upper end of the thalamus. This important integrating substation consists of interlacing neurons traversed by larger fibers carrying impulses to and from the higher and lower centers (Fig. 8–9).

If we could face someone with transparent skin, we would be looking at the ventral surface of the brain stem, the "front" side where the cranial nerves exit. When we look at someone's back, we direct our gaze toward the dorsal surface of the brain stem (Fig. 8–10).

The midbrain and pons have three distinct parts:

1. A roof plate, the *tectum,* lies behind (dorsal to) the ventricular system that contains the cerebrospinal fluid. In the midbrain it is the corpora quadrigemina. In the pons it is the cerebellum.

2. A central core, the *reticular formation,* sits just in front of (anterior to) the ventricular system. This mass contains a mix of nerve cell bodies, axons, and dendrites.

3. A large collection of ventral fibers come from the cerebral cortex (Fig. 8–11).

Gray matter (nuclei) lies close to the ventricular system compared with the white matter (nerve fiber tracts). The *tegmentum,* which includes the central

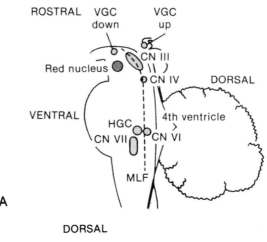
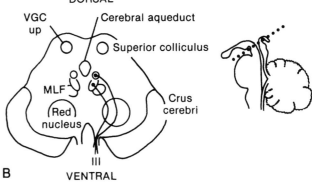
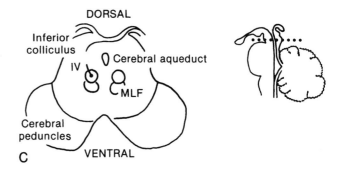
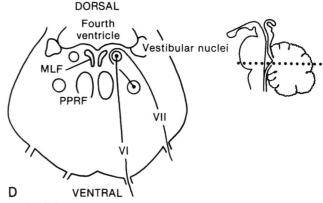

FIGURE 8–9. *A,* Midsagittal view of nuclei and structures in the brain stem important to visual function. *B,* Axial cut of brain stem at the level of CN III. *C,* Axial cut of brain stem at the level of CN IV. *D,* Axial cut of brain stem at the level of CN VI. MLF = medial longitudinal fasciculus, VGC = vertical gaze center, HGC = horizontal gaze center.

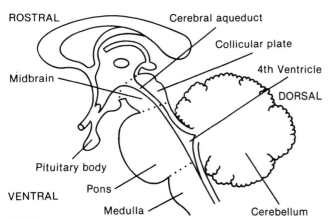

FIGURE 8–8. Midsagittal view of major areas of the brain stem.

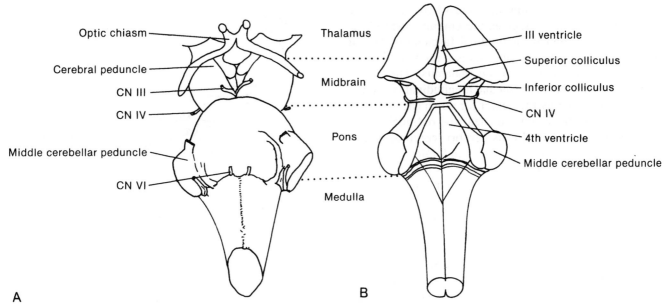

A

B

FIGURE 8–10. Brain stem. *A*, Ventral view. *B*, Dorsal view.

core, is a well-defined interwoven network of cranial nuclei plus brain stem tracts. The ventral fibers in the midbrain form the crus cerebri and part of the horizontal fiber bulge in the ventral part of the pons.

Midbrain

The midbrain (mesencephalon) is the smallest part of the brain stem, like a short pipe connecting the pons to the thalamus. Highly important for eye function, it contains reflex centers that interconnect the pretectum, tectum, and cerebellum. Except for the lateral rectus, the CNS III and IV innervate all the extraocular muscles (EOM), plus the levator, ciliary body and iris

sphincter. The complex CN III, like all the cranial nerves except CN IV, runs from its nucleus forward to exit the ventral (front) side of the midbrain. CN IV is the only cranial nerve that exits the brain stem on the dorsal (back) side at the junction of the midbrain and pons, then circles around the brain stem to run forward toward the orbit (Fig. 8–12). The nuclei of these two nerves are located in the tegmentum, the central core of the midbrain, just ventral (in front of) to the cerebral aqueduct. The cerebral aqueduct is a narrow tubular channel that funnels CSF from the 3rd ventricle in the diencephalon above to the 4th ventricle behind the pons below.

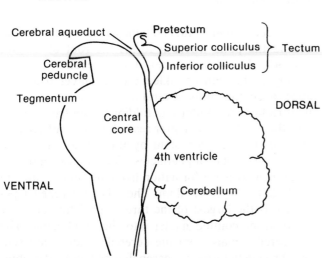

FIGURE 8–11. Parts of the brain stem.

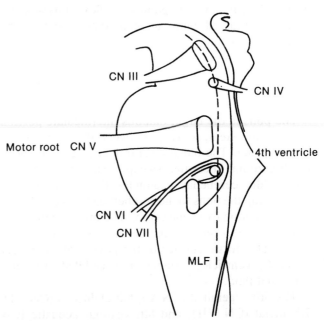

FIGURE 8–12. CN III through VII route out of the brain stem. MLF = medial longitudinal fasciculus.

Besides the 3rd (oculomotor) and 4th (trochlear) cranial nerve nuclei, the tegmentum contains the red nucleus and the medial longitudinal fasciculus. Among other functions, the red nucleus is a relay station between the cerebellum and the thalamus. The rostral interstitial nucleus of the medial longitudinal fasciculus (riMLF) is probably the center for down gaze, located above the 3rd nerve nucleus near the red nucleus.

The crescent-shaped crus cerebri (cerebral peduncles) forms the front base of the midbrain, containing corticospinal and corticopontine tracts with upper motor neurons descending for eventual innervation of skeletal muscle.

Above (behind or dorsal to) the cerebral aqueduct is the tectum, the roof, containing four bumps, the superior and inferior colliculi (also called the corpora quadrigemina or the collicular plate). The inferior colliculi analyze auditory signals. The superior colliculi are primary relay stations for the visual system. These large mounds of neurons receive the pupillary fibers from the optic tract, as well as fibers from the frontal, temporal, parietal, and occipital lobes. Frontal fibers from Brodmann area 8 arrive here from the midbrain tegmentum. This important control center for eye movements may contribute to head and eye movements used to localize and follow visual stimuli.

The posterior commissure lies in the pretectal area, just above the tectum. It connects the two superior colliculi; it marks the upper limit of the midbrain and is the final site for the afferent pupillary pathway, as well as the site of the vertical up-gaze center. Just above the tectum at the junction of the midbrain and the diencephalon is the pretectal area. Fibers for the consensual light reflex cross here. This midbrain center for the pupillary light reflex contains the termination of the afferent (sensory) pupillary reflex pathways and may be involved with accommodation and/or the vergence system.

Pons

The pons is the large, bulbous intermediate portion of the brain stem, a bridge between the medulla and the midbrain. The bulging ventral surface of the pons has horizontal fibers that sweep to each side, forming the middle cerebellar peduncles (brachium pontis). These strap the pons to the cerebellum behind it, bringing information from one cerebral hemisphere for regulation by the opposite cerebellar "computer" (Fig. 8–13). The dorsal surface of the pons forms the floor of the 4th ventricle, a triangular space filled with cerebrospinal fluid.

The 5th trigeminal (CN V), 6th abducens (CN VI), 7th facial (CN VII), and 8th vestibuloacoustic (CN VIII) cranial nerve nuclei all lie within the pons. CNs

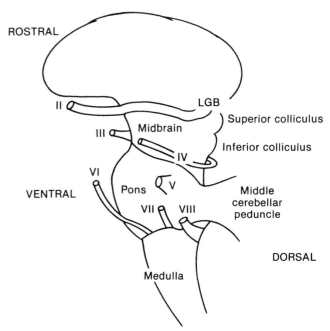

FIGURE 8–13. Lateral view of the right side of the pons.

V, VII, and VIII exit from the side of the pons. CN VI leaves the brain stem from the ventral midline at the junction of the pons with the medulla. The 6th nerve nucleus lies in the floor of the 4th ventricle, partially encircled by CN VII, which comes forward to exit from the side of the brain stem, before traveling forward toward the orbit. The reticular formation, referred to as the paramedium pontine reticular formation (PPRF) contains the horizontal gaze center (HGC). The HGC receives information from supranuclear centers and orchestrates the innervation of yoke lateral and medial recti by way of the medial longitudinal fasciculus (MLF).

• CEREBELLUM

The cerebellum is tucked beneath the cerebrum and behind the pons where it forms the roof of the 4th ventricle. The surface cortex of the cerebellum consists of gray matter with a crinkled, creased, layered appearance, accentuated by several deep fissures separating it into lobes. The patterns of folding are such that, when cut, the inside white matter resembles a cauliflower. It attaches to the brain stem by three heavy bands of fibers, the cerebellar peduncles. The inferior cerebellar peduncle brings information from the spinal cord and medulla to the cerebellum. The middle cerebellar peduncle is the largest of the three, consisting of many fibers from pontine nuclei into the cerebellum. The corrected signals from the cerebellar nuclei are sent out through the superior cerebellar peduncle, distribut-

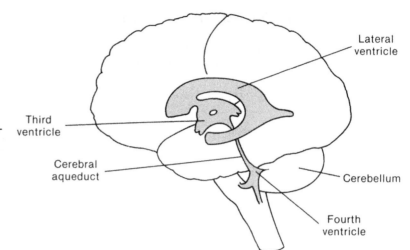

FIGURE 8–14. Ventricular cavities containing cerebrospinal fluid.

ing the analyzed information to the brain-stem motor-control centers. Some signals are sent to the red nucleus before descending to the spinal cord. Some signals bypass the red nucleus to ascend to the thalamus and then to the frontal lobe.

The cerebellum functions at a subcortical level as a closed loop system, interacting with the cerebrum, spinal cord, and brain stem. It times the action of muscle groups to produce smooth, strong, accurate movements, regulating equilibrium and posture and playing a critical role coordinating head and eye movement. The cerebellum does not originate commands, but once informed, it continuously monitors them by receiving feedback on existing conditions, correcting mistakes, returning signals to their origin, or adjusting for any error in the original information. It almost instantaneously analyzes information on body position and movements, determining how much, how fast, and how well these actions are performed.

• MEDULLA

The medulla oblongata, at the bottom of the brain stem, is an enlarged continuation of the spinal cord. The last four cranial nerves and several involuntary reflex centers help control body temperature, heart rate, blood pressure, breathing, swallowing, and digestion. Nerve fiber tracts both ascend to the brain and descend from the brain through the medulla.

• VENTRICULAR SYSTEM

The brain contains cavities filled with cerebrospinal fluid (CSF) that cushions the brain against injury. CSF is produced by the choroid plexus, which line the two lateral ventricles. CSF circulates to the 3rd ventricle, then through the tubular Sylvius's aqueduct into the 4th ventricle. From there it escapes into the subarachnoid space where it starts being reabsorbed (Fig. 8–14).

Excessive CSF in a newborn produces hydrocephalus, which results in an elevated pressure within the skull. This increased intracranial pressure (ICP) can be caused by overproduction of fluid, inadequate absorption, or most likely by an obstruction of outflow through the cerebral aqueduct. Optic nerve swelling, papilledema, seen during examination of the ocular fundus, is one method of detecting this.

• SUMMARY

Ocular function is most affected by the midbrain and pons. Brain stem control centers are located in the pons for horizontal gaze and in the upper end of the midbrain for vertical gaze. Pupil function for light has a control center in the posterior commissure. Pupillary function for near is located more ventrally. These control centers function subconsciously. The pons and midbrain are also where CN nuclei III to VIII originate. All have some effect on vision, the eye, the orbit, and the surrounding areas.

Bibliography

Angevine JB, Cotman CW: Principles of Neuroanatomy. Oxford, Oxford University Press, 1981.

Snell RS: Clinical Neuroanatomy for Medical Students, 3rd ed. Boston, Little, Brown, 1992.

Snell RS, Lemp MA: Clinical Anatomy of the Eye. Oxford, Blackwell Scientific, 1989.

Tortora GJ, Grabowski SR: Principles of Anatomy and Physiology, 7th ed. Hagerstown, MD, Harper & Row, 1992.

• CHAPTER 8 CENTRAL NERVOUS SYSTEM

1. The storage of information, storage of memory, planning, and execution of voluntary bodily functions take place in the
   a. cerebellum
   b. brain stem
   c. cerebral cortex
   d. autonomic nervous system
   e. ventricles.

2. The narrow tube containing cerebrospinal fluid that connects the third and fourth ventricles is found in the
   a. pons
   b. thalamus
   c. midbrain
   d. cerebellum
   e. medulla.

3. Recognition and interpretation of visual information occurs in
   a. Brodmann area 18
   b. the diencephalon
   c. Brodmann area 17
   d. Brodmann area 8
   e. the cerebellum.

4. The optic radiations are mostly located in the
   a. parieto-occipital junction
   b. frontal lobe
   c. thalamus
   d. parietal lobe
   e. temporal lobe.

5. Where are signals to coordinate head and body movements corrected and then sent to brain stem motor centers?
   a. cerebral cortex
   b. pons
   c. Brodmann area 19
   d. midbrain
   e. cerebellum

Supranuclear Mechanisms

LEARNING OBJECTIVES

- Identify four supranuclear eye movement systems.
- Discuss differences in function of the four supranuclear eye movement systems.
- Identify and locate two cortical supranuclear pathways.

- Identify and locate two subcortical supranuclear pathways.
- Identify and locate three gaze centers.
- Discuss eye movement syndromes occurring in the brain stem resulting from damage.

Four supranuclear eye movement systems (saccades, pursuit, vergences, vestibular) interrelate continuously, computing and feeding back visual data, allowing the body to relate to its environment visually. The eyes move synchronously, by the same amount, in the same direction (except for vergences) to quickly and accurately lock the image of the desired target onto both foveas, keeping it there, adjusting for head, body, and target movements. Two supranuclear cortical pathways for vision connect the frontal lobe, occipital lobe, and parietal lobe with the brain stem (midbrain and pons). They process visual information initiated by signals from the visual cortex (Brodmann area 17), the area involved in conscious vision where the sensory visual pathway ends. Brodmann areas 18 and 19, the visual association areas, recognize and interpret the visual information from area 17 and probably participate in sensory motor eye coordination from a frontal occipital pathway. Brodmann area 19, the peristriate cortex, straddles the border of the occipital and parietal lobes and is the major parietal center for integration of visual information.

Corticomesencephalic pathways from area 19 to the midbrain are responsible for accommodation and reflex (involuntary) eye movements, whereas pathways from the frontal cortical areas are for voluntary, intentional eye movements. All the pathways from the frontal cortex (frontomesencephalic tract) and from the occipital cortex (occipitomesencephalic tract) travel to vertical and horizontal gaze centers in the brain stem. The centers for vertical conjugate gaze are within the mid-

brain. The centers for horizontal conjugate gaze are within the pons.

Two supranuclear ocular pathways are subcortical. One is the nonoptic vestibular system that integrates equilibrium with vision. The other is the medial longitudinal fasciculus (MLF). This "interstate highway" of the brain stem links supranuclear eye pathways to infranuclear pathways.

Vestibular nerve fibers from the inner ear enter the brain stem to end in the cerebellum and in one of four vestibular nuclei in the medulla. The vestibular nuclei influence eye movements, especially nystagmus. Pathways from the vestibular nuclei, cerebellum, and cortex travel through the MLF both crossed and uncrossed to the 3rd, 4th, and 6th nerve nuclei, to muscles moving the head and neck, or down through the spinal cord to innervate lower motor neurons, influencing trunk and limb muscles for body balance and an upright position. Some fibers end in the tectal and pretectal areas (Fig. 9–1).

● EYE MOVEMENT SYSTEMS

Saccadic System

The saccadic system generates all fast eye movements (FEM). Saccades are primarily corrective refixation movements, are very fast (700°/sec), accurate, and voluntary. A moving object in the peripheral field triggers curiosity and a burst of innervational activity

FIGURE 9-1. Supranuclear pathways to the third (III), fourth (IV) and sixth (VI) nerve nuclei for eye movement. The saccadic pathways begin in the frontal eye fields (FEF). Fibers for horizontal movement descend to the pontine paramedian reticular formation (PPRF) and fibers for vertical movement descend to the rostral interstitial nucleus of the medial longitudinal fasciculus (riMLF) for down gaze and the superior colliculus (SC) for up gaze. The pursuit pathways begin in the region of the junction of the parieto-occipitotemporal area (POT). Fibers for horizontal movement descending to the same PPRF as for saccades, and fibers for vertical movement descending to the same riMLF for down gaze and the superior colliculus (SC) for up gaze. The diagram on the right summarizes the pathways within the brain stem for vertical gaze. The diagram on the left summarizes the pathways within the

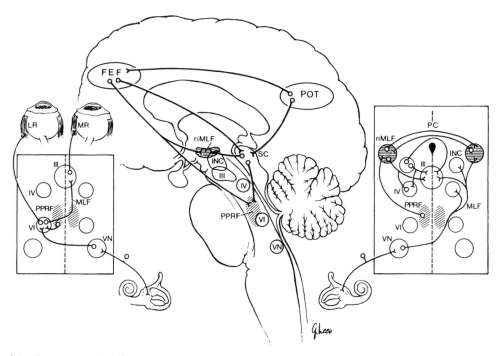

brain stem for horizontal gaze. LR = lateral rectus muscle, MR = medial rectus muscle, VN = vestibular nuclei, MLF = medial longitudinal fasciculus, INC = interstitial nucleus of Cajal, PC = posterior commissure, VN = vestibular nuclei. (From Miller NR: Walsh and Hoyt's Clinical Neuro-opthalmology, 4th ed. Vol 2, Section IV: The Ocular Motor System: Embryology, Anatomy, Physiology, and Topographic Diagnosis. Baltimore, Williams & Wilkins, 1985.)

that changes the angle at which the visual stimulus enters the eye through impulses to the extraocular muscles. The switch in fixation places the image of the moving object from the peripheral field to the fovea. This system functions as a homing device, guiding the eye until the image of the new target locks onto the fovea. Because the fovea is the most sensitive retinal area and possesses the highest resolving power for clearest focus, acute examination of the new target is possible.

Saccades originate in the frontal lobe in Brodmann area 8, also known as the frontal eye fields (FEF), descending as the *frontomesencephalic tract* to the upper end of the midbrain, where it splits into one pathway for vertical gaze and another for horizontal gaze. Horizontal gaze fibers descend through a corticospinal tract of the midbrain, cross at the level of cranial nerve 4, and descend on the *opposite side* to the horizontal gaze center (HGC) in the pons near the 6th nerve nucleus. Therefore, the left frontal lobe controls saccades into right gaze. A defect here produces a right gaze palsy on command and loss of the fast phase of optokinetic nystagmus to the right. Vertical fibers end on the *same side* in the medial posterior commissure for up gaze or in the rostral interstitial nucleus of the MLF (riMLF) for down gaze. The pathway for vertical saccades from the tectal area to the oculomotor nuclei is not known.

Often called command movements, the saccadic system is tested by requesting the patient to look in various directions on command. Reflex saccades also occur, e.g., looking toward a noise (Fig. 9–2).

Pursuit System

Slower following movements, or pursuits (30°/sec), maintain the image of a slowly but smoothly moving object on the fovea for tracking. Pursuit locks the fixated eye on the target as the target moves. Only when a moving target goes too fast (more than 40°/sec) for this involuntary slow eye movement (SEM) system does a saccade from the fast frontal pathway interrupt to reposition the target on the fovea, allowing slower smooth pursuit to continue following, or tracking. Both saccades and smooth pursuit are continuous monitoring systems.

Occipital centers for pursuit are independent of the frontal lobes for fast saccades. The center for smooth pursuit is at the junction of the occipital and parietal lobes, giving rise to the *occipitomesencephalic tract,* which descends to the upper area of the midbrain. Here the occipitomesencephalic splits into one pathway for vertical gaze and another for horizontal gaze. The vertical fibers end in the medial posterior commissure for up gaze or in the riMLF for down gaze. Vertical pursuit fibers mix with vertical saccadic fibers from the frontal tract. The horizontal pursuit fibers join the horizontal saccadic fibers from the frontal lobe, traveling through the tegmentum of the midbrain to the horizontal gaze center in the pons.

Pursuit pathways either cross twice or do not cross, so that fibers from one occipital lobe end in brain stem gaze centers on the same side, e.g., the left occipital lobe controls left gaze. A defect in this left pathway

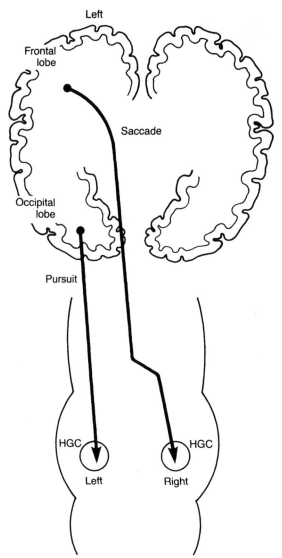

FIGURE 9–2. Schematic diagram for the frontomesencephalic pathway and the occipitomesencephalic pathway to the horizontal gaze center. Note that the frontomesencephalic pathway for saccades crosses from the left frontal lobe to the right horizontal gaze center (HGC). The occipitomesencephalic pathway for pursuit does not cross but travels from the left occipital lobe to the left HGC.

would affect left pursuit and the slow phase of optokinetic nystagmus. Smooth pursuit to the left would become jerky, a defect called "cogwheeling."

The pursuit system is tested by having the patient follow a fixation target into various positions while keeping the head still, as is also done when evaluating ductions or versions.

The occipitomesencephalic tract is probably involved with the near triad and vergence, but this circuitry remains uncertain. Involuntary eye movements initiated from the occipital cortex are known as optomotor reflexes.

Optokinetic Nystagmus (OKN)

This normal eye movement in response to a rotating striped drum or tape is controlled by both the saccade

and pursuit systems. The fast phase is a saccade, the slow phase is a pursuit. If the drum is rotated to the right, the eyes move right by pursuit for slow phase and quickly left by saccades for the fast phase (Fig. 9–3).

Vergence System

The vergence system angles the eyes away from parallelism, either apart or closer together, so that foveal alignment remains as the target changes its distance. Diplopia is the stimulus for a vergence movement, occurring whenever the target falls off corresponding retinal points. It generates the slowest eye movements, not more than 20°/sec. Comitant strabismus is a supranuclear imbalance of the vergence system at a cortical level.

The central nervous system pathways for vergence movements have not been precisely defined. They appear to originate in the occipital parietal cortex (Brodmann area 19) with a pathway that travels to the pretectal area and midbrain tegmentum.

Vestibular System

The vestibular system keeps the eyes fixed on a target as the head and body move, providing primitive stabilizing controls. As the head moves in one direction, the eyes move an equal amount in the opposite direction. Compensatory eye movements for a changing head position or from a moving object of regard are more important than for keeping the eyes looking straight ahead. Subcortical vestibular signals can override and modify messages to the ocular motor system, bypassing the gaze centers, enhancing the effort to keep a steady, fixed image on the foveas, especially responsive to changes in head and body position. The vestibular system is controlled by organs in the inner ear, the labyrinth and the otolith apparatus (Fig. 9–4).

The otolith apparatus is affected by gravity changes of position, such as a tilting away from the horizontal plane. The nerve fiber output pattern from the otolith end organ changes whenever the pull of gravity alters direction. If the head tilts, the eyes attempt tilting back to an upright position to maintain the vertical meridians. When the eyes attempt to right themselves they tilt in a direction opposite to that of the head. On right head tilt, the right eye makes a compensatory intorsion movement with both superior muscles, the right superior rectus (RSR) and the right superior oblique (RSO). The left eye makes compensatory extorsion movements with its inferior muscles, the left inferior oblique (LIO) and the left inferior rectus (LIR). This forms the basis of Bielschowsky's head tilt test.

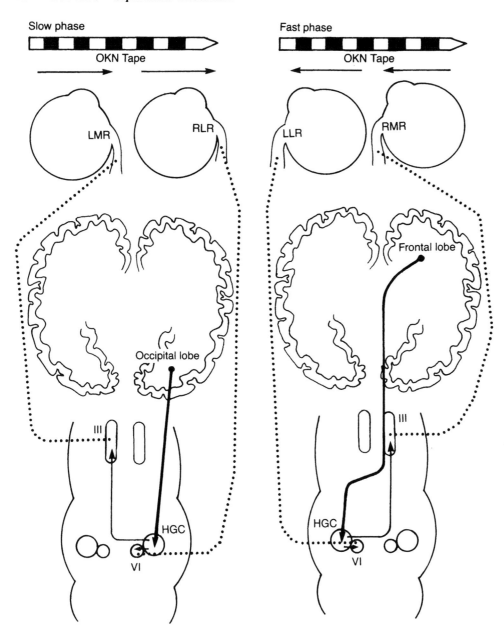

FIGURE 9–3. Biphasic innervation for optokinetic nystagmus (OKN). In this example, the OKN tape is moved to the right. The slow phase, initiated by the pursuit pathway from one occipitotemporo-occipital junction, follows one target to the right until the next target appears. Then a corrective, fast saccade to the left, initiated by the frontal lobe on the opposite side, fixates on the new target. HGC = horizontal gaze center, LMR = left medial rectus, RLR = right lateral rectus, LLR = left lateral rectus.

The doll's head, or oculocephalic, maneuver is one test of the vestibulo-ocular reflex. If the head is quickly turned sideways or vertically, the eyes move opposite to the head. In cooperative patients who can fixate a stationary object on request, the head is passively rotated. If command and pursuit are both affected by a defect, but the doll's head phenomenon is intact and version excursion full, then the vestibular system, nuclei, and infranuclear system are not affected. The defect is at the level of the brain stem gaze centers or higher in the supranuclear control centers or pathways.

Stimulation of the vestibular apparatus produces a false sense of motion or spinning. Motion sickness when traveling is the most familiar example of prolonged stimulation.

Gaze Centers

Brain stem gaze centers receive information from the frontal, occipital, and vestibular pathways. They transmit signals to the 3rd, 4th, and 6th nerve nuclei for eye movement. The HGC and vertical gaze centers (VGC) send commands by the same final pathway, the MLF, for both fast eye movements (saccades) and slow eye movements (pursuit or vestibular) to the III, IV, and VI cranial nerve nuclei for extraocular muscle innervations.

The HGC, pontine gaze center (PGC), or the pontine paramedian reticular formation (PPRF) (the three terms used interchangeably by most authors), is an ill-defined area near the 6th nerve nucleus in the pons where it functions as the horizontal conjugate gaze

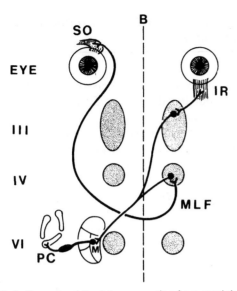

FIGURE 9–4. Example of the interconnection from semicircular canals to extraocular muscles. Fibers from the left posterior semicircular canal synapse in the left medial vestibular nucleus. Fibers then cross to the medial longitudinal fasciculus (MLF) on the right where they travel to the right fourth nerve nucleus (IV) to innervate the left superior oblique (LSO), and to the right third nerve (III) subnucleus to innervate the right inferior rectus (RIR). (From Miller NR: Walsh and Hoyt's Clinical Neuro-ophthalmology, 4th ed. Vol 2, Section IV: The Ocular Motor System: Embryology, Anatomy, Physiology, and Topographic Diagnosis. Baltimore, Williams & Wilkins, 1985.)

center. It may be the 6th nerve nucleus itself. Horizontal gaze requires firing of the 6th nerve on the same side as the gaze center and the subnucleus for the medial rectus (MR) on the opposite side. The 6th nerve nucleus appears to have two sets of neurons, one set for the LR on the same side, another set for interneurons that travel by way of the medial longitudinal fasciculus to the opposite subnucleus for the MR.

Two VGCs are located in the midbrain, one for up gaze in the posterior commissure and one for down gaze in the riMLF. The up-gaze center is close to where pupillary fibers synapse.

Notice the importance of the tectal and "pretectal" area, near or above the superior colliculus. Frontomesencephalic fibers for vertical saccades, occipitomesencephalic fibers for vertical pursuit, vestibular fibers, and pupillary fibers travel through here.

Medial Longitudinal Fasciculus

The MLF is the internuclear pathway, the "wiring mechanism" in the brain stem interconnecting the cranial nerves, linking information among and from the gaze centers, pupillary centers, and vestibular system to ocular motor cranial nerve nuclei. The MLF extends from the spinal cord to the thalamus, being most prominent in the brain stem. The MLF integrates reflex head and neck movement in response to visual stimuli, interconnects conjugate gaze signals between the 6th nerve nucleus on one side with the 3rd nerve medial

rectus subnucleus on the other side, and links contraction of the agonist muscle with relaxation of its direct antagonist muscle as required for a duction movement (Fig. 9–5).

Lesions

Supranuclear lesions produce gaze palsies but not strabismus (tropia) and not diplopia. The common exceptions are skew deviations and internuclear opthalmoplegias (INOs). A gaze palsy is a limitation of movement of both eyes in one direction. A complete horizontal gaze palsy is an inability to move either eye past the midline to the right or left. A vertical gaze palsy prevents both eyes from looking up or down. Damage to visual areas in the frontal lobe (Brodmann area 8), occipitoparietal area, and the vestibular system may cause temporary gaze palsies.

The position of the eye at any given time is a synchronous integration of the various levels of control. The higher the lesion, the more likely it will produce a gaze palsy. The defect is "higher" (more central) than the nucleus. If there is a gaze palsy, only the extraocular muscle function for that command is lost. The saccade, pursuit, and vestibular pathways need to be tested separately. With a supranuclear defect but an intact vestibular system (as in the normal doll's head maneuver)

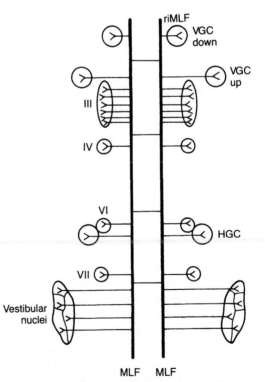

FIGURE 9–5. Medial longitudinal fasciculus interconnection from and among gaze centers and vestibular nuclei to cranial nerve nuclei. The two MLFs also interconnect with one another. VGC = vertical gaze center, riMLF = rostral interstitial nucleus of the medial longitudinal fasciculus.

the pontine pathways; the MLF; CNN III, IV, and VI; and infranuclear pathways still work. The extraocular muscles function whenever they receive a signal to do so. Only the functions affected by the defect, a damaged saccade or pursuit pathway or both, are absent.

• *Example. The eyes should roll up and out (Bell's phenomenon) when the patient is asked to close the eyes tightly. If up gaze is defective, the eyes remain in primary position. If the patient's chin is tipped down as a target is fixated, the eyes should rotate up (vestibulo-ocular reflex). When the eyes roll up with either test, it confirms an intact vestibular system and rules out any problem with the vertical muscles, their nerve supply, or the nerve nuclei.*

• *Example. A supranuclear lesion may produce a left gaze palsy so that no signals reach either the left lateral rectus (LLR) or the right medial rectus (RMR) to contract on attempted saccades. However, the RMR contracts along with the left medial rectus (LMR) when the eyes converge. When the doll's head maneuver is attempted, both eyes move into left gaze from contraction of the LLR and RMR when the head is moved to the right.*

All three systems will be out if there is a pontine brain stem lesion or a myopathy.

Skew deviation is a vertical strabismus associated with cerebellar or brain stem abnormalities. It is confused with other types of vertical strabismus, because no typical form is found. Skews may be concomitant, or mimic a paresis of a vertically acting extraocular muscle. Ductions are normal. The skew can be found on one side, or both sides, and the hypertropia may vary from right hypertropia (RHT) on one side to left hypertropia (LHT) on the other. One form is identified, the inferior rectus (IR) skew. Here both IR appear underactive, and the patient has an RHT on right gaze and an LHT on left gaze.

Internuclear

INO. An internuclear ophthalmoplegia (INO) is a sign of brain stem damage to the MLF after fibers leave CN VI on the same side but before reaching the CN III subnucleus for the MR on the opposite side. The signals destined for the MR subnucleus on the opposite side are damaged, producing an adduction deficit with diplopia. Convergence is usually intact, however, because its fibers are not affected. The laterality of the defect is named by the MR affected.

• *Example. A left INO reveals defective adduction into right gaze by the MR of the left eye and abducting*

nystagmus of the right eye. Exotropia and diplopia are seen in right gaze.

An INO in young adults is associated with multiple sclerosis, but in adults over 50 it is associated with vascular disease.

A variety of eye movement syndromes result from damage to ocular motor structures within the brain stem. These include the following.

Midbrain

Benedikt's Syndrome. This occurs from damage in the tegmentum of the midbrain affecting fibers from CN III, the red nucleus, and the corticospinal tract. If this occurs to fibers in the midbrain on the left side, a left exotropia and left ptosis from damage to the left CN III and tremor and irregular twitching of the right arm and leg result.

Parinaud's (Dorsal Midbrain) (Pretectal) (Sylvian Aqueduct) Syndrome. This occurs from damage in the pretectal area near the pupillary fibers and the vertical up-gaze center. Affects saccadic up gaze first, with eyelid retraction greater in up gaze. The eyelids work better than the eyes. Convergence retraction is noted when up gaze is attempted from cofiring of all the extra-ocular muscles. This can be tested by rotating an optokinetic nystagmus (OKN) drum downward. Convergence may be defective. Pupils are larger than normal with light-near dissociation. Vertical doll's head movement, tipping the head down so that the eyes move up, remains intact, as does Bell's phenomenon.

Weber's Syndrome. Affects the crus cerebri in the midbrain. Damage to the right corticospinal tract produces a spastic paralysis in the left arm and leg with a right eye exotropia, right eyelid ptosis, and dilated pupil on the right from damage to the right CN III.

Pontine

Millard-Gubler (Ventral Pontine) Syndrome. This is damage to the side of the pons near the ventral part. If on the right side, CN VI and CN VII damage results in a right esotropia and right facial palsy; damage to the right pyramidal tract results in a palsy of the left arm and leg.

Foville's (Dorsal-Lateral Pontine) Syndrome. This is similar to Millard-Gubler except that damage is to the pontine MLF so that the horizontal gaze to that side results rather than the CN VI palsy. Horner's syndrome may also be present.

Möebius' Syndrome. When complete, CN VI and CN VII on both sides are palsied, resulting in a droopy, mask-like, expressionless facial appearance with a marked esotropia from contraction of both MR. Neither eye can fix straight ahead. With a right face turn, the right eye can fix, and vice versa. The probable cause is a congenital absence or underdevelopment of the affected cranial nerve nuclei in the brainstem.

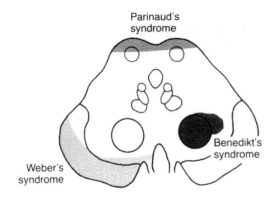

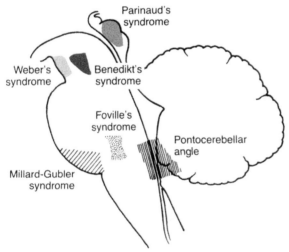

FIGURE 9–6. Brain stem locations where damage produces ocular motor dysfunction.

Pontocerebellar Angle. A slowly growing CN VIII tumor close to the attachment of the acoustic nerve to the brain stem exerts pressure on the pontocerebellar angle. At first, only the deafness from the CN VIII nerve damage is noticed. This progresses; abnormal labyrinthine responses appear, sometimes horizontal nystagmus. Damage to CN V then may develop, resulting in loss of corneal sensation and loss of pain and temperature sensation over the face on the side of the injury. When CN VII fibers become damaged, facial paralysis is noted, as well as LR palsy from damage to CN VI. Sometimes the diplopia from the esotropia from CN VI damage is the presenting complaint (Fig. 9–6).

Bibliography

Daroff RB, Troost BT: Supranuclear disorders of eye movement. In Glaser, JS (ed): Neuro-ophthalmology, 2nd ed. Hagerstown, MD, Harper & Row, 1990.

Dell'Osso LF, Daroff RB: Eye movement characteristics and recording techniques. In Glaser, JS (ed): Neuro-ophthalmology, 2nd ed. Hagerstown, MD, Harper & Row, 1990.

Miller NR: Walsh and Hoyt's Clinical Neuro-ophthalmology, 4th ed. Vol 2, Section IV: The Ocular Motor System: Embryology, Anatomy, Phsyiology, and Topographic Diagnosis. Baltimore, Williams & Wilkins, 1985.

Rosenberg, MA: Neuro-ophthalmology. In Peyman GA, Sanders DR, Goldberg MF (eds): Principles and Practice of Ophthalmology. Vol 3. Philadelphia, WB Saunders, 1980.

● CHAPTER 9 SUPRANUCLEAR MECHANISMS

1. Which choice defines voluntary corrective refixation movements?
   a. saccades
   b. doll's head maneuvers
   c. vergences
   d. pursuits
   e. vestibular movements

2. If an optokinetic drum is rotated to the right, the eyes move right by which of the following?
   a. saccade
   b. doll's head maneuver
   c. vergence
   d. pursuit
   e. vestibular movement

3. Which gaze center is located just above the superior colliculi?
   a. down gaze
   b. equilibrium
   c. horizontal gaze
   d. pursuit
   e. up gaze

4. Slow tracking movements are a function of the
   a. occipitomesencephalic pathway
   b. cerebellum
   c. medial longitudinal fasciculus (MLF)
   d. frontomesencephalic pathway
   e. vestibular system.

5. Which subcortical pathway interconnects the cranial nerve nuclei, gaze centers, and cerebellum?
   a. vestibular system
   b. medial longitudinal fasciculus
   c. frontomesencephalic pathway
   d. rostral interstitial nucleus of the MLF
   e. occipitomesencephalic pathway.

Barbara Cassin
Lindreth DuBois

Peripheral Nervous System

LEARNING OBJECTIVES

- Identify the cranial nerves by name and Roman numeral
- Describe the location of the cranial nerves that subserve the visual system
- Compare the functions of the cranial nerves that subserve the visual system
- Describe the infranuclear pathways of the cranial nerves that subserve the visual system
- Explain how the vestibular system interconnects with the ocular motor system

The peripheral nervous system is made up of cranial and spinal nerves and their associated ganglia. Included are both the input and the output part of the nervous system. It provides the route by which sensory (afferent) nerves transmit information from the world around us to the brain. Motor (efferent) nerves then send commands from the brain to muscles and glands. These nerves exit the brain and spinal cord and govern the reception of external stimuli and the reaction of the body's muscles.

This part of the nervous system below the level of the nerve nuclei contains the infranuclear pathways. It is also below the cortical level. In fact, the peripheral nervous system is below the level of the brain stem gaze centers, the vestibular system, and the medial longitudinal fasciculus.

The brain stem contains 12 paired sensory and motor cranial nerve nuclei, numbered with Roman numerals according to vertical location. Each one is also named according to function. The first two, olfactory and optic, have cell bodies located in their receptor organs (nose for smell and retina for sight). The rest have cell bodies in their nuclei. The nerve fiber tracts contain their axons. Some cranial nerves are purely sensory (afferent), some purely motor (efferent), some are mixed, and some also contain autonomic nervous system (ANS) fibers regulating involuntary body functions. In ophthalmology, the concern is with those cranial nerves that serve the eyes (Fig. 10–1).

● CRANIAL NERVES

Of the 12 cranial nerves (CNs), only seven are directly involved with the eye: CNs II to VIII (Table 10–1). The first two are not true cranial nerves, but sensory nerve fiber tracts whose cell bodies are at the site of origin: the first (olfactory) cranial nerve (CN I) in the nose for smell, and the second (optic) cranial nerve (CN II) in the retina for sight. A more detailed treatment of the optic nerves is found in Chapter 7. The rest of the cranial nerves have cell bodies in their nuclei.

The third (oculomotor) (CN III), fourth (trochlear) (CN IV), and sixth (abducens) (CN VI) are motor, innervating intrinsic and extrinsic eye muscles and the upper eyelid. *An infranuclear ocular motor defect affects the nerve before it innervates its designated muscle(s).*

The fifth (trigeminal) (CN V) and seventh (facial) (CN VII) are mixed, having both sensory and motor fibers. The trigeminal nerve is the largest; it originates in the pons and has fibers serving different areas of the face. CN VII innervates muscles of the scalp and face.

The eighth (acoustic/vestibulocochlear) (CN VIII) has two functions. The vestibular portion subserves body balance and equilibrium. The cochlear portion subserves the sense of hearing.

The ninth (glossopharyngeal) (CN IX) provides sensation for pain, touch, and temperature from the phar-

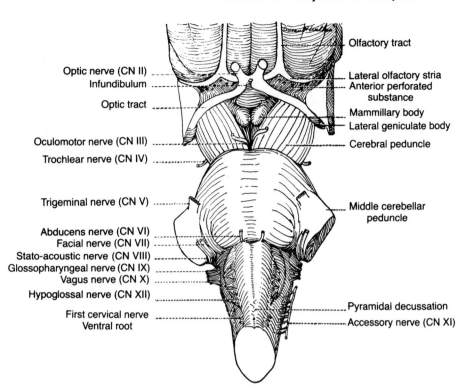

FIGURE 10–1. Ventral view of brain stem cranial nerves. (From Ranson SW, Clark SL: Anatomy of the Nervous System, 10th ed. Philadelphia, WB Saunders, 1959.)

ynx and back of the tongue; sensation for taste from the back of the tongue; and it carries motor fibers to the mouth for salivation and swallowing.

The tenth (vagus) (CN X) nerve connects sensory and motor fibers to the larynx, pharynx, and thoracic and abdominal internal organs (the viscera). It also has parasympathetic fibers to the heart, lungs, and gastrointestinal tract, including the esophagus. This highly important nerve slows the heart rate and increases the digestive process.

The eleventh (spinal accessory) (CN XI) serves major neck muscles and helps the vagus innervate the larynx.

The twelfth (hypoglossal) (CN XII) is the motor nerve with which the tongue moves.

The cranial nerves usually exit the brain stem in front of the ventricular system from the ventral surface and do not cross to the other side, except for the CN IV, which crosses after exiting dorsally (Fig. 10–2).

● OCULAR MOTOR SYSTEM

The ocular motor system contains the infranuclear pathways for the eyes. That part of the peripheral nervous system brings messages from the brain stem nuclei to the extraocular muscles (EOM) to move the eye, placing the image of a viewed target simultaneously on both foveas and retaining that image until a decision is reached to look at a different target.

The ocular motor system consists of the pathways of CNS III, IV, and VI as they leave the brain stem, travel along the base of the skull to enter the orbit, then innervate the extraocular muscles, levator, iris sphincter, and ciliary body (Table 10–2).

The extraocular muscles can only function if they receive a message from the ocular motor nerves. If an infranuclear pathway has a defect, then not all the muscles receive their signals, because some messengers are defective. No command from a higher control center can produce the desired eye movement. An incomitant eye misalignment results, producing diplopia.

If the infranuclear system has no defect, but a higher center does, the eyes do not produce the desired movement because the ocular motor cranial nerve nuclei do not receive the desired command. The messengers (ocular motor nerves) can transmit, but they need to

---

TABLE 10–1.

Mnemonic to Remember the Order of the Cranial Nerves

Location	Name	Mnemonic	CN
	Olfactory	ON	I
	Optic	OLD	II
Midbrain	Oculomotor	OLYMPUS	III
Midbrain	Trochlear	TOWERING	IV
Pons	Trigeminal	TOP	V
Pons	Abducens	A	VI
Pons	Facial	FINN or FAT	VII
Pons	(Acoustic) Vestibular-cochlear	AND VICIOUS	VIII
Medulla	Glossopharyngeal	GERMAN or GORILLA	IX
Medulla	Vagus	VIEWED	X
Medulla	Spinal accessory	SOME	XI
Medulla	Hypoglossal	HOPS	XII

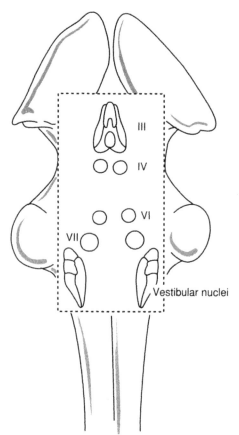

FIGURE 10–2. Dorsal view of cranial nerves involved in visual function. (Redrawn from Duane T: Biomedical Foundations in Ophthalmology, Volume I. New York, Harper & Row, 1989.)

get the command. With supranuclear palsies affecting horizontal or vertical gaze centers, defects of conjugate gaze occur, but diplopia does not occur.

● *For Example. With a left CN VI palsy, the left lateral rectus cannot move the left eye to the left even when the horizontal gaze center on the left stimulates the left CN VI to do so. Only the right eye moves to the left. The right horizontal gaze center can still stimulate both eyes to move to the right.*

TABLE 10–2.

Mnemonic Resembling a Chemical Formula for EOM Innervation

$$LR_6 \, (SO_4)^3$$

LR = Lateral rectus is innervated by the
6 = Sixth (abducens) cranial nerve
SO = Superior oblique is innervated by the
4 = Fourth (trochlear) cranial nerve
3 = Third (oculomotor) cranial nerve innervates all the other extraocular muscles and the levator:

MR (medial rectus)	IR (inferior rectus)
IO (inferior oblique)	SR (superior rectus)
Levator superioris	

An infranuclear ocular motor system defect may occur along the path of the nerve itself as it travels through the following structures:

1. Brain stem
2. Interpeduncular space separating the midbrain from the cavernous sinus
3. Cavernous sinus
4. Superior orbital fissure
5. Orbit

If more than one cranial nerve is involved, it raises the suspicion of a defect within the orbit or cavernous sinus, because of the proximity of the ocular motor cranial nerves to one another.

CN III

CN III nuclei are located in the center of the midbrain below the cerebral aqueduct at the level of the superior colliculi near the top of the midbrain. The CN IV (trochlear) nucleus lies just below it.

The CN III nucleus is actually a complex group of subnuclei (Fig. 10–3), supplying a pair of subnuclei for each extraocular muscle except the superior oblique and the lateral rectus. An unpaired subnucleus for the levator and an unpaired subnucleus, the Edinger-Westphal, sits on top, closest to the aqueduct in the midline, receiving pupillary and accommodation information and supplying parasympathetic motor innervation to the iris sphincter and the ciliary body. Superior rectus fibers are the only ones in the CN III nucleus that *cross*. Thus fibers from the right superior rectus subnucleus innervate the left superior rectus, and fibers from the left subnucleus innervate the right superior rectus. All the others are uncrossed, innervating extraocular muscles on the same side.

CN III leaves the midbrain, appearing on the front (ventral) surface near the midline junction with the pons. It crosses the interpeduncular space, slips into the cavernous sinus, runs through the outer wall near the top, enters the orbit through the superior orbital fissure within Zinn's annulus of the muscle cone, where it divides into superior and inferior branches. The superior branch innervates the superior rectus (eye elevation) and the levator (lid elevation), whereas the inferior branch innervates the medial rectus (eye adduction), inferior rectus (eye depression), and inferior oblique (eye elevation). Parasympathetic fibers (pupillary constriction) remain with the inferior division until the branches to the medial rectus and inferior rectus leave. They branch off, traveling to synapse in the ciliary ganglion. Postganglionic parasympathetic fibers enter the globe within the short ciliary nerves (Fig 10–4).

A complete CN III palsy leaves only the superior

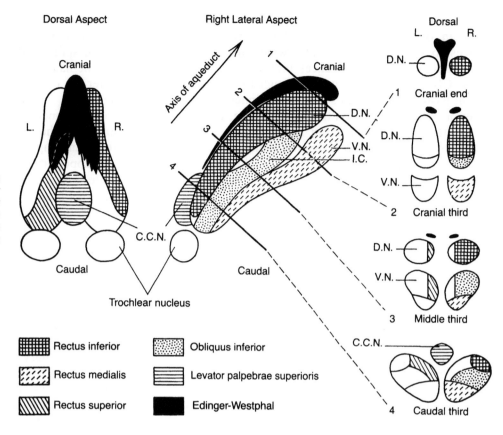

FIGURE 10–3. Third cranial nerve complex. Subnuclei, except for Edinger-Westphal, are labeled by the muscle they innervate. (From Warwick R: Wolff's Anatomy of the Eye and Orbit, 7th ed. Chapman & Hall, Hampshire, England.)

Rectus inferior

Rectus medialis

Rectus superior

Obliquus inferior

Levator palpebrae superioris

Edinger-Westphal

oblique and lateral rectus muscles functioning in the involved eye, causing the eye to deviate out and slightly down. The upper lid droops and the pupil dilates. The patient often does not complain of diplopia because the deviation is large, widely separating the images, and because the eyelid droop covers the image of that eye. A third nerve palsy is associated with four Ds:

Dilated pupil

Droopy eyelid

Down and out

Diplopia

CN III is sometimes called the *aneurysm* nerve, because cerebral aneurysms in the fifth to seventh decades of life commonly cause CN III palsies. Half of all CN III palsies that are vascular in origin produce pain. A widely dilated pupil with pain and palsy indicates an aneurysm in the circle of Willis. This is a semiemergency, usually requiring immediate hospital admission. If a CN III palsy has no change in pupil size, the usual cause is either diabetes or hypertension. Patients with these palsies usually recover in about six weeks. CN III palsies can also be caused by other vascular diseases, trauma, tumors, or inflammation.

CN IV

The CN IV (trochlear) nucleus arises just below the third nerve nucleus at the level of the inferior colliculi in the midbrain near its junction with the pons. This is

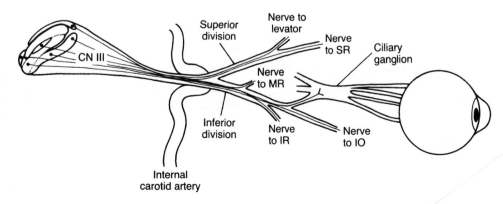

FIGURE 10–4. Route of the oculomotor nerve (CN III) from its nucleus in the brain stem around the internal carotid artery in the cavernous sinus to the eye.

the only cranial nerve that runs backward to exit the midbrain on the *dorsal* surface, however. It then crosses to the contralateral side, winds around the brain stem, and finally advances into the cavernous sinus. CN IV enters the orbit through the superior orbital fissure above Zinn's annulus to innervate the superior oblique muscle on the opposite side. For example, the CN IV nucleus on the *right* side of the midbrain innervates the *left* superior oblique.

As a consequence of crossing dorsally, this thinnest cranial nerve is more vulnerable than other cranial nerves to head injury. It is frequently called the *trauma* nerve. The trauma may be mild, like falling down, but if there is a pre-existing weakness, it is enough to cause paralysis. Nevertheless, congenital CN IV palsy is the most common cause. The second most likely acquired cause of a CN IV palsy is a vascular disease such as hypertension, or diabetes mellitus, especially in adults. Meningiomas are the most common tumors causing a CN IV palsy (Fig. 10–5).

CN IV palsies affect the superior oblique muscle, causing diplopia in opposite gaze, i.e., a *right* superior oblique palsy produces diplopia that is worse in *left* gaze. The head is often tilted to the opposite shoulder to maintain fusion, i.e., a patient with a *right* superior oblique palsy tilts the head to the *left* shoulder. And CN IV has opposite innervation, i.e., the *right* superior oblique is innervated by the *left* fourth nerve nucleus.

Note that the superior rectus and superior oblique are the only extraocular muscles whose nerve fibers cross in the brain stem area. All others have uncrossed (ipsilateral) innervation.

CN V

The trigeminal (CN V) is the largest cranial nerve. It originates in the pons and has both sensory and motor fibers serving different areas of the face. The nerve branches into three divisions: the ophthalmic (CN V$_1$), the maxillary (CN V$_2$), and the mandibular (CN V$_3$).

We are most concerned with the first division, the ophthalmic, which only has sensory function. The ophthalmic division splits in the cavernous sinus into three branches: the nasociliary, lacrimal, and frontal, all of which enter the orbit through the superior orbital fissure (Fig. 10–6).

The frontal branch of V$_1$ runs forward along the orbital roof above the levator muscle, splitting into the supraorbital and supratrochlear nerves. These supply the medial upper lid, conjunctiva, forehead, front half of the scalp, and side of the nose.

The lacrimal branch of CN V$_1$ runs forward above the lateral rectus, supplying the skin and conjunctiva of the upper and lower lids, as well as the lacrimal gland. It also carries parasympathetic fibers for reflex tearing to the lacrimal gland.

The nasociliary branch of CN V$_1$ supplies sensation to the eyeball, caruncle, and bridge and tip of the nose. Function of CN V$_1$ is assessed by testing corneal sensitivity. This branch splits off the long sensory root to the ciliary ganglion, carrying sensory fibers from the cornea, iris, and ciliary muscle that arrive at the ciliary ganglion through the short ciliary nerves. The nasociliary nerve also carries sympathetic fibers that innervate the iris dilator muscle. These fibers travel through the long ciliary nerves, bypass the ciliary ganglion, pierce the sclera, and travel forward between the sclera and choroid with the short ciliary nerves to form the ciliary plexus in the ciliary body (see Fig. 10–6).

The second branch of the trigeminal, the maxillary (CN V$_2$), contains fibers for pain, touch, and temperature on the cheek, lower eyelid, palate, upper jaw, teeth, and maxillary sinus.

The third branch, the mandibular (CN V$_3$), contains sensory fibers for pain, touch, and temperature from the lower jaw, teeth, lips, mouth, anterior tongue, and parts of the ear. It provides motor innervation for contraction of chin muscles and chewing. The Marcus Gunn syndrome, or jaw winking, occurs as an abnormal innervation involving the motor division of the trigeminal, which supplies the pterygoid muscles for chewing and inadvertently supplies the levator. In this syn-

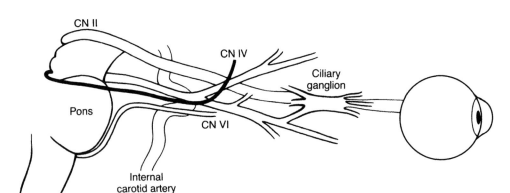

FIGURE 10–5. Route of the trochlear nerve (CN IV) from its nucleus in the brain stem around the internal carotid artery in the cavernous sinus to the eye.

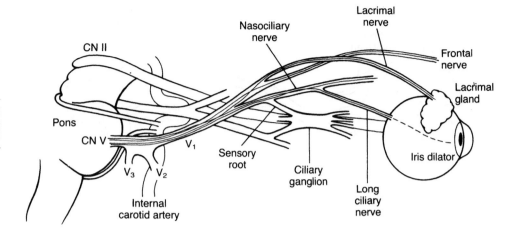

FIGURE 10-6. Route of the ophthalmic division of the trigeminal nerve (CN V₁) from its nucleus in the brain stem around the internal carotid artery in the cavernous sinus to the eye.

drome, whenever the patient chews, the eyelid blinks at the same time.

CN VI

The abducens (CN VI) nucleus arises in the ventral wall of the 4th ventricle in the pons. In close proximity is the horizontal gaze center responsible for sending impulses through the medial longitudinal fasciculus for horizontal versions. After running through the pontine paramedian reticular formation (PPRF), the CN VI exits the brain stem from the front (ventral) surface of the pons near the pons-medulla junction. It rises between the clivus bone and the pons before bending over the petrous ridge of the temporal bone on its way to the cavernous sinus, continuing through the superior orbital fissure into the orbit where it innervates the lateral rectus muscle on the same side. CN VI palsies affect the lateral rectus muscle, causing an esotropic (inward) deviation worse on the same side; e.g., a right CN VI palsy has the most esotropic deviation in right gaze (Fig. 10–7).

CN VI is sometimes referred to as the *tumor* nerve, because palsies result from pressure caused by growth of pontine gliomas in childhood or nasopharyngeal tumors in adults. Its passage over the petrous ridge makes

it particularly susceptible to injury from trauma or increased intracranial pressure. Children may develop a benign CN VI palsy following a viral illness. They usually recover. A CN VI palsy in an adult is more likely to be vascular in origin. CN VI palsies are more common than CN IV palsies, which are more common than CN III palsies.

CN VII

CN VII, the facial nerve, is a mixed nerve that arises in the center of the pons near its junction with the medulla. Its course is similar to that of CN IV in that it begins to leave the nucleus heading dorsally toward the fourth ventricle. It then loops around the CN VI nucleus and comes forward to exit the ventral surface of the pons, just medial to CN VIII nerve (Fig. 10–8).

Some parasympathetic fibers leave the pons within CN VII, synapse, switch to the zygomatic branch of the maxillary division (V₂) of CN V, and then switch back within the orbit to the lacrimal branch of the ophthalmic division (V₁) of CN V, to innervate the lacrimal gland for reflex tearing.

The facial nerve is mostly motor, producing facial expression by innervation of the muscles of the face and scalp. It also stimulates secretion by the lacrimal

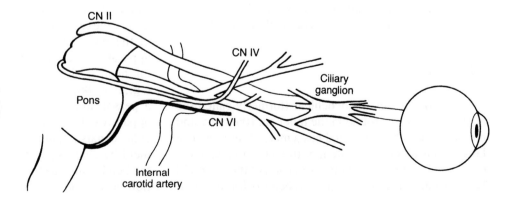

FIGURE 10-7. Route of the abducens nerve (CN VI) from its nucleus in the brain stem out through the cavernous sinus to the eye.

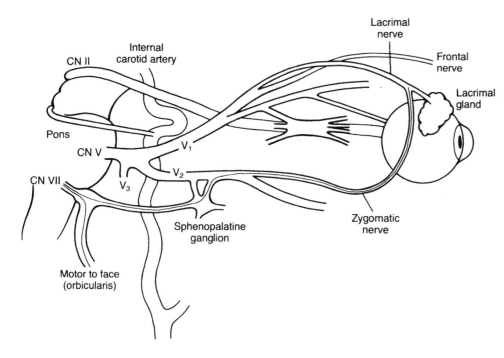

FIGURE 10–8. Route of the sensory portion of the facial nerve (CN VII) as it affects the eye and lacrimal gland from its nucleus in the brain stem to the orbit. The motor portion that innervates the orbicularis oculi is not shown.

gland. An important function of CN VII is innervation of the orbicularis oculi muscles, the oval sheet of concentric fibers circling the palpebral fissure. The peripheral orbital portion forcibly closes the eyelids as in sneezing. The central palpebral portion causes involuntary blinking.

Bell's phenomenon is an associated movement of the eye, eyelid, and surrounding facial muscles. The eyes involuntarily roll outward and upward when forcible efforts are made to close the eyelid against resistance. If this up-and-out movement of the eye is still present in those who cannot voluntarily elevate the eye, it confirms that brain stem pathways between the CN VII nucleus and that portion of the CN III nucleus responsible for eye elevation are intact. Ten percent of otherwise normal subjects do not have a normal Bell's phenomenon.

Bell's palsy is a pathological condition that interrupts the function of the facial nerve. It is a neuropathy of unknown cause that results in inability to close the involved eye. Bell's palsy is associated with elevation of the same eye on attempted eyelid closure. Most patients with Bell's palsy recover within 6 weeks.

CN VIII

CN VIII, the vestibulocochlear (formerly called the acoustic) nerve, is found in the inner ear (the bony and membranous labyrinth), and has a mixed function. The labyrinth is a delicate system of tunnels and chambers deeply imbedded in the petrous portion of the temporal bone. It consists of the cochlea (receptors for hearing),

the semicircular canals, and the otolith apparatus, similar to a small stone.

The cochlea, a spiral organ found at one end of the labyrinth, sends sound wave signals through imbedded sensory fibers in the cochlear branch of CN VIII to the brain for hearing.

With the help of the cerebellum, the vestibular system integrates information from all the senses in a constant effort to maintain body posture and adjust body position to stabilize the eyes, head, and body in space. One of its most important tasks is to keep the eyes on target by centering the image on the fovea and keeping it there as the head and body move. Another task is to issue continual commands to the appropriate cranial nerves so that the eyes, head, and body produce the correct movements at the correct time. Various pathways between the four vestibular nuclei, cerebellum, and cerebrum help the body maintain balance, smooth out body movements, and orient head position in space as the body moves.

The vestibular system of the inner ear has two divisions: (1) the semicircular canals, producing labyrinthine reflexes, are concerned with angular acceleration of the body and head movement; and (2) the otolith apparatus is concerned with linear acceleration, including head position with respect to the pull of gravity, e.g., in walking or running. The otolith apparatus keeps a person upright even with closed eyes. The otolith apparatus also produces righting reflexes. The semicircular canals maintain eye fixation despite head movement by changing eye and body posture, as in turning the head from side to side. Rotation (angular) acceleration of the body, for instance, occurs with rapid rota-

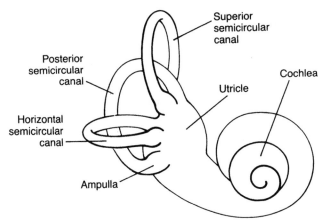

FIGURE 10–9. Labyrinth in the inner ear. A horizontal semicircular canal on one side is associated with the medial rectus on that side and the yoke lateral rectus on the other side. A posterior semicircular canal on one side is associated with the superior oblique on that side and the yoke inferior rectus on the other side. A superior semicircular canal on one side is associated with the superior rectus on that side and the yoke inferior oblique on the other side.

tion in a swivel chair and produces a characteristic rotational nystagmus (Fig. 10–9).

Each membranous labyrinth of a semicircular canal is oriented at right angles to the other two, forming a system of three coordinates (like the planes of movement of the extraocular muscles) for horizontal, vertical, and tilting functions. The output of any semicircular canal is maximal with movements in the plane of the canal, much as an extraocular muscle action is maximal when the eye is directed in the plane of the muscle. The semicircular canals interact with the extraocular muscles so that the eyes maintain their orientation in space regardless of changes in head position.

The semicircular canals and the otolith apparatus communicate both directly and indirectly with each other. The otolith moves with changing head position and stimulates tiny hairs in the canal walls. Receptors

for head position are in the semicircular canals. At the end of each canal is an expansion (ampulla) with hair cells which excite vestibular nerve fibers originating on the ampullae. A watery fluid, endolymph, in the semicircular canals is stimulated by accelerating or decelerating the motion of the head. Motion from the flow in the canal toward the ampulla stimulates sensory vestibular fibers. The motion is changed to electrical energy and transmitted to the appropriate vestibular nucleus in the pontine medullary junction and then to the cerebellum and the medial longitudinal fasciculus (MLF). Proprioceptive fibers for balance and equilibrium also relay information from the vestibular branch of CN VIII to the four vestibular nuclei in the pons and medulla.

The vestibular system is tested by the vestibulo-ocular reflex (VOR), which maintains images on the fovea despite head and neck movements. When the head is upright and stationary, input is balanced from the semicircular canals in both ears. Movement of the head causes disruption of this balanced input. When the head moves, the eyes are driven to move an equal amount but in the opposite direction. For example, as the head turns to the right, endolymph in the horizontal semicircular canal flows to the left, toward the right horizontal ampulla and away from the left horizontal ampulla, sending impulses through the MLF to the left sixth and the right third nerve nuclei to turn the eye to the left to maintain eye position. This VOR is the basis for the doll's head maneuver in ocular motility testing. The vestibulo-ocular reflex travels by way of the vestibular branch of the CN VIII from a semicircular canal on one side to vestibular nuclei, bypassing the brain stem gaze centers (Fig. 10–10).

In summary, the interconnections of CNs III, IV, V, VI, VII, and VIII integrate visual information from the brain stem centers for smooth eye movements, maintaining steady fixation on desired targets without diplopia. Interruptions in any of these interconnections

HEAD RIGHT

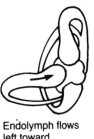
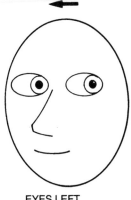
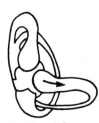
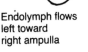

FIGURE 10–10. Doll's head maneuver tests the ability of the vestibular system. RMR = right medial rectus, LLR = left lateral rectus.

Endolymph flows left toward right ampulla

EYES LEFT
RMR Contraction
LLR Contraction

Endolymph flows left away from left ampulla

produce disruptions of normal visual function. The CN III (oculomotor) and CN IV (trochlear) nuclei are found in the midbrain. CN V (trigeminal), CN VI (abducens), CN VII (facial), and CN VIII (acoustic) nuclei are located in the pons.

A CN III palsy produces diplopia with the affected eye misaligned outward (exotropia) and down, a dilated pupil, and a droopy upper eyelid from the paresis of the levator muscle. A CN IV palsy results in a head tilt to the opposite shoulder from the affected superior oblique muscle. A defect in the ophthalmic (V_1) division of CN V results in reduced corneal sensation in the affected eye. A palsied CN VI produces an inward (eso) deviation in the affected eye from the weak lateral rectus. A defect in the vestibular system may result in nystagmus, defective balance and gait, or dizziness.

Bibliography

Glaser JS: Infranuclear disorders of eye movement. In Neuro-ophthalmology, 2nd ed. Hagerstown, MD, Harper & Row, 1990.

Miller NR: Walsh and Hoyt's Clinical Neuro-ophthalmology, 4th ed. Volume Two, Section IV: The Ocular Motor System: Embryology, Anatomy, Physiology, and Topographic Diagnosis; and Volume Two, Section V: Sensory Innervation of the Eye and Orbit. Baltimore, Williams & Wilkins, 1985.

Rosenberg MA: Neuro-ophthalmology. In Peyman GA, Sanders DR, Goldberg MF (eds): Principles and Practice of Ophthalmology, Volume III. Philadelphia, WB Saunders, 1980.

● CHAPTER 10 PERIPHERAL NERVOUS SYSTEM

1. If the sixth (abducens) cranial nerve (CN VI) is damaged near the superior orbital fissure, what is the defect?
   a. interpeduncular
   b. infranuclear
   c. supranuclear
   d. nuclear
   e. internuclear

2. The only cranial nerve that crosses from one side of the brain stem to enter the orbit on the other side innervates the
   a. superior oblique muscle
   b. lateral rectus muscle
   c. medial rectus muscle
   d. lacrimal gland
   e. levator muscle.

3. Sympathetic fibers that innervate the iris dilator reach the orbit by which nerve?
   a. facial
   b. oculomotor
   c. frontal
   d. nasociliary
   e. maxillary

4. Where is the cranial nerve that has a complex group of subnuclei that work on a three-coordinate system found?
   a. medulla
   b. midbrain
   c. cerebral aqueduct
   d. cerebellum
   e. superior colliculi

5. When the head moves to the left, the eyes move to the right in order to maintain fixation. What is this a function of?
   a. CN VII
   b. CN IV
   c. CN V_1
   d. CN VIII
   e. CN V_2

Barbara Cassin
Sidney Cassin

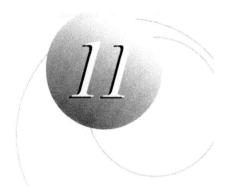

Autonomic Nervous System

LEARNING OBJECTIVES

- Compare the differences between the sympathetic and parasympathetic divisions of the autonomic nervous system
- Compare the differences between the adrenergic and cholinergic chemical transmitters
- Explain the role of the autonomic nervous system in relation to eye function
- Name four miotic drugs

- Name four anticholinesterase drugs
- Name three cycloplegic drugs
- Name three direct adrenergic-agonist drugs
- Name three beta-blocker drugs
- Trace the sympathetic nerve fiber pathways to the eye
- Trace the parasympathetic nerve fiber pathways to the eye

The autonomic nervous system (ANS) controls internal organ function as a self-preservation mechanism (Fig. 11–1). It controls contraction of the smooth and cardiac muscle as well as glandular secretion for regulation of body temperature, heart rate and output, arterial and venous pressures, regional blood flow, capillary filtration and exchange, airway resistance, gastrointestinal motility and secretion, bladder and ureteral motility, and several aspects of sexual function. Thus it contributes to maintaining the constancy of the internal environment (homeostasis). *Autonomic* refers to the fact that most of these activities function unconsciously and without direct voluntary control even though they can be strikingly influenced by psychological factors (blushing with shame, turning white with fear, sweating from anxiety, and nervous diarrhea). Pupil dilation can occur as an emotional response to fear, pain, and surprise.

● FUNCTIONS OF THE ANS

The ANS has two major divisions, sympathetic and parasympathetic. The hypothalamus controls the activities of both. Each division consists mostly of efferent fibers carrying impulses away from the central nervous system (CNS) to the effector organs. Most organs are innervated by both divisions, which usually function in opposition to each other, but work concurrently.

In general, the sympathetic system activates a variety of functions that achieve their maximum intensity in emergencies and stressful situations, the *flight or fight* system. Physical stress excites the sympathetic nervous system, providing extra energy for the body's self-preservation, permitting more strenuous physical exercise than would otherwise be possible. This reaction to challenge innervates many organs simultaneously. Most sympathetic reactions are energy-consuming activities. Cardiac output is redistributed with blood shifting to the brain, heart, lungs, and skeletal muscles. Heart rate, blood pressure, and breathing increase; pupils dilate; blood vessels to skeletal muscles dilate; and basal metabolic rate increases. Blood vessels to the skin and organs in the abdomen constrict, allowing more effort to be devoted to sudden reactions. Sweat glands moisten the skin. Adrenal glands secrete epinephrine and norepinephrine. The liver breaks down glucose, releasing it into the blood stream, thus increasing the amount of blood glucose needed for energy. The body mobilizes its fuel stores.

On the other hand, the parasympathetic system tends to be the resting, restoring, energy-conserving system. It has more localized reactions than the sympathetic; it is the *housekeeper* of the nervous system, concerned with daily body functions. It causes secretion of salivary glands; constriction of the bronchi in the lungs; and increased motility of the stomach, small intestine, and gallbladder. The latter tasks enhance digestion and

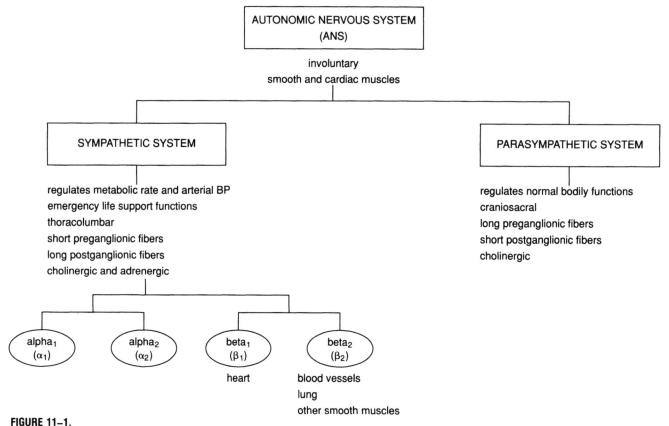

FIGURE 11-1.

absorption of food for future energy needs. The parasympathetic system also conserves energy by relaxing smooth muscles and by slowing the heart rate. Not all reactions fit this scheme, but it is a useful way of looking at autonomic function.

• ANS PATHWAYS

After leaving the CNS, fibers of the ANS synapse once before arriving at the effector cells (target tissues), making it a two-neuron chain. These synapses occur in cell body clusters called ganglia. White myelinated preganglionic axons travel from the CNS to a ganglion. Gray, nonmyelinated postganglionic axons pass from a ganglion to the effector organ.

Anatomic differences exist between the two systems. The sympathetic system has an outflow from the thoracolumbar part of the spinal cord. Sympathetic ganglia can be paravertebral (close to the spinal column) or prevertebral (in front of and further away from the spinal column). Fibers that supply the head travel through paravertebral ganglia that lie in a vertical row as the sympathetic chain, or trunk, on either side of the vertebral (spinal) column. The fibers continue to a prevertebral ganglion where they synapse, e.g., to the superior cervical ganglion located in the neck next to the internal carotid artery. This arrangement results in

a short preganglionic fiber and a longer postganglionic fiber (Fig. 11–2).

The parasympathetic axons have terminal ganglia not arranged in chains but found in or near the effector organ, e.g., the cilary ganglion in the muscle cone of the orbit. The cell bodies of the preganglionic fibers are found in the brain stem and their axons are distributed with the cranial nerves. Other cell bodies are found in the sacral part of the spinal cord. The parasympathetic system has a craniosacral outflow. The parasympathetic efferent limb consists of a relatively longer preganglionic and a short postganglionic fiber. After leaving the spinal cord, the preganglionic fibers travel with CNs III (oculomotor), VII (facial), and IX (glossopharyngeal) to the head, and with CN X (vagus) to the chest and upper abdomen. Probably 80% of all parasympathetic neural activity is transmitted in the vagus nerve, which innervates the heart, lungs, esophagus, digestive system, ureters, liver, gallbladder, and pancreas.

• NEUROTRANSMISSION

Excitation is conveyed from one cell to another by release of a chemical neurotransmitter at the nerve terminal. Acetylcholine is the transmitter that conveys excitation from the preganglionic to the postganglionic

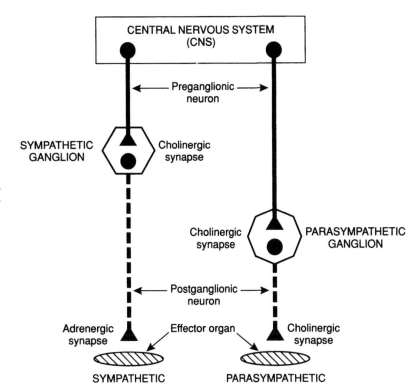

FIGURE 11–2. Anatomical differences between sympathetic and parasympathetic pre- and postganglionic fibers.

fibers for both sympathetic and parasympathetic systems. Fibers that release acetylcholine are called cholinergic. After the impulse is transmitted, the enzyme cholinesterase works quickly to inactivate the acetylcholine; therefore, cholinergic fibers tend to have a local, short-lived effect.

A second gap exists between postganglionic nerve terminals and the effector cells. Acetylcholine is also the transmitter between the parasympathetic postganglionic terminals and the effector cells that they supply, e.g., the iris sphincter. Acetylcholine is also the transmitter at certain sympathetic postganglionic terminals, e.g., sympathetic cholinergic fibers to skeletal muscle, blood flow vessels, and sweat glands.

Receptors that bind acetylcholine are present on the surface of skeletal, cardiac, smooth-muscle, and glandular cells. They are present in the levator, orbicularis, iris, ciliary body, and extraocular muscles. After receptor activation, a sequence of reactions causes contraction or relaxation of muscle or glandular secretion. Many synthetic substances can activate or block cholinergic receptors. Considerable variation exists, however, in the blocking action at different sites. As an example, atropine blocks smooth-muscle cholinergic receptors in doses that have little effect on ganglionic or skeletal neuromuscular transmission (Fig. 11–3). On the other hand, hexamethonium blocks only ganglionic transmission.

In the sympathetic nervous system, the transmitter to most effector organs, e.g., the iris dilator, is norepinephrine. Fibers releasing norepinephrine are adrenergic. The term comes from the older American and current British literature, in which epinephrine and norepinephrine are called Adrenalin. Most body parts have both sympathetic and parasympathetic innervations. Adrenergic (sympathetic) and cholinergic (parasympathetic) systems are mutually antagonistic. What one system stimulates, the other inhibits.

The response of any organ to norepinephrine depends on the relative activity of one of its two types of receptors, alpha (α) and beta (β). The combination of norepinephrine with smooth-muscle beta receptors leads to a relaxation. There appear to be two subtypes of beta receptor. These have been designated as beta$_1$ and beta$_2$ on the basis of their responses to synthetic agonists and antagonists. Beta$_1$ receptors are present in heart muscle. Activation by epinephrine, one of the hormones of the adrenal medulla, increases contraction of the heart and the rate of force development. Beta$_2$ receptors are found in vascular (blood vessel), bronchial, and other smooth muscle. Epinephrine can work through both alpha and beta receptors.

The counterpart of cholinesterase in the sympathetic system is catechol-O-methyl transferase (COMT) or monoamine oxidase (MAO). These enzymes work much more slowly than cholinesterase, allowing norepinephrine time to enter the blood stream. Therefore, sympathetic stimulation is longer lasting and more widespread than parasympathetic stimulation.

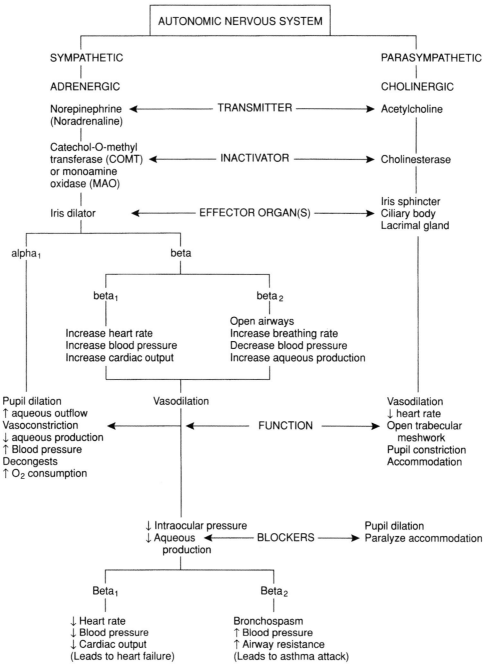

FIGURE 11–3.

• ANS INNERVATION TO THE EYE

The ANS is an important regulator of eye function. The diameter of the pupil is determined by an antagonism between radial muscle fibers enlarging the pupil opening and circular musculature closing the pupil opening. The radial fibers are innervated by sympathetic fibers from the superior cervical ganglion, whereas the circular fibers are innervated by parasympathetic fibers from the ciliary ganglion. Focusing of the lens is also regulated by parasympathetic fibers from the ciliary ganglion that control the ciliary muscle.

Secretion of tears is controlled by parasympathetic fibers from the sphenopalatine ganglion (Fig. 11–4).

• PARASYMPATHETIC NERVOUS SYSTEM

In ophthalmology, our concern is mostly with the parasympathetic fibers whose cell bodies are in the oculomotor (CN III) nerve. Long preganglionic fibers from the Edinger-Westphal nucleus exit the brain stem within the oculomotor nerve, continuing with its inferior division until the preganglionic fibers leave as the

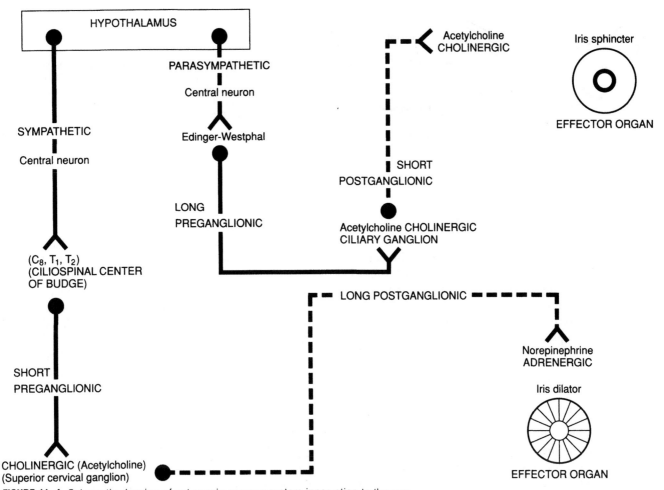

FIGURE 11–4. Schematic drawing of autonomic nervous system innervation to the eye.

motor root to the ciliary ganglion. Here they synapse. Short postganglionic fibers travel within the short ciliary nerves to the eye (Fig. 11–5).

These postganglionic parasympathetic fibers cause contraction of the iris sphincter. Like pulling purse-strings, this decreases pupil size and causes miosis. Small pupils in bright light protect the retina from being dazzled by too much light. They also cause contraction of the ciliary body, which produces accommodation of the lens for near vision and helps open the trabecular meshwork to decrease resistance to aqueous outflow by pulling on the scleral spur. Parasympathetic pregan-

glionic axons from the facial (CN VII) nerve synapse in the pterygopalatine ganglion, sending postganglionic axons to the lacrimal gland for tear secretion (Fig. 11–6).

You may remember this more easily if you associate the action of the parasympathetic system on the eye with four Cs:

1. Cholinergic (acetylcholine transmitter)
2. Constriction of pupil
3. Ciliary ganglion fibers synapse
4. Ciliary body causes accommodation

FIGURE 11–5. Parasympathetic innervation to the iris sphincter and ciliary body through preganglionic fibers from the Edinger-Westphal subnucleus, which provides the motor root to the ciliary ganglion with postganglionic fibers to the eye within the short ciliary nerves.

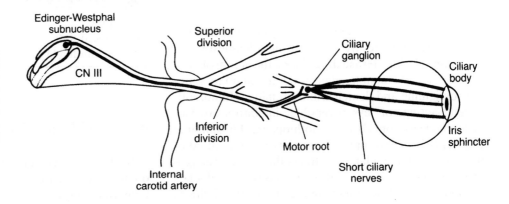

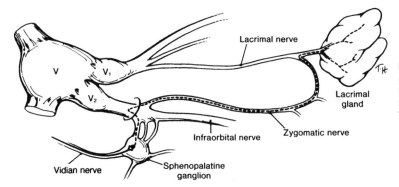

FIGURE 11–6. Parasympathetic innervation to the lacrimal gland for tear secretion. (From Miller NR: Walsh and Hoyt's Clinical Neuro-ophthalmology, 4th ed. Vol. Two, Section III: The Autonomic Nervous System. Baltimore, Williams & Wilkins, 1985, p. 465.)

Parasympathetic Pharmacology

Many commonly used drugs in ophthalmology act like ANS agonists or antagonists. An agonist drug stimulates or encourages the action. An antagonist drug blocks or prevents the action.

The activity of the parasympathetic system can be altered by drugs acting as:

1. Direct parasympathetic agonists (miotics)
2. Indirect parasympathetic agonists (anticholinesterases)
3. Parasympathetic antagonists (cycloplegics)

Direct parasympathetic agonists compete for the same receptor sites as acetylcholine on the motor endplate. They probably lower intraocular pressure by contraction of the ciliary body, exerting a pull on the scleral spur, opening the trabecular meshwork or Schlemm's canal. Side effects are headaches and decreased visual acuity from accommodative spasm, especially in young people, producing pseudomyopia. Night vision also decreases because miotics decrease pupil size.

Miotic Drugs

Acetylcholine (Miochol)
Carbachol (Miostat)
Methacholine (Mecholyl)
Pilocarpine

Indirect parasympathetic agonists permit acetylcholine to accumulate by inactivating cholinesterase. These anticholinesterase drugs block the action of cholinesterase. Reversible shorter-acting inhibitors are physostigmine and demelcarium bromide (Humorsol). Longer-acting, or less reversible, inhibitors are isoflurophate (Floropryl) and echothiophate (Phospholine Iodide) (PI). These indirect agonists have more common and severe ocular side effects than the direct agonists, including decreased night vision, headaches around the orbit, accommodative spasm that induces

pseudomyopia, and generalized visual field contraction. Systemic side effects are flu-like with a drippy nose, increased heart rate, sweating, diarrhea, increased urination, and behavioral changes such as dreams, delusions, hyperactivity, and anxiety. In addition, the longer acting anticholinesterases are highly toxic if taken by mouth, being closely related chemically to commercial organophosphate insecticides and chemicals used to "dip" dogs. They should be discontinued before general anesthesia because they are so long lasting that they can prevent resumption of spontaneous breathing.

Anticholinesterase Drugs

Demelcarium (Humorsol)
Echothiophate (Phospholine Iodide)
Edrophonium (Tensilon)
Isoflurophate (Floropryl)
Pyridostigmine (Mestinon)

Blockers of the parasympathetic system (parasympathetic antagonists) dilate the pupil by paralyzing the iris sphincter and eliminate accommodation by paralyzing the ciliary muscle. These parasympathetic antagonists, called cycloplegics, compete with acetylcholine for its receptors.

Cycloplegic Drugs

Atropine
Cyclopentolate (Cyclogyl)
Tropicamide (Mydriacyl)

• SYMPATHETIC NERVOUS SYSTEM

In the eye, sympathetic fibers dilate the pupil (iris dilator), elevate the lid slightly (Müller's muscle), and constrict blood vessels. When an individual is subjected to conditions of flight or fight, the eyes serve to place the image of potential sources of harm on the fovea for close scrutiny.

The sympathetic pathway to the eye begins in the posterior hypothalamus, the highest brain center involved. The central neuron leaves the hypothalamus, descends through the red nucleus, down the brain stem and cervical spinal cord to the ciliospinal Budge-Waller's center, located in the last cervical and first two thoracic segments of the spinal cord (C_8, T_1-T_2), where a synapse occurs.

Short preganglionic fibers exit the ciliospinal center, entering the sympathetic paravertebral chain alongside the spine. Fibers for the head continue around the lung and the subclavian artery, traveling along the internal carotid artery to the prevertebral superior cervical ganglion at the base of the neck for the second synapse (see Fig. 11-5).

Some long postganglionic fibers that leave the superior cervical ganglion, as a sympathetic plexus, entwine the internal carotid artery as it moves up into the skull until it reaches the level of the nasociliary branch of the ophthalmic nerve (CN V_1). Some sympathetic fibers then leave the sympathetic plexus to travel in the nasociliary nerve and exit the nasociliary to enter the long ciliary nerves as their route into the eyeball to innervate the iris dilator muscle. Contraction of the iris dilator muscle enlarges the pupil—similar to shortening the spokes on a wheel toward a fixed, outer rim (Fig. 11-7).

Some postganglionic fibers from the internal carotid artery plexus enter the orbit through the superior orbital fissure, pass through the ciliary ganglion without synapsing, then enter the short ciliary nerves to carry constrictor fibers to the blood vessels of the eye. Other fibers from the internal carotid plexus find their way

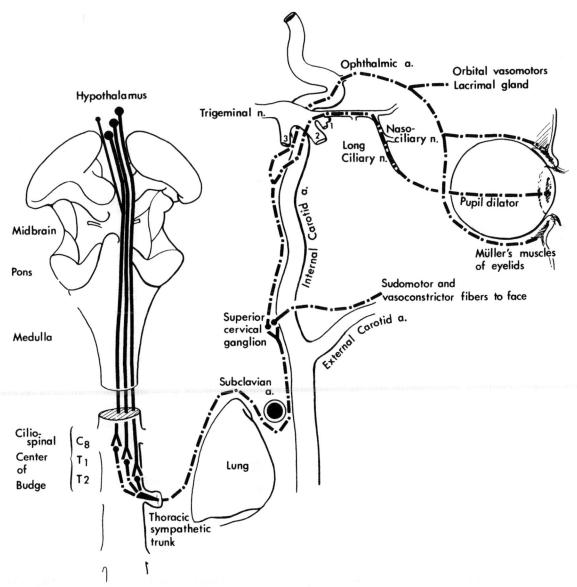

FIGURE 11-7. Sympathetic pathway from the hypothalamus to the iris pupil dilator, the tarsal muscle in the lower eyelid, and Müller's (tarsal) muscle in the upper eyelid. (From Glaser JS: The pupils and accommodation. In: Neuro-ophthalmology, 2nd ed. Hagerstown, MD, Harper & Row, 1990, p. 173.)

to muscles in the upper and lower eyelids. Sensory fibers from the eyeball pass through the ciliary ganglion and exit through the long sensory root to the nasociliary nerve.

If you use the aid to memory of associating the parasympathetics with the letter C, you may want to remember the association of the sympathetics with the letters A, B, D, and E:

A = Adrenergic; also alpha (receptors)

B = Beta (receptors)

D = Dilator (iris)

E = Epinephrine (and norepinephrine)

Sympathetic Pharmacology

The activity of the sympathetic nervous system can be altered by drugs acting as

1. Direct alpha and beta agonists (catecholamines)
2. Indirect agonists
3. Antagonists (alpha and beta blockers)

As described earlier, receptors for the adrenergic system include alpha- and beta-adrenergic receptors. Alpha receptors are more powerfully activated by norepinephrine than epinephrine. The opposite is true of beta receptors. Alpha receptors may be further subdivided into alpha$_1$ and alpha$_2$ subtypes. Alpha receptors increase blood pressure and constrict blood vessels. In the eye they produce mydriasis (iris dilator) and slight lid retraction (Müller's muscle), and they increase the speed at which aqueous flows out of the eye through the trabecular meshwork. Beta-adrenergic receptors increase aqueous outflow facility and generally cause vasodilation. Beta$_1$ (β_1) receptors predominate in cardiac tissues and are responsible for accelerating heart output and heart rate. Beta$_2$ (β_2) receptors predominate in smooth muscles and glands, producing bronchodilation, and slightly increasing aqueous production.

Many drugs influence adrenergic receptors. Adrenergic neurotransmitters, epinephrine and norepinephrine, are chemical derivatives of catecholamine. Norepinephrine stimulates mainly alpha receptors. The body produces epinephrine, also formerly known as adrenaline (stimulates both alpha and beta receptors), and norepinephrine (mostly alpha receptors, but a few beta). Phenylephrine is an alpha-selective sympathetic agonist that imitates the effects of norepinephrine. Tissue response is characterized as alpha if the order of potency is such that norepinephrine has a greater effect than isoproterenol (a synthetic beta agonist), whereas the order of potency for beta receptor stimulation is such that isoproterenol has a greater effect than norepinephrine. Phenylephrine is a pure alpha agonist,

whereas isoproterenol (Isuprel) is a pure beta agonist, used in the treatment of asthma because it dilates the bronchi in the lungs.

Catecholamines

Epinephrine
Norepinephrine

The exact mechanisms by which epinephrine reduces intraocular pressure are not known. Epinephrine has a high incidence of side effects, such as stinging, headaches, conjunctival redness, allergic blepharoconjunctivitis, cystoid macular edema in aphakia, arrhythmias, increased blood pressure, and increased anxiety. Because of the side effects, dipivefrin epinephrine (Propine) is often the drug of choice. Propine is a prodrug that remains inactive until it converts to epinephrine inside the eye. It also has better corneal permeability than epinephrine.

Indirect sympathetic agonists do not act directly on receptor sites to stimulate activity. For example, amphetamines cause an increase in sympathetic epinephrine release and therefore indirectly cause an increase in sympathetic activity. Cocaine interferes with norepinephrine uptake. Indirect sympathetics are rarely used clinically.

Indirect Sympathetic Agonists

Amphetamines
Cocaine

Sympathetic antagonists prohibit storage of norepinephrine, block its release from the neuron, or interfere with receptor sites. Some antagonist drugs specifically block one or another receptor and thereby prevent the action of the agonist. Phenoxybenzamine or phentolamine blocks the effects of adrenergic agents on the alpha receptors without influencing beta receptors. In contrast, the beta-receptor blocking agent propranolol prevents the action of all adrenergic agents on beta receptors but does not influence alpha receptors.

Alpha Blockers

Phenoxybenzamine
Phentolamine

Beta$_1$ blockers such as betaxolol (Betoptic) decrease both heart rate and blood pressure. They are contraindicated in patients with cardiac problems such as heart block or a slow heart rate. Beta$_2$ blockers produce pulmonary effects such as bronchospasm. They are contraindicated in patients with asthma and chronic obstructive pulmonary disease (COPD). Timolol is a beta$_1$ and a beta$_2$ blocker that decreases aqueous production. It does not cause mydriasis, miosis, or accommodation, being remarkably free of ocular side effects, but it can cause fatigue, confusion, and depression.

Another beta$_1$ and a beta$_2$ blocker is levobunolol (Betagan) (Fig. 11–8).

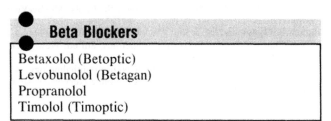

Beta Blockers

Betaxolol (Betoptic)
Levobunolol (Betagan)
Propranolol
Timolol (Timoptic)

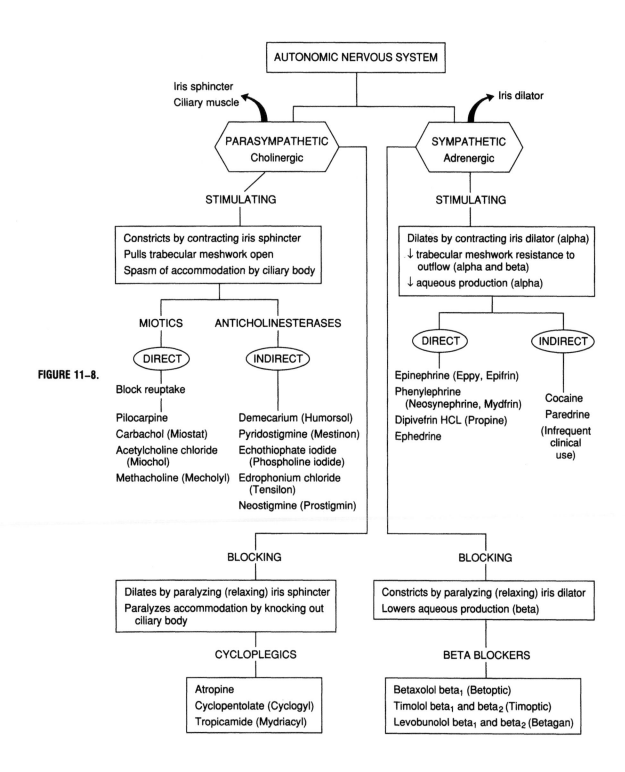

FIGURE 11–8.

Bibliography

Berne RM, Levy MN: Physiology, 3rd ed. St. Louis, Mosby-Year Book, 1993.

Gilman AG, Goodman LS, Rall TW, et al.: Goodman and Gilman's The Pharmacological Basis of Therapeutics, 8th ed. New York, Macmillan, 1990.

Miller NR: Walsh and Hoyt's Clinical Neuro-ophthalmology, 4th ed. Volume Two, Section III: The Autonomic Nervous System. Baltimore, Williams & Wilkins, 1985.

• CHAPTER 11 AUTONOMIC NERVOUS SYSTEM

1. The sympathetic part of the autonomic nervous system is associated with which of the following?
   a. craniosacral outflow
   b. long preganglion, short postganglionic fibers
   c. inferior division, CN III (oculomotor)
   d. adrenergic transmission
   e. lens accommodation

2. The parasympathetic part of the autonomic nervous system is associated with which of the following?
   a. ciliospinal center of Budge-Waller
   b. Müller's muscle
   c. fight or flight
   d. beta blockers
   e. synapse in the ciliary ganglion.

3. What are the direct parasympathetic agonists known as?
   a. anticholinesterases
   b. miotics
   c. beta blockers
   d. catecholamines
   e. cycloplegics

4. In the eye, what is the autonomic nervous system responsible for?
   a. closure of the eyelids
   b. size of the pupils
   c. corneal sensation
   d. tear drainage system
   e. color of the iris

5. Which of the following drugs constricts the pupil by contraction of the iris sphincter and opens the trabecular meshwork by traction on the scleral spur?
   a. Cyclogyl
   b. Propine
   c. Mydfrin
   d. Timoptic
   e. Pilocar

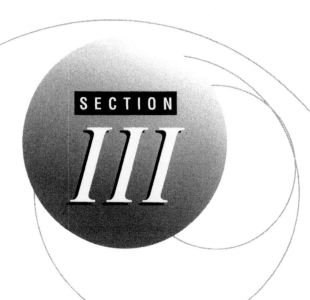

Optics

Physical Optics

LEARNING OBJECTIVES

- Understand the particle and electromagnetic theories about the propagation of light rays
- Explain the nature and properties of
  Polarization

Interference
Fluorescence
Lasers

The sun is the natural source for all the energy that moves from place to place by electromagnetic radiation, classified according to its specific wavelength. The higher the temperature of an energy source, the greater the percentage of short wavelength (high energy) light it will contain, such as gamma rays. Conversely, the lower the temperature of a light source, the greater the percentage of longer wavelength (low energy) light it will contain, such as microwaves or radio waves.

Energy appears in many forms: electrical, chemical, mechanical, thermal, magnetic, and sound. One form can be converted to another. We will study *light* energy, that tiny portion of the electromagnetic spectrum that is visible to the human eye. Its wavelengths vary from 400 to 800 nanometers (nm). Nanometers are 10^{-9} (0.000,000,001) m, or 10^{-6} (0.000,001) mm. One billion nanometers equals one meter. White light contains a mixture of all visible wavelengths in varying phases of their cycles, with variable frequencies that spontaneously radiate in random directions. The different lengths of light waves determine their color. Of those wavelengths in the visible spectrum, red (650 nm) has the longest and blue (450 nm) has the shortest. Rays of the same wavelength always have the same color and are called monochromatic (Fig. 12–1).

Light travels in space until it strikes an interface, at which time it undergoes reflection, transmission, or absorption. All three events occur in varying amounts, but together they account for all the incident light. The appearance of an object depends on the percentage of each one. Because optical surfaces are primarily transparent, the amount they absorb is insignificant.

1. Reflected light does not penetrate an interface but bounces back from its surface, e.g., a mirror.
2. Absorbed light enters, but does not leave, an opaque object. Its energy is often transformed into heat, e.g., sunlight on a black roof.
3. Transmitted light penetrates a transparent interface and emerges as refracted light. The light may strike perpendicularly and may produce no change in direction, e.g., light through a window. Alternatively, the light may strike nonperpendicularly, producing a change in direction, e.g., a ray of light through a prism.

• ELECTROMAGNETIC WAVE THEORY

Two theories have been proposed about the properties of light, as with all electromagnetic radiation. The electromagnetic wave theory is that light, like all matter, is composed of electric and magnetic charges that leave from a source in waves to radiate in all directions. The waves form concentric wave fronts, which vibrate up and down perpendicular to the line of travel. The light source acts like a pebble dropped in water that causes a series of ripples to circle out from the spot (Fig. 12–2).

The wave front represents an oscillating electric field and an oscillating magnetic field, perpendicular to each other, but with both perpendicular to the direction of

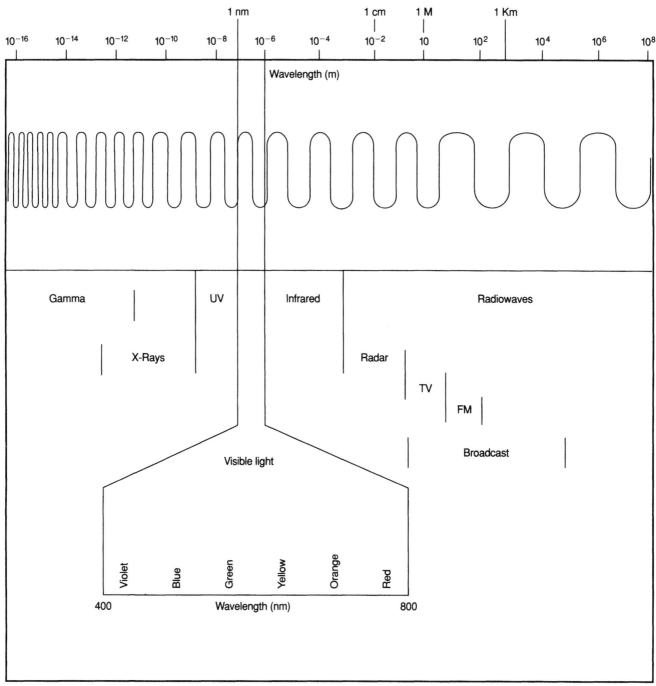

FIGURE 12-1. Electromagnetic spectrum.

travel of the wave. Both are zero at the same time, they reverse directions together twice during each cycle, and they depend on each other. Because physical optics can be explained by the electric wave alone, it is not necessary to discuss the magnetic wave component (Fig. 12-3).

A line connecting the wave fronts from the point source is called a ray, which is usually shown with an arrow indicating the direction of travel of the wave front. Geometric optics uses rays for analysis of reflection and refraction.

The wavelength of light is the distance light travels through one complete vibration cycle between the crest of one wave and the crest of the next. The amplitude is half the distance from the maxima (crest) to the minima (trough) of a wave; this determines the intensity of the wave, i.e., the brightness. Phase is a fraction of a wavelength. A complete cycle is a phase change of 360°. The frequency (energy) of the wavelength is the number of waves that vibrate through a given point in one second. The longer the wavelength, the more slowly it vibrates and the lower its frequency and en-

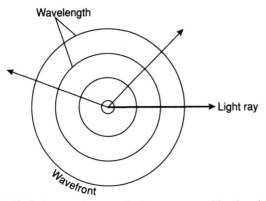

FIGURE 12–2. Concentric wave fronts as proposed by the electromagnetic wave theory.

ergy. Although frequency and wavelength vary, the speed with which light travels through a vacuum stays constant at 186,000 miles per second. Because wavelength times frequency equals speed, wavelength and frequency are inversely proportional. In other words, as one increases, the other decreases (Fig. 12–4).

● PARTICLE THEORY

Another theory about properties of light, the particle theory, states that light is composed of invisible particles called photons with characteristic frequencies. The photon's frequency determines its energy, which is constant.

An atom can be visualized as a miniature solar system. It has a nucleus and electrons that orbit around it in concentric shells. Usually, an electron neither gains nor loses energy. An electron may leap from one orbit to another, however, closer (downward) to the nucleus by releasing energy or further away (upward) by absorbing energy from some outside source. Usually electrons in an atom are most stable at their lowest possible energy level, when they are ready to absorb any photons that may hit them. Their internal vibrations are at their minimum. Resting state electrons absorb photons; higher energy (excited) electrons release photons. As electrons absorb photons, they pump to an excited state with increased vibrations and gain energy from the photon. As they lose (emit) photons, they return to their resting state and lose energy. When an electron drops to a less excited state, it releases energy by emitting a photon equal to the energy difference of the two states. An electron remains in an excited state for less than a microsecond, except on those occasions when the excited state does not change for a considerably longer time. Photons rearrange the structure of matter through interaction. Absorbed energy may be released as light.

An excited electron returns to its stable state by several pathways. It can decay by heat dissipation or by releasing photons, such as occurs with fluorescence. The electron can decompose, reacting with some substances to yield a chemical product, as occurs in the retina when the rods and cones absorb light.

Each of the two theories (wave versus particle) is useful. Short waves such as x-rays behave like particles. Long waves like radio waves behave more like waves. Light has the characteristics of both waves and particles. Sometimes one form predominates, sometimes the other. Light behaves as either, or both, depending on the circumstance. When light is absorbed, as occurs in fluorescence, it behaves as expected according to the particle theory. Light amplification in lasers behaves like that described in the particle theory, but the laser beam itself behaves like that described in the wave theory. Reflection, refraction, polarization, and interference also behave like waves when we attempt to calculate their activity.

● POLARIZATION

Most light waves are unpolarized. They vibrate perpendicular to the direction in which the light is traveling, but with no particular direction. They may vibrate up and down, sideways, or obliquely. Polarization is the process of restricting the vibration directions of the electromagnetic wave to only one direction. The most common mechanisms are by transmission, reflection, and scattering.

Polarizers, such as certain crystals or specially treated thin plastic sheets, act as filters, cutting off all light waves except those vibrating parallel to the molecular chain. After transmission through such a

FIGURE 12–3. Electric and magnetic fields are perpendicular to one another, although in-phase and travel in the same plane as the wave front.

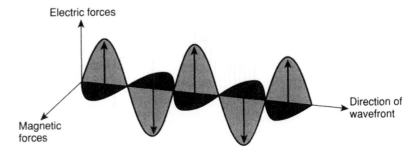

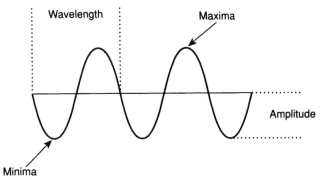

FIGURE 12–4. Illustration of motion of wave.

filter, all emerging waves are polarized in the direction of the axis of the filter. A second polarizer, parallel to the first one, also allows the light to pass through, until the second polarizer is rotated. It gradually cuts off the light until its axis is 90° to the axis of the first filter, when all the polarized light is absorbed. What one sheet does not absorb, the second one will. If one sheet allows vertically vibrating waves, the other allows horizontally vibrating waves. When two polarizing sheets with axes 90° apart are placed one in front of each eye, polarized pictures can be viewed wherein each eye sees only that part of the picture polarized for its filter. This is the basis of certain stereo acuity tests and projection charts in ophthalmology (Fig. 12–5).

When sunlight strikes horizontal surfaces such as pavement, snow, or water, what is reflected is partially horizontally polarized by scattering. The glare produced can be reduced by polarized sunglasses with a vertical transmission axis. The sky acts as a partial polarizer when light is scattered by molecules of air.

• INTERFERENCE

Any portion of a wavelength cycle is a phase. Most light has wavelengths of different frequencies going in different directions, with continuously changing phase

differences. These waves are incoherent. The energy falls as a blur. No pattern is produced. The effect is similar to choppy water (Fig. 12–6).

If two or more monochromatic (same wavelength) waves travel in the same direction (polarized), with no phase difference (in-step), they are in-phase. As long as they continue in-phase, they are coherent, e.g., laser beams. The wave maxima reinforce one another as do the wave minima, producing resultant amplitudes of brighter (higher intensity) light. Waves of equal wavelength with the same polarization, however, but out-of-step, are *out-of-phase*. Halfway phase difference waves, out-of-step by 180°, negate their amplitudes because maxima add to minima, cancelling out the light and decreasing the intensity. As long as the phase difference stays constant, however, out-of-phase waves are also coherent. Coherence, then, can occur *only* with light waves of the same wavelength and frequency, and only as long as neither changes (Fig. 12–7).

Interference is the superimposition of at least two light waves from two coherent beams traveling in the same region. Interference acts like two pebbles dropped into water adjacent to each other. When two waves collide (in-phase), they coincide to produce a higher wave. If one wave meets another's trough (out-of-phase), they cancel out, interfering to produce smoother water and neutralizing one another. Reinforcement is constructive interference; cancellation is destructive interference. The alternate reinforcement and cancellation produces alternating light and dark bands called interference fringes. No light is lost; it gains at constructive interference and loses at destructive. The total amount of energy is the same as with incoherent light.

Laser interferometry images these interference fringes onto the retina to test potential recovery of vision in patients with opaque media such as cataracts. As the slit separating the two beams decreases, the

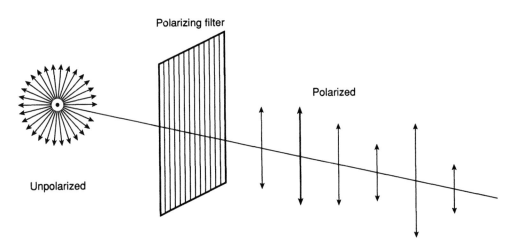

FIGURE 12–5. Unpolarized light waves from many different light sources travel in all different directions. Only light waves traveling in the same direction as the axis of the polarizing filter emerge from such a filter.

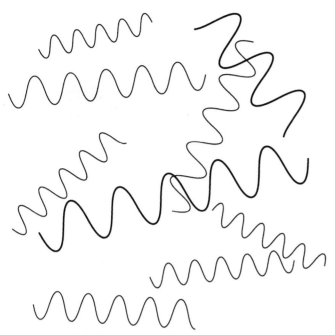

FIGURE 12–6. Incoherent light waves are a jumble of different wavelengths traveling in different directions with variable phase differences.

distance between fringes increases. The interference fringes bypass the eye's optical system (Fig. 12–8).

● FLUORESCENCE

When an electron absorbs photons of light, it pumps to an excited but less stable state. If it decays to a lower state that is higher than its resting one, an electron emits less energy than it had absorbed, but on a longer wavelength. Fluorescence is a property of some substances to absorb light of a shorter wavelength (with

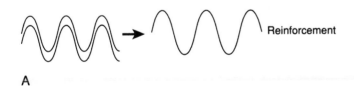

Reinforcement

A

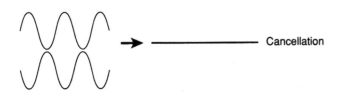

Cancellation

B

FIGURE 12–7. Constructive and destructive interference. *A*, Two coherent light waves in-phase superimpose to reinforce one another, thus increasing the intensity (brightness) of the light. *B*, Two coherent light waves 180° out-of-phase superimpose to cancel one another, decreasing the intensity (brightness) of the light to zero.

higher frequency), then to convert it immediately, thus emitting light of a longer wavelength (with lower frequency).

Sodium fluorescein is a water-soluble, orange-brown indicator dye producing a bright yellow-green fluorescent color in alkaline solutions, such as aqueous humor, and a yellow-orange color in more acid solutions, such as precorneal tear film. The dye is visible even at extreme dilution. In white light it is orange-brown when concentrated, yellow-green when diluted. When viewed using a cobalt blue filter, the dye glows (fluoresces) bright green, with the shade and intensity increasing with the thickness of the fluorescein layer. This technique is utilized with the slit lamp to evaluate the cornea. Intact corneal epithelium will not absorb fluorescein, but a break in the epithelial barrier turns the fluorescein bright green, because it binds to the epithelial basement membrane. This allows visualization of corneal epithelial defects. Aqueous leaks after surgery or trauma can also be visualized by instillation of fluorescein. A tiny stream of green fluid will flow down from the wound. Fluorescein is also selected in evaluation of contact lens fit and in applanation tonometry.

Fluorescein molecules absorb light best at a 490-nm wavelength in the blue part of the visible spectrum, increasing their energy levels and converting to an excited state, which emits light at 530 nm in the green part of the visible spectrum. If fluorescein is injected into the bloodstream, it can be followed as it circulates through the eye's blood vessels. By positioning a blue exciter filter in front of the illuminating beam of the fundus camera, only short (490 nm) wavelengths of blue light pass into the eye. This excites the fluorescein and momentarily changes its vibrational state to a higher energy level. All those structures and vessels containing fluorescein in the fundus will fluoresce by emitting longer (530 nm) green-yellow wavelength light. A second yellow barrier filter, placed in the optical system between the eye and the film, blocks shorter wavelengths of extraneous blue light from leaving the eye and permits only passage of the longer wavelength, emitted fluorescent light to be recorded on film. This technique is used in ophthalmic photography to diagnose retinal blood vessel diseases and tumors (Fig. 12–9).

● LASERS

Coherent light could be produced only at low intensities before lasers were invented. Lasers use the natural vibrations of atoms to amplify wavelengths in the visible spectrum, producing highly coherent, intense light.

Some excited electrons change orbits, dropping from a higher to a lower energy state just by chance but with

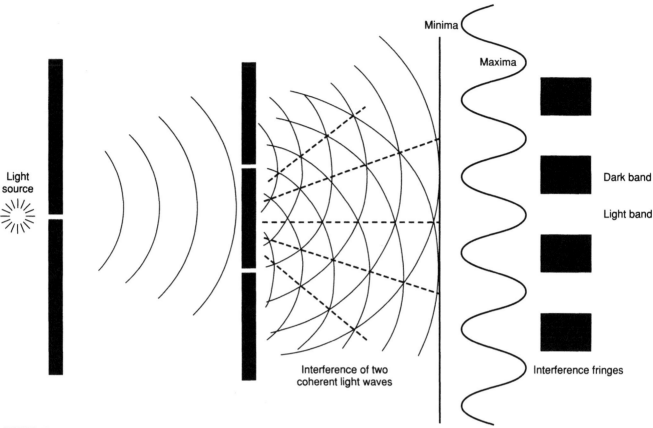

FIGURE 12–8. Production of interference fringes from two coherent light waves.

a certain probability. This is *spontaneous emission.* White light results. If a photon's frequency exactly matches the energy difference needed by an electron, it can strike that electron to cause a transition in either direction, i.e., photon emission with electron energy drop to a lower level or photon absorption with electron energy gain to a higher level. The probability of emission equals the probability of absorption. In atom populations, however, there are normally more electrons at a lower baseline state than at an excited higher one. Therefore more electrons are likely to absorb photons than to emit them. After a drop to a lower, less excited state, there are two identical photons, the striking one and the released one, and one electron at the less ex-

cited state. The released photon has exactly the same energy (wavelength), but not necessarily the same direction (nonpolarized), as the striking photon. An incoming light beam gradually weakens because it cannot find enough excited electrons to bump.

An amplification process using electrical discharges between electrodes pumps more electrons into a higher energy state than the resting state. This produces a condition known as population inversion. More electrons vibrating at higher than baseline levels increases the probability of more photons being released. With an inverted population, extra photons are produced as electrons are struck by photons, dropping those electrons from an excited to a resting state. As photons

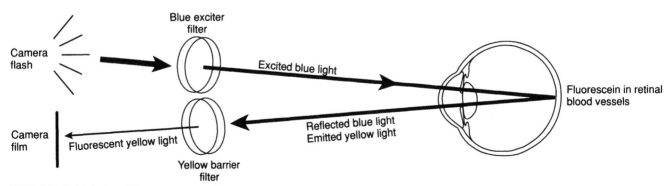

FIGURE 12–9. Emission of fluorescent light following excitation of fluorescein injected into the circulatory system.

are emitted, they bump other electrons and *stimulate* them to release photons of the same wavelength (monochromatic), direction (polarized), and phase. These waves meet the conditions for also being coherent. For this to occur, the electrons must remain excited longer than usual, to allow time before spontaneous emission. An incoming light beam will become brighter as its electrons find excited electrons to bump.

Lasers work by creating these quick movements among electrons. LASER is an acronym for *Light Amplification by Stimulated Emission of Radiation*. Lasers produce incredibly intense, monochromatic light from coherent, in-phase beams radiating parallel rays (collimated) in a narrow beam in or near the visible spectrum. A laser is composed of

1. A chemical substance (such as argon or krypton gas or a crystal such as yttrium-aluminum-garnet [YAG]);
2. A power source of excitation (electrical, optic, or heat energy)
3. A mirror system to amplify the generated light.

The power supply bathes the electrons in the chemical substance in an intense flash of incoherent white light and provides enough energy to produce a large number of excited electrons.

Lasers are designed and constructed with a mirror system in a tube with both ends having parallel mirrors but one partially silvered. The length separating the mirrors is a multiple of the photon's wavelength. The light entering the mirror system is reflected. Photons ricochet back and forth through the excitable substance from mirror to mirror many times, hitting new electrons and emitting extra photons. The reflected rays are in the same direction as the original i.e., polarized, as well as having the same wavelength. The extra photons set up a chain reaction by striking excited electrons, resulting in a drop of energy but release of more photons into the excited substance. One mirror reflects all its light back to the other mirror, which in turn reflects only part of its light. The rest escapes the system by

transmission to form the laser beam that flows out the tube end. The laser beam can travel for miles without scattering its light waves. For ophthalmic instruments, the created beam enters a fiberoptic cable for delivery to the eye (Fig. 12–10).

Because all the photons released by this stimulated emission are identical in phase, wavelength, and direction, the emerging beam has *coherence*. Any divergent photons are lost out of the tube, resulting in a thin laser beam with parallel light rays. The created light concentrates its brightness from the coherent light, increasing its amplitude by summation of its wavelength's maxima and minima. This effect produces phenomenal intensity when focused on a small area.

Pulsed laser energy has less effect on surrounding tissue than continuous wave energy. Continuous wave lasers *photocoagulate* tissue to "spot weld" tears and leaks. The duration of application, the power, and the spot size can be varied. Continuous laser light is absorbed by the tissue and converted to heat, which produces thermal damage. The resulting burns are commonly used for pan-retinal photocoagulation of diabetic retinopathy.

Continuous blue-green wavelength (488 to 515 nm) argon lasers produce heat wherever that wavelength of light is absorbed, burning the target tissue without increasing the temperature of the surrounding tissue. These wavelengths are not absorbed by the transparent ocular media, namely, the cornea, anterior chamber, lens, and vitreous. Thus burn depends on light absorption by xanthophyll and hemoglobin pigments mostly in the pigment epithelium, choroid, macula, and blood. Because it effectively destroys blood vessels, it is useful for treating the leaking blood vessels that lead to neovascularization. Argon laser is utilized for lower energy, lighter burns with larger spot sizes.

Krypton lasers emit continuous red wavelength (647 nm) beams that have excellent transmission through cataracts and hemorrhages, coupled with good absorption by melanin in the choroid and retinal pigment epithelium (RPE), but without absorption by retinal blood

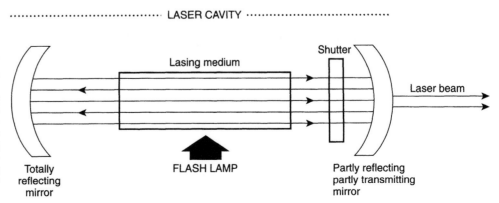

FIGURE 12–10. Schematic design of a laser. Flash lamp acts as an optical pump to excite electrons to throw off photons, which bounce back and forth between two mirrors, one of which only partly reflects and partly transmits the light. As the light reflects from one mirror to the other, it reinforces itself, becoming more and more intense. Because the reflected light has the same wavelength, direction, and phase as the original beam, the light is coherent. Some of the light shoots out of the partly transmitting mirror as a needle laser beam.

LASER CAVITY

Lasing medium

Shutter

Laser beam

Totally reflecting mirror

FLASH LAMP

Partly reflecting partly transmitting mirror

vessels. The krypton laser is employed for deeper choroidal coagulation and outer retina and macula burns. The RPE reaches the highest temperature for both argon and krypton lasers.

Contact lenses are often utilized for added magnification and plus power for converging the beam. Continuous wave gas lasers, such as the argon, have a slow production of energy compared with the extremely short duration pulsed laser, such as the YAG, which has an intermittent burst of energy output from a shutter mechanism. The YAG is a cold, "cutting" laser; the argon and krypton are hot, "welding" lasers.

Pulsed laser energy employs rapid, tiny bursts of energy to make openings in eye tissue. Very high temperatures are generated, but for so short a period that the effect of this temperature is negligible. A pulsed laser heats the target tissue so quickly and so high with its burst of energy that the target sustains vibrational and shockwave destruction. The power densities at the target produce intense electromagnetic fields that shear electrons to break up molecules to create a microexplosion, called optical breakdown or *photodisruption,* with subsequent vaporization of tissue by the shock wave from the sudden release of energy. The spark from the YAG laser as electrons rejoin atoms is like a lightning flash, only at much lower intensity.

The YAG solid laser is a hard, synthetic crystal, with excellent optical quality and the ability to withstand the high power densities of the laser beam. The YAG emits radiation in the infrared spectrum (1064 nm), just beyond visible light, at power densities 100,000 times greater than the argon laser. The YAG can focus down to extremely small spot sizes. The transparent ocular media absorb these infrared wavelengths and make the YAG useful for doing anterior segment surgery, cutting posterior lens capsules, severing vitreous adhesions, and performing iridotomies.

The new argon/fluorine excimer laser emits ultraviolet light. *Photoablation* is the effect on tissue of intense ultraviolet light when focused for brief, high energy pulses. Suggested uses are to remove corneal opacities or reshape the cornea to reduce refractive errors.

Bibliography

Campbell CJ, Koester CJ, Rittler MC, et al: Physiological Optics. Hagerstown, MD, Harper & Row, 1974.
Constable IJ, Lim ASM: Laser: Its Clinical Uses in Eye Diseases, 2nd ed. London, Churchill Livingstone, 1990.
Elkington AR, Frank HJ: Clinical Optics. Oxford, Blackwell Scientific, 1984.
Fried W: Physical optics. In Peyman GA, Sanders DR, Goldberg MF (eds): Principles and Practice of Ophthalmology, vol I. Philadelphia, WB Saunders, 1980.
Miller D: Physical optics. In Duane TD (ed): Clinical Ophthalmology, vol 1. Hagerstown, MD, Harper & Row, 1987.
Rubin, ML: Optics for Clinicians, 2nd ed. Gainesville, FL, Triad, 1974.
Schecter RJ: Laser physics. In Duane TD (ed): Clinical Ophthalmology, vol 1. Hagerstown, MD, Harper & Row, 1987.

• CHAPTER 12 PHYSICAL OPTICS

1. What describes visible wavelengths of light of different frequencies, with changing phase differences, that spontaneously radiate in different directions?
   a. white
   b. polarized
   c. fluorescent
   d. laser
   e. monochromatic

2. Half the distance from the crest of a light wave to its trough is known as
   a. frequency
   b. phase
   c. minima
   d. wavelength
   e. amplitude.

3. What describes concentric wave fronts radiating in all directions from a single light source, vibrating up and down perpendicular to the line of travel?
   a. particle theory
   b. interference
   c. electromagnetic wave theory
   d. polarization
   e. lasers

4. What are excited electrons that drop from a higher to a lower energy state called?
   a. fluorescent
   b. spontaneously emitted
   c. collimated
   d. amplified
   e. stimulated

5. What are two or more light waves with the same wavelength and frequency, traveling in the same direction?
   a. incoherent
   b. fluorescent
   c. interference fringe
   d. coherent
   e. polarized

Geometric Optics

LEARNING OBJECTIVES

- Understand how light rays are affected by prisms and lenses
- Understand the relationship between vergence power and focal length
- Convert from vergence power to focal length and vice versa
- Determine the power of prisms and lenses
- Understand the formation of images by light rays from objects traveling through an optical system
- Calculate the changes in vergence power of light rays entering an optical system
- Draw light-ray diagrams to graphically analyze image formation
- Understand and calculate magnification of objects and images
- Understand the optical differences between spheres and cylinders
- Record optical cross notations of spheres and cylinders

Geometric optics involves a theoretical concept in which all objects in space are considered as sources of light that emit divergent light rays. By convention, these light rays move from left to right. As they travel away from an object, these light rays become farther apart and may be affected by an optical system such as a lens, mirror, prism, or a combination of several. Such optical systems alter the direction of the light rays. Geometric optics is the study of image formation by these optical devices.

• SNELL'S LAW

Snell's law determines the speed of light through a substance by comparing it with the speed of light in air. This comparison is the index of refraction.

$$\text{Index of refraction} = \frac{\text{speed of light in air}}{\text{speed of light in the substance}}$$

The index of refraction of air, 1.00, is the standard. Every substance denser than air slows down the speed of light, producing a higher index of refraction. For example:

Substance	Index
vacuum	1.000000
air	1.000293
water	1.333
crown glass	1.517
diamond	2.416

Every optical effect we notice when looking through a transparent substance is a direct consequence of this change in the velocity of light. The angle at which the light waves strike the interface is equally important. If perpendicular light rays strike a medium of greater density than air, they will be slowed down according to Snell's law, but they would emerge unchanged in direction. If, however, light rays strike a medium obliquely, they will be bent by the surface of the material to emerge in a changed direction (Fig. 13–1). The imaginary line perpendicular to the interface of two optical media at the point where the ray strikes the interface is the *normal*. The higher the density of the new medium, the more reduced the speed of the light rays will be, and the more they will be bent (Fig. 13–2).

When light strikes an interface, some of its rays bounce off the surface as reflected light rays. The angle as the light approaches between the path of the incident

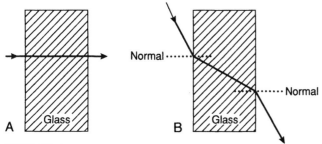

FIGURE 13–1. Behavior of light rays refracted by passing through a plane optical interface. Entering a denser medium slows down the wavefronts. *A*, Light rays strike the optical interface perpendicularly, on the normal. Rays are not bent. *B*, Light rays strike the interface obliquely. Entering a denser medium (air to glass) bends rays toward the normal. Entering a less dense medium (glass to air) bends rays away from the normal.

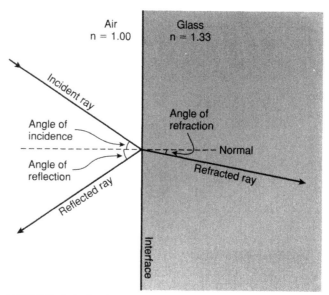

FIGURE 13–3. Reflection and refraction of a light ray as it strikes an optical medium.

light ray and the normal is the *angle of incidence*. The angle between the normal and the path of the reflected light ray as it departs from the surface, the *angle of reflection,* is equal to the angle of incidence. If the new medium is transparent and differs in density, and the light strikes at an angle, the rays that pass through the new medium are bent (refracted) as they do so. The angle between the normal and the path of the refracted ray is the *angle of refraction* (Fig. 13–3).

• INTERNAL REFLECTION

If the angle of incidence becomes too high when going to a less dense medium, a critical angle is surpassed after which all the rays are reflected internally and none escape (Fig. 13–4). This can be made to occur in an internal core of higher index of refraction optical glass or plastic fibers, sheathed in a transparent outer

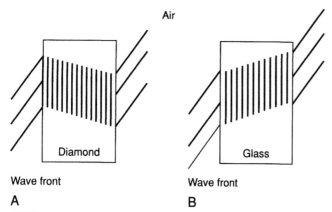

FIGURE 13–2. Amount of bending of light rays depends on the density of the new medium. The denser the new medium, the greater the bending of light rays. *A*, New medium, diamond, denser than glass. Light rays bent more. *B*, New medium, glass, denser than air but less dense than a diamond.

covering of lower index of refraction. Light enters one end, but does not shine out the sides because it is internally reflected. It zigzags down the rod to the other end, even when the rod is bent, before it exits by refraction. These transparent, flexible, fiberoptic probes provide a method of lighting up inner parts of the body or eye, such as the vitreous and retina (Fig. 13–5).

• PRISMS

For light rays to be bent, it makes no difference whether the ray itself is oblique, or the optical surface it strikes is sloped. A prism is a wedge-shaped optical device with a sloped surface. Light rays strike the sloped surface of the prism (which has an index of refraction greater than air) at an angle. This bends the light rays toward the normal of the interface, which happens to be toward the base (Fig. 13–6). Then, as the rays leave the denser medium of a prism at the second interface, they bend away from the normal, again toward the base. The images we see when looking through the prism are virtual, however. They are localized by the brain as coming from the apex of the prism (Fig. 13–7).

The magnitude of the prismatic effect depends on the size of the angle at the apex of the prism. The greater the angle at the apex, the more the sides of the prism slope, the more obliquely the rays strike, the greater the angle of incidence, and the greater the deflection of light rays (Fig. 13–8).

The power of a prism to deflect a light beam is ex-

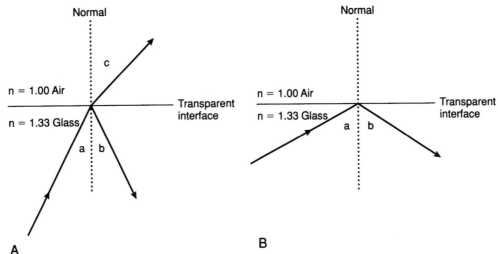

FIGURE 13–4. Angle of incidence below and above the critical angle when light moves from a more dense to a less dense medium. *A*, Angle of incidence (a) low enough so some light is reflected, some is refracted. The angle of reflection is b and the angle of refraction is c. *B*, Angle of incidence is so high that all light is reflected. None is refracted.

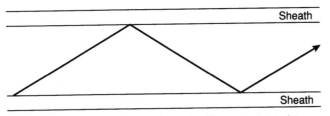

FIGURE 13–5. Internal reflection through a fiberoptic light pipe.

pressed in prism diopters (PD). One PD bends light rays by 1 cm at a distance of 1 m from the prism, 2 cm at a distance of 2 m, 1/3 cm at a distance of 1/3 m, and so forth. The relationship is a direct proportion. As the distance from the prism increases, the amount of deflection increases. A 5 PD bends light rays 5 cm at a distance of 1 m, 10 cm at a distance of 2 m, 5/3 cm at a distance of 1/3 m (Fig. 13–9).

FORMULA: P = C/D

P = prism power in PD

C = displacement of object in cm

D = distance from prism in meters (m)

 1 PD bends light by 1 cm at 1 m

 1 PD bends light by 2 cm at 2 m

 2 PD bends light by 2 cm at 1 m

10 PD bends light by 10 cm at 1 m

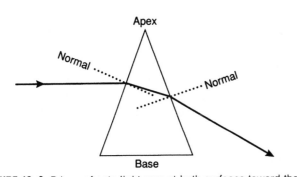

FIGURE 13–6. Prism refracts light rays at both surfaces toward the base.

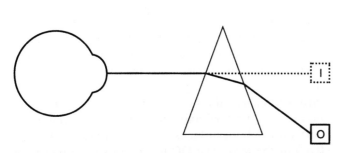

FIGURE 13–7. When a real object (O) is viewed through a prism, its virtual image (I) shifts toward the apex of the prism.

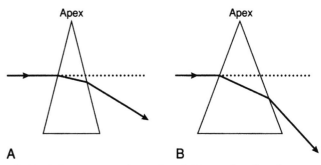

FIGURE 13–8. The greater the angle at the apex of a prism, the more the lights rays are bent.

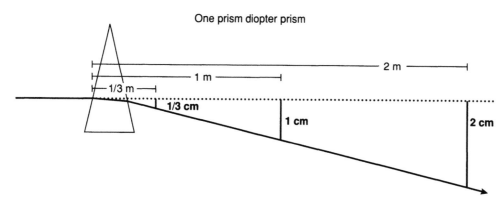

One prism diopter prism

FIGURE 13–9. The amount a light ray is bent by a prism depends on the strength of the prism and the distance at which the deflection is measured.

• VERGENCE

Light rays have one of three possible states:

1. Divergence: Rays that spread apart from an object point have minus (−) power. This is the natural state (Fig. 13–10A).

2. Zero vergence: Rays that are parallel (collimated) to each other have no power (Fig. 13–10B).

3. Convergence: Rays that come toward one another have plus (+) power. Light rays do not converge "naturally." All convergent rays have been changed in direction after passing through an optical system (Fig. 13–10C).

As light rays travel from their point source, they diverge in all directions until they strike a transparent interface (such as a lens). When these divergent rays enter an optical system obliquely, the divergence may be increased, decreased, or changed to convergence.

The vergence power (P) in diopters (D) of these light rays at the interface is inversely proportional to the distance (f) in meters (m) from the point source to the interface; i.e.,

$$P = 1/f.$$

The farther from the light source we measure, the lower the vergence power (P) of the light rays coming from that source. The light rays diverge less rapidly from one another (Fig. 13–11). Therefore at A, the rays from point X have a vergence of 1/.10, which equals −10 D. At interface B the vergence power would be 1/.50, or −2 D (Fig. 13–12).

• LENSES

A transparent spherical *lens* is an optical device that bends light rays with the same power in all directions. It has two surfaces, at least one of which is curved, and a common principal axis, also referred to as an optical or lens axis, which travels perpendicularly through the centers of curvature of both surfaces. The normals of both surfaces are parallel here. Because both lens surfaces are parallel, the direction of travel through this axis does not bend (Fig. 13–13). The portion of the principal axis that connects the centers of curvature of both surfaces represents the optical center (OC) of the lens. The OC has no prismatic power. A curved refracting surface has plus power if the middle bows away from the center, and minus power if it bows

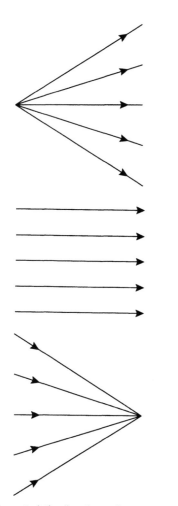

FIGURE 13–10. Characteristic directions of movement of light rays.

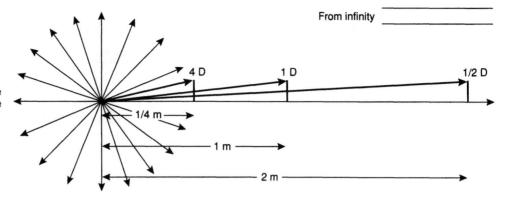

FIGURE 13–11. Light rays lose vergence power as they recede from their source.

toward the center. It has no power (plano) if it has no curve (Fig. 13–14).

If you hold a lens parallel to the floor at waist level and shine a light six inches above it aimed at the lens periphery, two light images are seen, one on each lens surface. As the light is moved so that it is aimed more toward the lens center, the images move closer and finally superimpose when the light is aimed at the optical center of the lens.

Lenses can be thought of as a combination of prisms. A convex lens theoretically consists of two prisms, base to base. It is a converging system, increasing the convergence (or decreasing the divergence) of light rays, and has plus power. This system adds vergence by bending the rays toward the principal axis. It is thicker in the middle and thinner at the edge (Fig. 13–15A).

A concave lens theoretically consists of two prisms, apex to apex. It is a diverging system, increasing the divergence (or decreasing the convergence) of light rays, and has minus power. The system subtracts vergence by bending the light rays away from the principal axis. It is thinner in the middle and thicker at the edges (Fig. 13–15B).

By viewing a near object through the lens, you can verify whether the lens has plus or minus power. If the object appears larger than its true size, the lens is plus. If smaller, the lens is minus. Moreover, if the lens is moved slightly to the right and the image also moves to the right (*with* movement), the lens is minus. If the image moves to the left (*against* movement), the lens is plus (Fig. 13–16).

The optical power (vergence) of a lens is the amount the vergence of the light rays is changed by that lens. When the lens is thin, the power is the sum of the vergence power of each surface (Fig. 13–17).

Just as vergence power can be determined for light rays leaving an object, it can be determined for the change in direction of light rays bent by an optical device, often forming an image. Parallel light rays that enter a lens are refracted to a point focus. The focal length of a lens (f) is the distance from the lens at which this focal point lies. The stronger the lens, the less distance it needs to focus. Therefore, focal length distance and lens power are inversely proportional. Vergence power for light rays as well as lenses can be compared only when both are converted to meters or, more commonly, diopters. Beware of comparing meters to diopters, because they are not similar.

Mathematically, the dioptric power of a lens (P) and its focal length (f) are reciprocal to each other. It is quantified by the formula

$$P = 1/f$$

P = vergence power in diopters (D)

f = focal length in meters (m)

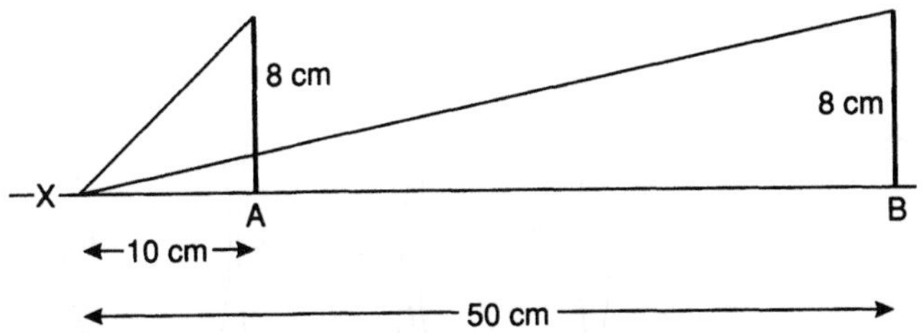

FIGURE 13–12. Light rays at shorter distance A diverge faster for same amount of deflection as light rays at longer distance B.

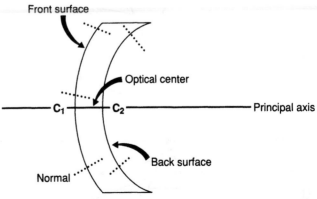

FIGURE 13–13. Light rays that travel through lens surfaces parallel to one another travel through the optical center of the lens.

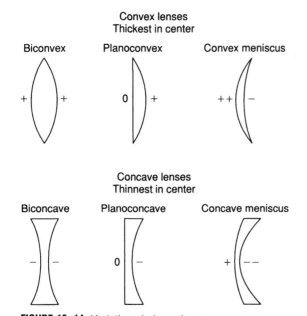

Convex lenses
Thickest in center

Biconvex   Planoconvex   Convex meniscus

Concave lenses
Thinnest in center

Biconcave   Planoconcave   Concave meniscus

FIGURE 13–14. Variations in lens shapes.

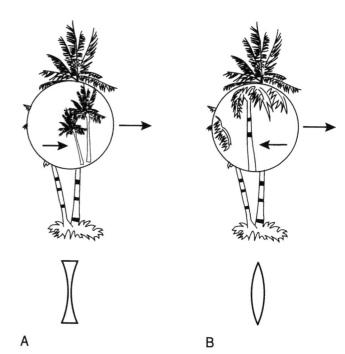

A   B

FIGURE 13–16. Effect of lenses on size and direction of movement. *A*, Minus lens reduces object that moves in same direction as lens. *B*, Plus lens magnifies object that moves in opposite direction as lens.

in similar fashion to the vergence power of light rays. Both are inversely proportional. The farther the light rays are from the light source when we examine them, or the longer the distance it takes to focus parallel light rays traveling through lenses, the lower the power (Fig. 13–18).

Optical power also depends on the steepness with which the sides of a lens or an interface slopes, which in turn depends on the radius of curvature. Compare a baseball with a basketball. The baseball has a smaller diameter and so a smaller radius of curvature than a basketball. The baseball's surface has a steeper curve than the basketball's surface. With lenses, the smaller the radius of curvature, the steeper the slope and the higher the refractive power. This principle is important

for the fit of contact lenses as well as for determining the power of lenses (Fig. 13–19).

● OBJECT-IMAGE RELATIONSHIP

Light rays, by convention, travel from left to right. Rays to the left (in front) of the lens are in minus space and rays to the right (behind) of the lens are in plus space.

Real Image. If diverging rays from an object point converge after refraction by an optical system, they meet to form an image point in plus space. This image will be inverted (upside down). Since it can be seen on a screen it is also real (Fig. 13–20*A*).

Virtual Image. If diverging rays from an object point are still divergent after refraction by an optical system, the image appears at a point in front of the lens in minus space. That is the only point where the rays can meet. The image is erect (right side up) but cannot

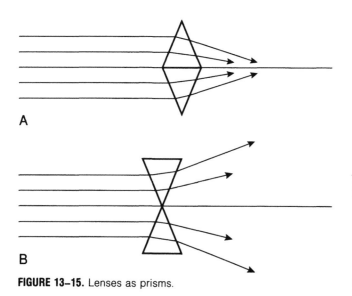

A

B

FIGURE 13–15. Lenses as prisms.

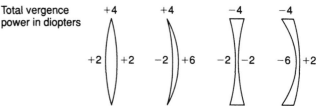

Total vergence power in diopters

+4   +4   −4   −4

+2 | +2   −2 | +6   −2 | −2   −6 | +2

FIGURE 13–17. Total thin lens power is the sum of both lens surfaces.

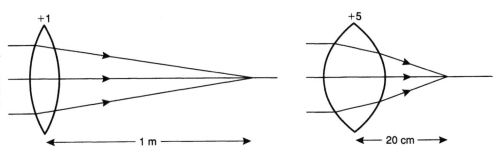

FIGURE 13–18. As lens power increases, focal length decreases. A weak +1 D lens has a 1 m focal length. The stronger +5 D lens has a much shorter 1/5 m (20 cm) focal length.

be seen on a screen; therefore, it is also virtual (Fig. 13–20*B*).

Parallel light rays from infinity are refracted by a lens to cross the principal axis at a point called the secondary focal point. The distance from the lens to the focal point is the focal length. The strength and the sign of a lens are determined by the position of its secondary focal point. The secondary focal point is behind a plus lens in plus space; it is in front of a minus lens in minus space (Fig. 13–21).

Lenses have two focal points, one in front (to the left) of the lens, and one behind (to the right of) it. Both are on the principal axis, equidistant from the lens (same focal length) if the medium on both sides of the lens is the same. The primary focal point of a plus lens is in front of the lens; of a minus lens, behind it. Light rays that *originate* or pass through the primary focal point leave the lens in bundles parallel to each other and the principal axis (Fig. 13–22).

The two focal points are conjugate, i.e., mirror images of one another. A light source emanating from the primary focal point emerges parallel from the lens. Parallel light rays striking a lens come to a focus point at the secondary focal point.

• IMAGE FORMATION

The object-image relationship can be understood by studying the vergence of light rays coming from an object, the change in direction caused by the power of the optical system, and the resulting vergence of light rays forming the image. The position of the image depends on the power of the lens and the distance of the object from the lens. The formula for the change in vergence when a lens or optical system interrupts light rays is as follows:

$$U + P = V$$

U = vergence of the object rays in diopters = 1/u

P = vergence power of the lens in diopters = 1/p

V = vergence of the image rays in diopters = 1/v

u = distance, in meters, of the object from the lens = 1/U

p = focal length of the lens in meters = 1/P

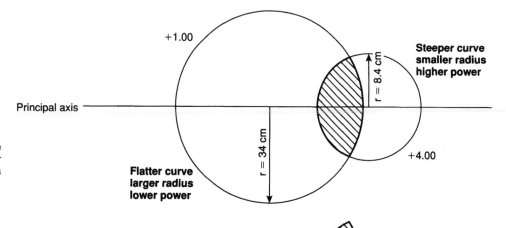

FIGURE 13–19. The steeper the curve of a lens surface, the higher the power and the lower its radius of curvature.

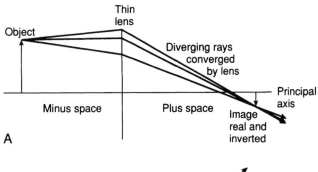

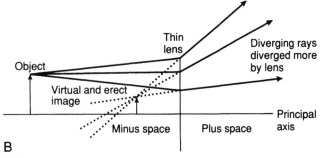

B

FIGURE 13–20. Types of images produced by lenses.

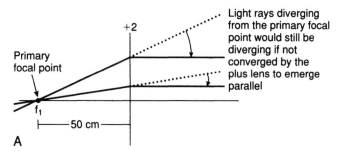

A

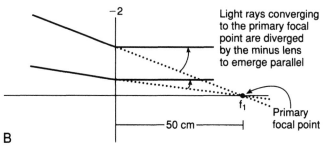

B

FIGURE 13–22. Primary focal points.

v = distance, in meters, of the image from the lens = 1/V

For calculation, diopters are more common units of measurement than meters. Convert to meters (or centimeters), if needed, for the answer after the problem is solved in diopters. Beware: Comparing diopters and meters is similar to comparing apples and oranges.

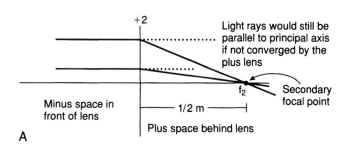

A

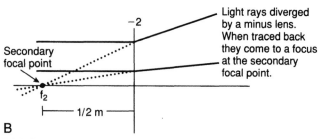

B

FIGURE 13–21. Secondary focal points.

• **Example 1.** *If we have an object 1 meter to the left of a +3D lens, we can find the location of the resultant image by knowing that:*

$$P = +3D \text{ (power of the lens)}$$
$$u = -1 \text{ meter (distance from object to lens)}$$
$$1/u = -1 D \text{ (conversion from distance to vergence power. Sign is minus because object is in front of the lens in minus space.)}$$

$$U + P = V$$
$$-1 + 3 = V$$
$$V = +2$$
$$v = 1/V$$
$$v = 1/2 \text{ m}$$

• *Because the vergence of the image light rays is +2D, the image is in plus space to the right of the lens. Whenever the object is in minus space, and the image is in plus space, a real inverted image is produced by the convergence of light rays leaving the lens. In this case, they focus 1/2 m (50 cm) behind the lens.*

• **Example 2.** *If we simply change the lens power to −3 instead of +3, the formula becomes as follows:*

$$U + P = V$$
$$-1 + (-3) = V$$
$$V = -4$$

Because:

$$V = 1/v$$
$$v = -1/4 \text{ meter.}$$

Now the image ray vergence brings the light rays to a focus at 1/4 m (or 25 cm) to the left (in front) of the lens. We have a virtual erect image because the divergent (minus) lens bends the incoming light rays away from the principal axis behind the lens. Only by an imaginary continuation of the divergent light rays back toward minus space do the refracted light rays come to a focus. If the object and the image are both in minus space, the image will always be virtual and erect.

• GRAPHICAL ANALYSIS

Another way to describe the object-image relationship is to draw a diagram. Selecting three specific rays, we can trace their pathways from the object through the lens to find the resultant image. This discussion will simplify the optics at this time, by making the lenses so thin that they appear to be a line that includes both interfaces and the space between them.

An image is composed of an infinite number of points, each coming from the corresponding point on the object. If we calculate where one image point is on its principal axis, and then calculate where the distal image point is, we can position the entire image and determine its size (Fig. 13–23A).

We could choose several of the many rays diverging from the distal object point to calculate the position of its corresponding distal image point (Fig. 13–23B). We choose to study three specific rays for the ease with which we can calculate their refraction:

1. The chief (or nodal) ray from the distal object point passes through the optical center of the lens without being changed in direction by the lens. With a thin lens, the optical center is found where the lens is crossed by the principal axis. All rays passing through the optical center pass through normals at both interfaces. Their direction of travel does not change (Fig. 13–24).

2. Another ray leaves the distal object point parallel to the principal axis. This ray, like all rays parallel to the principal axis, will be refracted by the lens to strike the principal axis at the secondary focal point.

3. The third ray leaves the distal object point in such a direction that it strikes the principal axis at the primary focal point. This ray will be refracted by the lens to emerge parallel to the principal axis. Sometimes this ray leaves the primary focal point to pass through the distal object point before it strikes the lens where it is refracted to emerge parallel.

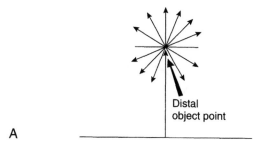

A

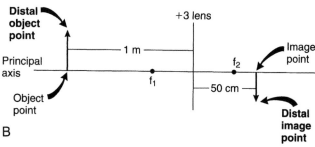

B

FIGURE 13–23. Calculation of the position of the distal image point from the position of the distal object point is all that is needed to position the entire image. *A*, An infinite number of rays diverge from the distal object point. *B*, Relationship of distal image point and the image point on the principal axis from distal object point and the object point on the principal axis.

• *Example 1. If we use:*

$$U + P = V$$
$$-1 + 3 = +2,$$

• *the primary focal point is 1/3 m (33 cm) in front of the lens, and the secondary focal point is 1/3 m (33 cm) behind the lens.*
• *we chose the following three rays diverging from the distal object point.*

1. The chief ray[1] leaves the distal object point and passes through the optical center of the lens without being refracted (Fig. 13–25A).

2. The second ray leaves the distal object point parallel to the principal axis, emerging from the plus lens converged toward the principal axis so that it passes through the secondary focal point of the lens (Fig. 13–25B).

3. The third ray leaves the distal object point to pass through the primary focal point until it strikes the plus lens where it will be converged toward the principal axis just enough to emerge parallel to it (Fig. 13–25C).

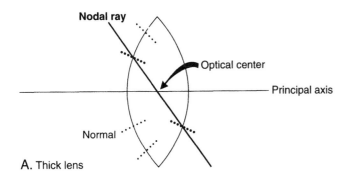

A. Thick lens

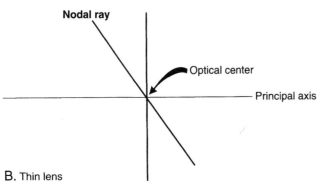

B. Thin lens

FIGURE 13–24. Nodal (chief) ray is not refracted by the lens.

- *Figure 13–25*D *combines the three light rays diverging from the tip of the distal object point to meet at the distal image point. We deliberately selected the three rays we know most about. In this case, all intersect 1/2 m behind the lens, locating the position of the distal image point.*

- ***Example 2.*** *If we take:*

$$U + P = V$$
$$(-1 -3 = -4)$$

- *and draw diagrams using the same three selected rays, the chief ray leaves the distal object point to pass through the optical center on the principal axis undeviated (Fig. 13–26A).*

  The second ray leaves the distal object point parallel to the principal axis. When this ray strikes the −3D lens, however, it diverges from the principal axis. The amount it diverges is as though it were coming from the secondary focal point one-third of a meter in front (to the left) of the −3D lens (Fig. 13–26B).

  The third ray leaves the distal object point, heading toward the primary principal focus one-third of a meter to the right of (behind) the lens. This ray is interrupted when it strikes the lens and diverges to emerge parallel to the principal axis (Fig. 13–26C). When this parallel ray is continued backward, it is

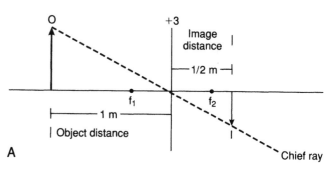

A

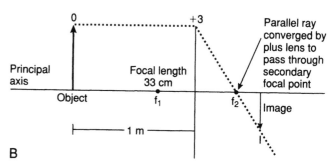

B

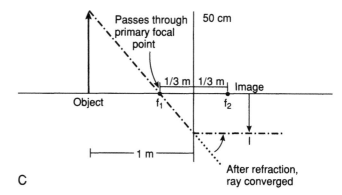

C

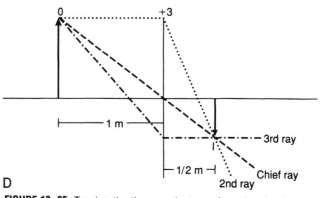

D

FIGURE 13–25. Tracing the three easiest rays from the distal object point that will come to a focus at the distal image point. Example shown is a plus (+3D) lens. *A,* Chief ray from distal object point passes through the optical center of the lens without refraction. *B,* Ray from distal object point that is parallel to principal axis is refracted by the lens to cross through the secondary focal point. *C,* Ray from distal object point that crosses through the primary focal point is refracted by the lens to emerge parallel to the principal axis. *D,* Combination of the three rays.

at the same height as the distal image point. All three rays are combined in one diagram (Fig. 13–26D).

Note that images are in the same direction (upright) as the object if they are located on the same side of the lens as the object, but are in the opposite direction

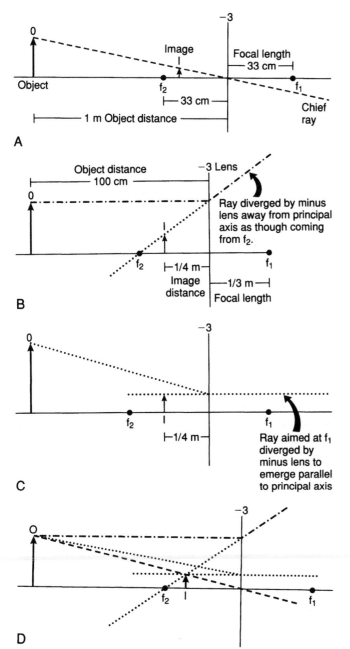

FIGURE 13–26. Tracing the three easiest rays from the distal object point that will come to a focus at the distal image point. Example shown is a minus (−3D) lens. *A*, Chief ray from distal object point. *B*, Ray from distal object point that is parallel to principal axis is refracted by the lens to cross through the secondary focal point. *C*, Ray from distal object point that crosses through the primary focal point is refracted by the lens to emerge parallel to the principal axis. *D*, Combination of the three rays.

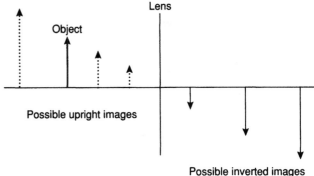

FIGURE 13–27. Direction of the image depends on the side of the lens on which the image is located.

(inverted) of the object if they are located on the opposite side of the lens (Fig. 13–27).

● LINEAR MAGNIFICATION

The relationship between the object size and its distance from the lens and the image size and its distance from the lens is directly proportional, in contrast to the inverse relationship between vergence power and focal length. The greater the distance from the lens, the larger the size of the object or image; the smaller the distance from the lens, the smaller the size of the object or image. Whichever is closer to the lens is smaller. If one of them is twice as far from the lens, it is twice the size. If the object and image are equidistant from the lens, they are the same size. We can determine the linear magnification by the formula:

$$M = \frac{Is}{Os} = \frac{Id}{Od}$$

$$\text{Magnification} = \frac{\text{image size}}{\text{object size}} = \frac{\text{image distance}}{\text{object distance}}$$

However, we can also describe linear magnification by the formulas:

$$\frac{Is}{Id} = \frac{Os}{Od}$$

$$\frac{\text{image size}}{\text{image distance}} = \frac{\text{object size}}{\text{object distance}}$$

Remember that image distance is v and object distance is u from our U + P = V formula explained previously.

• ***Example 1.*** *A 10-cm high object is 1 m from the lens. Its image is 0.5 m from the lens. The image size will be half the object size because the image distance is half the object distance.*

$$\frac{Os}{Od} = \frac{Is}{Id}$$

$$\frac{Os}{Od} = \frac{10\,cm}{1\,m} = \frac{Is}{Id} = \frac{x}{0.5\,m}$$

$$\frac{10\,cm}{1\,m} = \frac{x}{0.5\,m}$$

$$x = 5\,cm = Is$$

Alternatively, because $\frac{1\,m}{0.5\,m} = 2$

$$\frac{10\,cm}{x} \times 2,$$

$$x = 5\,cm$$

• ***Example 2.*** *An object is 10 cm high and its image is 2.5 cm high. If the object distance is 80 cm, the image distance will be 25% of that because the image size is 25% the object size.*

$$\frac{Os}{Is} = \frac{Od}{Id}$$

$$\frac{10\,cm}{2.5} = \frac{80\,cm}{x}$$

$$x = \frac{80 \times 2.5}{10} = 20\,cm = Id$$

Alternatively, $\frac{10\,cm}{2.5} = 4$

$$\frac{80\,cm}{x} = 4$$

$$x = 20\,cm$$

• MULTIPLE LENS SYSTEMS

So far, our lens problems have dealt with thin lens systems. More complex optical systems, such as telescopes and the eye, are multiple lens systems with thick lenses instead of thin. Moreover, plus and minus space frequently have different indices of refraction in multiple lens systems.

If we have a series of lenses in an optical system, the effect on incident light rays can be taken in turn, starting with the leftmost lens, and assuming that the object is even farther to the left. The optics problem for the leftmost lens is solved as for a single thin lens. The image from the first lens then becomes the object for the second leftmost lens, and so on. The problem is illustrated with two lenses, a +4D and a +1D, separated by 25 cm, acting on light rays coming from an object 50 cm in front of the first lens. Solving for the first lens (Fig. 13–28A):

$$u = -50\,cm = -1/2\,m \qquad U + P = V$$
$$1/u = U = -2 \qquad\qquad -2 + 4 = V$$
$$\qquad\qquad\qquad\qquad\qquad V = +2$$

The first image (I_1) has plus power from being refracted by the first lens to a position 25 cm behind the second lens. It is now the object (O_2) of the second lens.

The second problem becomes (Fig. 13–28B):

$$u = 25\,cm = 1/4\,m \qquad U + P = V$$
$$1/u = 4 = U \qquad\qquad +4 + 1 = V$$
$$V = 5 = 1/v \qquad\qquad V = +5$$
$$v = 1/5\,m = 20\,cm$$

Our solution indicates that the second image is 20 cm behind the second lens.

We could add a third −6D lens 10 cm, behind the second lens, so that the second image (I_2) becomes the third object (O_3) 10 cm from the −6D lens. Now we have:

$$U + P = V \qquad V = +4 = 1/v$$
$$+10 + (-6) = V \qquad v = +0.25\,m$$
$$\qquad = +4 \qquad\qquad = +25\,cm$$

This third image is 25 cm behind the third lens (Fig. 13–28C).

• CARDINAL POINTS

Fortunately, there is a simpler method of analyzing multiple lens systems by theoretically replacing the multiple lenses with six cardinal points to make it similar to a thin lens system. All the lens powers are combined, and the optical system is hypothetically dealt with as though it were one ''thick'' lens. Refraction through this thick lens is more complicated than through a thin lens.

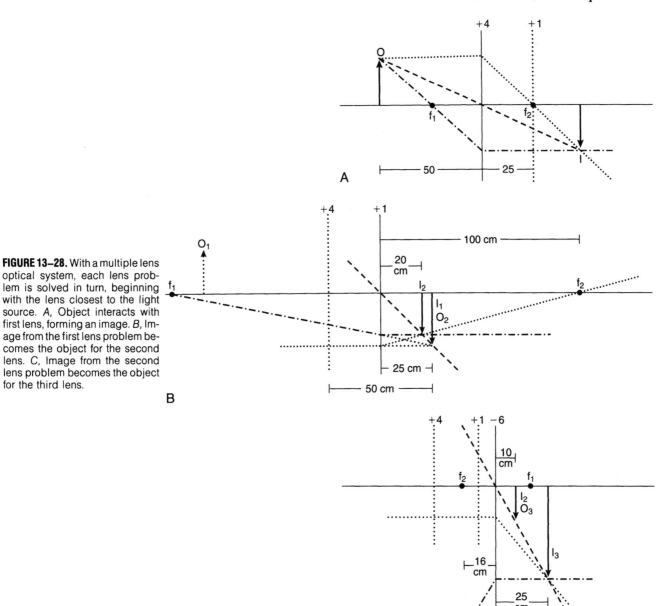

FIGURE 13–28. With a multiple lens optical system, each lens problem is solved in turn, beginning with the lens closest to the light source. *A,* Object interacts with first lens, forming an image. *B,* Image from the first lens problem becomes the object for the second lens. *C,* Image from the second lens problem becomes the object for the third lens.

This system uses two focal points, two principal points, and two nodal points. The similarity is that both thick and thin lenses have anterior and posterior focal points. The distance from the primary focal point to the primary principal point is the *front* or anterior focal length, and the distance from the secondary principal point to the secondary focal point is the *back* or posterior focal length. Both focal points are located on the principal axis where they would be for a particular set of multiple lenses. The thick lens has two refracting planes, the principal planes, which replace the two surfaces of our thin lens. The planes cross the principal axis at the principal points (Fig. 13–29).

All rays from the object parallel to the principal axis are refracted by the entire lens system at the secondary principal plane to strike the principal axis at the secondary focal point. All rays from the object that pass through the primary focal point strike the primary principal plane to emerge parallel to the principal axis. Notice that this discussion ignores the space between the principal planes as though it were not there. Any ray striking at some height on the first principal plane is transferred to the second principal plane at exactly the same height as though the space were not there.

What happens to the chief ray, the ray that traveled through the nodal point (optical center) of the thin lens undeviated? Well, there are actually two nodal points, each located at a principal point as long as the image space and object space are in the same media. In our thick lens system, the slope of the ray directed toward

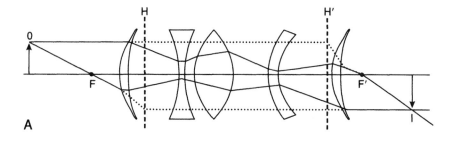

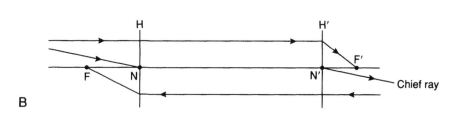

FIGURE 13–29. Alternate method for solving multiple lens optical system problem utilizes system of six cardinal points and treats the complex of lenses as one thick lens. *A,* Method of solving each lens problem in turn. *B,* Cardinal points include two principal points (H and H') representing the two principal planes, two focal points (F and F'), and two nodal points (N and N'). This simplifies optical problems dealing with a specific set of multiple lenses and indices of refraction, as occurs in the eye.

the first nodal point is the same as the slope of the ray leaving the second nodal point, as though the space between the first and second nodal points were absent.

The thin lens was a good way to begin studying image formation, because both principal points and both nodal points intersect where the lens crosses the principal axis. In our thin lens system, we considered air as the medium on both sides of our lens. In the eye, with its higher refractive index, the nodal points shift off the principal points.

• CYLINDERS

So far, all lenses are considered spherical, with equal vergence power in all directions. Rays striking spherical surfaces come to a point focus. In the space between

where the rays leave the spherical surface and where the rays come to a focus, they come closer and closer together, producing a conical configuration. Within this configuration the image begins to be seen as a blur in the shape of a circle. As these *blur circles* become smaller and smaller, the focus becomes sharper at the end of the cone. They reach the best, sharpest focus at the focal point (Fig. 13–30).

A cylindrical lens has a flat and a curved surface. Rays striking the curved surface are refracted by that surface's power. Rays striking the flat surface are not refracted, because that surface has no curve and therefore no power. This cylindrical lens has refracting power in one direction; the other direction 90° away has zero power and is called the cylinder axis. Light rays refracted by cylindrical lenses come to a sharp focus at a focal line instead of a focal point. The focal

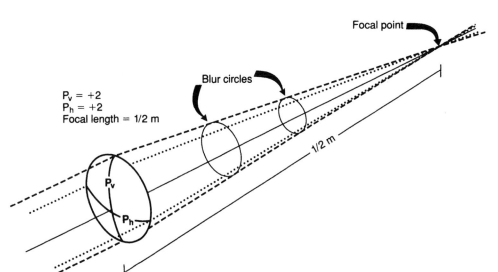

FIGURE 13–30. Spheres produce blur circles that come to a point focus.

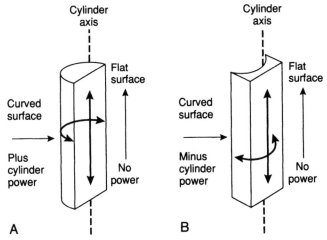

FIGURE 13–31. Cylinders have power in one direction, and no power in the direction 90° away. *A,* Plus cylinder. *B,* Minus cylinder.

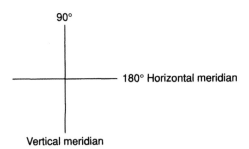

FIGURE 13–32. Most common directions of cylinder axes.

line is parallel to the cylindrical axis but perpendicular to the direction of cylindrical power. Cylindrical lenses are designated by their axis (Fig 13–31), not by their power meridian 90° away. The power may be plus or minus depending on whether the curved surface is convex or concave. The most common orientations of cylinders for the eye are at 90° and at 180°: 90° is the vertical meridian; 180° the horizontal meridian (Fig. 13–32).

● OPTICAL CROSSES

Because the power a cylinder possesses is 90° from its axis, a cylinder of $+5 \times 180°$ can be recorded on a cross like this:

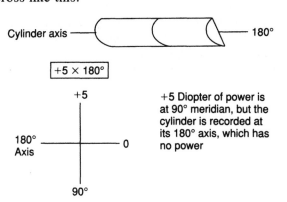

+5 Diopter of power is at 90° meridian, but the cylinder is recorded at its 180° axis, which has no power

The power is at the 90° meridian but the axis is at 180°.

There are two ways of recording a sphere on an optical cross. Because a $+2.00$ sphere has the same power in all meridians, we can have one resultant cross such as:

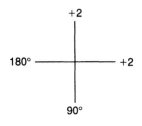

or we can record it on two crosses as two cylinders such as:

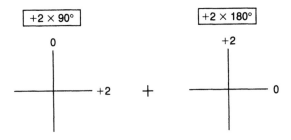

A spherocylindrical lens has one spherical and one cylindrical surface, giving it two unequally powered radii of curvature. This type of lens can be thought of as two cylinders, perpendicular to each other, with one direction having the maximal refractive power, and the other minimal. We can record a spherocylinder in several ways.

● *Example 1.*

● *For the spherocylinder $+3.00 + 1.50 \times 90$, the sphere is separate from the cylinder in plus form:*

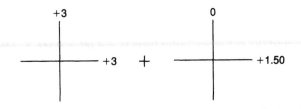

or separate the sphere from the cylinder in its minus form:

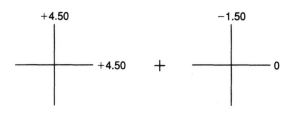

Think of it as two cylinders:

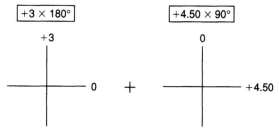

or as the resultant:

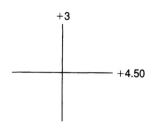

On a lensometer, the thin lines at 90° would be in focus at +3.00, and the wide lines at 180° at +4.50.

● *Example 2.*
● *Two cylinders, a +8 × 180 and a +4 × 90, can be diagrammed as:*

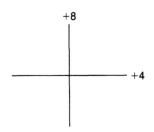

or on two crosses as a sphere and a plus cylinder:

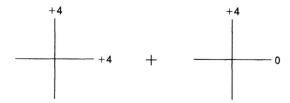

and the spherocylinder form is +4.00 + 4.00 × 180.
On a lensometer, the thin lines at 90° are in focus at +4.00, and the wide lines at 180° at +8.00.

● *Example 3.*
● *The spherocylinder +3.00 + 2.00 × 135 may be diagrammed as:*

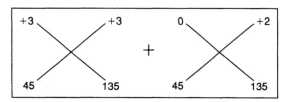

or as:

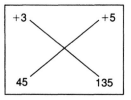

and may be written in minus cylinder form as:
+5.00 − 2.00 × 45.

On a lensometer, the 135° axis reading (thin lines) would be in focus at +3.00, and the 45° axis reading (wide lines) at +5.00.

● *Example 4.*
● *If we have the following cylinders in combination:*
(+2 − 4 − 8 + 5 = −5 at 90°)

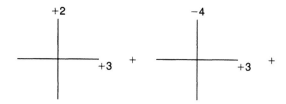

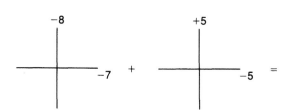

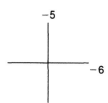

Resultant

(+3 + 3 − 7 − 5 = −6 at 180°)
The combined power in spherocylindrical form is −5.00 −1.00 × 90° in minus form or −6.00 + 1.00 × 180° in plus form.

● STURM'S CONOID

A spherocylindrical lens will not produce a point focus as does a sphere, but two line foci 90° from one another. We determine each one separately. The +1 cylinder axis 180° produces a horizontal focal line 100 cm from the cylinder, parallel to the cylinder axis (Fig. 13–33A). The +5 cylinder axis 90° produces a vertical focal line 20 cm from the cylinder parallel to its axis (Fig. 13–33B).

If we draw the combined spherocylinder showing both focal lines, one meridian comes to a line focus at a different distance than the line focus of the meridian 90° away. The horizontal line focus is formed by narrower and narrower horizontal blur ellipses just as the vertical line focus is produced by narrower and narrower vertical blur ellipses. The locations of the line images are determined in the same way as the location of an image point produced by a spherical lens, but the two line images are perpendicular to one another and parallel to their cylinder axes.

The space between the two line foci is called Sturm's interval. In the interval lies Sturm's conoid created by the light rays connecting the two line foci. The conoid has a peculiar, somewhat conical shape that contains the circle of least confusion, representing the position where the rays come closest to forming a spherical focus. The circle of least confusion, dioptrically halfway between the two focal lines, represents the axial position within the conoid at which the least blurry image is produced. The spherical power that produces this circle is called the spherical equivalent (Fig. 13–34).

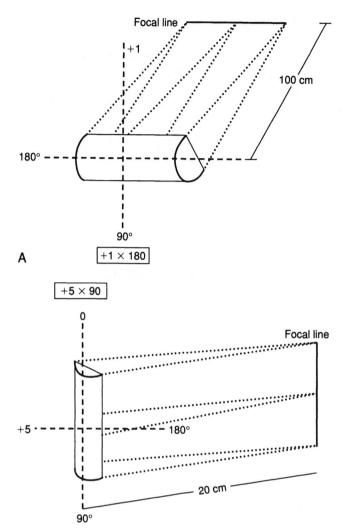

FIGURE 13–33. Spherocylinders produce two focal lines at two different distances, 90° away from one another. *A*, Cylinder at 180° axis produces horizontal focal line. *B*, Cylinder at 90° axis produces vertical focal line.

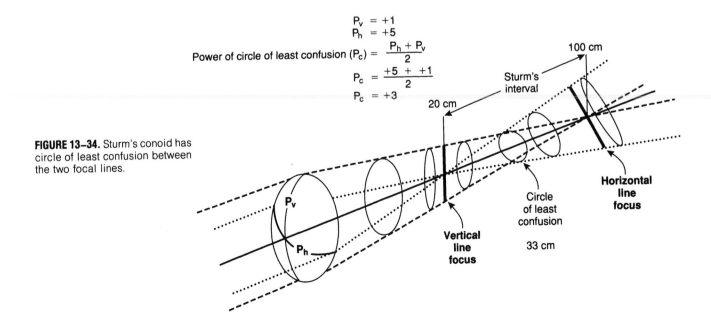

$$P_v = +1$$
$$P_h = +5$$

Power of circle of least confusion $(P_c) = \dfrac{P_h + P_v}{2}$

$$P_c = \dfrac{+5 + +1}{2}$$

$$P_c = +3$$

FIGURE 13–34. Sturm's conoid has circle of least confusion between the two focal lines.

Bibliography

Brooks CW, Borish IM: System for Ophthalmic Dispensing. Chicago, Professional Press, 1979.

Campbell CJ, Koester CJ, Rittler MC, et al.: Physiological Optics. Hagerstown, MD, Harper & Row, 1974.

Elkington AR, Frank HJ: Clinical Optics. Oxford, Blackwell Scientific, 1984.

Kuether CL: Geometric optics. In Duane TD (ed): Clinical Ophthalmology, vol I. Hagerstown, MD, Harper & Row, 1990.

Michaels DD: Visual Optics and Refraction, 3rd ed. St Louis, CV Mosby, 1985.

Mittelman D: Geometric optics and clinical refraction. In Peyman GA, Sanders DR, Goldberg MF (eds): Principles and Practice of Ophthalmology, vol I. Philadelphia, WB Saunders, 1980.

Rubin ML: Optics for Clinicians, 2nd ed. Gainesville, FL, Triad, 1974.

• CHAPTER 13 GEOMETRIC OPTICS

1. Which of the angles illustrated is the angle of refraction?

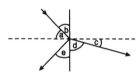

   a. a
   b. b
   c. c
   d. d
   e. e

2. Where is the secondary focal point of a −8 diopter (D) lens?
   a. 12 cm in front of the lens
   b. 8 cm in front of the lens
   c. 1/8 meter behind the lens
   d. 12 cm behind the lens
   e. 8 cm behind the lens

3. A 5 mm object is located 16 cm in front of a lens. Its real image is located 12 cm from the lens. What is the strength of the lens?
   a. −2 D
   b. +14 D
   c. +4 D
   d. −4 D
   e. +7 D

4. This lens has its power recorded on an optical cross. Its spherocylindrical notation is
   a. +2.00 + +7.00 × 180°
   b. +2.00 − +7.00 × 90°
   c. +2.00 + +5.00 × 90°
   d. +7.00 − +2.00 × 180°
   e. +7.00 − +5.00 × 90°

5. A spherocylinder has a vertical line focus 33 cm away and a horizontal line focus 100 cm away. Its circle of least confusion is found at
   a. 66 cm
   b. 133 cm
   c. 25 cm
   d. 50 cm
   e. 40 cm.

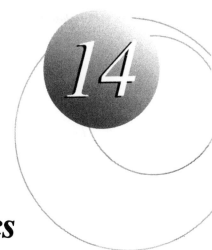

Physiological Optics

LEARNING OBJECTIVES

- Understand how the eye's natural lens provides a variable optical power, allowing objects to remain in focus at all distances, near and far
- Explain the relationship between accommodation and any refractive error
- Calculate the effects of age and refractive error on the near point of accommodation
- Describe the types of refractive error caused by abnormal axial lengths
- Understand how astigmatism affects the eye's ability to focus
- Calculate the prismatic effect produced by the relationship between the placement of the optical center of a spectacle lens and the interpupillary distance
- Describe how the eye functions as a reflecting mirror

• OPTICAL SYSTEM OF THE EYE

The optical system of the eye contains five interfaces and four optical media. Each successive medium has a change in refractive index from its predecessor (Fig. 14–1). This complex optical system can be replaced by six cardinal points, allowing analysis of the eye as a thick lens. Two principal points are less than a millimeter apart in the anterior chamber, and two nodal points are equally distant near the posterior surface of the lens. The anterior focal point is 15.7 mm in front of the eye; the posterior is on the retina.

The clarity of the retinal image depends on the eye's refractive surfaces and media. The front and back surfaces of the cornea, the front and back surfaces of the lens, and the retina are the refracting interfaces. The tear film, corneal stroma, aqueous, lens cortex, and vitreous are the refracting media. Each part of this multilens optical system has its own refractive index and some plus power. The cornea contributes about 43 diopters (D) and the lens about 15 D. This totals about 60 D, making the eye a powerful plus lens system. The refracting power of the cornea and the length of the eyeball (axial length) are the two most important elements in determining the total refractive power of an eye. Normal axial length is about 24 mm (Fig. 14–2).

A standardized, simplified model of the eye's optical system has evolved. It unifies the refracting surfaces and the indices of refraction of the intraocular media, allowing easier study. This *reduced* eye combines the two principal points and relocates it to the front surface of the cornea. This allows all 60 D of refracting power to take place at this one interface. The optical center is found near the posterior surface of the lens where the two nodal points combine 5.55 mm from the cornea. An anterior focal point is located 17 mm in front of the cornea and a posterior focal point 17 mm behind the nodal point on the retina. In order to reduce the optics to this simple model, the eye is shortened to 22.5 mm and given a uniform index of refraction of 1.33.

• ACCOMMODATION PHYSIOLOGY

The lens provides variable focusing power, *accommodation*, for the eye's optical system. In the unaccommodated state, the ciliary muscle is at rest, stretching the zonular fibers and keeping the lens as flat as possible. The refractive power of the lens is at its minimum, with about 10 D of plus power, but exerting 0 D of accommodation. This resting state results in clear vision when looking at infinity, which is clinically determined at 20 ft and beyond (Fig. 14–3).

Accommodation is this variable focusing power (up to 18 D) supplied precisely and instantaneously by the flexibility of the ocular lens. This enables the eye to

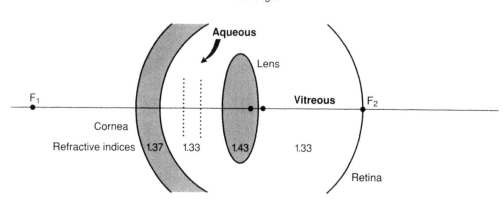

FIGURE 14–1. Optical system of the eye. Refractive interfaces and refractive media with different refractive indices.

keep images in focus on the retina. Without accommodation, our eye would focus on an object at a specific fixed distance. Any object we wanted to see clearly would need to be put at this distance. The image of an approaching object would blur, because it would focus behind the retina. Accommodation is stimulated by this blurred image. As the eye accommodates, its plus power increases, *pulling* the focused image back onto the retina. It does this by steepening the curve of its natural lens. This increases the lens power and keeps an object in focus as the distance from the eye decreases.

Age and Accommodation

The lens change from unaccommodation to maximum accommodation is the amplitude of accommodation (A), measured in D. This remarkable capacity of the eye is greatest in childhood. It works so well under age 20 that we are not even aware of its functioning until it starts to fail our near needs over age 30. Accom-

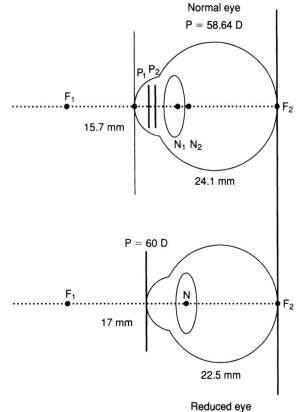

FIGURE 14–2. Simplified optical system. The reduced eye loses 1.6 mm of axial length and replaces the two principal points with one refracting interface at the front corneal surface. The two nodal points are replaced with one in the middle of the lens. The anterior focal point is 17 mm in front of the corneal surface and the posterior focal point is 17 mm behind the nodal point on the retina.

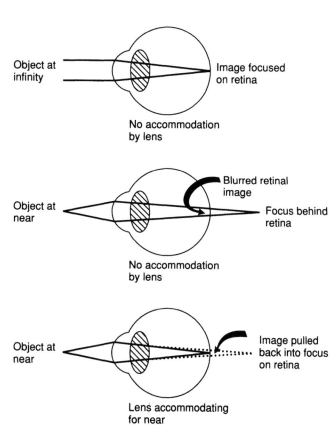

FIGURE 14–3. Mechanics of maintaining a clear image on the retina as a viewed object approaches.

modation gradually decreases with increasing age. Becoming more rigid decreases the len's ability to become spherical. Donder's table gives age norms for loss of accommodation. Memorize a few examples. Note that at age 10, the average amplitude is 14 D; at age 20, it is 10 D; at age 44, it is 4 D; and at age 60, it is 1 D (Table 14–1).

Another guideline for average *normal* accommodation is:

Age 40—6 D.   For each 4 years under 40, add 1 D.
Age 44–4 D.
Age 48–3 D.   For each 4 years over 48, subtract ½ D.

• *For example:*
  1. A 32-year-old woman would have
     6 D + 2 D = 8 D.
  2. A 56-year-old man would have
     3 D − 1 D = 2 D.

Loss of accommodation with age is called presbyopia. Because it arrives at different ages, using a standard chart could lead to mistakes in prescribing reading glasses. The process begins at birth and becomes clinically evident by a receding near point of accommodation around age 40, when the remaining power approximates the amount required at the average reading distance. At first, reading material is held farther away. Finally, the arms are not long enough. For a 44-year-old emmetrope, all the remaining 4 D of accommodation is used to clear images seen at the near point of 25 cm (¼ D = .25 m), leaving no reserve. The eyes tire from this maximal effort.

Presbyopia can be corrected by replacing the focusing ability of the lens with plus correction, whether in reading eyeglasses or in the lower segment of a bifocal lens. Most patients are comfortable using about half their reserve.

Optical Relationships

As an object nears, the capacity of the lens to increase its power (i.e., accommodate) is finally exceeded and the image blurs. The near point of accom-

modation (n) is the closest point to the eye at which an object's image is focused on the retina. It occurs when the lens is maximally accommodating. The younger individual has a greater ability to accommodate, a higher amplitude of accommodation, and a closer near point. Amplitude decreases with age and results in the near point receding from the eye.

This can be written as a formula:

$$N = 1/n,$$

where N is the increase in focusing power of the eye in diopters when the lens is maximally accommodating at the near point, and n is the near point distance in meters. Beware of substituting meters for diopters. The distance in meters of an object from the eye is inversely proportional to the amount of accommodation in diopters that the eye exerts as vergence power to focus that object. Converting from one unit of measurement to the other is common. If an object is 0.33 m distant, it requires 3 D of the eye's natural lens' accommodation to focus the image on the retina; an object 2 m away requires ½ D of accommodation; an object at infinity requires no accommodation in a normal, or *emmetropic,* eye with no refractive error.

The *far point of accommodation* (f) is the greatest distance at which an object's image can be focused on the retina. The ciliary muscle is relaxed, the eye is not accommodating, and the lens has its minimum power. The eye's refractive error (F) is its dioptric equivalent, e.g., so if f is 0.5 m in front of the eye, F is −2.00 D. If the far point is somewhere in front of the eye, but closer than infinity, it is in minus space. All points between the eye and infinity are minus numbers. All points behind the eye are in plus space. If we know the refractive error in diopters of lens power, we can calculate the position of the far point in meters. Put into another familiar formula relating diopters to meters:

$$F = 1/f$$

where f is the far point distance in meters, and F is the refractive error measured in diopters

---

TABLE 14–1.

Donder's Table for Amplitude of Accommodation Norms

Age (yr)	1	5	10	15	20	25	30	40	44	50	60	75
Accommodation (diopters)	18	16	14	12	10	8.5	7	4.5	4	2.5	1	0

• ***Example 1.*** *A patient has a far point 1 m in front of the eye. What is the refractive error? The far point is in minus space.*

$$F = 1/f$$
$$F = 1/1\,m$$
$$= -1\,D$$

• ***Example 2.*** *If the far point is 1 m behind the eye, what is the refractive error? The far point is in plus space.*

$$F = 1/f$$
$$= +1/1\,m$$
$$= +1\,D$$

• ***Example 3.*** *If the far point is at infinity, what is the refractive error?*

$$f = infinity$$
$$F = 1/infinity$$
$$= 0\,D$$

A theoretical concept of "beyond" infinity explains plus space, which starts at infinity and goes "around the world" to end behind the retina. Once you accept this somewhat illogical theory for plus space (and consider the distance from the eye to infinity as being in minus space), far points, near points, refractive errors, and their symptoms and corrections become easier to understand.

• REFRACTIVE ERRORS

Our optical system refracts light so that images are focused onto the retina. When the eye's optical system is emmetropic, light rays from distant objects refract to a clear, focused, retinal image without accommodation. The eye has no refractive error (F = 0). Its far point is at infinity (Fig. 14–4). Eyes with refractive errors, *ametropia,* cannot refract distant objects to a clear focus on the retina without using some reserve

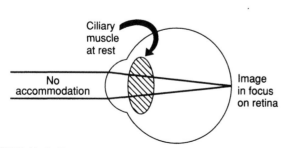

FIGURE 14–4. Emmetropic eye looking at distance object has its image focused on the retina.

accommodative power or wearing corrective lenses in eyeglasses or contact lenses, which correct the defect in the eye's optical system. An optically corrected eye has become artificially emmetropic. Although there are other causes of refractive errors, this chapter next explains the most common, the axial length, the distance from the center of the front surface of the cornea to the center of the retina at the posterior pole.

Hyperopia

If an eye has too short an axial length (less than 22 mm), the eye is hyperopic (farsighted). Without accommodation, parallel light rays come to a focus *behind* the retina, at the eye's far point in plus space. Because children have smaller eyes, their eyes are also short, so that most of them are far-sighted. An uncorrected (e.g., F = +2D) hyperope has an optical system with too *little* plus power, that is, not strong enough to produce a clear image of a distant object without accommodation. Of course, the patient can see clearly at a distance by wearing a refractive correction, in this case +2 D, in eyeglasses or contact lenses. However, he or she has another option. The patient can *cheat* and use some of his or her accommodative ability to increase the eye's plus power. The patient pulls the image onto the fovea by *adding* plus (in this example 2 D) from his or her own lens. He or she makes up for the diopters of the refractive error with some of his or her accommodative reserve. Because the patient uses some of this reserve to clear distant objects, he or she has less for the near point than the emmetrope. An uncorrected hyperope ultilizes the amount of accommodation required for clear near vision by the emmetrope, *plus* the amount of his or her hyperopia.

A 5-year-old child easily *cheats* because he or she has a large accommodative reserve. A 20-year-old patient can also, unless he or she has a hyperopic error greater than +4. By age 35, with the dwindled accommodative reserve, most hyperopes prefer at least some error corrected by eyeglasses or contact lenses.

Because the far points for hyperopes are behind the retina, they are *beyond* infinity and thus are plus numbers. All uncorrected hyperopes have a far point in plus space (Fig. 14–5).

Myopia

If the axial length of the eye exceeds 24 mm, the optical system will refract parallel rays of light from infinity to a focus in *front of* the retina, producing *myopia.* Children often become nearsighted as teenagers when their eyeballs reach mature size. An uncorrected (e.g., F = −3 D) myope has an optical system

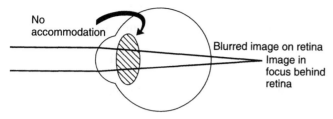

Uncorrected hyperope looking at distance

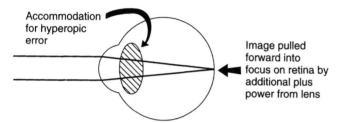

Uncorrected hyperope looking at distance

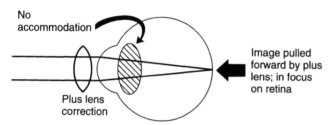

Corrected hyperope looking at distance

FIGURE 14–5. Effect of accommodation and plus lenses on hyperopia.

amount of the myopia. The patient has more accommodative reserve left for his or her near point than the emmetrope (Fig. 14–6).

At any age, an uncorrected myope has a closer near point, and an uncorrected hyperope a farther near point, than an emmetrope. All uncorrected myopes have a far point in minus space. An uncorrected hyperope has both near and far points *farther* away than the emmetrope of the same age, and the uncorrected myope has the far and near points *closer* to the eye than an emmetrope of the same age (Fig. 14–7). The uncorrected hyperope needs reading glasses earlier than the emmetrope and the uncorrected myope later. The corrected myope, to avoid bifocals, can remove his or her eyeglasses for near work as he or she ages.

In summary, the eye can *increase* its plus power by accommodation to help the hyperope, but it cannot *decrease* its plus power to help the myope. An eye will accommodate only enough to keep approaching objects in focus. An emmetrope, or a patient wearing refractive error correction, can accommodate the amount of diopters dictated by the distance in meters of the approaching object from the eye. An uncorrected hyper-

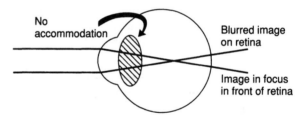

Uncorrected myope looking at distance

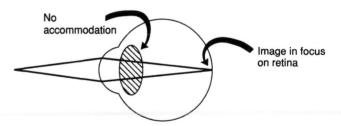

Uncorrected myope looking at far point

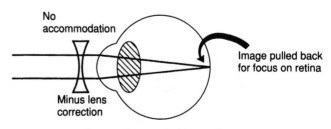

Corrected myope looking at distance

FIGURE 14–6. Effect of accommodation and minus lenses on myopia.

with too much plus power. An object from infinity comes to a focus in front of the retina. The myope cannot produce clear images from distant objects because he or she cannot decrease the eye's plus power. The far point is between the eye and infinity, in minus space. The higher the myopia is, the closer the far point is to the eye. The myope without eyeglasses cannot clear anything farther away from the eye than his or her far point. As an object is brought from infinity closer to the eye, it reaches the far point distance, in this case 0.33 m in front of the eye, at which distance the diverging light rays can be focused to form a clear image on the retina. All uncorrected myopes have a far point in minus space.

Myopia is corrected by reducing the eye's excessive plus power with minus lenses. There is no other option to reduce the power in this eye to bring a distant object in focus on the retina, except by wearing its refractive correction (or having keratorefractive surgery). The myope does not use any accommodation until objects are closer than the far point. An uncorrected myopic patient maintains clear near vision by using the amount of accommodation required of an emmetrope, *less* the

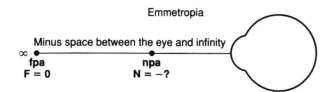

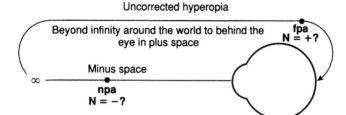

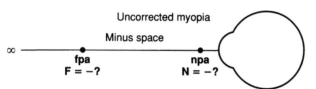

FIGURE 14–7. Relationship of refractive error on far point and near point distances.

ope has to accommodate as much as the emmetrope, *plus* the amount of the hyperopia. The uncorrected myope has to accommodate as much as the emmetrope, *less* the amount of the myopia (Table 14–2).

● *Example 1*. A patient has 4 D of myopia. How much accommodation will he exert if he is:

1. Uncorrected (F = −4) and fixates at 20 cm. He accommodates the amount dictated by the 20 cm (Y5 m) distance for an emmetrope (5 D) less his myopia (−4 D), 5 D − 4 D = 1 D.

2. Uncorrected and fixates at 10 cm. He accommodates as an emmetrope would at 10 cm (10 D) less his myopia (−4 D), 10 D − 4 D = 6 D.

● *Example 2*. A patient has 2 D of hyperopia. How much accommodation will he exert if:

1. He is uncorrected and fixates an object at 0.33 m?

TABLE 14–2.

Amount of Accommodation Required (diopters)

Distance	Emmetropic Patient	Uncorrected +2 Hyperopic Patient	Uncorrected −3 Myopic Patient
Infinity	0	0 + 2 = 2	0 but blurred
0.33 m	3	3 + 2 = 5	3 − 3 = 0
0.20 m	5	5 + 2 = 7	5 − 3 = 2

0.33 m = 1/3 m
at 1/3 m he accommodates 3 D plus the hyperopic error
3 D + 2 D = 5 D

2. He is uncorrected and fixates an object at infinity?

Zero accommodation at infinity plus the hyperopic error.
O D + 2 D = 2 D

● AMPLITUDE OF ACCOMMODATION

The amplitude of accommodation is the maximum plus power that can be added to the plus refractive power of the unaccommodated eye and is age dependent only. The far point depends on the refractive error or on the lack thereof; the near point depends on both the refractive error and the amplitude.

The relationship follows this equation:

$$A = F - N = 1/f - 1/n$$

where

A = amplitude of accommodation in diopters
F = refractive error in diopters
F = dioptric equivalent of the far point
F = 1/f
f = far point in meters
N = dioptric equivalent of the near point
N = 1/n
n = near point in meters.

For calculation purposes, it is usually preferable to work in diopters rather than in meters. Since the amplitude is in diopters, the far point (f) in meters is changed to its dioptric equivalent (F), and the near point (n) in meters to its dioptric equivalent (N).

● *Example 1*. The dioptric equivalent for a near point at 5 cm (1/20 meter) is found by

$$n = 0.05 \text{ m} = 1/20 \text{ m}$$
$$1/n = N = 20 \text{ D}$$

● *Example 2*. The dioptric equivalent for a far point at 33 cm (1/3 meter) is found by

$$f = 0.33 \text{ m} = 1/3 \text{ m}$$
$$1/f = F = 3 \text{ D}$$

● *Since the far point for all emmetropes is at infinity, f = ∞, F = 0; therefore, A = F − N = 0 − N = N.*

The near point distance in meters is reciprocal to the amplitude in diopters. With their refractive corrections worn, both hyperopes and myopes become emmetropic, optically.

• **Example 1.** *A 20-year-old emmetrope has 10 D of amplitude. To find her near point*

$$A = F - N$$
$$10 = 0 - N$$
$$N = -10\ D$$
$$n = -1/10\ m = -10\ cm$$

• **Example 2.** *An 11-year-old has 14 D of amplitude and uncorrected hyperopia of +6 D. To find his near point*

$$A = F - N$$
$$14 = +6 - N$$
$$N = -8\ D$$
$$n = 1/8\ m = -12\ cm$$

• *However, if he is corrected with glasses, his near point improves to*

$$14 = 0 - N,\ N = -14\ D$$
$$n = -1/14\ m,\ n = -7\ cm$$

• **Example 3.** *A 50-year-old has 3 D of amplitude and an uncorrected myopia of −4 D. His near point is*

$$3 = -4 - N,\ N = -7,\ n = 1/7\ m,\ n = 14\ cm$$

• *However, if he wears his glasses, without bifocals, his near point recedes to*

$$3 = 0 - N,\ N = -3,\ n = -1/3\ m,\ n = 33\ cm.$$

Range of accommodation is the distance between the far point and the near point of accommodation through which the eye, can see clearly, expressed in m. It is the eye's depth of focus. The range of accommodation (r = f − n) is from the near point to infinity for emmetropes; from the near point past infinity, around the world, and behind the eye to the far point for hyperopes; and in front of infinity from the near point to the far point in myopes. One usually refers to the range as going from the near point to the far point, giving the actual distance at which this occurs. The range is the reciprocal of the amplitude.

$$r = 1/A \qquad r = f - n$$
$$f = 1/F \qquad r = 1/F - 1/N$$
$$n = 1/N$$

If f is 33 cm from the eye and n is 10 cm, we know from the equation D = 1/f that

$$F = 1/f \qquad\qquad N = 1/n$$
$$ = \frac{1}{1/3} \qquad\qquad = \frac{1}{1/10}$$
$$ = -3\ D \qquad\qquad = -10\ D$$

We can now find a and A.

$$a = f - n \qquad\qquad A = F - N$$
$$a = -33\ cm - (-10\ cm) \qquad A = -3\ D - (-10\ D)$$
$$ = -23\ cm \qquad\qquad\qquad = 7\ D$$

Range of accommodation gives a depth of focus from 33 cm to 10 cm for a 23 cm distance and an amplitude of accommodation of 7 D.

Astigmatism

Normally, the cornea is spherical, like a slice from a basketball. The refractive surfaces are equally curved in all directions. Astigmatism is a refractive error caused by the nonspherical (toroidal) surface of the cornea or lens, or in combination. Like a football, it is more curved in one direction than in the direction 90° away (Fig. 14–8). It has different curvatures in its two principal meridians. An eye with uncorrected astigmatism cannot refract focal points on the retina. It refracts two line foci, one horizontal and one vertical, at different locations on or near the retina depending on the type of astigmatism. Sturm's conoid separates the two. Simple hyperopic astigmatism has one focal line on the retina and the second behind the retina. Compound hyperopic astigmatism has both focal lines behind the retina (Fig. 14–9). Simple myopic astigmatism has one focal line on the retina and the second in the vitreous. Compound myopic astigmatism has both focal lines in the vitreous. Mixed astigmatism has one in the vitreous and the other behind the retina.

Spherocylinders correct for astigmatism. They can be written in plus or minus cylinder form. The most

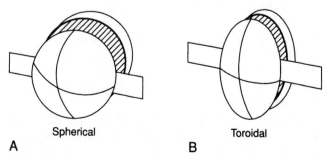

FIGURE 14–8. *A* and *B*, Difference in curvature between spherical and toroidal surfaces.

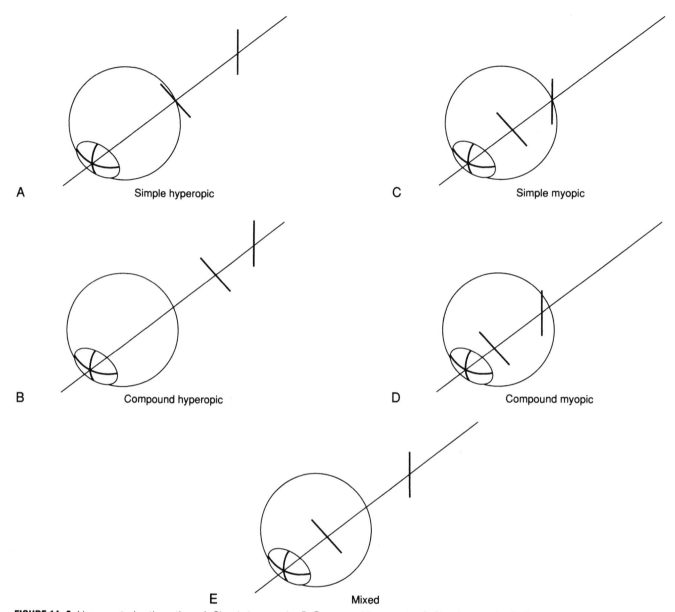

FIGURE 14–9. Uncorrected astigmatism. *A*, Simple hyperopic. *B*, Compound hyperopic. *C*, Simple myopic. *D*, Compound myopic. *E*, Mixed.

common directions for astigmatic correction are at 90°
(vertical meridian) and 180° (horizontal meridian).
More astigmats need plus cylinders at 90° than at 180°,
so that toric lenses with plus cylinders at or near 90°
are *with the rule*. Uncorrected astigmatism with the
rule always has the horizontal focal line in front of the
vertical focal line. The eye's vertical corneal meridian
has the steeper curvature (Fig. 14–10). The refractive
correction steepens the horizontal meridian to negate
the eye's error.

Those at or near axis 180° are *against the rule*. Uncorrected astigmatism against the rule always has the
horizontal focal line behind the vertical focal line. The
eye's horizontal meridian has the steeper curvature.

The refractive correction steepens the vertical meridian to balance the eye's error.

When retinoscoping astigmatism with plus cylinder
phoropters, the front focal line is moved to the retina
with the spherical correction, then Sturm's conoid is
collapsed when the cylinder correction puts the other
focal line also onto the retina (Fig. 14–11).

When retinoscoping astigmatism with minus cylinder
phoropters, the back focal line is moved to the retina
with the spherical correction, then Sturm's conoid is
collapsed when the cylinder correction puts the other
focal line also onto the retina (Fig. 14–12). The system
designating the direction of the cylinder axis is shown
in Figure 14–13.

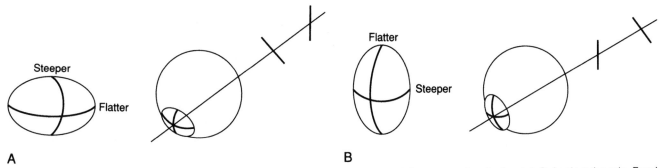

FIGURE 14–10. Uncorrected astigmatism. *A*, With-the-rule. Eyes' vertical corneal meridian steeper then horizontal. *B*, Against-the-rule. Eyes' horizontal corneal meridian steeper then vertical.

• INDUCED PRISMATIC EFFECT BY LENS DECENTRATION

As in geometric optics, the light rays passing through the lens's optical center are not bent. All rays passing through the lens other than through the optical center

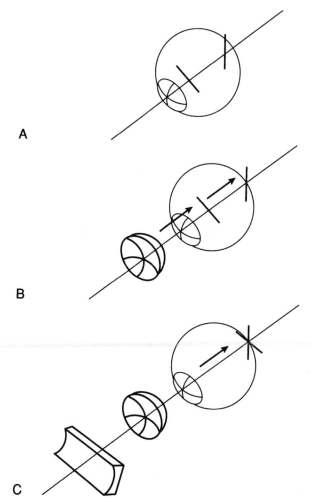

FIGURE 14–11. Steps in correcting compound hyperopic astigmatism with-the-rule with plus cylinder. *A*, Uncorrected. *B*, Correcting plus sphere repositions both focal lines forward just enough so that front horizontal line focus is on retina. *C*, Correcting plus cylinder at 90° axis collapses conoid of Sturm, superimposing both focal lines on the retina.

FIGURE 14–12. Steps in correcting compound myopic astigmatism with-the-rule with minus cylinder. *A*, Uncorrected. *B*, Correcting minus sphere repositions both focal lines backward so that back vertical line focus is on retina. *C*, Correcting minus cylinder collapses conoid of Sturm, superimposing both focal lines on the retina.

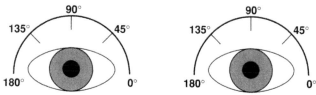

FIGURE 14–13. System designating cylinder axis notation.

deviate to pass through the focal point. This produces a prismatic effect whenever an eye is *not* looking through the optical center of a lens. Prism may be *induced* in a lens by positioning its OC so that the eye is looking through one of the prisms that make up the lens. The direction of the prism induced depends on the kind of lens (− or +) and the direction of the displacement of the optical center from the visual axis. Consider plus lenses as prisms base to base and minus lenses as prisms apex to apex.

Under normal conditions, patients have lenses prescribed with the optical centers of the two lenses positioned so that the distance between them is equal to the patient's interpupillary distance (PD). Sometimes the distance between the two optical centers and the patient's interpupillary distance, however, unintentionally induces a prismatic effect. Diplopia or eye discomfort may result (Fig. 14–14). Other times, it is deliberately changed to induce a prismatic effect, alleviating diplopia or eye discomfort. Decentering the len's optical center produces prismatic correction without adding extra weight, bulk, or expense to the prescription. A lens with a ground-in prism has extra weight and bulk and is considerably more expensive. Temporary plastic *press-on* Fresnel prisms over 10 PD decrease vision and scratch easily.

Be careful to note in which direction the optical center deviates from the corneal reflex. If there is no deviation, decentration will produce one (Fig. 14–15). Whatever that base corrects, the deviation produced will be opposite. For instance, BO prisms are used to correct an esodeviation. If the decentration results in BO effect, an orthophoric patient will artificially test as an exotropia. Base-down prisms correct a hyperdeviation (upward). If decentration has an unnecessary BD effect, an orthophoric patient will screen a hypodeviation (downward).

Prentice's rule is a formula used to evaluate prism production by decentration of the optical center of lenses. The power of the prism induced (pd) depends on the power of the lens in diopters (D) and the amount of the optical center (OC) displacement in cm (d). When determining the amount of prism induced, the cylinder is taken into account as part of the power of the lens. The meridian where the cylinder has power, as depicted on an optical cross, is the lens power used to evaluate any induced prism.

Prentice's Rule

Induced prism = lens power × OC displacement
(in prism diopters) (in diopters)   (in cm)

When the lens is plus, the decentration shifts with the lens, i.e., if the lens is decentered *out*, the induced prism is *base out* (Fig. 14–16). If the plus lens is decentered *up*, the induced prism is *base up*.

When the lens is minus, the decentration shifts opposite from the lens, e.g., if the lens is decentered out (temporally), the induced prism is base in (Fig. 14–17). When a minus lens is decentered up, the induced prism is base down.

When determining the amount of prism induced, the cylinder is counted as part of the lens's power. The power at the vertical meridian is used for any vertical displacement. The power at the horizontal meridian is used for any horizontal displacement.

• *Example 1.*   Rx: + 12.00 Sph OD
                       + 10.00 Sph OS

• *If the optical centers are both displaced 5 mm temporally (decentered out), the induced base-out prism (BO) is:*

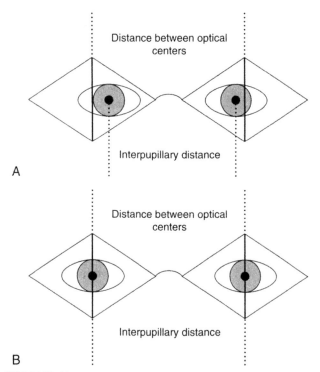

FIGURE 14–14. Whenever optical centers of lenses do not coincide with interpupillary distance of lens wearer, as in *A*, prism is induced. No prism is induced when optical centers of lenses are coincident with interpupillary distance of lens wearer, as in *B*.

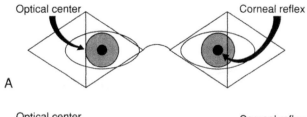

Optical center   Corneal reflex

A

Optical center   Corneal reflex

B

FIGURE 14–15. *A* and *B,* Be careful not to mistake optical center of lens from corneal reflex position.

$$OD = +12.00\,D \times 0.5\,cm \quad BO = 6^\Delta\,BO \quad 5^\Delta + 6^\Delta = 11^\Delta\,BO$$
$$OS = +10.00\,D \times 0.5\,cm \quad BO = 5^\Delta\,BO$$

● **Answer.** *11$^\Delta$ BO*

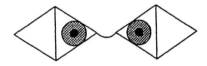

● **Example 2.** *Calculate the induced base-down (BD) prism when a patient looks 5 mm above the optical center when wearing:*

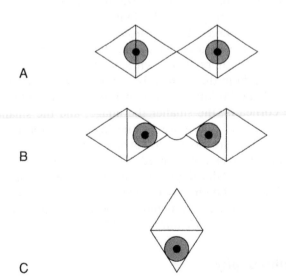

A

B

C

FIGURE 14–16. Plus lenses work as prisms base to base. *A,* No prism induced when optical centers of lenses coincident with interpupillary distance. *B,* Base out prisms induced when lenses are decentered out. *C,* Lens decentered up induces base up prism effect.

$$Rx: \ + 4.00 \quad 4 \times .5 = 2.0^\Delta \quad BD\,OD$$
$$+ 2.00 \quad 2 \times .5 = 1.0^\Delta \quad BD\,OS$$

● **Answer.** *Difference is a net 1$^\Delta$ BD OD induced.*

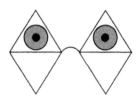

● **Example 3.** *Patient needs −4.00 Sph OU. The right lens needs to be decentered 2$^\Delta$ BO. How much decentration is there and in what direction?*

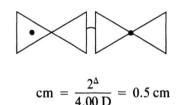

$$cm = \frac{2^\Delta}{4.00\,D} = 0.5\,cm$$

● **Answer.** *OD lens decentered "in" by 5 mm.*

● **Example 4.** *Calculate the induced base-up (BU) prism when a patient looks 5 mm below the optical center when wearing:*

$$Rx: +4.00 \quad +1.00 \times 90$$
$$+1.50 \quad +1.50 \times 180$$

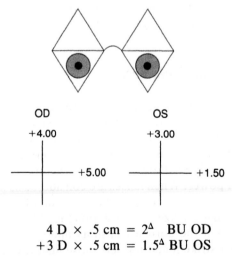

OD   OS
+4.00   +3.00

+5.00   +1.50

$$4\,D \times .5\,cm = 2^\Delta \quad BU\,OD$$
$$+3\,D \times .5\,cm = 1.5^\Delta \quad BU\,OS$$

● **Answer.** $+2^\Delta - 1.50^\Delta = 0.5^\Delta\,BU\,OD$

When a horizontal prism is base-out (BO) over both eyes, or base-in (BI) over both eyes, the power is additive, e.g., 2$^\Delta$ BO OD + 4$^\Delta$ BO OS = 6$^\Delta$ BO, as to correct 6$^\Delta$ esotropia (ET), or induce 6$^\Delta$ exotropia (XT).

Vertical prism power is additive when the bases are opposite over either eye, e.g., 2$^\Delta$ BU OD + 3$^\Delta$ BD

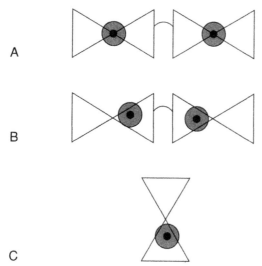

FIGURE 14–17. Minus lenses work as prism apex to apex. *A*, No prism induced when optical center of lenses and interpupillary distance are coincident. *B*, Base in prism induced when lenses are decentered out. *C*, Lens decentered up induces base down effect.

OS = 5^Δ BD OS or 5^Δ BU OD, as to correct 5^Δ left hypertropia (LHT), or induce 5^Δ right hypertropia (RHT).

Usually, decentration is negligible in small refractive errors. With lens strengths greater than 4 D, however, slight changes in optical centers from measured PDs can solve, but may also create, problems. Whenever one eye has a plus lens correction and the other a minus lens correction, prismatic effect creates problems when the patient looks above or below the optical centers. One lens will have BD effect, but the other is BU, thus creating an additive vertical discrepancy.

• PURKINJE'S IMAGES

Convex mirrors act in exactly the opposite fashion as convex lenses. Because the angle of incidence equals the angle of reflection, convex mirrors diverge light rays and produce images behind the mirror at a focal length equal to half the radius of curvature, equivalent to $-2/r$ power. When lenses are considered as mirrors, the radius of curvature can be calculated from the reflected image's size and location (Fig. 14–18).

Although the cornea transmits almost all the light rays that strike it and refracts those light rays because of its convex surface, it does reflect some of the light as a spherical convex mirror does. The reflections, called Purkinje's images, are from four of the optical components of the eye, one each from the anterior and posterior surfaces of the cornea, and one each from the anterior and posterior surfaces of the lens. The brightest is the first Purkinje's image from the anterior surface of the cornea, clinically called the corneal reflex. Because the radius of curvature of the cornea is almost 8 mm, the reflection is located almost 4 mm

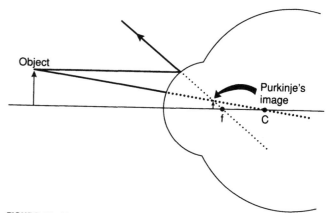

FIGURE 14–18. Eye reflects some light as a mirror, producing Purkinje's images. First Purkinge's image shown.

behind the anterior surface. An 8 mm cornea would have

$$2/r =$$
$$2/.008 =$$
$$-250 \text{ D of power as a mirror,}$$

but only

$$n - 1/r =$$
$$1.337 - 1/.008 =$$
$$.337/.008 =$$
$$+42 \text{ D of power as a refracting lens.}$$

Two applications of the corneal reflex are measurement of strabismus and determination of the radius of curvature of the anterior corneal surface for contact lens calculation.

The corneal curvature is calculated by comparing a projected target of known size and position with the size of its corresponding Purkinje's image. In a keratometer, the target mire is projected onto the cornea; then its images are doubled in the observing microscope. This mire of known size, focused at a fixed distance from the cornea, is compared with the exact size of the Purkinje's image it produces. The steeper the cornea is, the smaller the image, and the smaller the radius of curvature is, the higher the refractive error. The mires lock into correct alignment when the corneal images are focused. The keratometer is calibrated to read the dioptric power directly. Keratometer readings are commonly referred to as the K readings, or simple Ks. By convention, the flatter meridian is recorded first. For example, 43.00/44.00 at 90.

Bibliography

Campbell CJ, Koester CJ, Rittler MC, Tackaberry RB: Physiological Optics. Hagerstown, MD, Harper & Row, 1974.
Corboy JM: The Retinoscopy Book. Thorofare, NJ, Charles B Slack, 1979.

Michaels DD: Visual Optics and Refraction, 3rd ed. St Louis, CV Mosby, 1985.

Milder B, Rubin ML: The Fine Art of Prescribing Glasses, 2nd ed. Gainesville, FL, Triad Scientific, 1991.

Rubin ML: Optics for Clinicians, 2nd ed. Gainesville, FL, Triad Scientific, 1974.

● CHAPTER 14 PHYSIOLOGICAL OPTICS

1. A 45-year-old man has an uncorrected refractive error of −2.00 D. His near point is at _____ cm.
   a. 25
   b. 50
   c. 33
   d. 16
   e. 8

2. Where is the anterior focal point of the reduced eye?
   a. 17 mm in front of the cornea
   b. 5.5 mm behind the cornea
   c. at the front surface of the cornea
   d. on the retina
   e. 22.5 mm in front of the cornea

3. When looking at distance, an uncorrected mild hyperope has
   a. > 60 D power
   b. < 60 D power
   c. < 40 D power
   d. < 44 D power
   e. < 15 D power.

4. What is the type of astigmatism shown?
   a. simple myopic
   b. compound hyperopic
   c. simple hyperopic
   d. mixed
   e. compound myopic

5. A patient is wearing: +6.00 OD and −3.00 OS. His glasses keep slipping down his nose so that he looks 3 mm above both optical centers. How much induced prism does he have?
   a. 3$^\Delta$ BD OD
   b. 2.7$^\Delta$ BU OD
   c. .9$^\Delta$ BD OD
   d. 9$^\Delta$ BU OD
   e. 2.7$^\Delta$ BD OD

Ophthalmic Technical Skills

Basic Skills

HISTORY TAKING

LEARNING OBJECTIVES

● Explain the importance of obtaining an accurate and a concise history
● Outline the order of topics covered in obtaining a history

● Discuss examples of questions designed to provide pertinent information

History taking is one of the first tasks taught to the ophthalmic medical assistant. Often considered easy to learn, it is actually one of the hardest to master. An accurate concise history, taken quickly, is essential for patient evaluation. With it alone, a skilled evaluator can deduce the diagnosis most of the time. Its importance cannot be overemphasized.

History taking develops skills in communication and disease recognition. Questions will vary with each patient. There are no hard and fast rules. Some patients need to be encouraged to give more information whereas others need to be discouraged from giving irrelevant information. Knowing what information to elicit and include and what to discard as extraneous takes much experience. You must sort out the data and reassemble it to reconstruct the progression of the disorder. Is the available information compatible with a tentative diagnosis? Develop skills in combining information until it makes sense. Obvious background history includes previous surgery, previous and current medication, and previous injury to the eye and orbit. Other injuries, medications, and operations may or may not be contributory. Many chronic diseases, e.g., diabetes and hypertension, are known to produce vision problems. Only through experience can questioners focus on pertinent information.

Information volunteered by the patient is unedited. Your job is to edit. Try to verify your interpretation of what the patient says because the patient may not repeat the same history in the same way to the next examiner. Misinterpretations and variations are com-

monplace. For example, blurriness may mean a visual field defect, distortions, ghosting of images, or diplopia. You know that blurriness and diplopia are two distinct entities. Many patients do not make the same distinction. Be as professional as you can. Make the patient feel comfortable about divulging confidential information. *Never* repeat this privileged information other than to your ophthalmologist-employer.

If subsequent examination discloses unexpected abnormalities, ask additional questions. Go back and forth between history and examination until the two sources of information match. Discrepancies indicate an unidentified problem or a wrong tentative diagnosis. The technologist is never responsible for the diagnosis, but must know enough about eye abnormalities to make tentative diagnoses in his or her mind. Otherwise, no progress will be made in history taking in subsequent patients.

A framework for history taking includes:

1. Greeting
2. Chief complaint
3. History of present illness
4. Past ocular history
5. Ocular medications
6. Past medical history
7. Systemic medications
8. Social and vocational history
9. Family ocular history
10. Allergies
11. General information

• GREETING

Call the patient by name. Introduce yourself, explaining that you are an ophthalmic technologist/technician/assistant helping Dr. _____. Explain that you will be obtaining preliminary information and taking measurements. Only when asked should you inform the patient that you can neither diagnose nor provide information about the test results, but that Dr. _____ will do this when all tests are complete. If the patient volunteers the name of a previous consultant, record it. Ask about the referring doctor. If seen previously by someone else, is this a second opinion? Does the patient want a report sent to anyone?

• CHIEF COMPLAINT

You want to obtain a concise and accurate description in one sentence or less of the reason for the visit stated in the patient's words. Your typical question would be:

"What brought you to the office today?"

"What problem are you having with your eyes?"

"How are your eyes bothering you?"

A typical answer would be:

"I have gunk oozing out of my left eye."

"My right eye hurts."

"I need new glasses."

"The doctor scheduled this follow-up visit."

The chief complaint is your guide. It should conjure up a series of questions on your part for pertinent information. Decide from the chief complaint on the urgency of the required care. Is this an emergency situation for the doctor's immediate attention? Before the patient leaves the office, your ophthalmologist must explain to the patient why he or she has the complaint, what it means, and how it should be managed. Technical personnel usually do not have this responsibility.

• HISTORY OF PRESENT ILLNESS

The history is the supporting data for the chief complaint with enough detail to make sense. Write it down in the correct time sequence: how and when it began and in what order the following events occurred.

How has the patient's vision changed? Intermittently, gradually, in one or both eyes? Does the vision appear blurred, double, worse in the dark, with less color? Does the patient have floaters, haloes, rainbows, lightning flashes, rings? Is there pain in the eye around it, behind it? Is it a foreign body sensation on the surface, or deep in the eye or orbit? If the eye is itchy or burning, does the patient have allergies, or wear make-up? Mild headaches may be eye-related. Where are the headaches located? Does the pain radiate? What relieves the pain? Incapacitating headaches are usually not from the eye, unless caused by trauma. Is there a discharge from the eye? Watery, purulent, only in bright light? Eye matted shut in the morning? Crusting on eyelashes? Are the symptoms constant or transient? Has there been trauma? Illness? Is it getting better or worse?

Repeating an unsuccessful treatment usually does not work the second time either. Therefore, record what has already been done. Has the patient taken any medication, had any surgery, had eyeglasses changed recently? Obtained any other advice? By whom (pediatrician, optometrist, family practice physician, another ophthalmologist)? What medications and diagnostic tests were ordered and what were the results?

Ask questions designed to develop tentative diagnoses. Begin to guess possibilities in your mind. The more you know about disease, the more critical the questions you ask.

• PAST OCULAR HISTORY

Ask about eyeglasses. Does the patient have any? Does the patient wear them? How long ago were they prescribed? When were they last changed? Has the patient had this problem before? What other eye problems has he or she had in the past? Trauma? Glaucoma? Lazy eye? Does the patient wear contact lenses? What type, wearing schedule, problems? Any previous eye infections? Surgery?

• OCULAR MEDICATIONS

Determine the names of all ocular medications with dosages, and why they were prescribed. Be specific as to the name and dose of the medication, and ask whether the patient has faithfully used it. Ask about any allergies, side effects, or toxicities to these drugs. Many times patients do not know the drug names. Ask for cap colors. Some types of drugs have specific colors and knowing the color may thereby help identify the drug. Do they need a prescription for this drug?

• PAST MEDICAL HISTORY

Ask about the patient's past medical history, about other illnesses, hospitalizations, chronic conditions, and accidents. With an older patient, add questions about high blood pressure, diabetes, heart problems, strokes (CVAs), transient ischemic attacks (TIAs), arthritis, thyroid dysfunction, seizures, tumors, and how long the patient has been sick. Ask which operations the patient has had and when. With a pediatric patient, ask the parent about pregnancy, birth, and developmental history.

● SYSTEMIC MEDICATIONS

Ask the names of all other medicines and dosages, and why? Tranquilizers? Hormones? For women of childbearing age, ask about birth control pills. Ask about any allergies, side effects, or toxicities with these drugs. What over-the-counter drugs, such as decongestants or antihistamines, is the patient taking? Many elderly patients take too many drugs to remember all the names. Encourage them to write them down at home and carry the list with them at all times. This helps us greatly, but also can be important if the patient suddenly has to go to the emergency room.

● SOCIAL AND VOCATIONAL HISTORY

Obtain information about smoking, alcohol consumption, or drug abuse. Ask the patient for a current job description, including past jobs, e.g., construction worker, arc welder, or tennis player.

VISUAL ASSESSMENT

● FAMILY OCULAR HISTORY

Because many eye problems are hereditary, the family ocular history is pursued. Has anyone in the family had a similar problem? Ask about siblings, children, or parents with glaucoma, blindness, cataracts, retinitis pigmentosa, eye deviations, retinal detachments, diabetes, tumors, or allergy. Expect to have difficulty knowing when to stop asking. All major eye problems in family members are relevant. In African-Americans or patients of Mediterranean origin, ask about sickle cell history.

● ALLERGIES

What allergies or reactions has the patient had to what drugs, dyes (e.g., fluorescein), or contact lens solutions? Does the patient have seasonal allergies to pollens? Describe the reactions, e.g., nausea, vomiting, or hives.

● GENERAL INFORMATION

The fact sheet identifies the patient: name, address, telephone number, age, sex, race, marital status, occupation, and insurance. Each piece of paper added to the chart, e.g., a visual field test, or an ultrasound A scan, must have written on it the patient's name, number, and the date the test was performed.

LEARNING OBJECTIVES

- Understand the necessity for and how to measure vision
- Discuss various methods of measuring visual acuity
- Understand why and when vision is retested with a pinhole
- Understand how to record visual acuity
- Understand when and how to test for potential visual acuity in the preoperative patient with decreased vision
- Explain contrast sensitivity and glare

The brain *sees* only what the eye's optical system can produce as a retinal image. The cornea, aqueous, lens, and vitreous are collectively referred to as the ocular media, the transparent tissues of the eye that have optical power. Cloudiness, opacities, or distortions of these tissues may prevent the eye's optical system from producing a clear retinal image. In addition, transmission from the optic nerve through the optic chiasm, tracts, and radiations to the occipital cortex must not be damaged for accurate interpretation of vision. Excellent vision is proof of normal processing of incoming information along the entire sensory visual pathway.

When asked to look at a vision chart, a normal eye shifts position to image the chart's symbols, called optotypes, directly onto the fovea. This shift results in central fixation because the fovea's ability for fine spatial discrimination produces especially sharp perception of shapes. So for maximum visual acuity there must be a normal fovea, densely packed with cones, within a normal macula.

Normal vision, 20/20 or better, either with correction or without, indicates that the:

1. Cornea, lens, aqueous, and vitreous are clear.
2. Cornea, lens, aqueous, and vitreous have normal resolving power.

3. Fovea is being used for fixation.

4. Foveal cones have normal function.

5. Optic nerve is conveying useful information to the occipital cortex.

6. Visual cortex and its adjacent processing centers have normal function.

Best corrected visual acuity (BCVA) less than 20/25 is abnormal. A major task of an eye examination is to find the cause.

The size of a retinal image depends on the size of the object and its distance from the viewer. The smaller the object we can recognize, or the greater the distance at which it can be recognized, the better the eye's optical system. Twenty feet (six meters) is the standard test distance because rays of light from optical infinity are almost parallel there. (Rays are acutally diverging very weakly with one-sixth of a diopter [D.] of power.) At that distance, virtually no accommodation is required if the patient has no refractive error.

Visual acuity is a measure that evaluates the resolving power of the eye through its cone and rod function, especially in the macula. It is a measure of form vision, distinguishing details and shapes of objects. Vision is usually tested in a darkened room by projecting charts onto a wall screen using a standardized lighting system. This maximizes the contrast of very black symbols (optotypes) on a very white background. Results are tabulated by how well shapes are perceived under these ideal conditions of contrast. Automated instruments such as the Mentor B VAT (Mentor O + O, Inc., Norwell, MA) have almost unlimited changes of optotypes in each size.

Most ophthalmic practices have examination rooms about 12 feet long. A mirror system on the far wall enables the patient looking through to visualize a Snellen chart that has been projected on the wall behind the patient. This works well for most patients except preschool children, who are often confused by this setup.

The minimum angle of resolution (MAR) for eyes in normal observers varies between 30 seconds and one

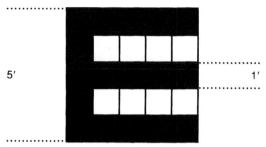

FIGURE 15–1. One minute of arc subtended on the retina is the standard measure of the resolving power of the eye. Each line or space on an optotype subtends 1 minute of arc. The entire optotype subtends 5 minutes of arc.

minute of arc subtended on the retina. If the resolving power of the observer's eye is 30 seconds of arc, he or she can see 20/10. If it is one minute of arc, the observer can see 20/20. Some eyes have better optical systems than others. One minute of arc has become the standard. Each line and each space of an optotype subtend one minute of arc on the retina (Fig. 15–1).

The thickness of each line of a optotype such as a Snellen letter is one-fifth the size of the letter. At a distance of 20 feet (six meters), the 20/20 size letters subtend an angle of five minutes of arc. At 40 feet, the 20/40 size letters subtend an angle of five minutes of arc. At 20 feet, the 20/40 size letters subtend an angle of 10 minutes of arc, and so on (Fig. 15–2).

Visual acuity is measured as a fraction, comparing what should be seen at the testing distance to what is seen, measured by standard clinical tests and distances. The patient with 20/20 vision sees at 20 feet what the average individual sees at 20 feet. If the patient's vision is 20/40, then the patient sees at 20 feet what the normal person theoretically sees at a 40-foot distance, and so on. The numerator is the distance at which the patient is tested, usually 20 feet. The denominator is the distance at which the test object subtends an angle of five minutes of arc on the retina. The denominator is marked on most charts near one end of each line containing optotypes of a given size.

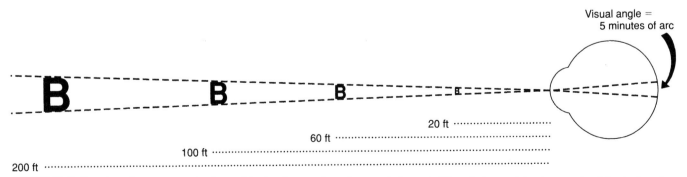

FIGURE 15–2. The size of an optotype is dictated by its distance from the eye. Letters of different sizes subtend an angle of 5 minutes of arc at the specific distance designated. This distance is the denominator when vision is recorded as a fraction. A 20/200 optotype at a 20-foot testing distance is 3 inches overall. Each unit is 5/8 of an inch.

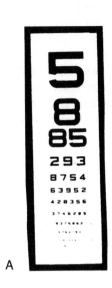

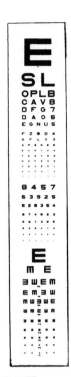

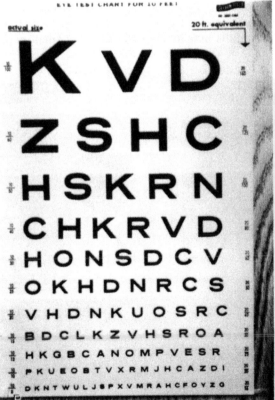

FIGURE 15–3. Examples of visual acuity charts. *A,* Snellen letter and number charts for vision. *B,* Good-lite Sloan letter chart for vision. *C,* Mentor B Vat. (*A,* Redrawn Courtesy of Reichert Ophthalmic Instruments, Buffalo, NY. *B,* Courtesy of Good-lite Co., Forest Park, IL. *C,* Courtesy of Mentor O + O, Inc., Norwell, MA.)

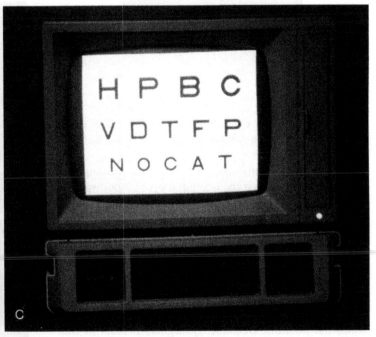

• TESTING STRATEGY

Visual acuity is evaluated at the beginning of each examination on each visit. Exceptions are children with strabismus and emergency patients with chemical burns. Each eye is tested independently while the fel-low eye is covered (occluded). The top segment of bifocal glasses contains the optical correction for distance vision. Testing without spectacle correction is usually not necessary. Only repeat the vision test without the glasses if vision is less than 20/20 with them. If both eyes have excellent vision, approximately

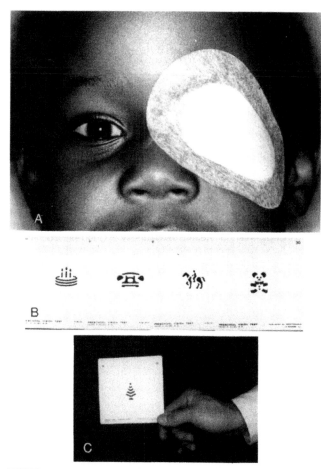

FIGURE 15–4. Allen cards test for preliterate children. *A,* On-the-face patch prevents child from peeking. *B,* Set of Allen cards. *C,* Card presented singly.

is often a better indicator of visual function in patients with latent nystagmus.

By convention, the right eye is tested first, but if one eye has markedly poorer vision, that better eye is often tested first. If you suspect optotypes were memorized with the "good" eye, simply test the "bad" eye with a different chart. During testing, note abnormalities in the manner with which the patient reads the letters. Does the patient miss all the letters on one side (possible field defect)? Are the letters read quickly and correctly on one line, with the next line reported to be completely blurred (possible malingerer)? Some optotypes are easier to recognize than others. Charts using the recommended Sloan letters (D S R K V O H N Z C) make for better uniformity of difficulty (Fig. 15–3).

Especially for children, test a whole line of optotypes rather than isolated test objects whenever possible. Only when vision cannot be otained otherwise are isolated optotypes used, e.g., Allen cards. A patient with amblyopia resolves smaller letters with isolated optotypes better than with a whole line of optotypes (Fig. 15–4).

If the vision is less than 20/30 without correction, the vision is retested using a multiple pinhole. Each 1.5-mm pinhole acts as an artificial, very small pupil,

20/20, the binocular acuity is often one line better than the vision in each eye independently; in this case, maybe 20/15. Test a whole line of optotypes, not isolated ones.

Patients, especially children, may be reading the chart with both eyes if the occluded eye is incompletely covered. The occluder before the eye not being tested should rest against the nose to prevent peeking. Suspect peeking or nystagmus with a null point when the patients adopts an unusual head posture. To avoid peeking, children should be tested whenever possible with a stick-on patch rather than a hand-held occluder.

If a patient with nystagmus has a preferred abnormal head posture, vision is tested with the head in this abnormal positon. Because nystagmus is least in that position, vision is best. Sometimes, if there is nystagmus, additional latent nystagmus may decrease monocular vision. When tested binocularly (both eyes at the same time), the latent component disappears. Vision often improves dramatically. The nystagmus may dampen, and vision may improve when the patient is tested with both eyes open. This is an exception to the rule that each eye is tested independently because it

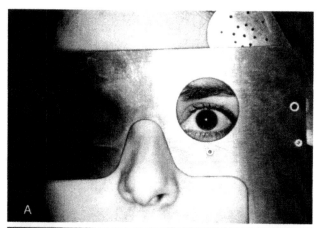
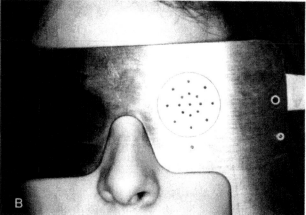

FIGURE 15–5. DaLaur occluder. *A,* with pinhole lifted out of the way. *B,* With pinhole in place.

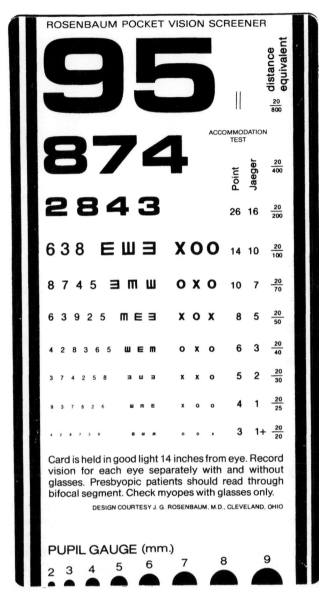

FIGURE 15–6. Near vision card.

comparatively large change in the visual angle subtended on the retina. If near vision is 20/20 but distance vision is poorer than 20/40, suspect myopia. If near vision in an adult is poorer than distance vision, suspect presbyopia. All patients over the age of 40 years need a near vision assessment. Poor vision with a pinhole, approximately 20/200 or less, both distance and near, indicates a nonrefractive cause of the decreased vision. Your ophthalmologist will investigate for an opacity or a disease (Fig. 15–6).

Best corrected vision (BCV) is what is obtained with the refractive correction that gives the best resolution of the smallest letters.

Best corrected vision less than 20/200 in the better seeing eye is part of the definition of legal blindness. With no corneal or lens irregularity, it indicates that central vision is lost. Many abnormalities of the eyes and visual system produce undetected painless progressive loss of vision.

Certain psychological factors, such as attention, motivation, and intelligence, affect vision test results. Patients may see better than they admit. They see only as well as they want to, or try, because it is a subjective test. Obtaining an accurate visual acuity in an adult patient with normal vision and average intelligence is easy. If there is mental immaturity, senility, subnormal intelligence, or visual deficit, it becomes more difficult. If a patient reads the 20/50 line easily with no mistakes and no hesitation, then claims he or she can see no further, your interpretation should be that the next line is not as clear, the patient is not sure of what he or she sees, and wants to avoid making a mistake. Your job is to encourage the patient to read the smaller optotypes. Patients often say they cannot see letters when they mean they are not sure they can recognize them. Strategies such as: "Try this next line anyway" or "Tell me what you *think* you see," are warranted. If the 20/20 line is read correctly, do not stop. Continue farther down the Snellen chart until the patient no longer correctly identifies more than half the letters on a line. Only when the patient attempts to recognize optotypes but misses more than half the line has the limit been reached. Now you can record the visual acuity. Children and the elderly need the most prodding in the gentlest manner you can manage.

● PRELITERATES

Whole line Snellen chart is the most universal method for accurate assessment of vision. Since the advent of Sesame Street on TV, many preschool children can recognize Snellen letters. For most patients over the age of four, test using these standard charts.

Many children respond better at a 10-foot distance. A standard chart held at 10 feet changes the numerator

increasing the depth of focus. Only parallel rays from the viewed object that are not refracted enter the eye. The blur circles from this uncorrected lens system are made smaller, thus more in focus. Improved vision through a pinhole indicates a refractive error, a defect in the power of an eye's multiple lens system that can be corrected by eyeglasses or contact lenses. A corrective lens will improve the vision at least to the level obtained through the pinhole. Vision can often be improved an additional line or two over the pinhole vision (Fig. 15–5).

If vision is still poor at distance with a pinhole, the decrease is probably not caused by a refractive error in the eye's optical system. Test near vision. Use the exact testing distance indicated on the near vision chart, usually 14 inches from the eye. A small change in the distance at which the near card is held has a

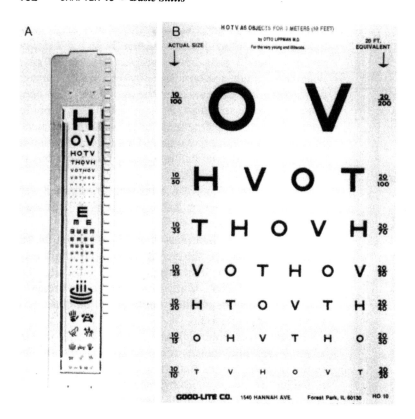

FIGURE 15-7. HOTV vision test. *A*, Slide for projector. *B*, Ten-foot distance wall chart. (Courtesy of Good-lite Co., Forest Park, IL.)

but not the denominator. The 20/20 line, identified at 10 feet, is recorded as 10/20 (equivalent to 20/40). In preschoolers, 20/40 is acceptable as normal vision. Comparison of vision between the eyes is more important than obtaining 20/20 (Fig. 15-7).

Preschool children are often not able to discriminate their letters and numbers well enough for testing purposes. Less accurate methods are available. In all children older than two and a half years, an attempt is made to teach them the HOTV matching game. The child need not verbalize. He just points at the matching optotype on the master card he holds. If the child needs single optotypes and is verbal, try the four plastic Allen cards where the patient has to name the picture on the card. It does not matter whether the birthday cake is called a boat, as long as the child is consistent. With these cards the denominator is 30, the numerator the farthest distance (in feet) that the cards are recognized. Testing with either Allen cards or HOTV begins one foot away. The examiner backs away a few feet each time he changes cards. Over 20 feet away, HOTV charts can be used in similar fashion to Snellen charts.

The illiterate E is falling out of favor. Although the test appears to have four options, up, down, right, and left, it often has only two options. Preliterate children have not mastered their directions. The examiner often has to settle for the child's recognition of a vertical or a horizontal orientation only.

• FIXATION TESTS

If a child is too immature for visual acuity to be subjectively tested, but there is a strabismus present, difference in vision is assessed using the following binocular fixation pattern descriptions. The descriptions are central (C), steady (S), and maintained (M). Central and steady may be determined with either eye separately. Maintained refers to which eye keeps fixing straight at the target when neither eye is covered (Fig. 15-8). When a child with a deviation spontaneously alternates, vision is equal. This is designated as CSM in either eye. With the first look, decide which eye is the straight fixing eye. That eye's vision is CSM. When that eye is covered, the other eye should straighten to look at your target. That is worth C. If the eye steadily stays straight, that is worth S. If this second eye fails, either by being UC (for UnCentral), or US for (UnSteady), then this second eye will redeviate as soon as the cover is removed. That is worth UM (for UnMaintained). Even if this second eye is CS, it may not maintain when the first eye is uncovered. To earn the designation M, this second eye has to stay straight while the first eye remains deviated through a blink, about six seconds. If this occurs, you have forced the child to alternate, because now the previously deviated second eye is straight. Vision is probably equal.

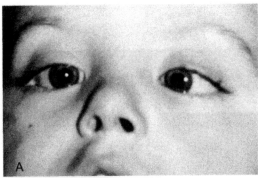

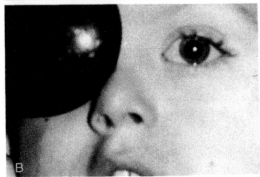

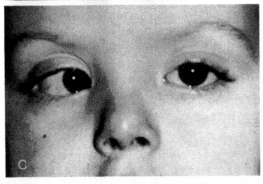

FIGURE 15–8. Assessment in a preverbal child for equal vision in both eyes using the fixation preference technique. *A,* On first look, the child is fixing with the right eye. Therefore, VOD = CSM, C = CENTRAL, S = STEADY, M = MAINTAINED. *B,* When the right eye is occluded, the child fixes steadily with the left eye. Therefore, VOS = CS. No assessment of MAINTAINED possible. *C,* when the right eye occluder is removed, the child continues to fix with the left eye. That is MAINTAINED. Therefore, VOS = CSM.

If vision in the poorer eye is UCUSUM, vision is thought to be less than 20/200. If CSUM, vision is thought to be about 20/200. If the poorer eye holds fixation briefly, a few seconds, vision is approximately 20/70. If fixation is maintained to a blink, about five seconds, vision is considered to be about 20/40. Distinguish between picking up fixation (CS) when the preferred eye is covered, and maintaining fixation (M) when the preferred eye is uncovered.

In preferential looking testing, an infant is held in front of a gray screen with a window. Infants are tested 38 cm from the screen, toddlers 55 cm away, and preschoolers 84 cm away. A gray rectangle, with black and white grating pattern stripes toward one side, is placed so as to obstruct the window. The theory is that the infant prefers the pattern of black and white stripes, if perceived, to the blank screen. A peephole in the middle allows the observer to note whether the child looks at the black and white grating pattern. Vision is estimated using the card with the narrowest stripe width that attracts the infant's attention. The narrower the black and white stripes are, the greater the cycles per degree. Visual acuity is estimated by converting the cycles per degree of the gratings to Snellen equivalents. With this test vision is often 20/100 by 12 months of age, 20/50 by 18 months, and 20/25 by 24 months. The advantages are the speed that the patterns can be evaluated and the young age that can be quantitated (Fig. 15–9).

CLINICAL VISUAL PSYCHOPHYSICS
Tom M. Maida

Decreased vision can have many causes. Finding the cause of poor vision is often difficult if a cloudy cornea or lens prevents viewing the retina or optic nerve. If the optical defect in the cornea or lens is eliminated, vision will improve if the retina can still produce a clear image and the sensory visual pathway is intact. Vision will not improve if the retina or optic nerve is defective, no matter how well the image is focused or how well the optical system is corrected. Various tests may help predict preoperatively what the patient may see postoperatively following removal of an opacity (e.g., cataract surgery).

• INSTRUMENTATION

The clarity of the view of the retina through a direct ophthalmoscope provides a rough measure of expected image degradation. Multiple pinhole testing, especially when the patient's pupils are dilated, is another measure, often improving vision if the deficit is caused by a corneal or lens defect.

Laser interferometry is a more sophisticated technique designed to bypass optical media defects in an attempt to establish the degree of impairment caused by opacities. This technique produces a clear image on the retina by bypassing the eye's optical system and any media opacities, focusing through the clearest remaining optical path. The size of the gratings is decreased and the number per unit area (spatial frequency) is increased until the subject can no longer detect them. This size is then converted into a Snellen equivalent. When performing interferometry, each eye

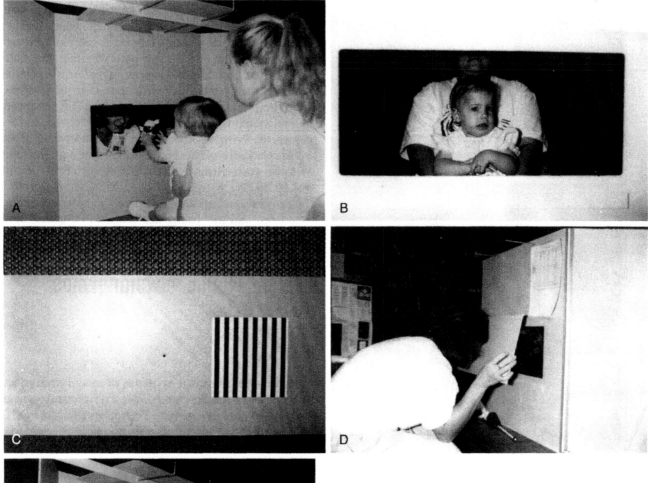

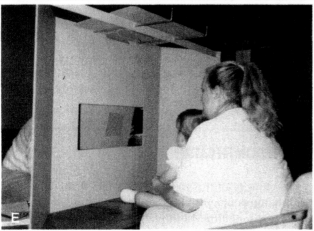

FIGURE 15–9. Assessment in a preverbal child of retinal grating acuity using the preferential looking technique. *A,* The examiner catches the child's attention with a puppet. *B,* The examiner's view behind the window. *C,* Card with a central peephole for the examiner and 0.64 cycles/cm (0.49 cycles/degree) stripe width. When viewed 38 cm away, (toddler distance), this is equivalent to 20/1200 Snellen. *D,* Examiner presenting the card while looking through the central peephole for the child's reaction. *E,* The child prefers to fixate stripes (when large enough to detect) rather than gray background. (Teller Acuity Cards, Courtesy of Vistech Consultant Services, Dayton, OH.)

is tested separately. By testing the ability of the retina to send information into the nervous system independent of the ocular refractive media, it estimates potential visual acuity in the presence of opacities (e.g., cataracts). Gratings (striped graded pattern) are projected optically onto the retina from a safe, low power, helium-neon laser beam. The gratings may be presented vertically, horizontally, or obliquely. The patient identifies the orientation. It is often useful to allow the patient to ''look for'' the pattern after describing the procedure. Most patients understand if you tell them to look at the center circle, looking for alternating red and black stripes.

Laser interferometers optically divide one light ray into two beams close together, then focus the two pinpoints of coherent laser light through the pupil into the anterior segment of a patient's dilated eye. All entering light is focused through these two pinpoints. Only 2% of the light from the interferometer has to reach the retina for an interference fringe to be projected onto it.

Testing Procedure: Visual Acuity (VA)

1. Test with glasses or contract lenses on, if the patient wears them.
2. Seat the patient twenty feet (six meters) from the chart.
3. Instruct the patient to cover, not press, the left eye with an occluder.
4. Ask the patient to read the largest letter with the uncovered right eye.
5. Ask the patient to read two or three letters that you randomly select on every other line down the chart until the patient slows down or begins missing letters.
6. The number at the end of the smallest line where more than half the optotypes were correctly identified is recorded as the denominator.
7. Record 20 as the numerator.
8. If acuity is less than 20/20, repeat the test without glasses. If no improvement, test with a multiple pinhole before the right eye, keeping the left eye covered.
9. Repeat procedure for the left eye with the right eye covered.
10. If the patient's vision is too poor to recognize the largest optotypes, usually 20/200 or 20/400:
    a. Hold a 20/200 size "E" (3" letter) at 20 feet.
    b. Walk closer to the patient one foot at a time until the direction of the "E" is recognized.

The numerator is the distance in feet where the "E" is recognized. The denominator is 200.

c. If vision is so poor that the "E" is not recognized at five feet from the patient, hold differing numbers of fingers three or four times at 15 inches from the eye for recognition of counts fingers (CF) vision. Fingers are about the same size as the 20/200 E.
d. If the patient cannot accurately count fingers, move your hand either in a horizontal or vertical direction at 15 inches for recognition of hand movements (HM) vision.
e. If the patient cannot assess hand movements, turn a fixation light on and off from the left, from the right, from below and above, for detection of light perception (LP) vision, with (LP + P) or without projection.
f. If the patient cannot tell whether the light is on or off, there is no light perception, recorded as NLP.

11. If needed, near acuity is measured at 14 inches, (35 cm) with the near card. The procedure is the same. *The near chart distance is critical.* Near acuity is recorded in Snellen ratios or the Jaeger notation found on the card.

Because mild to moderate cataracts are not uniformly opaque throughout the lens, the examiner attempts to shine the light through any clear areas in the opacity.

Concentric wavefronts from the coherent beams diverge and interfere, resulting in high contrast, striped light and dark interference fringe patterns falling on the retina. A light band has an *in-phase* fringe with a low frequency. A dark band has an *out-of-phase* fringe with a high frequency. By changing the separation between the two beams, the images move closer together or farther apart. A 1.1 mm spacing of images produces a grating that subtends one minute of visual angle, or

Helpful Hints

1. Test vision (V) before all other tests, except for children with misalignments and patients with emergency chemical burns.
2. If vision is 20/20 or better with glasses worn, testing without them is not indicated.
3. Encourage patients to read the smaller optotypes.
4. Do not stop with the 20/20 line. Many patients can see 20/15, and some can see 20/10.
5. Suspect peeking or nystagmus when the patient attempts reading with an unusual head posture.
6. Improvement in vision tested through a pinhole (ph) indicates a refractive error. If no improvement, record as NI (no improvement).
7. Visual acuity is a ratio. The numerator is the testing distance. The denominator refers to the size of the smallest optotype the patient identifies.
8. Record which test is used at each evaluation and whether the patient is tested with refractive correction, cc (cum correctio), or without refractive correction, sc (sine correctio).
9. The right eye, OD (oculus dexter), is recorded first. The left eye, OS (oculus sinister), below it. For example:

    VOD cc 20/200 ph NI
    VOS sc 20/40 ph 20/20−
    or
    VOD   20/70   20/25
         sc   ph
    VOS   20/50   20/25

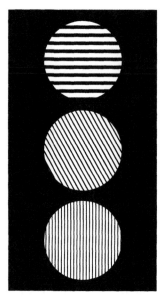

FIGURE 15–10. Retinal grating acuity as tested by laser interferometry.

the equivalent of 20/20. Laser acuity, determined by the finest stripe pattern the patient can identify, is a measure of retinal grating acuity. Optimum retinal grating acuity as measured by interferometry is about one minute of arc (Fig. 15–10).

As the lens changes with cataract development, the refraction changes frequently. These changes in refraction are not usually prescribed, but a best-corrected visual acuity is found on each visit. The patient need not wear his or her correction for testing, however, because refractive errors do not influence the interference fringes. Pupillary testing and fundoscopy with its bright lights should be done enough in advance so that the patient has no after images that might interfere

with interpretation of the fringes. Pupils are dilated, especially with opacity in the center of the lens or cornea. Results are most accurate when only partial lens opacities are present. Patient cooperation and understanding are limiting factors.

Another method to estimate how well the patient may see after cataract extraction is the potential acuity meter (PAM). This instrument attaches to the slit lamp and projects a tiny beam of light containing a brightly illuminated Snellen acuity chart through the less dense areas of a cataractous lens, essentially bypassing the cataract. Depending on how well the Snellen letters are perceived, postoperative acuity can be predicted. The test is easier to perform than laser interferometry.

Serous macular detachments, cystoid macular edema, retinal pigment epithelium (RPE) atrophy, central scotomas, early retinal detachments, macular cysts or holes, and amblyopia have been reported to provide a falsely positive potential visual acuity. The method may produce erroneous results in the presence of certain types of pathology, such as macular disease, or very dense opacities. If the patient has been diagnosed with one of these clinical conditions, the interferometer results will not reliably predict postoperative acuity. The potential acuity meter does not overpredict postoperative vision with age-related macular disease. If the patient does not have one of these conditions, but does have a mild cataract or an opaque membrane requiring a capsulotomy, the acuity estimate is highly reliable.

The acuity visual evoked potential (VEP) is similar to laser interferometry with a difference in the recording site. It picks up the electrical response from the surface of the skull as viewed on the face of a video monitor instead of a verbalized response by the patient. It is most useful in young children with dense cataracts.

Technique for Laser Interferometry

1. Test the better eye first.
2. Instruct the patient to identify the direction of the striped pattern by moving his or her hand in the same direction, allowing the eye and head to remain as still as possible.
3. If the patient begins to describe disorganized stars, worms, dots, or wavy lines, listen to the description but then instruct that they be ignored.
4. Focus the beam in the center of the pupil at the plane of the iris.
5. Ask the patient to indicate the direction of the alternating light and dark stripes seen in the central circular field, ignoring outer spirals of light.
6. Continue to the narrowest stripes the patient can identify for each meridian.
7. If the patient cannot identify the widest stripes, move the beam around in the pupil to improve the penetration of the striped pattern, with the patient's help.
8. Instruct the patient to concentrate on the clearest stripes in the brightest areas of the vision field.
9. Repeat the test on the patient's poorer eye.

• CONTRAST SENSITIVITY

Contrast sensitivity testing determines the retina's ability to detect subtle differences in brightness or shading of gray between targets and their backgrounds. The difference in brightness between the target and its background can be barely discerned. Under these conditions, contrast is low and contours indistinct. The test measures the contrast necessary to detect the luminance of alternating light and dark stripes (sinusoidal gratings) at various sizes. Clinical and laboratory research suggests that contrast sensitivity may be a more sensitive indicator of visual dysfunction than standard visual acuity. This method of evaluating vision more closely mimics real life visual demands. Instead of measuring maximum resolution at very high contrast, like a Snellen chart, this measures the minimum contrast necessary for resolution of each target size.

Contrast sensitivity changes, especially for the smallest sizes (high spatial frequencies), can sometimes be detected before visual deficits affect acuity. Because it is frequently abnormal when Snellen vision remains normal, it has been advocated for early screening for ocular disorders. Several ocular conditions, including multiple sclerosis, glaucoma, cataracts, and retinal and optic nerve disease, can alter contrast sensitivity function. Conditions that alter clarity or curvature of the cornea such as corneal edema, keratoconus, and refractive keratoplasty can also cause reduction in contrast sensitivity. Contrast sensitivity tests often detect and document subtle visual loss from optic nerve disease and neurological disease as well as immature cataracts. The loss is similar for all types of visual pathology. Because decreased contrast sensitivity is a nonspecific sign, it cannot differentiate disease processes. By itself it cannot be used to justify cataract extraction.

Visual acuity decreases when contrast decreases, especially at low light levels. That is why some patients complain they cannot see as well outside the examining room as when tested inside the examining room. An elevation of contrast threshold occurs at higher spatial frequencies in some amblyopes. Even when a patient has relatively good acuity of better than 20/30, with retinitis pigmentosa or rod-cone dystrophy, there is relative loss of sensitivity to smaller gratings (middle to higher spatial frequencies). An overall response effect is usually caused by optic neuritis and multiple sclerosis.

Testing

Most contrast sensitivity tests use sinusoidal wave gratings that vary in both contrast and spatial frequency. In a grating, one cycle has two elements, a light stripe and a dark stripe. With 30 cycles per degree (CPD) of visual angle, 60 elements are present. Because a degree is 60 minutes, each element of a 30 cpd pattern subtends one minute of arc. Their spatial frequency is expressed as the number of cycles per degree, i.e., the number of times the pattern of light and dark bars repeats in the space of a degree of visual space. At low spatial frequencies, the bars are wide and widely spaced. At higher spatial frequencies, the bars are narrower and closer together.

Early contrast sensitivity tests, presented vertical sine wave bars of various frequencies that slowly increased in contrast. The patient responded when the bars first become visible. These tests provided no means by which the examiner could determine patient reliability. An overly anxious patient might respond before the bars are actually visible. A hesitant patient might wait until the bars are dark enough to be "absolutely sure." All this despite the fact that patients are asked to scan the targets because low contrast targets disappear if stared at.

To avoid this pitfall, contrast systems began to incorporate *forced choice* testing, presenting gratings at various angles. The patients are encouraged to guess even if they are not sure. The last correct choice is recorded for each spatial frequency. The simplest and most common test of this type is the Vistech VCTS wall chart (Vistech Consultants, Inc., Dayton, OH) with grids of various sizes and contrast. The gratings in each of the five rows are of a different spatial frequency. The level of normal contrast sensitivity varies depending on the spatial frequency of the characters. Contrast sensitivity is greatest on midrange spatial frequency (five to ten cycles/degree) and less at high and low spatial frequencies.

In each of the tests that include both the contrast and spatial frequency, patient responses to the two variables are plotted on a graph and compared with a normal curve. Pelli Robson contrast charts eliminate the variable of spatial frequency. The lettered charts of 20/100 characters decrease in contrast only. This has the added advantage of presenting the familiar format of lettered charts. This type of testing is undergoing rapid advances. How soon before the tests mentioned will be supplanted is speculative, but it will not be surprising.

• GLARE

Projected visual acuity charts provide a means of determining a patient's vision in nearly optimal conditions. Yet some patients complain about disability in bright surroundings such as sunlight outdoors. Glare is a light stimulus not near a fixation target that can raise the threshold of the macula and decrease visibility of the target.

Technique for Mentor BAT

1. Darken the room illumination.
2. Fit the patient with best corrected distance correction.
3. For testing the right eye, occlude the left eye, and have the patient hold the BAT vertically against the spectacles or eyebrow.
4. With the BAT turned off, instruct the patient to read the smallest line of optotypes possible.
5. Record.
6. Turn the BAT to its lowest illumination, wait at least 30 seconds, and repeat testing vision, preferably from a different chart.
7. Record.
8. Repeat with the BAT at its medium, and then high, illumination.
9. Now occlude the right eye, and test the left eye.

Glare is produced by scattering of light caused by material in the light's path. A common glare source in the eye is caused by protein particles in the anterior chamber (*flare*). Patients with intraocular lenses, cataracts, other media opacities, and postoperative radial keratomies are likely to be disabled by glare. Glare in bright sunlight, or while driving at night, is particularly noticeable.

Glare disability, the decrease in vision or contrast sensitivity caused by sources of glare, is generally not detected in routine vision testing. Real world vision requires recognition of details against an infinitely variable background, hardly the ideal high-contrast condition. Glare testing is more specific for visual disability from immature cataracts than contrast sensitivity. A glare tester measures contrast discrimination in less than ideal conditions, i.e., in the presence of glare. No standard method for measuring glare disability exists among the various instruments currently available.

With the Mentor BAT (Brightness Acuity Tester), the patient is tested in the dark, seated at the 20-foot distance from a standard, illuminated, projected acuity chart. Visual acuity is tested four times in succession under different lighting conditions while the eye being tested views the chart through the 12-mm opening in the BAT. The test is performed before dilation with the patient wearing his or her best correction. The first test is with the BAT turned off, simulating normal visual acuity testing conditions. The second test is with the BAT on its lowest setting, equivalent to conditions in a room with overhead fluorescent lighting. The third test is at the BAT medium setting, equivalent to lighting conditions out-of-doors on a concrete sidewalk on a cloudy day. The fourth test is at the BAT highest setting, equivalent to lighting conditions out-of-doors on a concrete sidewalk with direct overhead sunlight.

Not more than a one line difference should occur in patients without ocular opacities or distortions. Often mild posterior subcapsular cataracts will reduce vision from 20/20 under standard testing condition to 20/50

with high illumination. If vision improves, suspect a residual refractive error.

Visual Assessment

1. When visual acuity is 20/40, the smallest size letter recognized on the retina subtends which angle?
   a. 5 minutes of arc
   b. 1 minute of arc
   c. 40 seconds of arc
   d. 10 minutes of arc
   e. 20 seconds of arc

2. When recording visual acuity as a ratio, what does the second number represent?
   a. testing distance from eye
   b. rod function
   c. minimum angle of resolution of retina
   d. distance where optotype subtends 5 minutes of arc on retina
   e. best corrected visual acuity

3. When visual acuity improves using a multiple pinhole, what does it indicate that the patient has?
   a. macular defect
   b. presbyopia
   c. refractive error
   d. legal blindness
   e. nystagmus

4. How can vision be tested in most preverbal children?
   a. binocular fixation preference
   b. Snellen letters
   c. Allen cards
   d. contrast sensitivity
   e. HOTV chart

5. What does contrast sensitivity test?
   a. ability to detect minimal brightness differences with alternating light and dark gray stripes
   b. color vision by two different methods
   c. visual acuity decrease as contrast sensitivity increases
   d. ability to detect maximal differences in spatial frequencies
   e. change in spatial frequency as glare increases

PUPIL FUNCTION

The pupil, the circular opening in the middle of the iris diaphragm, is the keyhole of the eye. It acts much like the aperture of a camera, regulating the amount of entering light by changing its opening's size. In dim illumination, the pupil enlarges. Pupil dilation is called mydriasis. In bright illumination, the pupil gets smaller. Pupil constriction is called miosis. Two muscles of the iris, the sphincter pupillae and the dilator pupillae, control pupil size. The sphincter dominates. Both pupil size and pupil reaction are controlled by the autonomic nervous system (ANS). Both the central and peripheral nervous systems stimulate pupil function.

• AFFERENT PUPIL PATHWAYS

The outer segments of the rods and cones are the receptor organs both for vision and for pupillary light reflex. Stimulation by light excites the rods and cones, sending signals to the bipolar cells, then to the ganglion cells. Ganglion cell axons constitute the nerve fiber layer that exits the eye as the optic nerve. Eighty percent of the axons in the optic nerve are for vision. Twenty percent are for pupil function. Visual and pupillary fibers appear identical. Axons for vision have different pathways and connections than axons for pupil function however. The incoming information to the brain from the afferent pupillary fibers follows the same course back from the optic nerve to the optic tract, as does the incoming information from the sensory visual fibers. As each optic tract swings around from the front of the midbrain to the back, it keeps the incoming visual fibers but the pupillary fibers go their separate ways, entering the brain stem above the superior colliculus to synapse in the pretectal nucleus (Fig. 15–11).

Some interconnecting interneurons cross through the posterior commissure to the opposite pretectal nucleus, whereas some interneurons run around the cerebral aqueduct to the ipsilateral Edinger-Westphal (E-W) subnucleus, where another synapse occurs. The E-W subnucleus is the sphincter center of the pupillary light reflex as well as the center for accommodation, with more fibers for accommodation than for light reaction. No pupillary fibers transmit messages higher than the posterior commissure in the midbrain. None travel to any of the cerebral lobes, making *the system for response to light entirely subcortical.*

• EFFERENT PATHWAY

The returning motor pathway for the light reflex, as well as accommodation, is with parasympathic fibers that leave the E-W nucleus, traveling to the orbit as

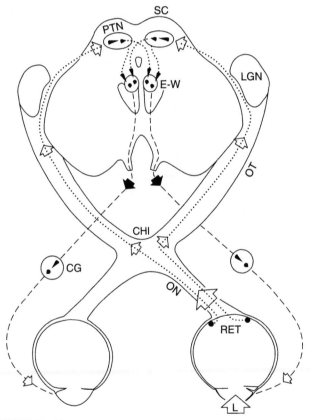

FIGURE 15–11. Pupillary pathway for light. Light (L) entering eye stimulates retinal nerve fibers (RET) that travel in optic nerve (ON) to chiasm (CHI). Temporal fibers travel uncrossed in left optic tract (OT), whereas nasal fibers cross to the right optic tract. Light fibers leave the optic tract before it ends in the lateral geniculate nucleus (LGN) to enter the pretectal nuclei (PTN) where they synapse. Crossed and uncrossed fibers travel around the cerebral acqueduct to enter both Edinger-Westphal (E-W) nuclei. Parasympathetic motor fibers leave the midbrain within the third (oculomotor) cranial nerve (CN III). In the orbit, the nerve fibers for light leave the oculomotor nerve as the motor root to the ciliary ganglion (CG). After synapsing, postganglionic nerve fibers enter the eye through the short ciliary nerves. (From Glaser JS: Neuro-Ophthalmology. Hagerstown, MD, Harper & Row, 1978.)

part of the oculomotor CN III. The inferior division of this nerve first loses the medial rectus fibers, then the inferior rectus fibers. It then loses the pupillary light fibers that travel to the ciliary ganglion where they synapse before entering at the back end of the eyeball through the short ciliary nerves. These motor pupillary fibers innervate the sphincter pupillae muscle of the iris, a circular band of unstriated muscle fibers surrounding the pupil, which tighten as they contract, like pursestrings, thus decreasing pupil size (pupil constriction), allowing less light to enter. Other parasympathetic fibers reach the ciliary body, providing innervation for accommodation.

Innervation to the iris dilator muscle comes from sympathetic nerve fibers in the nasociliary nerve. These fibers enter the eye through the long ciliary nerves, bypassing the ciliary ganglion. The iris dilator contains radial muscle fibers, like spokes on a wheel, which originate in the peripheral iris and extend nearly to the pupil margin. Contraction of the dilator pupillae enlarges pupil size, allowing more light to enter. The balance between antagonistic sympathetic and parasympathetic innervation to the pupil constantly fluctuates. As one relaxes, the other contracts (Fig. 15–12).

• SYNKINETIC NEAR REFLEX

A relationship known as the synkinetic near response is a triad of simultaneous but separate reactions to approaching objects that is controlled by the oculomotor CN III. The three responses are miosis, accommodation, and convergence. Although convergence and miosis exist independently, accommodation always occurs in conjunction with the other two. As an object is brought closer to the eyes from infinity, both accommodation, to keep the image clear, and convergence, to keep the image single, are necessary. As fixation is moved from a distance to a closer position, innervation travels to the iris sphincter, the ciliary muscles, and the medial recti, to trigger simultaneous pupillary con-

striction, accommodation, and convergence. As the object gets closer, the image falls behind the retina, and appears blurred. This signals the ciliary muscle to contract, increasing accommodation. The image also falls on disparate temporal points, which produces double vision. This signals convergence by contraction of the medial recti to bring the image back onto both foveas, eliminating the double vision. At the same time, the iris sphincter contracts, decreasing pupil size. Pupillary constriction increases the depth of focus, maximizing the eye's resolving power and helping to achieve optimal stereoacuity. Current opinion is that miosis is coupled with convergence more than with accommodation. It is not known how these three mechanisms are linked.

The occipitomesencephalic pathway for accommodation is probably similar to the pursuit pathway from the occipital lobe to the midbrain. The tract runs from the occipital cortex into the upper part of the brain stem. However, this tract for near then travels through the ventral portion of the midbrain to the E-W portion of the CN III nucleus, not through the dorsal superior colliculi as do the fibers for light. The final common motor pathway for the synkinetic near reflex is through the oculomotor CN III with convergence from medial rectus fibers and accommodation and miosis from parasympathetic fibers (Fig. 15–13).

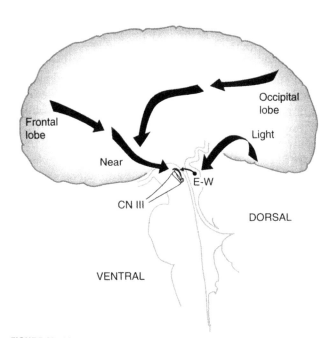

FIGURE 15–13. Pupillary pathways for light and for near are separate. Near nerve fibers from the frontal and occipital area for accommodation enter the Edinger-Westphal (E-W) nuclei from the ventral side of the midbrian. Nerve fibers for light enter the pretectal nuclei from the dorsal side of the midbrain. (From Thompson HS: The Innervation of the Pupillary Sphincter, Section 5. Neuroanatomy and Neuroophthalmology; Ophthalmology Basic and Clinical Course, 1974, p 57.)

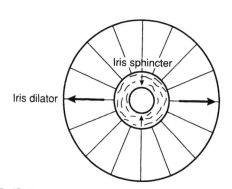

FIGURE 15–12. Schematic diagram of function of iris sphincter and iris dilator muscles.

● FUNCTION

Pupil size in older children is about 4 mm; in infants and older people it is smaller, about 2 mm; in adults it is about 3 mm. Blue and myopic eyes have larger pupils than brown and hyperopic eyes. The sphincter maximally constricts pupil size to 1.5 mm. The dilator maximally dilates pupil size to 8 mm.

Ten percent of the population has anisocoria (difference in pupil size). It is physiological (within normal limits) if the difference is less than 1 millimeter. It is essential anisocoria (benign anisocoria, central anisocoria) if the difference is more than 1 millimeter but pharmacological drug testing (e.g., pilocarpine) reveals no defect. Both physiological and essential anisocoria have a +4 reaction to light in both eyes. The difference in pupil size is maintained under normal room light and in the dark.

● SWINGING FLASHLIGHT TEST

Two types of light reaction, direct and consensual, work in tandem. A bright light, such as that from an indirect ophthalmoscope, is held at cheek level to one side as the patient looks into the distance to prevent interference from accommodation. The light beam should be small enough to stimulate only one eye as it is crisply moved from one eye to the other, about every three seconds. A second dim light may be held to the side of the nonstimulated eye for improved observation of both pupils. Both pupils should stay the same size. When a normal eye is illuminated, both eyes respond briskly with a marked decrease in pupil size to about 1.5 mm (Fig. 15–14). The second eye, when illuminated, should stay the same small size. Direct light stimulation of one eye tests the impulses from one eye traveling by the afferent pathway to the E-W nucleus, then back

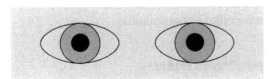

Pupils mid-dilated in dim illumination

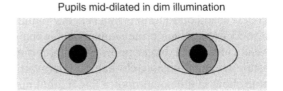

Pupils mid-dilated in dim illumination

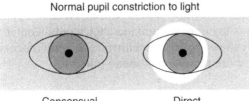

Normal pupil constriction to light

Consensual   Direct

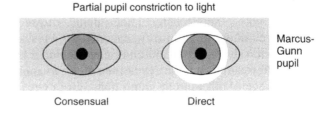

Partial pupil constriction to light

Consensual   Direct

Marcus-Gunn pupil

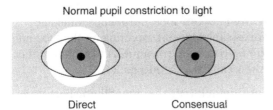

Normal pupil constriction to light

Direct   Consensual

A. Normal response

Normal pupil constriction to light

Direct   Consensual

B. RAPD in left eye

FIGURE 15–14. Response to light stimulation. When one eye is stimulated by light, that eye's pupil constricts directly. The other eye constricts at the same time (consensual). When this other eye is then stimulated by light, it is already constricted and stays so (directly). It affects the other eye to stay constricted consensually. A relative afferent pupillary defect (RAPD) exists when one eye dilates on direct stimulation. When it does, the other eye dilates consensually. A normal response is demonstrated on the left; RAPD of the left eye is demonstrated on the right.

through the efferent pathway to the sphincter of the same eye. The consensual response to light is the reaction seen simultaneously in the nonilluminated eye.

This equal response from the contralateral eye is due to impulses that cross in the optic chiasm and, again, at the superior commissure in the brain stem. The amount of stimulation to the left eye for the consensual response is dictated by the amount of stimulation to the right eye for the direct response. Whenever this direct response of the stimulated eye and consensual response of the nonilluminated eye are equal, it signifies an intact afferent system of the stimulated eye. The same intensity signal reaches both E-W subnuclei.

In summary, when a bright light stimulus to the right eye results in both pupils constricting briskly, the right eye directly, the left eye consensually, it indicates a normal pupil pathway for the right eye.

A relative afferent pupillary defect (RAPD), or Marcus Gunn pupil, is a difference in pupil response to direct light stimulation from each eye. This swinging flashlight test requires observation of first one eye, then the other, for direct reaction to light in a dimly illuminated room. A difference in pupil constriction indicates decreased conduction from sensory pupillary fibers to the E-W nucleus on the same side as the eye that constricts less well (larger pupil). This larger pupil results from a weaker signal sent back by parasympathetic motor fibers in the oculomotor CN III that innervate the iris sphincter.

When a defective eye is illuminated, neither eye responds in the same normal fashion. *Both* are larger. The defective eye responds better to consensual stimulation than to direct. It is easier to detect the crisp constriction when the better eye is stimulated than the dilation of the eye with a subtle defect. Each pupil is tested at least three times. An arbitrary scale of 0 to +4 is used to describe the pupil dilation and constriction as the light is alternated from one eye to the other. No anisocoria is seen with Marcus Gunn pupil. Both eyes respond by the same amount at all times. The amount is less when the defective eye is stimulated, but both eyes are affected equally.

To summarize, when decreased information is sent *in* by the sensory pupillary pathway to the E-W nucleus, a decreased response is sent *out* directly to the eye sending decreased information, and consensually to the other eye.

A relative afferent pupillary defect is most often caused by an organic visual loss. If the eye with the lesser reaction has a decrease in visual acuity, color vision brightness, visual field, or optic disc color, the finding is corroborated. This may or may not occur. Optic nerve disease produces a significant RAPD (Marcus Gunn); retinal disease, a small one at best. An opaque media (e.g., a cataract), a refractive error, and a hysterical decrease in vision do not produce an afferent pupillary defect. Detection of a relative afferent pupillary defect is an important finding during examination of the eyes.

The response to near is then evaluated by having the patient look at the light. The near response is compared with the light response. All pupil responses should normally be greater for light, especially bright light, than near.

• PUPILLARY ABNORMALITIES

Abnormalities in pupil function aid in the diagnosis of eye and nervous system dysfunctions. These abnormalities can be caused by an iris muscle defect or by a paresis of autonomic nerves that controls pupil function. In the weeks following destruction of an autonomic nerve, for some unknown reason, the affected organ becomes more and more sensitive to norepinephrine or acetylcholine. A much lower concentration than usual of the drug, when applied as drops, will mimic the reaction of the chemical transmitter. This phenomenon is called denervation supersensitivity. By grading the response of the eye to very low concentrations of certain drugs, an autonomic nerve can be proved to be at fault in some pupil abnormalities.

Sympathetic Pupil Defects

Sympathetic pupil defects have increased anisocoria in *dim* illumination. Because the iris dilator muscle is defective, the *smaller* pupil is the abnormal one. It stays small when it should enlarge, because the radial muscle fibers that should contract to enlarge the pupil cannot because they are paretic. Called Horner's syndrome, this is the only situation in which a pupil defect is caused by the sympathetic pathway. Several defects are caused by the parasympathetic pathway.

Horner's Syndrome

This may result from a lesion anywhere in the sympathetic nervous system. It is usually unilateral. Characteristics are:

1. Miosis because the iris dilator does not contract
2. Ptosis from lack of tone in Mueller's muscle
3. Anhydrosis (absence of sweating on the face and neck) on the involved side from affected sympathetic fibers from the external carotid plexus

If sweating is intact, then the sympathetic fibers traveling with the external carotid arteries are intact, suggesting Horner's syndrome with 3rd neuron (postganglionic) damage, because a central or preganglionic Horner's syndrome effect would destroy the sympathetic fibers before they branch off to the external carotid arteries. Review the section on autonomic nervous system in Chapter 11 for more detail.

A photograph often does not show a Horner's pupil, because the bright light from the flash attachment causes the sphincter to contract, which it does because the parasympathetic innervation is intact. The defect is readily apparent only in dim illumination where the dilator muscle should contract to enlarge the pupil, but it cannot do it.

Drug testing can detect where the sympathetic pathway is defective. When a 4% cocaine solution is dropped on the cornea, a normal pupil dilates as the cocaine prevents reuptake of norepinephrine. More norepinephrine stays in the synaptic cleft. A Horner's pupil will not dilate with cocaine instillation. No norepinephrine has been released for it to act upon, regardless of which neuron is damaged. So cocaine proves the diagnosis, but not which of the three neurons has the defect. A 1% hydroxyamphetamine (Paredrine) solution dropped on the cornea stimulates the release of norepinephrine stored in postganglionic nerve terminals in the iris dilator muscle, however, which is only possible if the postganglionic neurons have normal nerve endings. A postganglionic Horner's pupil has no norepinephrine to be released. Therefore, hydroxyamphetamine dilates a Horner's pupil when the damage is central or preganglionic, but not when the damage is postganglionic (3rd order neuron). All other pupil abnormalities involve parasympathetic innervation.

Parasympathetic Pupil Defects

Parasympathetic pupil defects have increased anisocoria in *bright* illumination. Because the iris sphincter muscle is defective, the *larger* pupil is the abnormal one. The pupil stays dilated when it should constrict because the sphincter fibers that should contract are paretic.

Third Nerve Palsy

When caused by compression of the nerve, the pupil is usually involved because the pupillary fibers are found near the outside edge of the nerve. When a compressed nerve recovers, aberrant regeneration is often found. When caused by a blocked blood vessel, the pupil is usually spared because the blood supply affects the center of the nerve. When such an ischemic palsy recovers, no aberrant regeneration occurs.

Tonic Pupil (Adie's Syndrome)

In most instances, the cause is unknown although nonspecific viral illnesses, or trauma to the orbit, can cause this efferent defect to one eye. The damage occurs at the ciliary ganglion or to postganglionic parasympathetic fibers serving the iris sphincter. In daylight only the normal pupil constricts. The other slightly irregular pupil remains large, with a delayed or diminished constriction to the light. A slow, decreased pupil contraction to prolonged near-effort is noted, along with segmental irregular movement of the iris border. Decreased accommodation results in a recessed near point of accommodation compared with the unaffected eye. It is usually unilateral, associated with diminished deep tendon ankle and knee jerks, and is more common in females.

Because of denervation supersensitivity, pupil size is compared in both eyes 30 minutes after instillation of pilocarpine 1/8% in both eyes. This dose is enough to stimulate the tonic iris sphincter to constrict, even though it is too weak to constrict a normal pupil. If the problem is to distinguish a pupil dilated from instillation of atropine from a dilated Adie's pupil, 1% pilocarpine is used. It will constrict the tonic Adie's pupil but will still be too weak to constrict the atropinized pupil.

Argyll Robertson Pupil

Both pupils are small and almost unresponsive to light (either direct or consensual) but responsive to accommodation. This is called light-near dissociation. The small pupil is more striking in the dark, where it does not dilate. It does not constrict in the light either. There is no drug test to prove its presence.

The lesion is thought to occur in the interneurons in the pretectal region where afferent pupillary fibers synapse, making it a midbrain defect. Reaction to light is defective because the affected fibers are on the dorsal side of the E-W nucleus, whereas the near reaction is intact because its fibers arrive at the E-W nucleus from the ventral side. Because the pupils are commonly irregular and eccentric, it can be mistaken for Adie's. Now that syphilis has been controlled by readily available medication, the major causes of light-near dissociation are chronic alcoholism and diabetes.

Parinaud's Syndrome

Like Argyll Robertson pupil, this defect occurs in the pretectal region of the midbrain, with light-near dissociation. However, unlike it, there is no miosis. Characteristic signs are:

1. Paralysis of upward gaze, and sometimes downward gaze
2. Lid retraction (Collier's sign)
3. Defective convergence with convergence retraction nystagmus on attempted up gaze
4. Both accommodative paresis and accommodative spasm (failure or relaxation of accommodation following near effort) may be found
5. Enlarged pupil (mid-dilated).

Parinaud's syndrome is also called the dorsal midbrain syndrome, tectal midbrain syndrome, or tectal aqueductal syndrome.

Amaurotic Pupil

A blind eye (no light perception) does not transmit information to the E-W subnucleus. No efferent impulse to produce miosis returns to the blind eye from direct light stimulation. Its normal fellow eye does not constrict as a consensual response. When the normal eye is stimulated it constricts, and the blind eye constricts as the consensual response. Both eyes always match in size, but there is a large relative afferent pupillary defect (RAPD). The response to near is normal and equal in both eyes (Fig. 15–15).

Fixed Dilated Pupil

A fixed, dilated pupil may be the result of a ciliary gangion lesion, a CN III palsy, or the instillation of a cycloplegic drug, e.g., atropine. The affected eye has a *blown* pupil, i.e., the affected eye stays larger than the unaffected eye even for the consensual response. The atropinized eye cannot constrict because the iris sphincter is paralyzed. When the reaction to light is tested in an atropinized eye, the information is transmitted to the iris sphincter in the normal eye for its consensual response, even without direct response in the affected eye. Because the normal eye constricts, it proves that the entire pupillary system is functioning and that the affected eye has vision.

The amaurotic (blind) pupil will constrict to a 1% pilocarpine solution, as will a normal eye, a dilated eye from a CN III palsy, or an Adie's tonic pupil. An atropinized eye will not constrict with a 1% pilocarpine solution, which is too weak to overcome the stronger effects of atropine.

Pupil Function

Perform test in dim illumination.

Size

1. Have patient look at distant target with eyeglasses.
2. Shine light from below so that both pupils are equally, but not directly, illuminated.
3. Observe whether the pupils are round, regularly shaped, and equal in size. If in doubt, observe with slit lamp.
4. Measure and record each pupil size in millimeters.

$$\frac{\text{OD size in mm}}{\text{OS size in mm}}$$

5. If pupil size differs, patient has anisocoria. Re-evaluate in light.

Afferent pupillary evaluation; i.e., "Swinging flashlight test"

1. Have patient look at distant target.
2. Shine light directly into one pupil—normally it should constrict.
3. Quickly shine light directly into other pupil—normally it should already be constricted (consensually) and should remain constricted.
4. Note if either pupil *dilates* with direct illumination after initially having been constricted. If it does, it has a relative afferent pupillary defect (Fig. 15–16).
5. Record.

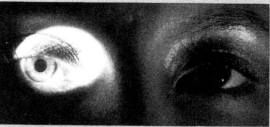
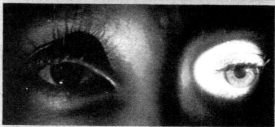

FIGURE 15–16. Normal response to the swinging flashlight test with either eye stimulated.

OD size in mm	Direct light response 0 to +4	Consensual response 0 to +4
OS size in mm	Direct light response 0 to +4	Consensual response 0 to +4

Near reaction

1. Have patient look at distant target.
2. Note pupil size.
3. Ask patient to look at near target and note pupil constriction when fixation changes from distance to near.

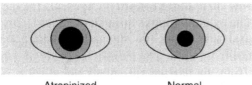

Fixed dilated right pupil

Atropinized   Normal

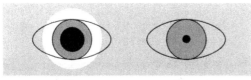

No   Normal
direct response   consensual response

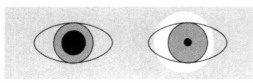

No   Normal
consensual response   direct response

FIGURE 15–15. Unilateral fixed dilated pupil. When the normal pupil is stimulated, it constricts directly no matter what caused the other pupil to be dilated. The dilated pupil constricts consensually unless that pupil has had instillation of a cycloplegic agent such as atropine. All fixed dilated pupils do not constrict to direct stimulation. The consensual response in the normal pupil is reduced unless the dilated pupil is from a cyloplegic agent. In that case, the consensual response is normal in the normal pupil.

Pupil Function

1. To where do pupillary fibers travel along with visual fibers in the sensory visual pathway?
   a. occipital cortex
   b. just before the lateral geniculate body
   c. Edinger-Westphal nucleus
   d. just before the chiasm
   e. optic radiations

2. What does the synkinetic near reflex interrelate to?
   a. mydriasis, convergence, and accommodation
   b. constriction, accommodation, and miosis
   c. miosis, convergence, and accommodation
   d. constriction, mydriasis, and accommodation
   e. divergence, accommodation, and miosis

3. What does the swinging flashlight test evaluate?
   a. difference in response to direct light stimulation from each eye
   b. anisocoria
   c. defective response to near stimulation
   d. refractive error
   e. difference in response to indirect light stimulation from each eye

4. What is increased anisocoria in dim illumination often caused by?
   a. Adie's syndrome
   b. Argyll-Robertson pupil
   c. amaurotic pupil
   d. third nerve palsy
   e. Horner's syndrome

5. When is an afferent pupillary defect found?
   a. consensual eye constricts
   b. direct eye dilates
   c. both eyes constrict
   d. near response is greater
   e. direct eye constricts

BIOMICROSCOPY
Donna McDavid

LEARNING OBJECTIVES

- Describe the operation of the slit lamp
- Describe six methods of illuminations and an example of when to use each one
- Identify common signs of inflammation, scars, lens and cornea changes, and abnormal tissue formation

The slit lamp, or biomicroscope, is a table-mounted, binocular microscope with its own lighting system (Fig. 15–17). The microscope can be adjusted with a joystick to move up, down, sideways, forward, or backward on the table. The lighting system can be adjusted to vary the beam width and the angle at which it strikes the eye. Controls on the illuminating arm can change the beam of light to a narrow slit, vary the length of

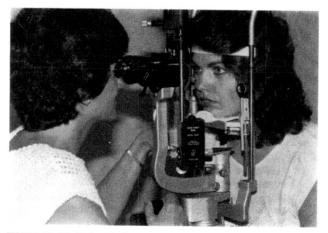

FIGURE 15–17. Patient being examined with the slit lamp.

terior lens capsules. The patient looks straight ahead. A narrow slit is aimed toward the eye from the temporal side. The examiner looks through the microscope from the nasal side. Both the slit and the biomicroscope are sharply focused. The pattern is observed when the angle from the narrow slit equals the angle it reflects into the slit lamp. The technique tends to be difficult to master. Most examiners find it easier to focus monocularly. Specular reflection is especially good for details of the mosaic pattern of corneal endothelial cells.

the slit to a small pinpoint of light, add green or deep cobalt blue filters to the beam, rotate the slit, and adjust the angle between the slit beam and the microscope's line of sight. The slit lamp and slit beam are focused so that the area to be studied is simultaneously illuminated and magnified. Many different views of the same area can be obtained. Most slit lamps can vary magnification from 6× to 40×.

The following lighting variations are in common use.

1. *Diffuse illumination.* A wide beam of light, slightly out of focus (diffuse illumination), is directed from the side at low (10×) magnification. The eyelids, eyelashes, bulbar and palpebral conjunctiva, sclera, and iris are scanned for gross abnormalities (Fig. 15–18).

2. *Direct focal illumination.* This most common technique for the slit lamp adjusts the beam to be narrow and high, with the slit beam and slit lamp both focused in a specific area of interest, first on low magnification, then on higher magnification. Details can be observed. Slit beam width and angle can be varied to decrease reflections and to determine the depth of lesions (Fig. 15–19).

Parallelopiped illumination is a variation with a wider beam presenting a three-dimensional view of a block of cornea from the precorneal tear film to the posterior endothelial surface.

3. *Retroillumination.* Good for corneal opacities or defects in the iris. The illumination comes from behind the structure to be visualized, giving shape and visibility to abnormalities in areas that should be clear. Light is reflected from the iris to view the cornea, from the posterior capsule of the lens to view the iris, and from the fundus to view the iris or lens. The microscope stays focused on the structure to be visualized.

4. *Specular reflection.* This technique uses the mirror-like reflections from smooth surfaces such as corneal epithelium and endothelium and anterior and pos-

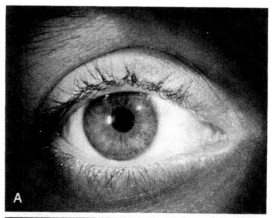
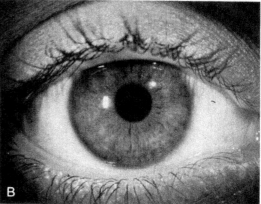
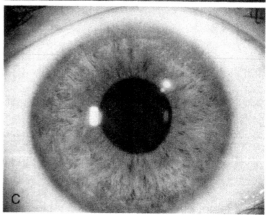

FIGURE 15–18. Different diffuse views on slit lamp examination. *A,* Diffuse illumination at lowest 6× slit lamp magnification. *B,* Diffuse illumination at 10× slit lamp magnification. *C,* Diffuse illumination at higher 16× slit lamp magnification.

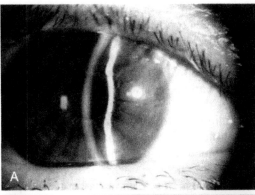
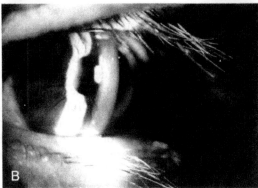

FIGURE 15–19. Different focal views on slit lamp examination. *A*, Focal illumination with thin beam. Dark interval indicates normal anterior chamber depth. *B*, Focal illumination with wide beam. Note the white specks at the upper corneal edge that denote normal debris.

5. *Sclerotic scatter illumination.* A narrow slit under low (10×) power is directed toward the temporal limbus from a wide angle while the microscope is focused on the center of the cornea. The light exits the nasal limbus by internal reflection. Normally, no light is seen. Abnormalities will obstruct the internal reflection and become illuminated. The technique is excellent for evaluating any adverse corneal effect from contact lenses.

6. *Indirect illumination.* The slit beam is directed to an area adjacent to the structure to be visualized. The adjacent area should show only some scattered light, but irregularities next to it will be illuminated.

● EXTERNAL EXAMINATION

When the eye is open, the upper eyelid covers the top millimeter of cornea. If more cornea is covered, there is ptosis (droopy upper eyelid). The lower eyelid lies at the lower border of the cornea. The eyelid margin should tightly abut the front surface of the globe. There is ectropion if the eyelid margin projects outward, away from the eyeball and entropion if the eyelid margin points inward against the globe. (See Color Plates 30

to 32.) Any abnormality of eyelid structure can cause corneal exposure, excessive dryness, tearing, or irritation. Eyelid abnormalities to note are scaling, oozing, redness (increased number of blood vessels, dilated blood vessels), elevations, and pigmentation.

Tiny openings of the sweat- and oil-secreting glands are visible on the eyelid margins. The oil-producing meibomian glands within the eyelid tarsus have ducts that open onto the eyelid margin just behind the gray line. These glands secrete the outer portion of the tear film, which retards tear evaporation and tear overflow, and provides airtight eyelid closure. A chronic inflammatory granuloma of these glands is a *chalazion.* (See Color Plate 29.) The inflammatory swelling plugs the gland and causes it to rupture. In the acute stage, it presents as a tender red area within the tarsal plate. Sometimes it resolves completely; sometimes it leaves a firm nodule. An acute inflammation is an internal *hordeolum,* caused by bacteria that form an abscess containing a small amount of pus. An acute inflammation of the short Zeiss's glands found in the hair follicles is a *stye.*

The roots of the eyelashes at the margins of both upper and lower eyelids are examined for excessive secretions from these oily sebaceous glands. *Blepharitis* is a chronic inflammation of the eyelid margin. The usual symptoms are a sandy or itchy feeling. The base of the eyelash is caked with greasy, flaky scales. The eyelid margins are red, thickened, and vascularized. If eyelashes are misdirected and turn inward to touch the globe, *trichiasis* is present.

The tear-film liquid bathes the cornea and conjunctiva. Because matter moves with a blink, look for debris in the tear layer when the patient blinks.

The conjunctiva is a thin, transparent mucous membrane lining the inner surfaces of the eyelids and the outer surface of the eyeball. It is usually white, quiet (i.e., noninflamed), and nonpigmented in caucasians but may be highly pigmented in African-Americans. Examination of the fornices may reveal foreign bodies, e.g., eyelashes, clumps of make-up, or discharge.

The palpebral conjunctiva that lines the eyelids can best be examined when the lids are everted (flipped inside out). To do so, have the patient look down, firmly grasp the base of the upper eyelashes and gently pull upward while pushing down into the lid fold with a cotton-tip applicator. *Conjunctivitis* is any irritation or inflammation of the conjunctiva, characterized by grittiness, swelling, discharge, or overall redness (hyperemia). The condition may be allergic, viral, bacterial, chronic, or acute in origin. (See Color Plate 18.) A papillary reaction, seen in many forms of conjunctivitis, is noted as tiny elevations of the conjunctiva that contain a central blood vessel. Polygonal red mounds of papillae are signs of inflammation. Giant papillary conjunctivitis (GPC) is an allergic type with hard, flat papillae forming a cobblestone pattern. GPC is associated with prostheses, contact lenses, and exposed suture ends. Follicular conjunctivitis, on the other hand, has follicles, tiny glistening translucent elevations without blood vessels. Follicles are seen primarily in viral and allergic conjunctivitis, or that caused by an irritant (Fig. 15–20).

Subconjunctival hemorrhages may arise spontaneously, appearing as a bright red patch of pooled blood extending to the limbus. (See Color Plate 17.) Usually it follows an episode of coughing, sneezing, or vomiting, or after flying or mild trauma. Despite its ominous appearance, it is benign, subsiding in seven to ten days. Some forms of viral conjunctivitis may show subconjunctival hemorrhages as part of the clinical picture.

• ANTERIOR SEGMENT

The cornea should have uniform thickness with a smooth ground-glass appearance. The smoothness of its outer surface, any abnormalities from scarring such as thinning, the homogeneity of the stroma, and the depth of the cornea can be observed. Localization of a specific abnormality can be estimated from its distance

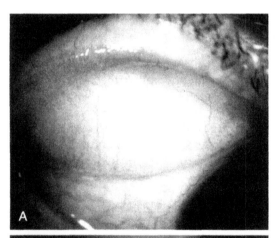
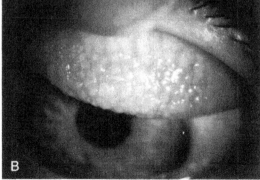

FIGURE 15–20. Upper eyelid viewed under slit lamp magnification. *A,* Upper eyelid everted in patient with normal palpebral conjunctiva. *B,* Upper eyelid everted in patient with follicles in the palpebral conjunctiva.

relative to the anterior or posterior surface. With swelling (edema) the corneal beam appears thicker than normal. It may be cloudy near a lesion, such as that surrounding an ulcer, or cloudy all over (diffuse) such as in acute-angle closure glaucoma (Fig. 15–21).

Opacities can be seen with retroillumination; as can dystrophies that affect the corneal epithelium, stroma, or endothelium; patterns of corneal ulcers in the epithelium; and folds in Descemet's membrane.

Parallelopiped illumination allows a three-dimensional view of a block of cornea from the anterior surface face through the stromal layer to the posterior surface face. The bulk of the observed depth comes from the stroma. Before the stroma, the precorneal tear film is noted, then a darker epithelial layer, then a brighter Bowman's membrane. Behind the stroma is the somewhat brighter Descemet's membrane and finally the darker endothelium. The anterior surface face, the epithelium, is examined for defects such as superficial punctate keratitis (SPK) and microcystic edema. Corneal infiltrates, consisting of white blood cells under the epithelium, are a response to inflammation and hypersensitivity.

The epithelium is the only corneal layer that cannot form a scar when damaged. Instead it heals by replacing and realigning its cells. This occurs secondary to corneal wounds, including grafts and radial keratotomies. (See Color Plates 8, 11, and 15.) The cornea can lose its transparency from edema (swelling), drying, deposition, infiltration, vascularization, and scarring. (See Color Plates 12 to 15.) The regular arrangement of collagen fibers in the stroma becomes disorganized, causing light to be scattered, and producing a hazy view. Vascularization in the stroma is a sign of active inflammation.

Corneal ulcers result from bacterial, viral, and fungal infections. The epithelium breaks down, requiring prompt, vigorous, medical therapy. Otherwise, the cornea may perforate. (See Color Plates 15 and 19.)

Use the blue cobalt filter after instilling fluorescein in the lower cul-de-sac to evaluate the extent of an abrasion, (see Color Plates 23 and 24) a superficial punctate lesion, or a corneal ulcer. Wherever there are breaks in the corneal epithelium, the underlying basement membrane stains bright green. SPK produces pinpoint staining seen in many conditions such as dry eyes or toxic keratopathy.

The basement membrane and Bowman's layer are so thin that they cannot be distinguished separately and are viewed together. Bowman's membrane cannot repair itself from trauma except by forming a fibrous white scar. Scarring under the epithelium (subepithelial) can be detected in the beam just in front of the stroma. The stromal layer, composed of layered collagen fibrils and cells, forms 90% of the cornea. It also scars during healing. Most corneal opacifications

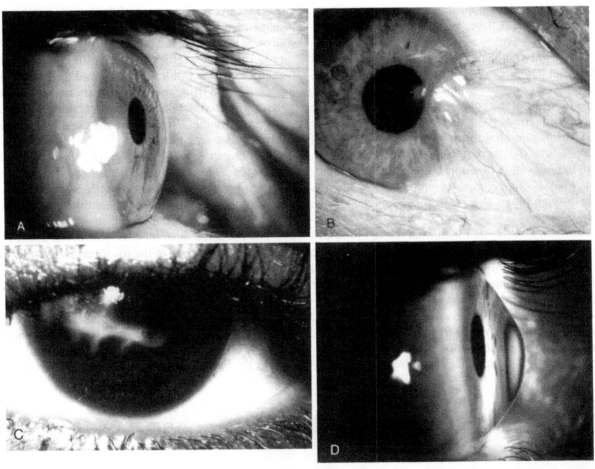

FIGURE 15–21. Cornea viewed under slit lamp manification. *A,* Normal appearance of the cornea. *B,* Pterygium in medial canthal area impinging on cornea. *C,* Corneal scar residual caused by trauma. *D,* Cornea with keratoconus.

(scars) are caused by corneal infections or trauma. Scarred tissue is usually thinner.

Descemet's membrane is the basement membrane of the endothelium and posterior limiting membrane of the cornea. The tissue is very strong, elastic, and in a constant state of tension. The endothelium, a single layer of cells, has an active transport pump mechanism that normally keeps excess water out of the stroma. Descemet's membrane cannot be visualized unless it is altered by pathology. It scrolls up when torn or folds with marked corneal swelling because the anterior limiting membrane stays taut. Folds are from trauma, inflammation, or surgical processes. (See Color Plate 22.) Actual tears occur in Descemet's membrane with keratoconus. If the endothelium is damaged, the pump mechanism fails, and swells and clouds the cornea. Endothelial cells do not regenerate. The cells enlarge but do not increase to compensate for lost or damaged cells. If the membrane becomes weak from too much cell loss, guttata form. Guttata appear as "pits" in the endothelium. They are best seen with indirect retroillumination, looking at the area next to the bright backlight from the iris.

When the endothelium is examined, the back surface should be clean and free of deposits. Keratic precipitates (KPs), representing collections of inflammatory cells on the back of the cornea, appear white when active or recent, but become pigmented with time. They are best seen with parallelopiped or retroillumination.

The depth of the anterior chamber can be estimated by comparing the width of the corneal section (white interval) to the aqueous section (dark interval). The high thin beam is placed at the limbus at a 60° angle. If the anterior chamber angle is deep, the dark aqueous interval should be approximately one-quarter to one-half the width of the white corneal section. If the width of the dark aqueous interval is less than one-quarter the width of the white interval, the angle is narrow. If the two beams meet, the angle is closed.

Because the aqueous and the cornea are transparent, they provide a window to peer into the anterior chamber for observation of active inflammation. Normally the aqueous contains a very small amount of protein. If an inflammatory response such as uveitis or iritis is present, the protein content increases. Leaking intraocular blood vessels spill a high concentration of plasma proteins, which appear as a haze, into the anterior chamber. This is flare. Usually found in the presence of cells, flare often remains after the cells disappear. When this happens, flare represents persisting blood vessel damage rather than active inflammation. To best observe this haze reflected by the light beam, look just in front of the beam in the aqueous, using fine oscillating movements with the light source to show the contrast from one area to the other. Appreciation of flare depends on the use of the thin, high-intensity beam on high magnification in contrast to the dark pupillary border. Flare is often compared with a car's headlights cutting through fog or to a projection beam in a movie theater.

Inflammation induces an increased white blood cell passage through blood vessel walls out into the aqueous. The number of white blood cells (leukocytes) depends on the amount of inflammation. Cellular elements may include red blood cells, appearing yellowish; white blood cells, appearing like white flakes; or pigment cells from the uvea, appearing dark brown, as they float through the beam of light. Gently oscillating the arm of the illuminating beam from side to side

makes cells easier to see. Fibrin (inflammatory cells suspended in a clot) are found if the inflammation is severe. Hypopyon is a collection of pooled white blood cells (pus) that settles to the bottom of the anterior chamber. (See Color Plates 20 and 21.) Hyphema is pooled blood from an iris or a ciliary body hemorrhage that settles to the bottom of the anterior chamber, usually from trauma. Both hypopyons and hyphemas usually resolve with time.

Sometimes exudates *glue* part of the back of the iris to the lens. These scar together, in a posterior synechia. A peripheral anterior synechia (PAS) scars part of the front of the iris to the cornea near the anterior chamber angle. Synechiae often form with iritis. (Fig. 15–22).

The iris is the most forward part of the uvea. Expansion and contraction of the iris form circular pleat lines, or furrows, visible on the surface. Record any elevated lesions (nevi) on the iris surface, irregularities in the shape of the pupil, any new blood vessel formations (iris rubeosis), and any additional holes (removal of iris tissue, surgical iridectomy, laser iridotomy). (See Color Plate 34.) Iris atrophy is best seen with retroillumination because the light reflected back from the pos-

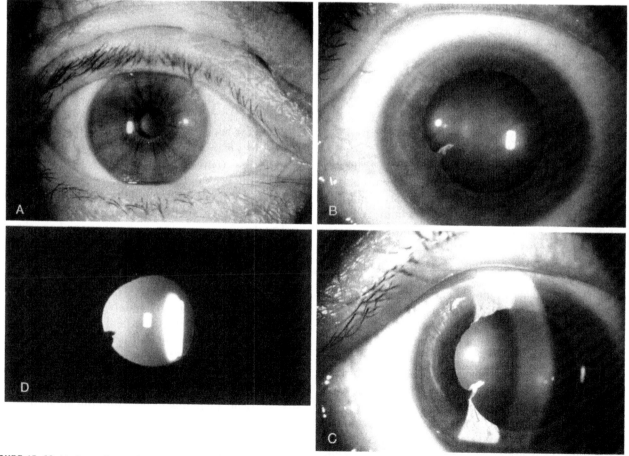

FIGURE 15–22. Various views of a patient with posterior synechia. *A*, Undilated diffuse illumination. No defect noted. *B*, Diffuse illumination when the eye is dilated reveals synechia at 8 o'clock. *C*, Better view of the extent of synechia under wide beam focal illumination. *D*, Synechia outlined in retroillumination with light bounced off the retina.

terior capsule of the lens comes not only through the pupil, but any less pigmented (atrophic) areas of iris.

Use a narrow beam through the lens, preferably in a dilated eye, to look for opacities, water clefts, or color changes. In the lens center is the embryologic nucleus with two "Y" sutures just before and just after it. The posterior Y is inverted. The cortex is formed of the young adult fibers just outside the adult nucleus. Slice through the lens with your beam to find which zone level has the changes. (See Color Plates 1 to 7.)

Technique

1. Position the patient comfortably in the chin rest with no need to stretch up, down, or sideways.

2. Correct the angling of the machine so the patient's forehead rests against the headrest.

3. Align the eye marker on the headrest to the lateral canthus of the eye to be observed.

4. Set your interpupillary distance on the binoculars.

5. Adjust the refractive error adjustment on the binoculars. The setting should be at "0" if you are emmetropic.

6. Ask the patient to look at your right ear when examining the right eye, and vice versa.

7. Set the slit lamp to the lower (10×) magnification.

8. Turn on the control box, switching the power to its lowest voltage.

9. Swing the lamp housing unit (which contains the light source) on the temporal side of the right eye.

10. Place the microscope binoculars straight ahead and look through the oculars.

11. Adjust the slit aperture on the lamp housing unit to its widest opening, using the vertical control on the joystick to position this light onto the eye. You have grossly adjusted the light.

12. Push the joystick forward, toward the patient, until the cornea comes into focus. If you cannot focus, check to see if the patient's forehead is still on the headrest, or use the vertical controls at the joystick.

13. Use the neutral density filter to reduce discomfort caused by the brightness of the wide beam for the patient.

14. Try to use one hand for the joystick and the other for eyeball control, such as when you hold an eyelid everted, or when you hold the eyelids apart for applanation tonometry.

Biomicroscopy

1. A high narrow beam of light focused in the area of interest where the slit lamp is also focused is which type of illumination?
   a. retro
   b. direct focal
   c. parallelopiped
   d. diffuse
   e. indirect

2. A light beam reflected from behind the area of interest with the slit lamp focused on the area of interest is which type of illumination?
   a. retro
   b. direct focal
   c. parallelopiped
   d. diffuse
   e. indirect

3. What are the hard flat papillae, resembling cobblestones, on the palpebral conjuctiva called?
   a. chalazion
   b. blepharitis
   c. giant papillary conjunctivitis
   d. trichiasis
   e. hyperemia

4. Excess cells in the aqueous are called
   a. flare
   b. synechia
   c. hyphema
   d. inflammation
   e. subconjunctival hemorrhage.

5. The active transport pump mechanism of the cornea is a function of which of the following?
   a. the endothelium
   b. Descemet's membrane
   c. the epithelium
   d. the stroma
   e. Bowman's membrane

TONOMETRY

LEARNING OBJECTIVES

• Discuss the principal difference between applanation and indentation tonometry

• Identify three commonly used tonometers

Indentation

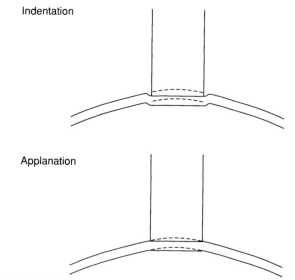

Applanation

FIGURE 15–23. Schematic illustration of the difference in design between indentation and applanation tonometry.

Tonometry is the measurement of intraocular pressure (tension within the eye). Three types of instruments (tonometers) are used clinically for this measurement: indentation, applanation, and noncontact. All methods are based on the application of pressure to the center of the cornea and the measurement of the eye's resistance to this external pressure (Fig. 15–23).

Eyelids and lashes must be held so that they do not touch the tonometer. It is best when the patient can voluntarily keep his eyes wide open. If the examiner holds the lids apart, however, care must be taken not to exert pressure on the eyeball (i.e., restrain the lids against the bony orbit). The tonometer surface must be free of all cleaning solvents or oily residues from handling. During the measurement, the tonometer must remain perpendicular to the plane of the front of the cornea. The patient remains relaxed in a comfortable position; the examiner cautions the patient to breathe normally and remain still. Successive measurements can artificially lower intraocular pressure, especially with indentation-type tonometers.

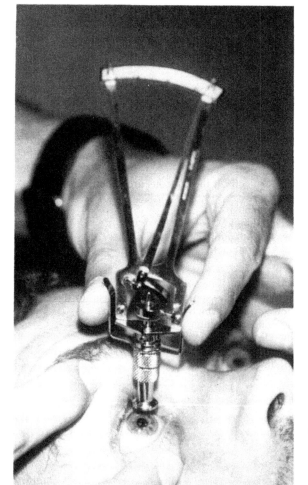

Calibration Scale for Schiotz Tonometers
(Revised 1955)

Scale Reading	Plunger load (in g)			
	5.5	7.5	10.0	15.0
0	41	59	82	127
.5	38	54	75	118
1.0	35	50	70	109
1.5	32	46	64	101
2.0	29	42	59	94
2.5	27	39	55	88
3.0	24	36	51	82
3.5	22	33	47	76
4.0	21	30	43	71
4.5	19	28	40	66
5.0	17	26	37	62
5.5	16	24	34	58
6.0	15	22	32	54
6.5	13	20	29	50
7.0	12	19	27	46
7.5	11	17	25	43
8.0	10	16	23	40
8.5	9	14	21	38
9.0	9	13	20	35
9.5	8	12	18	32
10.0	7	11	16	30
10.5	6	10	15	27
11.0	6	9	14	25
11.5	5	8	13	23
12.0		8	11	21
12.5		7	10	20
13.0		6	10	18
13.5		6	9	17
14.0		5	8	15
14.5			7	14
15.0			6	13
15.5			6	11
16.0			5	10
16.5				9
17.0				8
17.5				8
18.0				7

FIGURE 15–24. Technique and conversion scale for Schiotz measurements Technique for Schiotz tonometry (left). (Courtesy of Sklar, West Chester, PA) Tonometer plunger touches central cornea on the perpendicular. Calibration scale (right). Conversion from scale reading to intraocular pressure.

● INDENTATION TONOMETER

Indentation tonometry measures how much force must be applied to the cornea to indent it. The Schiotz tonometer is an indentation type. It has been used for decades. As the footplate rests on the cornea, the movable central plunger indents a small area by a given weight, which the attached scale needle indicates. The depth that a given weight indents depends on the intraocular pressure (IOP) (Fig. 15–24). The higher the IOP the less that weight indents. The numbers on the extra weight discs represent the cumulative weight as each is added in sequence. The scale reading conversion to millimeters of mercury (mm Hg) is on a separate chart provided with the tonometer. The pressure is inversely proportional to the scale reading, i.e., the lower the scale reading, the higher the intraocular pressure. The readings are accurate in the usual range of normal measurements. A scale reading below four is inaccurate meaning the reading must be repeated with an additional weight on the plunger.

The Schiotz tonometer has the advantages of portability, ease of use, and low cost. Its major disadvantage is that weight reading can be affected by either the improper manipulation of the instrument or the rigidity (distensibility) of the sclera. A falsely low estimate of IOP may be produced in young or highly myopic eyes by the Schiotz tonometer indenting the eye and pushing fluid out, thereby decreasing the ocular volume. Comparing intraocular pressure measurements with two different weights will indicate whether or not scleral rigidity is a factor. If it is not, the two pressure measurements will be equal. This instrument is still used widely in hospital emergency rooms and for screening IOP (Fig. 15–25).

Dismantle the Schiotz tonometer for thorough cleaning between patients. Disengage the weight disc by snapping it off to release the plunger and allow it to slide from the instrument. Holding the plunger at its

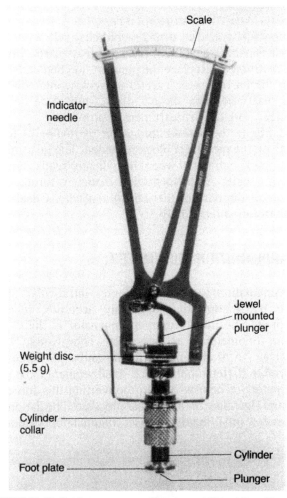

FIGURE 15–25. Schiotz tonometer. (Courtesy of Sklar, West Chester, PA)

notched end, wipe the shaft clean with an alcohol swab or another recommended solvent. Clean the instrument barrel by passing the wet plunger, or a pipe cleaner wet with alcohol, through it several times. Swab the footplate and set all parts aside on a clean surface to

---

Method

1. Have the patient lie down, without a pillow, and with collar or necktie loosened to allow unobstructed breathing.

2. Instill a drop of ocular anesthetic (e.g., proparacaine) into each eye.

3. Have the patient view a target on the ceiling directly above the patient's eyes.

4. With the thumb and forefinger of one hand resting against the bony orbit, hold open the upper and lower lids of the eye to be examined.

5. Take care not to obstruct the patient's view of the target seen with the other eye.

6. Hold the tonometer so that the scale faces you, and lower it gently onto the patient's cornea.

7. Hold the cylinder collar midway between the scale base and the footplate, neither raising nor lowering the instrument.

8. Note the number marked by the indicator needle on the scale. If less than four, add the next weight disc and remeasure.

9. Use the conversion chart provided to change the scale reading to mm Hg of intraocular pressure.

air dry. When the instrument is *completely* dry (alcohol in contact with the cornea's epithelial cell layer will cause a painful keratitis), reassemble its parts. Invert the instrument. Replace the plunger, notched end first, into the barrel, being careful to avoid contaminating the shaft and snap the 5.5 g disc into place on the plunger notch. The instrument is now ready.

Calibrate the Schiotz tonometer by resting its footplate on the metal test block provided. The instrument is properly calibrated when the indicator reads zero (0) on the scale. Adjustments are made by turning the screw at the base of the indicator needle. Check the calibration at least daily.

• APPLANATION TONOMETER

Applanation tonometry assesses intraocular pressure by a sophisticated, highly accurate, reliable method. The most common applanator is the Goldmann tonometer (Carl Zeiss, Inc., Thornwood, NY), attached to a slit lamp. This measures the force required to flatten (applanate) a small segment (3.06 mm diameter) of central cornea, converting this force to an mm Hg value for intraocular pressure. The flattening of such a small segment causes minimal fluid displace-

ment. Less corneal displacement, causing less change in ocular volume, negates scleral rigidity as a factor.

The face of the methylmethacrylate applanator is a prism system that splits the image of the circle of compressed tear film, converting it into two semicircles. Anesthetic and sodium fluorescein are instilled on the cornea to be applanated, then viewed through the beam splitter of the applanating unit with a cobalt blue slit-lamp beam. The mires' pattern is actually the tear meniscus. When the flat, round end of the applanator tip contacts the tear film, the examiner sees two equal but opposite semicircles centered in the field of view. If the semicircular mires are apart, the force is increased by moving the applanator knob clockwise until the mires overlap with a space separating the inner edges. The force is decreased until the mires align at their inner edges. The reading is taken from the pressure indicator (Fig. 15–26). The truest reading occurs when the pressure is set a little high with overlapped mires, then the applanator is released slightly, and the pressure decreased until the mires just align. Normal, minute fluctuations centering in the mires' pattern are caused by blood vessel pulsations. The midpoint reading is recorded. When the inner edges touch, the critical segment has been flattened.

Each number represents a gram of weight. When multiplied by 10 it corresponds to mm Hg of intraocular pressure. The readings are accurate, reliable, and reproducible (Fig. 15–27). Even with the Goldmann tonometer, there are a few sources of error. A too-wide, indistinct fluorescein ring results from too much fluorescein contact with the lid, or an unclean tonometer face to produce an artificially high reading. A too-thin fluorescein ring results from too little fluorescein, or corneal drying, producing a falsely low reading. If too much of the upper semicircle is seen compared with the lower, the applanator is too low.

Corneal irregularities such as scars, pterygia, grafts, or keratotomies alter the smooth surface of the epithelium, often rendering Goldmann tonometry inaccurate. Because it requires a slit lamp and an anesthetic, it is impractical for nonophthalmologically trained personnel. It is also expensive. Nevertheless, it has been the instrument of choice for over 30 years.

Thorough cleaning and calibration of applanation tonometers are generally performed by the manufacturers. Routine cleaning is accomplished by gently swabbing the applanation surface with alcohol or another appropriate solvent.

Calibration can be monitored using the balance rod supplied with the instrument. Each mark on the applanator's pressure indicator corresponds to 2 mm Hg, so that each number on the indicator knob is multiplied by 10. The calibration rod and its holder are affixed to a knob on the side of the instrument. The rod has been marked with five concentric rings. The center

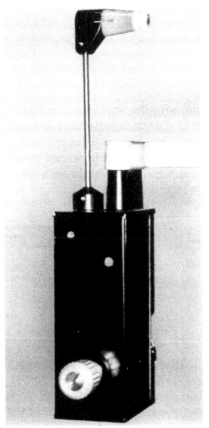

FIGURE 15–26. Goldmann applanator. (Courtesy of Haag Streit, Berne, Switzerland.)

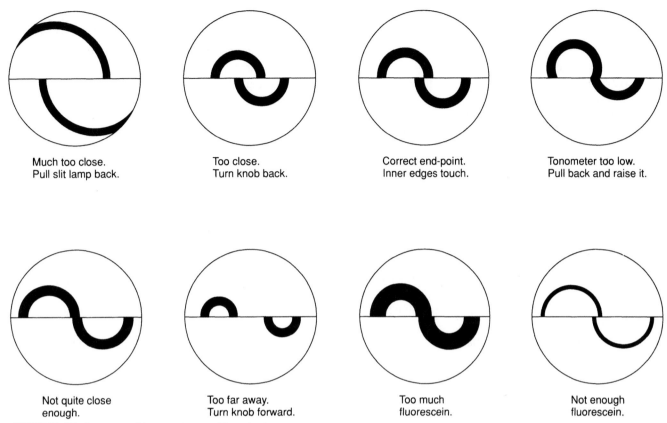

Much too close.
Pull slit lamp back.

Too close.
Turn knob back.

Correct end-point.
Inner edges touch.

Tonometer too low.
Pull back and raise it.

Not quite close
enough.

Too far away.
Turn knob forward.

Too much
fluorescein.

Not enough
fluorescein.

FIGURE 15–27. Correct and incorrect opposition of mires.

ring corresponds to the zero setting. When this ring is aligned with its holder, the applanator should rock forward and backward as the pressure indicator knob is turned plus or minus 2 mm Hg (i.e., around the first mark on the pressure indicator). If the rod is aligned on the next ring so that its weight counterbalances the applanator, the same procedure can be performed at 20 mm Hg (the applanator rocks back and forth between 18 and 22). The last ring on the rod is for 60 mm Hg (where it rocks between 58 and 62). All three test weights should be checked. As long as the applanator is handled gently, calibration checks can be done on a weekly basis. If the calibration check reveals an inaccurate instrument, it must be returned to the manufacturer (Fig. 15–28).

• TONO-PEN

The tono-pen (Intermedics Intraocular, Pasadena, CA) is a portable, hand-held, compact, reliable, accurate, easy-to-use, easy-to-calibrate tonometer with disposable latex probe covers for sterility. It is especially helpful for screening IOP, for measuring pressure on irregular corneas, and for examinations during rounds.

The action is between that of indentation and applanation principles. It is more reliable for accurate pressures than the Schiotz or noncontact. The principle behind the tono-pen is similar to that of the Mackay-Marg tonometer in use in the 1970s. It measures the force required to flatten the plate of the central plunger flush with its surrounding sleeve as it is pushed against the cornea to flatten it. The effect of scleral rigidity is transferred to the sleeve. This tonometer measures the force required to flatten a small segment of the cornea against a 1.5-mm plunger protruding just beyond the surface footplate. The probe plunger is a solid state strain gauge. It has a stationary ring surrounding a 1.2-mm post that makes minute movements as it is applied to the cornea (Fig. 15–29).

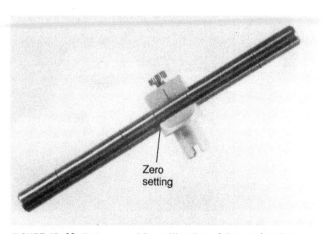

Zero
setting

FIGURE 15–28. Balance rod for calibration of the applanator.

Method for Applanation Tonometry

1. Instill one drop of ocular anesthetic (e.g., proparacaine) into the eye to be tested followed by touching the lower cul-de-sac with the orange end of a fluorescein strip.

2. Position patient at slit lamp, with forehead flat against the headrest bar, and chin in the chin rest.

3. Move the applanator into correct position on the slit-lamp base, aligned with the center of the cornea.

4. Insert the cobalt blue filter, adjust the slit-lamp beam for full intensity, and keep one hand on the joystick.

5. Set slit lamp on low power viewing (10×).

6. Caution patient to breathe regularly, remain motionless, and hold eyes wide open.

7. Scan cornea with blue light for any epithelial defects.

8. Position blue light source at 45 to 60° angle on patient's right side to take pressure of patient's right eye, so that the blue light strikes the applanator tip.

9. Lock tonometer unit applanator arm in straight ahead position.

10. Set applanator knob at mark #1.

11. Move tonometer toward right eye until it almost touches cornea.

12. Ask the patient to blink so that the fluorescein is distributed across the cornea.

13. Raise or lower the slit lamp until the mires are the same size.

14. View through left ocular as joystick moves the applanator to make contact with the cornea.

15. Center the mires' pattern with fine movements of the joystick.

16. Turn the applanator knob until the fluorescein pattern looks like Figure 15–27 (see *Correct end-point. Inner edges touch*), with the inner rim of the top circle touching the inner rim of the bottom circle.

17. Slowly move the slit lamp with attached tonometer straight away from eye.

18. Check applanator knob setting for pressure reading.

19. Move tonometer unit out of straight ahead locked position.

20. Reposition light source at 45 to 60° angle on patient's left side to take pressure of left eye.

21. Repeat steps 9 through 17 for left eye.

The cornea is first anesthetized with one drop of 0.5% proparacaine. The gauge is activated when the tip touches the cornea. Increased force is applied until the cornea is flattened by the footplate. The force on the strain gauge, representing the IOP, is transmitted as an electrical signal, amplified and transmitted to a microprocessor in the handle. Each pressure value is shown on a digital readout. Audible clicks indicate a valid reading.

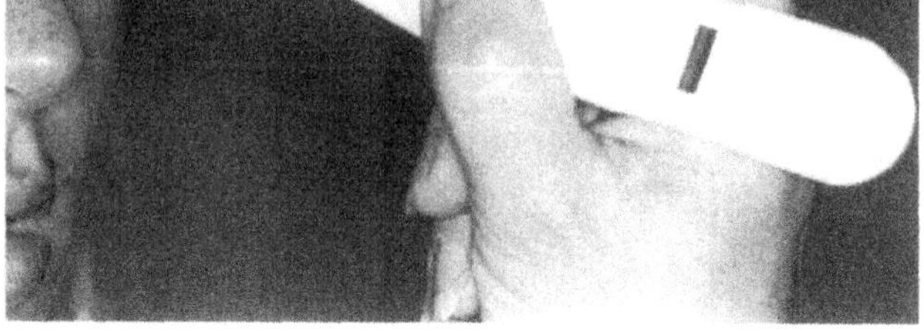

FIGURE 15–29. Tono-pen. (Courtesy of Intermedics Intraocular, Pasadena, CA.)

• NONCONTACT TONOMETER

All of the preceding tonometers contact the cornea, requiring both anesthesia and trained personnel to perform the test. A noncontact (*air-puff*) tonometer, technically an applanation-type instrument, registers the steadily increasing force of a burst of air required to flatten the cornea, converting this to an mm Hg recording of intraocular pressure. It is moderately accurate as a screening device; it becomes increasingly less accurate as intraocular pressure increases beyond the normal upper limit. The loud puff cannot be tolerated by some patients.

Tonometry

1. The most accurate and reliable method of measuring intraocular pressure uses which of the following?
   a. air puff tonometer
   b. applanation tonometer
   c. Tonopen
   d. Schiötz's tonometer
   e. indentation tonometer

2. Which of the following mires patterns is most accurate for an intraocular pressure reading?
   a. 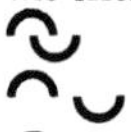
   b.
   c. 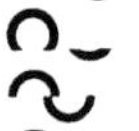
   d.
   e.

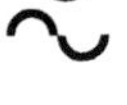

REFRACTOMETRY

LEARNING OBJECTIVES

- Recognize with motion, against motion, and neutrality of the retinoscopic reflex
- Describe the process of retinoscopy in sequence
- Explain the use of the cross cylinder, astigmatic dials, and duochrome test
- Estimate your working distance and calculate its effect on the results of your retinoscopy
- Convert retinoscopy results to spherocylinder notation
- Calculate the spherical equivalent of a spherocylindrical lens

The eye has a complex, multiple-lens optical system that focuses images of viewed objects onto the retina for close scrutiny. Sometimes differences in the length or shape of the eye do not allow comfortable, clear vision. Refractive errors caused by these differences however, can be entirely corrected by eyeglasses or contact lenses. Patients with eyeglasses or contact lenses should not be considered to have *bad* eyes because such eyes see within normal limits for comfortable clear vision as long as refractive correction is worn. *Bad* eyes have defective vision even with refractive correction.

Refractometry is the clinical procedure for determining a patient's refractive error. Ophthalmic medical personnel measure by refractometry. The ophthalmologist prescribes the refraction using clinical judgment to modify the results from refractometry. From the patient's symptoms, previous refractions, and occupation, he or she bases the new prescription for lenses by what is judged to be for the best benefit of the patient.

A streak retinoscope, such as an Op Tech 360 (Optec, Inc., Chicago, IL), allows technical personnel to measure objectively the optical power of the eye. The corrective lens needed can be quickly approximated. The retinoscope projects a streak of light into the eye. The examiner evaluates the light reflected back off the retina. In some instances, particularly with children, this is the only refracting method available, because subjective responses by the child are often not possible (Fig. 15–30).

In most patients, the retinoscopic refraction is refined by using subjective responses to obtain the *best corrected visual acuity* (BCVA or BVA). Usually the retinoscope is employed in conjunction with an adjustable refractor, a Phoropter (Fig. 15–31). By this refining procedure, the manifest refraction (M) is measured while the patient views a fixation point located at optical infinity (six meters away for clinical purposes). *Manifest refraction* is refractometry without cycloplegic drugs. BCVA is the best vision detected on that patient by manifest refraction on that day. It is subject to improvement after cycloplegia.

When a patient accommodates during retinoscopy or refinement, he or she invalidates the results by appearing to need too much minus power. Cycloplegia paralyzes accommodation, allowing the full refractive error to be more easily determined, especially in hyperopia. This method is the *cycloplegic refraction* (C). A changing reflex during retinoscopy indicates incomplete cycloplegia. The patient can still accommodate.

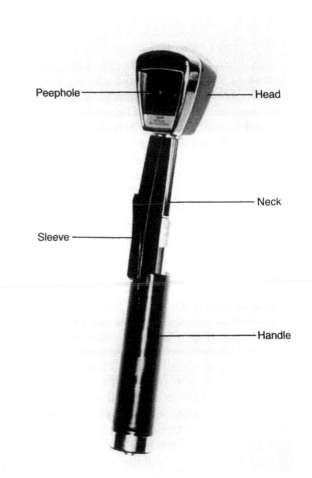

FIGURE 15–30. Streak retinoscope. (Courtesy of Optec Inc., Chicago, IL.)

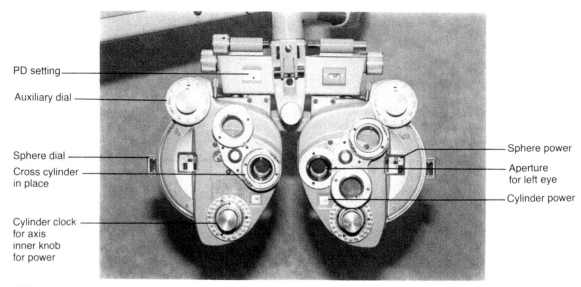

FIGURE 15–31. Phoropter. (Courtesy of Reichert Ophthalmic Instruments, Buffalo, NY)

• RETINOSCOPY

A common method of retinoscopy uses plus cylinders and *with* motion. The retinoscope projects a linear beam of light through the pupil. When testing the right eye, hold the retinoscope in your right hand, sit on the patients's right side, and fixate with your right eye. Reverse when testing the left eye. Look through the peephole at the streak of light which rotates as you rotate the sleeve of the instrument. Keep the sleeve in the up position. The beam of light is projected into the pupil and rotated 360°. You may see the same amount of *with* motion with no narrowing of the streak in all meridians, indicating a spherical error. With astigmatism, the reflex thins when the streak is on axis. This locates one major meridian. The other major meridian is 90° away. Read these meridians off the Phoropter axis clock. To assess the power of each meridian, move the light back and forth, keeping the beam parallel to that meridian.

• ***For example,*** *if the axis is set at 90°, the beam of light will be positioned vertically and moved from side to side (Fig. 15–32).*

As you wiggle the retinoscope, note whether the linear beam of light in the pupil moves in the same direction (*with*) as the retinoscope or in the opposite direction (*against*). Lenses from a Phoropter, or in a trial frame, placed in the light path, act to converge or diverge the light rays until the light is focused on the retina. Light focused in front of the retina will be converging, exhibiting *against motion*. This needs more

minus power to weaken the convergence of the light rays, placing the focus farther back onto the retina. Similarly, light that is focused behind the retina will be diverging, exhibiting *with motion*. This needs more plus power to increase the convergence of the light rays, bringing their focus forward onto the retina.

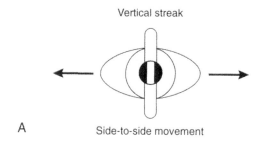

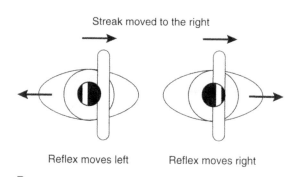

FIGURE 15–32. Streak movement during retinoscopy. *A,* Streak movement is perpendicular to streak orientation. *B,* Streak moves to the right. AGAINST movement is recorded if the retinal reflex moves left. WITH movement is recorded if the retinal reflex also moves right.

Start with no lens. As you wiggle the retinoscope, you may see the same amount of *with* motion in all meridians, indicating a spherical error. If the amount of motion varies in different meridians, it indicates astigmatism. No single lens power will bring neutrality in all meridians. If you see *against* motion in any meridian, add lenses by clicking in enough minus power on the sphere dial until you see with motion in all meridians.

Start with the streak in the meridian where the band is widest and with motion is slowest. If all meridians had *with* motion at the beginning, start by adding plus. If you added minus lenses at the beginning to convert all meridians to *with* motion, start by reducing the minus. Most likely, this will occur at the vertical (90°) meridian or the horizontal (180°) meridian. Neutralization, the end point, is reached when the pupil fills with light and motion is no longer detectable. If you continue past neutrality, the *with* motion converts to *against* motion. Neutrality is the reversal point from *with* to *against* motion. When in doubt, err on the side of *with* motion.

The power of the lens placed in front of the eye that neutralizes the motion in the first meridian is the spherical refractive error. If you turn the retinoscope beam 90°, you should still have neutralized the motion if the refractive error is spherical. You will still see *with* motion 90° away if there is a cylinder.

When you refract in plus cylinder, always approach neutrality from the *with* motion side. Add clicks from the cylinder dial until neutrality is reached. You will need more "plus" for the cylinder if the first meridian was correctly neutralized. The most common meridian for plus cylinder is at 90° (Fig. 15–33). Therefore, when plus cylinder is found at 90°, as expected, it is with-the-rule. Recheck both meridians. If the retinoscopic reflex scissors, check the axis.

A retinoscopic refraction can be difficult to obtain when a poor or dull reflex is encountered. You might be near neutrality. If that is so, leaning 6 inches toward the eye will change the reflex away from neutrality. This can also be caused by an unclear media such as a cataract, an irregular corneal surface as is seen with

keratoconus, or a high refractive error, either spherical or cylindrical. Begin with a +6.00 D lens and a −6.00 D lens to see if the reflex becomes more definite and recognizable. It will if there is a high refractive error. If the reflex improves with the +6, you have a patient with high hyperopia; if it improves with a −6, you have a patient with high myopia. If the reflex stays poor or dull, usually it is from unclear media.

● WORKING DISTANCE

Because you use the retinoscope at arm's length from the patient, not at infinity, you add some additional plus power greater than the refractive error to reach neutrality. The optical working distance equal to your arm's length must be subtracted from the retinoscopy before testing vision. Decrease the retinoscopic refraction by reducing the plus, or increasing the minus, by 1.50 D (or 6 clicks) if your arms are long, 2.00 D (or 8 clicks) if your arms are short, or if you sit closer than arm's length to the patient. Decreasing the retinoscopy by the 1.50 or 2.00 you added by not being at infinity requires subtraction.

● *For Example.*

   −4.00 +1.00 × 90 becomes −6.00 +1.00 × 90

   +3.00 +1.50 × 90 becomes +1.00 +1.50 × 90

● *Vision should improve as you take away your working distance. It should be best with 1.50 or 2.00 less if your retinoscopy was accurate.*

● REFINEMENT

After retinoscopy has been completed for both eyes, the subjective refinement begins. A Phoropter, an adjustable refractor with a series of discs containing plus and minus spheres and cylinders in 0.25 D increments, a cross cylinder, and a pupillary distance setting, is an instrument commonly used for refinement. The large outside dial of the Phoropter controls spherical lenses. The cylinder controls are near the center. Black numbers are plus corrections; red numbers are minus corrections. If the retinoscopic reflex is unclear, the patient's subjective response is vague. If the prescription is a recent one, begin with the patient's present prescription dialed into the Phoropter (Fig. 15–34).

The sphere is refined to find the least minus, or most plus, that maintains the best visual acuity. The patient quickly chooses between two alternatives for better

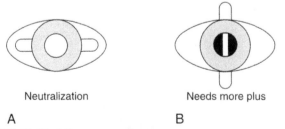

Neutralization   Needs more plus

A   B

FIGURE 15–33. Different neutralization of retinal reflexes in each principal meridian with astigmatism. *A,* Neutralization found at horizontal meridian. Recorded as the sphere. *B,* Vertical meridian needs more plus. When neutralized, will be recorded as the cylinder at 90.

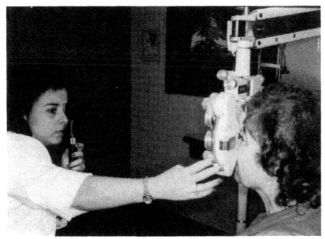

FIGURE 15–34. Examiner dialing the patient's present correction into the phoropter.

vision: +0.25 spheres are added to the retinoscopic result until vision blurs. If blur occurs with the first +0.25 sphere, add a −0.25 sphere in an attempt to improve vision. Avoid over-minusing, which indicates accommodation. If this is the case, the letters often appear smaller.

Last, the Duochrome test is performed on each eye independently to verify the refined spherical power, but only if the visual acuity of both eyes is within one line of being equal and better than 20/40 in either eye. A red-green filter in the projector splits the chart into a red and a green half. The green wavelength is shorter than the red wavelength by about .75 sphere. Therefore, the green wavelength focuses in front of the red. Both halves of the chart should appear equally clear. If letters on the green half appear blurred, add minus lenses; if letters on the red half appear blurred, add plus lenses. You should now have equal clarity.

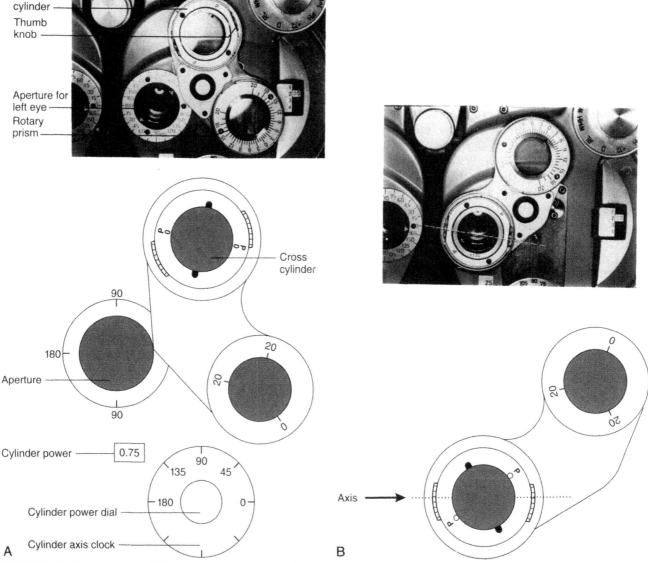

FIGURE 15–35. Placement of 0.25 D Jackson cross cylinder. *A,* Before placement. Not in place before aperture for left eye. *B,* Orientation for cylinder axis. Rotated into place before aperture for left eye. Position of AXIS orientation is imaginary line connecting both thumb knobs.

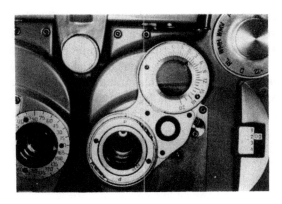

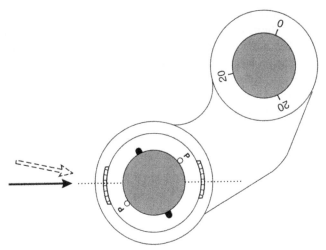

FIGURE 15–36. Cylinder axis rotated 10° toward the direction of the least blur.

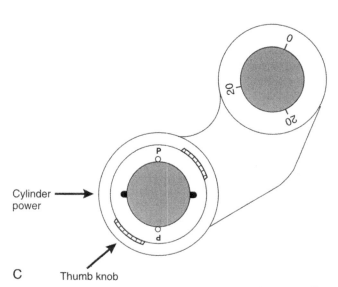

Cylinder power

C   Thumb knob

FIGURE 15–35 *Continued C,* Determination of cylinder power. Rotated into place before aperture for left eye to determine POWER fo cylinder. Thumb knob moved 45° off axis.

Next, the cylinder for the astigmatic correction is refined. To do so, a Jackson cross cylinder that has minus in one meridian and plus in the other is used. Cross cylinders have either +/− 0.25 D or +/− 0.50 D. If vision is better then 20/40, the 0.25 D is utilized. If vision is less than 20/60, use the 0.50 D cross cylinder. The red dot is minus; the white dot is plus. Refine the cylinder axis before you refine the cylinder power (Fig. 15–35).

The axis is tested with the thumb knob aligned with (parallel to) the axis. The thumb knob acts as a handle. As the *handle* is turned, the cylinder axis flips to straddle what you had chosen. Both flips should equally blur the vision if the axis was correctly aligned. If not, the axis is rotated 5 to 10° in the direction of least blur. Retest until there is equal blur when the cross cylinder is flipped (Fig. 15–36).

The cylinder power cannot be found without finding the correct cylinder axis first.

The cylinder power is tested with the thumb knob 45° away from the axis. This places the cross-cylinder power at the axis. One flip adds (white dot) 0.25 D

power to the cylinder. The other flip reduces (red dot) the cylinder by 0.25 D. If the added 0.25 D is clearer, add 0.25 D power to the cylinder dial. If the vision is clearer when 0.25 D is reduced, take 0.25 D away from the power in the cylinder dial. When the correct cylinder power is dialed in, there is equal blur with successive flips of the cross cylinder. If the power changes more than 0.50 D with refinement, the sphere must be changed by half the amount in the opposite direction, e.g., if +0.50 D is added, the sphere is reduced by 0.25 D.

● BALANCING

Once the manifest refraction is completed, a trial frame holding the results allows the patient to try the prescription. This can be especially important if a change has been found in the cylinder axis or power (Fig. 15–37).

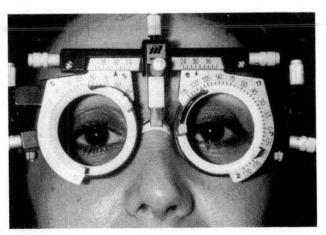

FIGURE 15–37. Patient wearing a trial frame.

Slightly fog both eyes with +0.75 spheres and occlude them alternately. Equal blur should be noticed by the patient. If the blur is not equal, fog the clearer eye by adding +0.25 until both eyes are equally blurred. Balance should be obtained within +0.25 of where you began.

Balancing can also be accomplished by using a 4$^\Delta$ prism with the base up or down, dissociating the eyes by producing vertical diplopia. A +0.25 sphere in front of either eye should blur that eye compared to the other eye. Whatever produces equal blur should be dialed in, the prism removed, and simultaneous +0.25 reductions are made until the fog decreases to best vision. You should be within +0.25 of where you began.

Retinoscopy in Plus Cylinder

1. Seat the patient behind a Phoropter (or place a trial frame in front of the patient's eyes and follow only steps 22 to 26).

2. Change all spherical and cylindrical lens settings to read zero (0).

3. Position patient, making sure:
   a. Phoropter is level.
   b. Patient's forehead rests on Phoropter.
   c. Patient is comfortable, not stretching up or down or sideways.
   d. P.D. setting is correct.
   e. Phoropter is aligned correctly, vertically and horizontally, so that patient can simultaneously view through both apertures.
   f. Lock the Phoropter arm.

4. Use your right eye to use the retinoscope on the patient's right eye as you sit slightly to patient's right, holding the retinoscope in your right hand.

5. Instruct patient to look at distance 20/200 *E*, even if examiner's head blocks view.

6. Raise the retinoscope sleeve.

7. Look for the light reflex in the pupil through the retinoscope.

8. Shift the reflex to the horizontal position, noting whether reflex motion is *with* or *against* by wiggling the retinoscope and your head up-and-down.

9. Repeat with the reflex in vertical position, wiggling the retinoscope and your head side-to-side.

10. If either meridian has *against* motion, add minus sphere lenses by moving the sphere dial up until all meridians have *with* motion.

11. Add plus to the meridian with least *with* motion by rotating the sphere dial down to the least plus (most minus).

12. Check periodically that there is still *with* motion at the meridian 90°.

13. Record the power at which you neutralize the least plus (or most minus) meridian. This is the sphere.

● **For Example.** +3.50, found at 180°

14. Set the Phoropter cylinder axis perpendicular to your first streak.

15. Rotate your retinoscope streak 90°. It now parallels the Phoropter cylinder axis.

16. Neutralize this new meridian with plus cylinders. The axis arrows should line up with the streak.

17. Record the power found on the cylinder dial as the plus cylinder power.

● **For Example.** +4.50 Power is +1.00 more than in Step 12; therefore, cylinder power is +1.00

18. Record the axis in this second meridian.

● **For Example.** Cylinder axis is 90°

19. Repeat Steps 4 to 17 on the other eye.

● **For Example.** +3.50 +1.00 × 90 found in other eye also

20. Remove working distance from both eyes.

● **For Example.** Working distance of 66 cm produced extra +1.50
● Now subtract from sphere to correct for infinity:
  +2.00 +1.00 × 90

21. Test vision for improvement.

22. If using a trial frame, neutralize each major meridian with a spherical lens.

23. Subtract your working distance from both lenses.

24. Record the least plus or most minus power as the sphere.

25. The difference between the two powers is the plus cylinder power.

26. The axis is the meridian of the higher plus (least minus) power.

27. Use your left eye to examine the patient's left eye with the retinoscope in your left hand as you sit slightly to the left of the patient.

Refinement with Jackson Cross Cylinder

1. Occlude the left eye.
2. Determine best visual acuity in the right eye with the *retinoscopic refraction*
3. Refine the spherical power:
   a. By adding +0.25 D steps until visual acuity blurs.
   b. If +0.25 D blurs vision, add −0.25 D to improve vision (clearest, blackest, sharpest image).
4. Be careful not to over-minus.
5. Refine the cylinder *axis*.
   a. Tell the patient this procedure will blur the vision slightly.
   b. Place the handle of a .25 D or .50 D Jackson cross along the axis of the cylindrical lens. A red dot will appear on one side of the axis and a white dot on the other.
   c. Flip the Jackson cross and ask which flip provides the sharper, blacker, clearer letter—"better, 1 or 2?"
   d. Turn the cross cylinder axis 10° toward the direction of the *white* dot.
   e. Continue with steps b. and c. until the preferred axis *reverses* direction.
   f. Flip the cross cylinder again, changing the axis only 5° toward the *white* dot.
   g. Continue to change the axis until the flip of the cross cylinder produces no difference in clarity.
   h. If the axis moves back and forth over the same 10°, set the cross cylinder in the middle.
   i. Confirm by rotating the axis to deliberately blur vision, then refine the axis again to the position with best vision.
   j. The cylinder *axis* is now refined.
6. Refine the *cylinder power:*
   a. Line up the "P" on the dial with the axis.
   b. Rotate the Jackson cross so that one of the dots aligns with the axis.
   c. Flip the Jackson cross—"better, 1 or 2?" If patient sees better when the *white* dot is over the axis, add .25 D of *plus* cylinder. If the *red* dot is over the axis, add .25 D of *minus* cylinder or subtract *PLUS* cylinder.
   d. For every +.50 D of cylinder added, −.25 D is added to the spherical correction. If −.50 D of cylinder is added, +.25 D is added to the spherical correction.
   e. Repeat until patient sees no difference between the two choices.
7. Repeat steps 1 to 5 for left eye.

Duochrome Test

1. Adjust projector to next larger Snellen line than the best visual acuity.
2. Slide the red-green filter into place.
3. Ask patient if letters are sharper, clearer, and more distinct on red or green side.
4. If red, add −0.25 D and repeat question 3. If green, add +0.25 D and repeat question 3. If neither, add +0.25 and repeat 3. Patient should answer red.
5. Leave patient even, or slightly into green, if prepresbyopic. Leave patient even, or slightly into red, if over 50 years old.
6. Remove red-green filter and ask patient which is better for seeing letters, with or without −0.25 D.

Balancing

1. Both the patient's eyes should look through the holes at the Snellen chart.
2. Isolate one line of print on the chart, usually the 20/40 line.
3. Blur patient to 20/40 or more by adding +1.00 D (4 clicks of plus spheres) simultaneously to both eyes.
4. Ask which eye sees clearer with alternate occlusion or, preferably, placing 3$^\Delta$ base down (3$^\Delta$ B.D) oculus dexter (right eye) (O.D.) and 3$^\Delta$ base up (B.U.) oculus sinister (left eye) (O.S.).
5. If no difference, eyes are balanced.
6. If any difference, add + sphere in .25 D increments to clearer eye until eyes are equally blurred, or the opposite eye becomes the clearer eye.
7. Remove .25 D (1 click) at a time, spheres simultaneously, from both eyes, approaching the original refraction.
8. Recheck visual acuity in each eye. Usually, it will be at least as good as before balancing.
9. If sphere or cylinder is more than 4 D, put refraction into trial frame and remeasure vision and vertex distance because the effective power of a lens varies with its distance from the eye. Vertex distance is the distance between the cornea and the spectacle lens.

Bifocal Adds in Presbyopes

1. Add +3.00 to the refractive error to get the presbyope on the Prince rule, somewhere around 35 cm.

2. Measure closest point where patient sees clearly on near vision card.

3. Convert to diopters, using P = 1/f (one divided by distance in meters). In this case, one divided by the closest point where the patient sees clearly on the near vision card.

4. Subtract +3.00 from the number in step 3. This is the patient's binocular amplitude of accommodation.

5. Divide the amplitude of accommodation in half. This is to be used by the patient for best vision and comfort at 16 inches in addition to any lenses you give for near vision.

6. Measure the bifocal add in the old eyeglasses.

7. Discuss patient's visual needs for occupation, working conditions, and hobbies. If the patient has no complaint, beware of changing the amount or shape of the bifocal add.

To summarize, refractometry measures the refractive error of the eye in three steps:

1. Retinoscopy. Objective neutralization of the retinoscope's streak of light in the pupil, using lenses in a Phoropter or a trial frame.

2. Refining. Modification of the retinoscopy findings using subjective patient responses to refine the sphere, and a Jackson cross cylinder to refine cylinder axis and cylinder power.

3. Balancing. Modification of the results to produce equal clarity to each eye.

• MEASUREMENT OF THE AMPLITUDE OF ACCOMMODATION

Testing the amplitude of accommodation is done subjectively, employing patient verbal responses. Whenever there is a dependency on patient cooperation, the endpoint is difficult to assess. The amplitude of accommodation, therefore, is at least as good as the patient admits to but may be better than obtained through testing.

The amplitude is measured monocularly to compare the two eyes. The measurement should be the same, unless one eye has had trauma or is diseased. If a patient is emmetropic, or is tested while wearing his or her refractive error (artificially emmetropic), the patient's far point should be infinity. The near-point distance of all emmetropes is the maximum accommodative capability when converted to diopters. While the refractive error is worn, the nearpoint distance is determined quickly, with the target in normal room illumination and with target size near the limit of patient recognition.

Three common methods measure the amplitude of accommodation.

1. *Push-up method.* This quick method produces a reasonable approximation of the amplitude of accommodation. An emmetrope, or a corrected ametrope, views 6 point type targets being moved toward him or her. If the type blurs at 12 cm (1/8 meter), the amplitude of accommodation is 8 D. If the refractionist uses a smaller or larger target size, the amplitude might differ slightly.

2. *Prince rule method.* The Prince rule is a half-meter scaled accommodative rule, marked off in centimeters as well as diopter equivalents. When the rule is combined with the push-up method, an examiner can measure both the near point and the far point of accommodation. The patient's far point needs to be moved from infinity onto the rule to make measuring possible. To do so, a +3.00 sphere is added to the patient's correction to pull the accommodative range within the half-meter range of the rule's scale. A standard reading card with small print is moved toward the patient's eye to locate the near point and away from the patient's eye to locate the far point, i.e., the farthest and nearest distances where the print is clear. When necessary, the distances are converted to diopters by P = 1/f.

• *For Example. While wearing a +3.00 sphere, the reading card blurs beyond 33 cm and closer than 8 cm. Using P = 1/f, the far point at 33 cm (1/3 m) is equivalent to −3 D. The near point at 8 cm (1 1/12 m) is equivalent to −12 D.*

$$A = \text{amplitude of accommodation in diopters}$$
$$F = \text{far point (in meters) converted to its dioptric equivalent}$$
$$N = \text{near point (in meters) converted to its dioptric equivalent}$$

$$F = -3, N = -12$$
$$A = F - N$$
$$= -3 - (-12)$$
$$= 9 \text{ D amplitude of accommodation}$$

• *The difference of these two refractive powers (dioptric equivalent) of the eye equals the accommodative amplitude.*

3. *Spherical add method.* The patient focuses on a stationary target as plus spheres are gradually added to relax accommodation until the patient reports the target is blurred. The amount of plus is recorded, and the spheres are removed. Minus spheres are added to stimulate accommodation until the target again blurs.

The difference between the greatest amount of plus and the greatest amount of minus equals the amplitude of accommodation. Always relax accommodation with plus lenses before stimulating it with minus lenses, because most patients cannot relax accommodation well after exerting maximal accommodative effort.

● Helpful Hints

1. When the patient arrives with current eyeglasses, use them as a starting point. If the patient is satisfied with them, beware of making changes, especially in the amount or axis of the cylinder.
2. When refining the refraction, ask about sharper, clearer letters, not brighter ones.
3. If vision improves with a pinhole, expect to find a significant refractive error.
4. The higher the refractive error, the more important the vertex distance, increasingly critical as the power becomes higher than $+/-4.00$ D.
5. For preschool children, record the unrefined cycloplegic refraction. Hyperopic children usually do not need their correction unless their distance vision is decreased, they have asthenopic symptoms, or they have an eso deviation. Cylindrical corrections of 0.75 D or more are usually prescribed. If there is a difference in the amount of hyperopia in each eye, the difference is prescribed, not the full plus.

- *For Example.*
- *Unrefined cycloplegic refraction:*

$$+2.50 + 1.25 \times 90$$
$$+3.75 + 1.25 \times 90$$

- *The sphere difference is 1.25*
- *Eyeglass prescription:*

$$\text{Plano} + 1.25 \times 90$$
$$+1.25 + 1.25 \times 90$$

- *Both spheres are reduced by 2.50*

---

6. For myopic patients, the uncorrected vision corresponds to the amount of refractive error. Each 0.25 D is approximately equal to one line on the visual acuity chart. Expect vision to decrease to:
   a. 20/40 if patient has approximately an uncorrected -1.00 D error.
   b. 20/80 if patient has approximately an uncorrected -2.00 D error.
   c. 20/200 if patient has approximately an uncorrected -3.00 D error.
   Uncorrected myopes have much better vision at near, usually 20/20.
7. Be careful about adding minus after a patient can read the 20/20 line easily. It is easy to over-minus. If you find -2.50 on a 20/40 patient, you have over-minused.
8. Preadolescents usually will not wear a myopic correction of -1.00 D or less if it is prescribed. They prefer to squint for its pinhole effect.
9. When the patient notices minification, you will have a clue about excess minus power.
10. Forget correcting a small 0.25 D cylinder if the axis is indefinite and the patient is indecisive.
11. Forget the duochrome test if the best visual acuity is less than 20/60.
12. Forget balancing if the:
    a. Difference in acuity is more than two lines.
    b. Best visual acuity is less than 20/50.
    c. Patient cooperation is poor.
    d. Patient is aphakic.
13. The bifocal segment of eyeglasses has additional plus power to aid near vision in patients who have decreased accommodative ability. The amount of additional plus power of the bifocal reading add should be equal for both eyes as long as:
    a. Equal adds are before the two eyes.
    b. Neither eye has a disease that limits accommodation.
    c. Neither eye is under the influence of miotic or cycloplegic drugs.
    d. Neither eye has an optical aberration that would influence the reading position.

● SPHERICAL EQUIVALENT

Sometimes we need a ball-park figure for the amount of dioptric power in a spherocylinder. It is a substitute sphere that represents the best correction the patient with astigmatism can obtain without the cylinder. This substitute is obtained by keeping the sphere and algebraically adding half the cylinder to it. When obtaining this spherical equivalent, it does not matter whether you start from a minus cylinder form or plus cylinder form. Because it is the dioptric equivalent of the circle of least confusion from Sturm's conoid, it is the dioptric midpoint of the two astigmatic line images (Table 15–1).

Refractometry

1. Best corrected visual acuity is obtained by which of the following?
   a. manifest refraction
   b. retinoscopy
   c. working distance
   d. neutrality
   e. cycloplegic refraction

2. With astigmatism, first refine
   a. against motion
   b. amplitude of accommodation
   c. cylinder axis
   d. working distance
   e. cylinder power.

TABLE 15–1.

Spherical Equivalent

Method	Plus Form	Minus Form
Record the spherocylinder Half the cylinder	$-4.00 + 3.00 \times 90$ $\dfrac{+3.00}{2} = +1.50$	$-1.00 \ -3.00 \times 180$ $\dfrac{-3.00}{2} = -1.50$
Keep the sphere but forget the axis	-4.00	-1.00
Add the halved cylinder to the sphere	$-4.00 + 1.50 =$	$-1.00 - 1.50 =$
ANSWER:	-2.50 sph. equiv.	-2.50 sph. equiv.

3. How is balancing the refraction performed?
   a. before retinoscopy
   b. with the cross cylinder
   c. after refining
   d. before refining
   e. with the Prince rule

4. What is the Prince rule used to measure?
   a. retinoscopy
   b. add in old glasses
   c. distance correction
   d. cylinder power
   e. near point of accommodation

5. The amplitude of accommodation compares the dioptric equivalent of the
   a. retinoscopy and far point
   b. far point cc and near point cc
   c. cycloplegic refraction and working distance
   d. cylinder power and near point
   e. far point cc and near point sc.

LENSOMETRY

LEARNING OBJECTIVES

● Explain the technique for measuring the power, cylinder, axis, bifocals, and prisms incorporated in an eyeglass presciption on a lensometer

● Convert minus cylinders to plus cylinders and vice versa by transposition

Technical personnel routinely measure and record the power of eyeglass correction currently being worn on new patients as well as any recently purchased eyeglasses on return patients (Fig. 15–38). Automated lensometers are readily available. After the lens is placed in position, pushing a button produces a reading that is displayed on a screen or printed on paper. No skill is required, but these instruments are much more costly than nonautomated ones. This chapter explains how to obtain accurate measurements on nonautomated lensometers. Fortunately, this task is one of the easier ones for technical personnel to master, requiring minimal understanding of optics.

Lenses are either spheres, cylinders, or a combination (spherocylinder or toric). Cylinders correct for astigmatism. A lensometer enables the technician to quickly measure the combination of lens surface powers in diopters. The instrument is calibrated for distance. No accommodation is required by the technician for focusing the mires. Yet, psychologically, the technician is aware that the mires are a matter of inches from the eyepiece. This may stimulate unwanted accommodation. If so, over-minused measurements will be recorded. A little experience eliminates this source of measurement error (Fig. 15–39).

● INSTRUMENTATION

When a patient presents with a complaint about a new pair of eyeglasses, the accuracy of the prescription is verified on the lensometer. Then the patient's interpupillary distance (PD) is checked. The PD and the distance between the optical centers of the two lenses

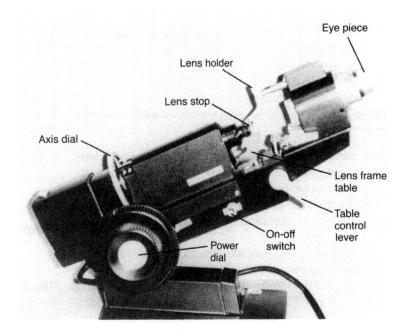

FIGURE 15–38. Example of nonautomated lensometer in common usage. Reichert lensometer. (Courtesy of Reichert Ophthalmic Instruments, Buffalo, NY.)

should be the same. The easiest method to do this is to center the lenses in the lensometer and mark the centers with the built-in marker, then measure the distance between the markings. If the inkwell does not have a fresh supply of ink, touch the center marker point with a *washable* felt tip pen. Alternatively, place the frames on the patient's face and use a washable felt-tip marker to dot the patient's PD. These dots should appear in the center ring when viewed through the lensometer. If so, it verifies that the distance between the optical centers of the lenses equals the distance PD. If not, prism is induced by decentration. How much is induced can be calculated by use of Prentice's rule found in Chapter 14 on physiological optics.

Because of the thickness and meniscus form of eyeglass lenses, the vertex power is usually measured from the back surface curvature of a lens. The spherical and cylindrical power, the cylindrical axis, the optical center (OC), the strength and direction of prisms in a

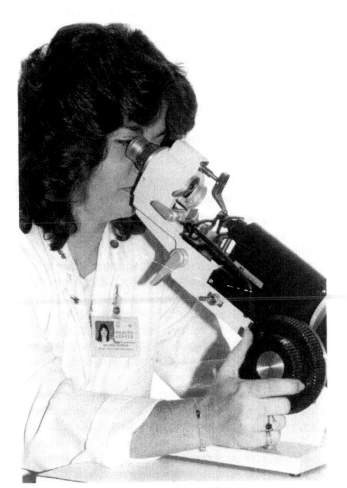

FIGURE 15–39. Technician rotating power dial on lensometer to measure amount of sphero-cylinder correction ground into spectacles.

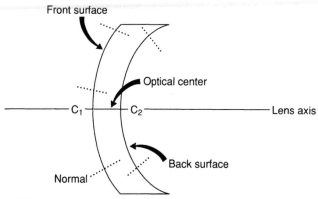

FIGURE 15–40. Lens axis connects the centers of curvature (C_1 and C_2) of both lens surfaces.

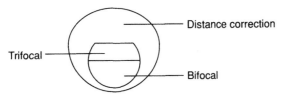

FIGURE 15–41. Spectacle lens with bifocal and trifocal segments for added plus power.

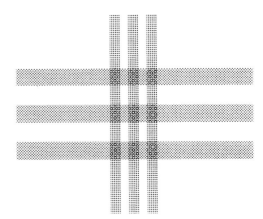

FIGURE 15–42. Common mires pattern found in a lensometer.

lens can be determined. The optical center of a lens lies at the point of zero prism where the lens axis connects the centers of curvature of both lens surfaces (Fig. 15–40). The normals of the two surfaces are parallel here. Further explanation is found in Chapter 13 on geometric optics.

Multifocal lenses provide a means of additional help at near distances. A bifocal has additional plus power ground onto the lens for patients to focus more clearly at near (about 15 inches from the bridge of the nose). A trifocal usually has half the strength of the bifocal to better focus at distances three to five feet away (Fig. 15–41).

Mires' patterns vary somewhat from one instrument to another. We chose a common pattern, three thin lines close together 90° from three thicker lines spaced further apart. The middle thin line crosses the middle thick line at the optical center of the lens (Fig. 15–42). By focusing the luminous mires in the lensometer, one can determine the power of each lens component. If the lens is a sphere, both sets of three lines will be in sharp focus at the same setting of the diopter dial. If the lens is a spherocylinder, only one set of three lines will be a sharp focus at any one setting. When the first set of lines comes into focus, that dial setting is the sphere power in diopters. Usually the intersections of

the lines will appear broken until the axis dial is rotated to eliminate the breaks. The diopter dial is again rotated in the same direction until the other set of lines comes into focus at a different diopter dial setting. The *difference* of the two diopter dial readings is the cylinder, and its axis is read from the axis dial setting previously obtained.

Spherocylinders can be measured in either minus cylinder form or plus cylinder form. Converting from one form to another is called transposition, covered at the end of this chapter. After becoming familiar with transposition, focusing on the thin lines and turning the dial either toward or away from you will result in the correct prescription of the pair of glasses. The method described in this chapter measures lenses in plus cylinder form. The set of lines representing the sphere is brought into focus first at the most minus (or least plus) power.

Technique for Measuring Spectacle Lens Power in Plus Cylinder Form

1. Test the eyepiece reticle (black rings) focus by pulling it toward you until it blurs. Then push it away until the black rings on the cross lines just come into sharp focus. Avoid placing fingerprints on the eyepiece. On some machines the eyepiece reticle is turned counterclockwise to blur and then clockwise to focus (Fig. 15–43).

2. Once a week, test the calibration by rotating the diopter dial without a lens in place on the frame table. It should read plano (zero).

3. When beginning to use the lensometer, place and measure the right lens of the eyeglasses on the lensometer frame table first, by convention.

4. Place eyeglasses firmly on moveable frame table with the ear pieces facing away from you (you read the back vertex power of the lens). The bottom of both lenses should touch the frame table platform to ensure that both are level (Fig. 15–44).

5. Hold the right lens against the lens stop, centered in place by the lens holder. Unless there is ground-in prism in the lens, the luminous mires composed of three thin lines crossed by three wider lines will be centered on the eyepiece reticle. Either one or both sets of lines may be blurred (Fig. 15–45).

6. Turn the top of the *diopter dial* away from you to read high minus power, around −10 D. On many lensometers, minus numbers are red (Fig. 15–46).

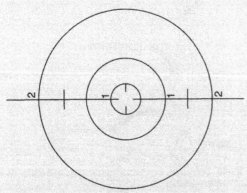

FIGURE 15–43. Eyepiece reticle.

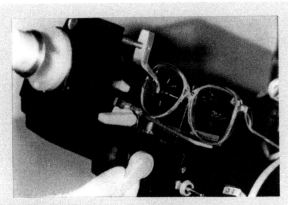

FIGURE 15–44. Right lens held by a lens holder in place on a frame table.

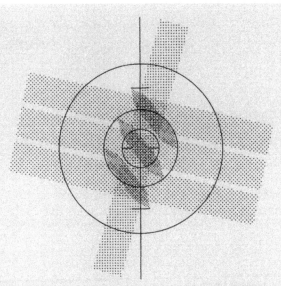

FIGURE 15–45. Mires pattern blurred out of focus for both sphere and cylinder.

7. Decrease the minus on the *diopter dial* by rotating the top of the dial toward you to bring the three thin luminous lines into sharp focus, simultaneously rotating the *axis dial* to straighten the thin lines where they break as they cross the wide lines, until they appear unbroken (Fig. 15–47).

8. Record the diopter dial reading as the sphere power portion of the prescription.

● *Example:*   +1.00 Sph

---

9. When you rotate the axis dial to form unbroken lines, the wide lines may mistakenly come into focus. If so, change the axis dial 90° to bring the three thin lines into unbroken focus (Fig. 15–48).

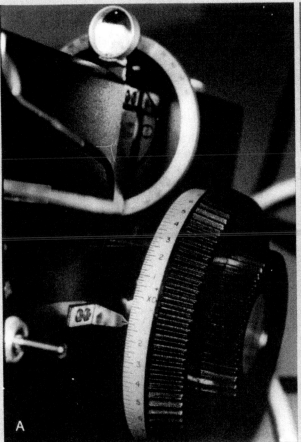
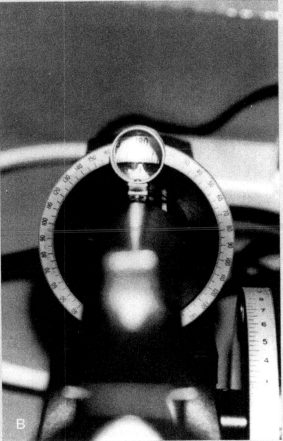

FIGURE 15–46. *A*, Diopter dial found on the side of a lensometer. *B*, Axis dial found at the rear of a lensometer.

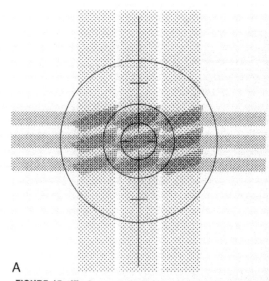
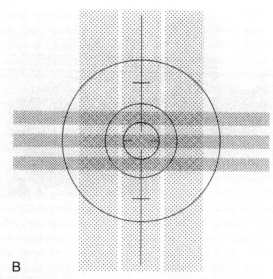

A

B

FIGURE 15–47. Correction of axis cylinder by rotation of axis dial while sphere lines are in sharp focus. *A,* Thin sphere lines almost in focus. Broken sphere lines indicate the need to shift the axis dial from an 80° setting. Cylinder lines out of focus. *B,* Thin sphere lines in focus. Unbroken sphere lines indicate axis dial at correct setting at 90°. Cylinder lines out of focus.

10. If both the thin and the wide lines are in focus with the same reading, the lens is a sphere (Fig. 15–49).

11. If so, record and repeat steps 6 through 10 on for the left lens. Otherwise, leave the *axis* dial at its setting but continue to rotate the top of the *diopter* dial toward you (towards "plus") to bring the three wide luminous lines into sharp focus. The wide lines run in the same orientation as the axis setting (Fig. 15–50).

12. The *difference* between the first diopter dial reading (thin lines in focus) and this second diopter dial reading (thick lines in focus) is the power of the cylinder.

13. You already have a record of the sphere from the first reading. Now record the plus cylinder from the second reading, then note axis dial reading.

- *Example:*
- *Thin lines focus at +1.00 power dial setting, axis dial at 90°*
- *Thick lines focus at +4.00 power dial setting, axis dial at 90°*
- *Record prescription as: +1.00 +3.00 × 90°*
- *(To get from +1 to +4, you have to algebraically add a +3.)*

- *Example:*
- *Thin lines focus at −5.00 power dial setting, axis dial at 135°*
- *Thick lines focus at −4.00 power dial setting, axis dial at 135°*
- *Record prescription as: −5.00 +1.00 × 135°*
- *(To get from −5 to −4, you have to algebraically add a +1.)*

- *Example:*
- *Thin lines focus at −2.00 power dial setting, axis dial at 180°*
- *Thick lines focus at +1.00 power dial setting, axis dial at 180°*
- *Record prescription as: −2.00 +3.00 × 180°*
- *(You have to add 2 to get from −2 to 0, then add another 1 to get to +1. You have added a total of +3.)*

For further help on this calculation, refer to the section on number lines in the Appendix.

---

14. Move the eyeglasses on the lens frame table so that the left lens is held in place and repeat steps 3 through 11.

15. Bifocals: Raise the lens frame table until the optical center of the bifocal add is centered in the lensometer reticle. Rotate diopter dial toward plus until the thin lines are in focus. The difference between this reading and the original sphere power (from step 6) is the power of the bifocal. Measure trifocal similarly; it is usually half the bifocal power.

- *Example:*
- *Thin lines in focus above bifocal at +4.00*
- *Thin lines in focus through bifocal at +6.00*
- *Power of bifocal is +2.00, the difference from +4.00 to +6.00*

---

16. Prism
   a. If you cannot center the crossing of the thick and thin lens in the lensometer eyepiece reticle (black rings), the lens has ground-in prism.

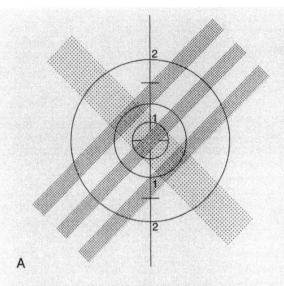

A

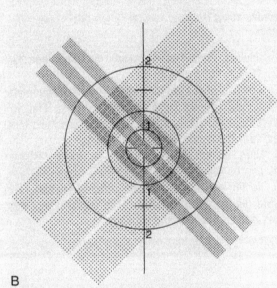

B

FIGURE 15–48. Changing focus from wide to narrow lines. *A,* When rotating axis and power dials, wide lines come into focus first. *B,* Rotation of axis dial by 90° brings thin lines into focus.

Place the area of the lens in the assumed center of the lensometer field. Each black ring in the eyepiece reticle measures 1$^\Delta$. Note that the three line mires are off-center. Depending on the brand of lensometer, up to five (5$^\Delta$) of prism can be measured directly through the viewing screen. The number of rings from the center of the reticle to the crossing of the white lines is the amount of prism.

The prism base is determined by the direction of displacement of the thin lines-wide lines mires. If the displacement is toward the nose piece, it is base in. If the displacement is toward the temple, it is base out (Fig. 15–51). If the amount of prism is greater than the limits of the lensometer, loose prisms included with a lensometry set can be added by opposing the base in the lens to neutralize the

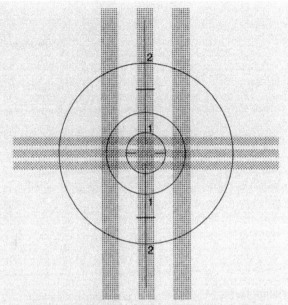

FIGURE 15–49. When the lens has no cylinder, both sets of lines come into focus simultaneously as the power dial is rotated.

prism to zero. Then measure the lens through the viewing screen. Horizontal prism is recorded as base-in (BI) or base-out (BO); vertical prism is recorded as base up (BU) or base down (BD).

b. Horizontally induced prism by optical center decentration can be measured by placing the glasses on the patient, marking the corneal light reflex position (patient's PD) with a *washable* felt-tip marker, and placing this PD mark in the center of the lensometer field. If the position of the mires is not also centered, the mm difference determines how much prism and in what direction (see Prentice rule).

c. Vertical induced or ground-in prism is measured by centering the mires in the lensometer reticle

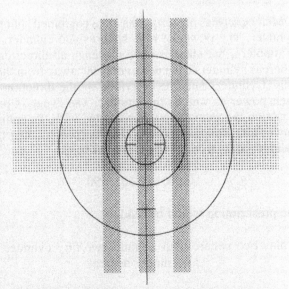

FIGURE 15–50. Cylinder lines in focus at 90°. Axis orientation is also at 90°.

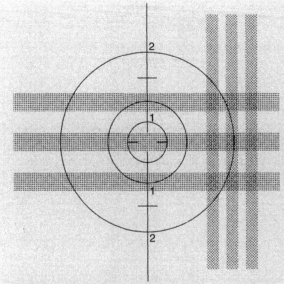

FIGURE 15–51. 2$^\Delta$ of base in (BI) prism ground into right lens (or 2$^\Delta$ base out (BO) prism ground into left lens).

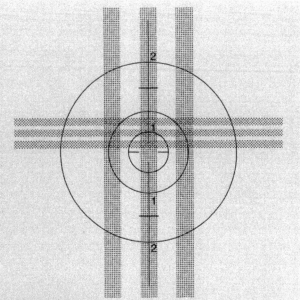

FIGURE 15–52. Ground in prism measures 1$^\Delta$ base up (BU).

for one lens. If you then move the eyeglasses to view the other lens, but it cannot be centered without moving the table up or down, there is vertical prism.

Measure the second lens without changing the vertical position of the eyeglasses. (*Do not move the lens frame table up or down*). The amount of displacement of the mires above or below horizontal measures the amount of prism. For each ring displaced on the reticle, there is one prism diopter induced. If the crossing of the mires is displaced downward, the induced prism is base down. An

upward displacement would be base up (Fig. 15–52).

17. Aphakic lenses are held in place on the lensometer reversed, with the earpieces towards you so that you measure the front vertex power. Then, to read the bifocal power, turn the lenses the usual direction.

18. Hard contact lenses or gas-permeable contact lenses can be read by holding the *front* curved surface, similar to the position of high plus aphakic lenses. You measure the front vertex power. The contact lens must be held by hand against the lens stop.

● TRANSPOSITION

Many eyeglass prescriptions are a combined spherocylinder. The power of both spheres and cylinders is in diopters, but spheres have power in all directions, whereas cylinders have power only 90° away from their axis. Cylinders must be described by the direction of their power as well as the amount. The eyeglass prescription, by convention, is recorded with the sphere power first, followed by the cylinder power, then the cylinder axis. In the example listed below

$$+2.00 \ -2.50 \times 90$$

the prescription would be read as:

a plus two sphere with a minus two fifty cylinder at axis ninety degrees

Eyeglass prescriptions may be written in either plus or minus form. Even though many ophthalmologists

prefer to measure cylindrical lenses in "plus" form, technical personnel have to measure in either "plus" or "minus" forms. Plus form is converted to minus form, and vice versa, by transposition (Table 15–2).

TABLE 15–2.

Transposition

1. Record the glasses prescription. EXAMPLE: Sphere = +2.00 Cylinder = −2.50 Cylinder direction = × 90°	+2.00	−2.50	× 90°
2. Add the sphere and cylinder powers: +2.00 −2.50 = −0.50	−0.50		
3. Reverse the sign of the cylinder: −2.50 changes to +2.50		+2.50	
4. Rotate the cylinder axis by adding 90° to it if the axis is 90° or less; or subtracting 90° from it if the axis is more than 90°: 90° + 90° = 180°			×180°
5. Our transformed resultant prescription is now in plus form	−0.50	+2.50	×180°

Lensometry

1. When a lens is centered in place against the lens stop by the lens holder, where does the middle thin line usually cross the middle thick line?
   a. at the bottom circle of the reticle
   b. at zero on the axis dial
   c. in the center cross hair of the reticle
   d. at zero on the diopter dial
   e. at the farthest left number of the reticle

2. What do you do when transposing a spherocylinder from plus to minus form?
   a. change the cylinder sign
   b. halve the cylinder power and change its sign
   c. keep the cylinder axis unchanged
   d. change the sphere sign
   e. halve the sphere power

KERATOMETRY

LEARNING OBJECTIVES

- Understand the relationship between keratometer (K) readings and astigmatism
- Describe in sequence the measurement of corneal curvature
- Identify three examples of clinical use of K readings
- Explain interpretation of K readings

Not only is the cornea a powerful refracting surface for the eye's optical system, its reflections from its front surface function as though the cornea were a high powered (-250 D), curved convex mirror. The keratometer provides an objective measure of the radius of curvature, in millimeters, of this corneal "mirror," then converts the millimeters to diopters of corneal optical power. These measurements are of the central 3 mm, the apical zone, of corneal curvature. Whereas the keratometer is calibrated in diopters, the inside curve of a contact lens is recorded in millimeters. Conversion tables are available.

- *For example:*

K reading (D)	Corneal radius (mm)
47.00	7.18
45.00	7.50
43.00	7.85
41.00	8.23

Keratometry is invaluable for detecting quickly and precisely the amount and direction of corneal astigmatism. It provides a baseline when refracting a postoperative patient following a corneal transplant or cataract extraction. These measurements are widely used to select the power of contact lenses as well as for determining the power for an intraocular lens implantation following an extracapsular cataract extraction (ECCE). Keratoconus patients must be measured at the cone's location, usually not in the central three millimeters.

• CORNEAL MEASUREMENT THEORY

If an object of specific size is illuminated at a fixed distance from a mirror, we can calculate the radius of curvature of the mirror from the size of the reflected image from the illuminated object. In the keratometer, a luminous target mire is projected onto the cornea (Fig. 15–53). The mire pattern is tripled by the optical system of the keratometer to appear as three rings. The lower right ring is doubled when out of focus. The focusing knob moves the keratometer closer or farther from the cornea to reach a fixed distance when the ring becomes single and in focus. Then it is compared with the size of its image reflected from the corneal surface. The mires reach correct alignment by turning the horizontal and vertical drums on each side of the keratometer. A hole in the center of the target allows the patient to see an image of his or her own eye, helping to hold fixation centered.

The flatter the cornea, the longer the radius of curvature, and the larger the image mire, the lower the power of the eye will be. The steeper the cornea, the shorter the radius of curvature, the smaller image mire, the higher the power of the eye. The average corneal curvature measures 44 D. High (steep) corneal curves (e.g.,

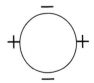

FIGURE 15–53. Mire pattern.

48 D) are associated with myopia and low (flat) curves (e.g., 40 D) with hyperopia.

Mires vary from one keratometer to another. Often, plus signs are used for horizontal alignment, and minus signs for vertical alignment. Sometimes, plus signs are used for both alignments. If the vertical and horizontal signs are superimposed and aligned at the same setting, no corneal astigmatism exists. With an astigmatic cornea, the vertical and horizontal signs do not superimpose at the same setting. The difference between the horizontal and vertical settings is the amount of corneal astigmatism.

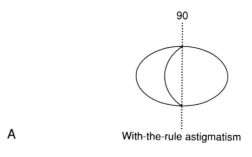

A   With-the-rule astigmatism

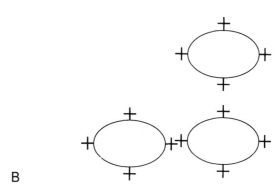

B

FIGURE 15–55. *A,* Oval shape of the cornea found in with-the-rule astigmatism. *B,* Oval mires found in with-the-rule astigmatism.

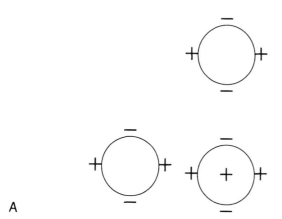

A

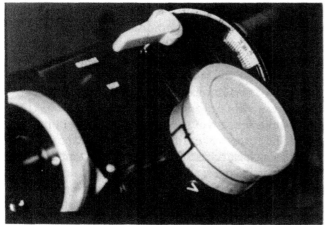

B

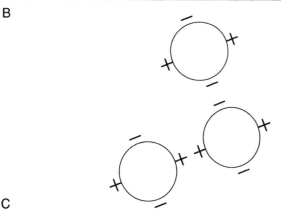

C

FIGURE 15–54. *A,* Horizontal plus signs out of alignment. *B,* Mires pattern aligned by rotating the keratometer body to axis 135°. *C,* Horizontal plus signs aligned.

• *For example:*

$$43.50/45.50 \times 90$$

• *43.50 is the flatter meridian at 180*
• *45.50 is the steeper meridian at 90*

Although the major axis of astigmatism is usually close to either the 90° or 180° meridian, the exact axis can be found by rotating the entire keratometer tube to align the rings so that the horizontal lines of the plus signs are on a straight line from one another (Fig. 15–54).

With significant astigmatism, the mire appears oval rather than circular. The more common with-the-rule astigmatism has the steeper (more plus) meridian at 90°, and the flatter at 180° (Fig. 15–55). The steeper meridian is at 180° in the less common against-the-rule astigmatism.

Distorted mires indicate corneal disease, but they are also seen with poor contact lens fits. Keratometer readings are commonly referred to as the K readings, or simply Ks (Fig. 15–56).

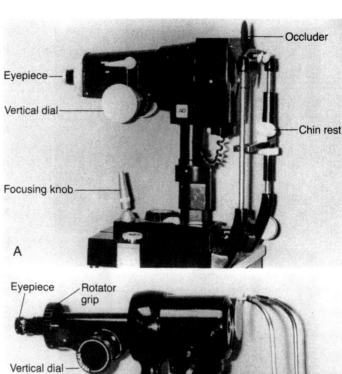

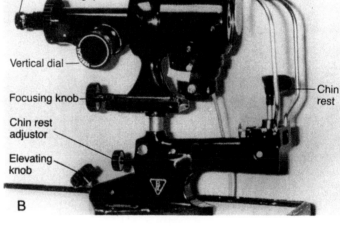

FIGURE 15–56. Two examples of keratometers in common usage. *A,* Reichert Ophthalmic Instruments, Buffalo, NY. *B,* Bausch & Lomb, Rochester, NY.

Measurement Technique

1. Turn the eyepiece counterclockwise (to the left) until the target blurs. Now turn the eyepiece clockwise (to the right) until the target just clears.

2. Instruct the patient to place the chin on the chin rest with the forehead firmly against the head rest (Fig. 15–57).

3. Grossly align instrument before right eye by adjusting the chin rest up or down, turning the tube horizontally to point toward the right eye, while moving the vertical knob.

4. Occlude the left eye.

5. View the eye through the keratometer eyepieces.

The corneal image of the circular mire can be seen on the cornea.

6. Instruct the patient to look at his or her own eye reflection in the keratometer.

7. Adjust the focusing knob until the doubled lower right rings become single (Fig. 15–58).

8. All three rings should be well separated. If not, rotate horizontal and vertical drums until they are.

9. Rotate keratometer body itself until the horizontal plus signs of the lower and center rings are on the same plane. Note the cylinder axis reading on the axis scale.

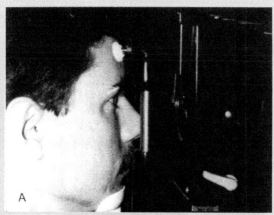

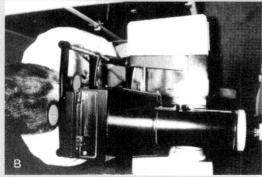

FIGURE 15–57. *A*, Patient positioned at the keratometer with the chin in the chin rest and the forehead against the head rest. *B*, Keratometer shifted toward the right eye with the left eye occluded.

10. Adjust the power of the left horizontal drum until the central plus signs superimpose. Read the power from the scale (Fig. 15–59).

11. Adjust the power of the right vertical drum until central minus signs superimpose (some keratometers have plus signs for vertical alignment). Read the power from the scale.

12. Fine tune the focus during the measurements to keep the right lower ring sharply single.

13. By convention, the flatter (lower) meridian is recorded first. Record the results for plus cylinder form as follows:

Lower of 2 readings/greater of 2 readings at the axis corresponding to the drum which has the greater of the 2 readings. *For example: 43.50/44.50 × 90*

14. Repeat steps 3 through 13 for the left eye, while occluding the right eye (Fig. 15–60).

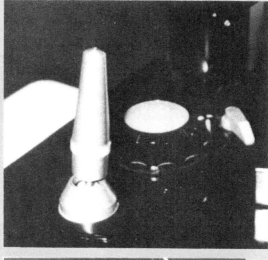

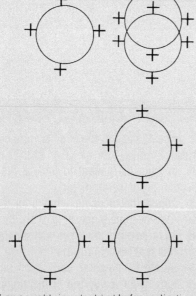

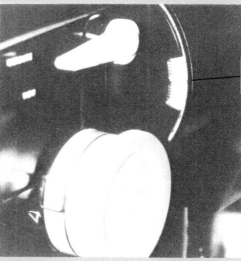

No rotation required axis set at 90°

FIGURE 15–58. *A*, Lower right ring doubled before adjusting with focusing knob. *B*, Focusing knob. *C*, Lower right ring single. Three rings separated. Horizontal plus signs aligned. *D*, No rotation of keratometer required.

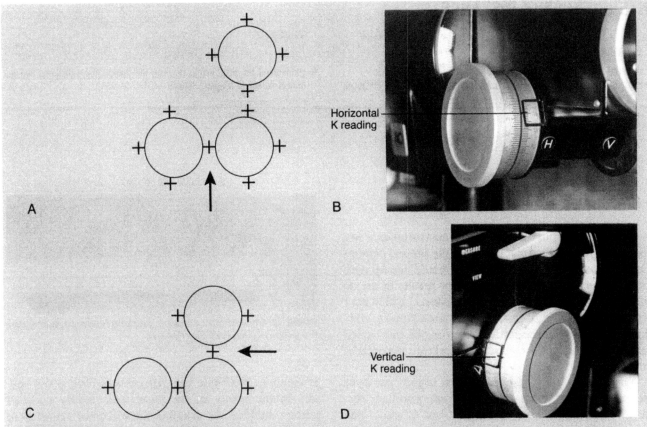

FIGURE 15-59. *A*, Central horizontal plus signs superimposed. *B*, Horizontal dial. *C*, Central vertical signs superimposed. *D*, Vertical dial.

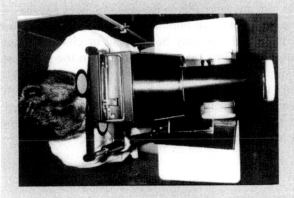

FIGURE 15-60. Keratometer aligned toward the left eye with the right eye occluded.

Keratometry

1. Steep corneal curvatures are associated with which of the following?
   a. average corneas
   b. flat corneas
   c. hyperopia
   d. myopia
   e. large image mires

2. What is the problem when the horizontal and vertical signs are not on a straight line from one another?
   a. axis is incorrect
   b. fixation is off center
   c. cylinder power is incorrect
   d. keratometer is out of focus
   e. sphere is incorrect

3. Where do horizontal signs superimpose?
   a. cylinder axis
   b. steepest meridian
   c. sphere power
   d. keratometer focus
   e. cylinder power

INTERPUPILLARY DISTANCE

LEARNING OBJECTIVES
- Understand common errors in measuring interpupillary distance
- Explain the difference between distance and near interpupillary distances
- Understand the relationship between the interpupillary distance and the optical center of eyeglass lenses

• RATIONALE

Accurate interpupillary distance measurements are necessary for correct placement of the optical centers (OC) of lenses. The optical centers should line up with the visual axes. Incorrect placement results in an induced prism producing an induced phoria, which may produce patient discomfort with prescription eyeglasses. The higher the refractive error, the more critical the placement of the optical centers (see the section on Prentice's rule.)

When viewing an infinitely distant object, the eyes are parallel. For most adults, the interpupillary distance (PD) will measure between 55 and 65 mm. Children are often 10 mm less. When viewing a near object the eyes assume a convergent position, decreasing the interpupillary distance by about 3 mm. When measuring PD with a millimeter rule, you simulate the patient's parallel eye position for distance viewing. Errors result if your head, or the patient's head, moves during the measurement (Fig. 15–61).

The interpupillary distance should be the measurement between the visual axes of a person's eyes when an infinitely distant object is viewed. The point along the visual axis on the cornea is located by the position of the corneal reflection of the fixation light the patient

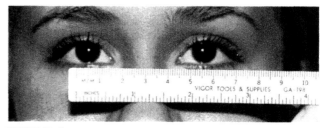

FIGURE 15–61. Millimeter scale set with zero reading exactly below the temporal limbus of the right eye.

is viewing. Note that the corneal reflection is not usually in the center of the pupil, but slightly nasal of center, making the distance between the visual axes smaller by at least 1 mm than the limbal interpupillary distance. Because the limbal PD is so much easier to obtain, it is usually substituted.

Do not measure the temporal pupillary border of one eye to the nasal pupillary border of the other eye because pupil size may be unequal or change during the measurement. Do not measure from the center of one pupil to the center of the other because of the lack of any accurate landmark. Do not measure with both of your eyes open because parallax will cause errors. The patient keeps both eyes open, but changes the viewed target at your direction.

Distance PD by Corneal Reflex

1. Position yourself in front of the patient so that your right eye is opposite the patient's left eye, and your left eye is opposite the patient's right eye.

2. Close your right eye.

3. Hold a millimeter rule on the patient's nose, just under the middle of both pupils.

4. Ask the patient to shift his or her view to your open left eye as you rest a fixation light aimed at the patient's right eye on your left cheek.

5. Set the zero scale reading exactly below the corneal light reflection on the patient's right eye.

6. Holding the rule steady, open your right eye while closing your left eye.

7. Shift the fixation light, now aimed at the patient's left eye, to your right cheekbone.

8. Ask the patient to shift his or her view to your open right eye.

9. Read the distance to the corneal reflection on the patient's left eye with your right eye.

10. Check that the rule has not moved from its starting position by observing the patient's right eye corneal reflection position after reopening your left eye as you reclose your right eye (Fig. 15–62).

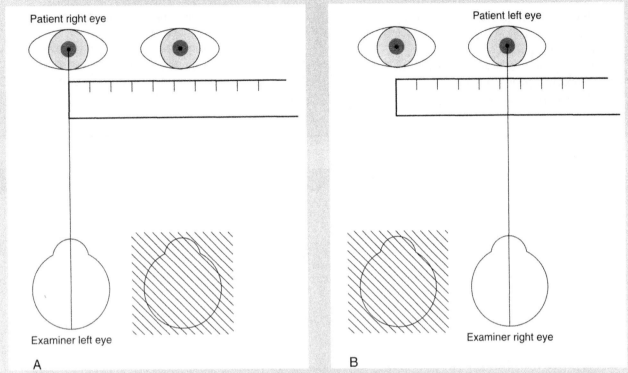

FIGURE 15–62. Distance PD by corneal reflex. *A*, Your left eye observes corneal reflex of fixation light on the patient's right eye. You set the zero reading on the millimeter scale exactly below the right corneal reflex. *B*, Your right eye observes the corneal reflex of fixation light on the patient's left eye. You read the millimeter scale exactly below the patient's left corneal reflex.

Distance PD by the Limbus

1. Position yourself in front of the patient so that your right eye is opposite the patient's left eye, and your left eye is opposite the patient's right eye.

2. Close your right eye.
3. Hold a millimeter rule horizontally on the patient's nose, just under the middle of both pupils.

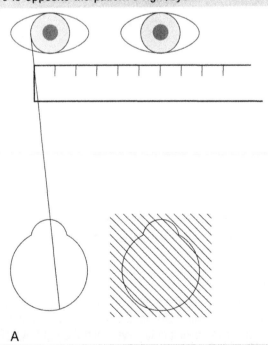

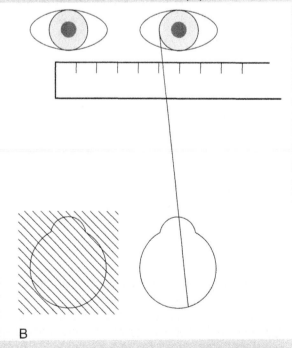

FIGURE 15–63. Distance PD by limbus. *A*, Your left eye observes the patient's right temporal limbus as you set the zero reading of the millimeter scale exactly below it. *B*, Your right eye observes the patient's left nasal limbus as you read the millimeter scale exactly below it.

4. Ask the patient to look at your open eye.

5. Set the zero scale reading exactly under the patient's *right eye temporal* limbus.

6. Holding the rule steady, open your right eye while simultaneously closing your left eye.

7. Ask the patient to shift his or her view to your open eye.

8. Read the distance to the *nasal* limbus of the patient's *left eye* with your right eye.

9. Check that the millimeter rule has not moved from its starting position by observing the patient's right eye limbus position after reopening your left eye while reclosing your right eye (Fig. 15–63).

Near PD

1. Measure the same as that for the distance PD by limbus for steps 1 through 4.

2. Keep your left eye open, right eye closed, and *do not move*.

3. Remind the patient to keep looking at your open eye.

4. Read the distance to the nasal limbus of the *patient's* left eye with *your* left eye (Fig. 15–64).

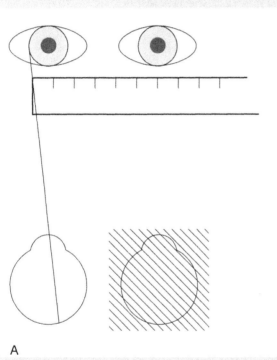
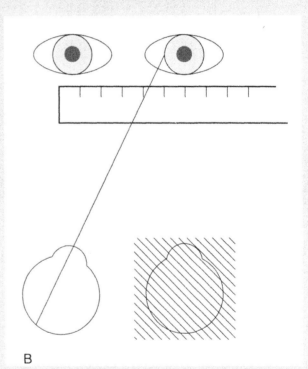

A

B

FIGURE 15–64. Near PD. *A,* Your left eye observes the patient's right temporal limbus as you set the zero reading of the millimeter scale below it. *B,* Your left eye observes the patient's left nasal limbus as you read the millimeter scale below it.

PD with Strabismus

1. Close your right eye as you rest the fixation light on your right cheekbone.

2. Cover the patient's left eye, asking him or her to look with the right eye at your open left eye.

3. Set the zero scale reading exactly below the corneal light reflection on the patient's right eye.

4. Open your right eye and close your left eye as you shift the fixation light to rest on your right cheekbone.

5. Without moving the millimeter rule, shift the cover to the patient's right eye, asking him or her to look at your open right eye.

6. Read the distance to the corneal reflection on the patient's left eye.

7. Because this method requires three hands simultaneously, you will need an assistant or you might ask the patient to cover the left eye, then the right eye (Fig. 15–65).

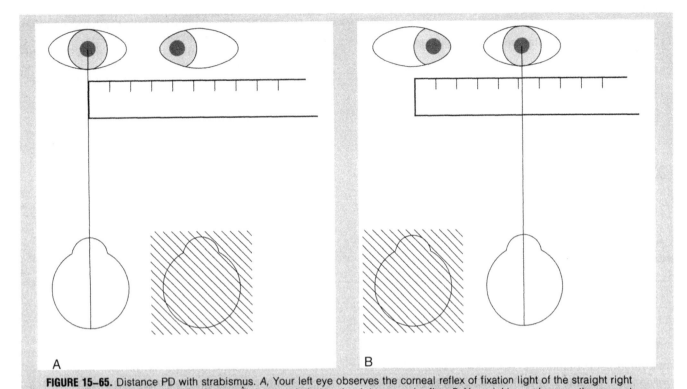

FIGURE 15–65. Distance PD with strabismus. *A,* Your left eye observes the corneal reflex of fixation light of the straight right eye as you set the zero reading of the millimeter scale below the right corneal reflex. *B,* Your right eye observes the corneal reflex of the fixation light on the straight left eye as you read the millimeter scale exactly below the left corneal reflex.

Monocular PD

1. Measure from the patient's pupil center in the right eye to the middle of the bridge of his nose, as he or she looks at your open left eye.

2. Measure from the center of the pupil in the patient's left eye to the middle of the bridge of his or her nose, as the patient looks at your open right eye (Fig. 15–66).

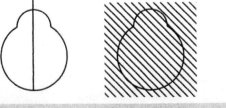

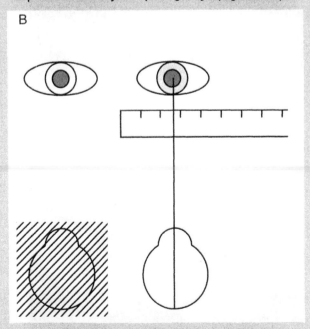

FIGURE 15–66. Monocular PD. *A,* Your left eye observes the center of the patient's right pupil as you set the zero reading of the millimeter scale below it. You read the scale at the middle of the bridge of the nose. *B,* Your right eye observes the middle of the bridge of the patient's nose as you set the zero reading of the millimeter scale below it. You read the scale at the middle of the center of the patient's left pupil.

Interpupillary Distance

1. What is the average interpupillary distance (mm) for adults?
   a. 50
   b. 60
   c. 70
   d. 80
   e. 90

2. How is the interpupillary distance best measured?
   a. from the temporal pupillary border of one eye to the nasal pupillary border of the other eye
   b. from the temporal limbus of one eye to the temporal limbus of the other eye
   c. from the nasal limbus of one eye to the nasal limbus of the other eye
   d. from the center of the pupil of one eye to the center of the pupil of the other eye
   e. from one visual axis to the other

EXOPHTHALMOMETRY

LEARNING OBJECTIVES

● Understand how to measure eye protrusion

Forward displacement of the eye in its bony socket, making the eyeball bulge is called *exophthalmus* or *proptosis.* The most common cause is Graves' disease. Graves' disease may also cause lid retraction, which pulls the lids away from the limbus, making the eye appear exophthalmic even when it is not. Abnormal prominence of the eye can be assessed by standing behind and above the patient, inspecting the eyes from above. Sometimes what appears to be a protrusion of an eye is not verified by measurement (Fig. 15–67).

Some patients may have *enophthalmus,* a backward displacement of the eye into the orbit, making the eyeball seem very small. Enophthalmus also causes ptosis because the eye is not in its normal position to maintain the normal lid shape or palpebral fissure height. Enophthalmus may be simulated by a true ptosis.

Whenever one eye is more prominent than the other, it is important to determine whether one eye is exophthalmic or the other enophthalmic. This can usually be done by actually measuring the prominence of the eyes with an exophthalmometer.

An exophthalmometer measures how many millimeters the anterior surface of the cornea is forward from the lateral orbital rim. The sides of the exophthalmometer have mirrors at 45° angles with a superimposed scale millimeter. A mirror system on a Hertel exophthalmometer (Bausch and Lomb, Rochester, NY) allows the measurement to be taken accurately even though the anterior corneal surface is not directly in front of the lateral orbital rim. The normal protrusion from the lateral orbital margin to the corneal apex aver-

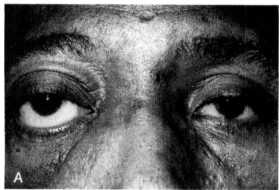
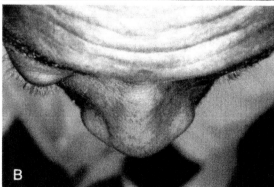

FIGURE 15–67. Proptosis of the right eye. *A,* The right eye appears larger than the left eye. *B,* Inspection from above reveals the right eye protruding further out of the orbit than the left eye.

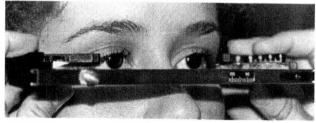

FIGURE 15–68. Hertel exophthalmometer (Bausch & Lomb, Rochester, NY) resting on both lateral orbital rims.

ages 16 mm with a range from 12 to 20 mm. It often measures 20 mm in African-Americans because their orbits tend to be shallow. A measurement of 21 mm is considered to be mild proptosis, whereas more than

28 mm is marked. Successive measurements on successive visits may need to be compared. For this, the bar reading should remain the same, usually within 10 mm of a 100-mm separation (Fig. 15–68).

Technique

1. Hold the exophthalmometer with one hand on each side of it and place it on either side of the patient's lateral bony orbital rims.

2. Widen the exophthalmometer bar greater than the outer canthal distance.

3. Change the separation of the two sides of the exophthalmometer until the sides rest comfortably on both lateral orbital rims.

4. Avoid too narrow a bar reading. The exophthalmometer should not rest against either eye.

5. Record the separation in millimeters between the lateral orbital margins.

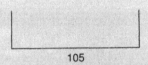

6. View the right cornea in the instrument's left mirror with your left eye, holding your head 12 to 18'' away.

7. Note the position of right anterior corneal surface on the millimeter scale just above the mirror.

8. Record the measurement.

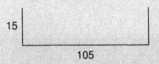

9. Using your right eye, line up the left cornea with its scale in the instrument's right mirror.

10. Note the position of the left anterior corneal surface and record.

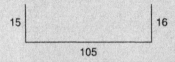

11. Some examiners line up the zero reading on the corneal protrusion scale with the edge of the mirror. This is unnecessary because it does not change the measurement.

Exophthalmometry

1. What is the normal protrusion (mm) of the corneal apex from the lateral orbital margin?
   a. 8
   b. 11
   c. 16
   d. 21
   e. 27

BIOMETRY

David Hodgetts

LEARNING OBJECTIVES

- Understand how ultrasound echoes are used to measure axial length
- Name four ocular structures that reflect ultrasound echoes
- Describe the best position for holding the probe to obtain the highest spikes
- Understand the effect of compression on axial length measurements

---

Sound travels in much the same way as light, with many of the same properties, e.g., absorption, reflection, and refraction. Sound travels at different speeds depending on the type and density of the tissue or substance through which it passes. The changes in the velocity of sound when traveling in different media help characterize the medium (i.e., tissue) through which it passes.

sound probe, it travels into and through the surrounding media (in this case the eye). The interface between two structures with different sound transmission properties produces echoes or spikes. Partially reflected sound waves from the echoes return to the probe. These are detected, absorbed, filtered, and amplified by the machine, then displayed on a small television or oscilloscope-type screen as vertical spikes from baseline. The greater the difference in sound velocities at an interface, the greater the reflected signal. The greater the amount of sound reflected, the higher the spike.

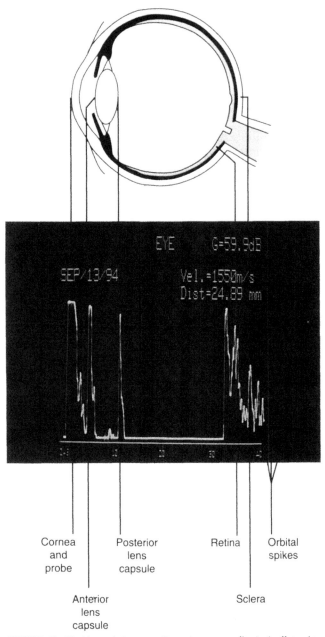

FIGURE 15–69. Normal A scan. Sound waves reflected off ocular tissues are represented as spikes, which are proportional in amplitude to the blunting of the sound wave by the interface.

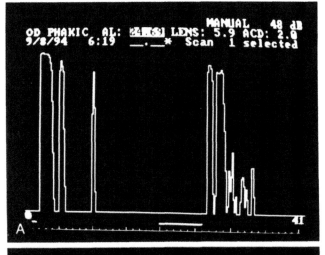

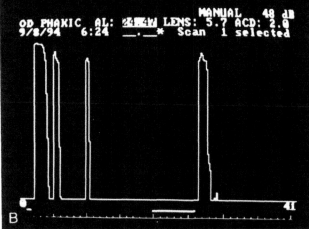

FIGURE 15–70. *A,* Normal A scan. *B,* Off axis A scan. Only one posterior spike is present. Although it is steeply rising and relatively high, suggesting perpendicularity, the retina/sclera combination and the orbital echoes are absent. The probe was incorrectly aimed at the optic nerve.

Inaudible high frequency sound waves, or ultrasound, are adapted for clinical use by the instrumentation and techniques known as ocular echography, a discipline designed to differentiate ocular structures. The technique is similar to that in radar and sonar systems. When a beam of sound is emitted by an ultra-

Ophthalmic ultrasound can be divided into biometric and diagnostic types. Biometry utilizes the one-dimensional, time-amplitude A-scan system. "A" stands for amplitude, the height of the characteristic echoes produced that provide landmarks from which measurements can be made. Diagnostic ultrasound makes possible detection of abnormalities within the eye that cannot be visualized because of media opacities in the cornea, anterior chamber, lens, or vitreous. Diagnostic ultrasound can be further defined into A scan and B scan and into standardized and nonstandardized. Two-dimensional B scans display multiple A scans as dots rather than spikes. B scans show a cross section of a slice of tissue, not unlike computerized tomography (CT) scans. Similar to CT scans, B scans are used to show the shape and location of abnormal tissue. In this text we discuss only biometry.

Biometry measures distances between structures. Measurements of the eyeball can be used to monitor progression of diseases such as congenital glaucoma, phthisis bulbi, and orbital tumors. In addition, the anterior chamber depth, lens thickness, and effects on eyeball size of microphthalmia and myopia can be determined. Most commonly, however, it is employed to measure the eye's axial length, that is, the distance from the cornea to the retina along the visual axis. The length of the eyeball is calculated by measuring the time for the sound signals to travel through the ocular tissues of known sound velocity. Four primary echoes, from which such measurements are calculated, are from the anterior cornea, anterior lens, posterior lens, and vitreoretinal junction.

The echoes produced during normal A-scan ultrasonography represent the acoustic interfaces where the sound velocity changes (Fig. 15–69). Spacing between echoes depends on the time needed for the sound beam to travel from one interface to the next. By knowing the sound velocity and the time required for the echoes to return to the probe, it is possible to calculate the distance the sound wave has traveled. Most modern A-scan units measure this almost instantaneously and display the results in millimeters. Sound velocity through some materials and structures is as follows:

Average lens	1641 m/sec
Average cataractous eye	1550 m/sec
PMMA	1550 m/sec
Aqueous and vitreous (aphakia)	1532 m/sec
Silicone	1486 m/sec

Acoustic interfaces produce the best echoes (those with the highest and sharpest-rising spikes) on the screen when the sound beam strikes the interface perpendicularly, thus maximizing the amount of reflected sound energy. This phenomenon is taken advantage of in producing an accurate axial length measurement. The sound beam must travel along the eye's visual axis from the center of the cornea to the macula. An off-axis scan will not yield the most accurate measurement. By positioning the probe to maximize spike height and to produce a sharply rising retinal spike, we ensure perpendicularity and remove one of the variables that might compromise the scan's accuracy (Fig. 15–70).

In a normal A scan, both the lens spikes and the retinal spike are as high as possible. The retinal spike is followed by a scleral spike, with a descending collection of orbital tissue spikes. The choroid does not create a distinct spike. The operator's ability to determine the quality of a scan is of major importance.

● PROCEDURE

Seat the patient comfortably with the chin rest at an appropriate height and position the machine so that you can easily glance from the patient's eye to the screen. Locate the foot pedal so that you can freeze the image conveniently. Some A-scan units automatically freeze the image on the screen when an *acceptable* scan is obtained. The acceptability of such a scan, however, is based on parameters programmed by the manufacturer, which may not be optimal on your inspection. As with all A-scan measurements, multiple consistent readings should be obtained before the axial length of a patient's eye is recorded.

After a brief explanation of the procedure, with mention that both eyes will be scanned for comparison, topical anesthetic drops should be given to both eyes. Encourage the patient to blink the eyes between scan attempts to prevent corneal drying, because the tear film meniscus is vital for optimal transmission of the sound waves between the probe and the eye. For this reason, each attempt should not last longer than 15 seconds. Methylcellulose products should not be applied for A scans when utilizing this contact method.

With the patient and machine in place, ask the patient to look straight ahead and blink once or twice. The probe is then aligned as closely as possible with the center of the cornea and moved forward until contact with the cornea occurs. Be sure that the patient does not fixate slightly above or below the horizontal, because this position will make it more difficult to achieve perpendicularity. Echo spikes will appear on the screen. By gently adjusting the probe position (up, down, left, and right), the echoes will shift and change. Some experimentation is required before perpendicularity is achieved and the characteristic spike configuration displayed.

• POTENTIAL PROBLEMS

Fixation

Some probes have an internal fixation light on which the patient can concentrate if visual acuity is good. It may be helpful to occlude the fellow eye. Some patients do well after being asked to "look straight ahead and try not to move your eyes around." In other cases you may need to have the patient fixate on some object with the fellow eye. When vision is poor in both eyes, or when strabismus is present, more ingenuity may be required on your part.

Media Opacity

Any media opacity that denies an adequate view of the posterior pole of the eye is an indication to perform a diagnostic ultrasound examination (combining A- and B-scan techniques) to alert the physician to any pathology before performing proposed surgery. Other indications for diagnostic scanning include difficulty in obtaining a steeply rising retinal spike (possibly from a posterior staphyloma or preretinal membrane), extra spikes along the vitreous baseline (possibly from a vitreous hemorrhage), or a difference in length between the two eyes.

Occasionally, a routine axial length scan can be marred by the appearance of extra spikes in the region of the posterior lens in a cataractous eye or just behind the intraocular lens (10 L) in a pseudophakic eye. Reverberations of the sound waves by these dense structures cause these extra spikes.

Compression

Having developed the skill necessary to locate and refine spikes with the probe, it becomes necessary to address compression. Obviously, by pressing horizontally too hard with the probe, the globe can be distorted vertically, artificially shortening the eye. A 1 mm compression may result in a 3 D calculated IOL power error. Prevent this problem by slowly backing off with the probe until the echoes disappear, indicating loss of contact, then gently move forward again just enough to re-establish contact. On comparison with scans obtained from a unit that records anterior chamber depth, as many now do, the scan with the deepest anterior chamber manifests the least evidence of compression.

• CONTACT VERSUS NONCONTACT TECHNIQUES

The contact method, in which the probe actually touches the cornea, is probably more widely utilized because it is regarded as easier, quicker, and cleaner. Many experts, however, believe that the results by noncontact methods are superior because the compression factor is eliminated and the reproducibility is high. Current, noncontact techniques employ some form of sleeve or tube filled with methylcellulose or saline being placed on the anesthetized eye of a supine patient. The probe is then immersed in the fluid, which acts as a medium through which sound travels. The probe itself does not touch the eye. All bubbles must be excluded from the sleeve because they will distort the sound beam and render the resulting echo pattern almost unrecognizable. The echo pattern produced by this method differs somewhat from that observed with the contact technique (Fig. 15–71). In the noncontact scan, corneal echoes are not obscured within the probe tip and two distinct spikes demonstrate the anterior and posterior corneal surfaces.

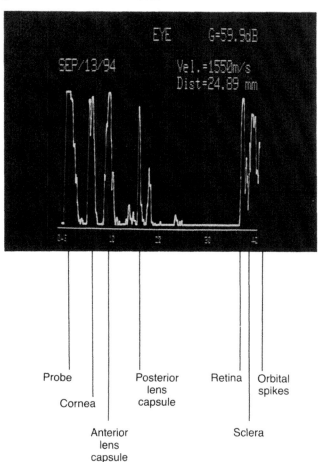

FIGURE 15–71. Noncontact A scan. Since the probe does not touch the cornea, there are separate echoes for the probe and the cornea. Because of the extra distance from the probe to the cornea, some orbital spikes are cut off from the display.

Both methods can provide acceptable scans. Regardless of the method, multiple, consistent, high-quality scans should be obtained from each eye and the axial length determined by choosing the best of these.

● CATARACT EXTRACTION

Cataract extraction with the implantation of an IOL is the most commonly performed surgical procedure on the eye. Precise determination of the dioptric power for an IOL ensures a desirable postoperative refractive state. The measurement of the eye's axial length is one of the primary factors in determining the optimal IOL power. A scan biometry is the method of choice for its accuracy and lack of risk.

The presence of a cataract, absence of a lens (aphakia), or presence of an IOL (pseudophakia) will affect the sound velocity and thus the axial length. The biometry unit must be adjusted for these parameters, which is usually a matter of selecting an appropriate setting from the unit's menu.

● INTRAOCULAR LENS POWER

Having obtained an accurate axial eye length measurement, most modern units are capable of calculating the IOL power required for an eye of that specific length. Many will generate a range of IOL powers capable of producing various postoperative refractive states. This information is helpful because the surgeon may aim for a postoperative refraction other than emmetropic, based on the preoperative refraction and visual needs of the patient. Many formulas have been developed and modified over the years. The specific formula used in a particular practice will depend on the surgeon's preference.

In order to perform the IOL calculations, two other pieces of information are required. Both must be accurately determined and entered into the unit.

Keratometer Readings. The cornea provides approximately two thirds of the refractive power of the eye. Accurate readings are imperative to attain the desired postoperative refractive state.

A-Constant. This number is usually supplied by the manufacturer for each IOL. It is generated according to a specific formula and is largely dependent on the proposed location of the lens within the eye, i.e., anterior versus posterior chamber.

In summary, measuring the ocular axial length and calculating the desired IOL power is relatively complex, requiring both skill and judgment on behalf of the examiner. Familiarity with the ultrasound unit and the techniques can only be acquired and maintained with practice.

Biometry

1. At ocular landmarks, what produces biometric ultrasound spikes?
   a. sound beams striking acoustic interfaces obliquely
   b. sound velocities increasing speed
   c. sound velocity changes at acoustic interfaces
   d. sound beams being absorbed by tissues
   e. sound beams striking opacities

2. Which eyeball measurement provides the axial length?
   a. precorneal tear film to the posterior vitreous face
   b. anterior corneal surface to the macula
   c. anterior corneal surface to the optic disc
   d. posterior corneal surface to the posterior scleral surface
   e. anterior pole to the posterior pole

Bibliography

History Taking and Visual Assessment
Comerford JP: Vision evaluation using contrast sensitivity functions. Am J Optom Physiol Optics 60:394, 1983.
Faulkner W: Laser interferometric prediction of postoperative visual acuity in patients with cataracts. Am J Ophthalmol 95:626, 1983.
Fish GE, Birch DG, Fuller DG, et al.: A comparison of visual function tests in eyes with maculopathy. Ophthalmology 93:1177, 1986.
Hirsch R, Nadler MP, Miller D: Glare measurements as a predictor of outdoor vision among cataract patients. Ann Ophthalmol 16:965, 1984.
Holladay JT, Trujillo J, Prager TC, Ruiz RS: Brightness acuity test (BAT) and outdoor visual acuity in cataract patients. J Cataract Refract Surg 13:67, 1987.
Jaffe N: Glare and contrast: indications for cataract surgery. J Cataract Refract Surg 12:372, 1986.
Minkowski J, Guyton D: New methods for predicting visual acuity after cataract surgery. Ann Ophthalmol 16:511, 1984.
Sloan LL: New test charts for the measurement of visual acuity at far and near distances. Am J Ophthalmol 48:807, 1959.
Westheimer G: Visual acuity. In Moses RA, Hart WM (eds): Adler's Physiology of the Eye, 8th ed. St Louis, CV Mosby, 1987.
Pupil Function
Burde RM, Savino PJ, Trobe JD: Anisocoria and abnormal pupillary light reactions. In Clinical Decisions in Neuro-ophthalmology, 2nd ed. St Louis, CV Mosby, 1992.
Glaser JS: Neuro-ophthalmology: The Pupils and Accommodation, 2nd ed. Hagerstown, MD, Harper & Row, 1990.
Miller NR: Disorders of pupillary function, accommodation, and lacrimation. In Walsh and Hoyt's Clinical Neuro-ophthalmology, 4th ed. Volume II. Baltimore, Williams & Wilkins, 1985.
Rosenberg MA: Neuro-ophthalmology. In Peyman GA, Sanders DR, and Goldberg MF: Principles and Practice of Ophthalmology. Volume III. Philadelphia, WB Saunders, 1980, p 1946.
Thompson HS: Afferent pupillary defects: pupillary findings associated with defects of the afferent arm of the pupillary light reflex arc. Am J Ophthalmol 62:860, 1966.
Thompson HS: The pupil. In Moses RA, Hart WM: Adler's Physiology of the Eye, 8th ed. St Louis, CV Mosby, 1987.
Thompson HS, Pilley SFJ: Unequal pupils: a flow chart for sorting out the anisocorias. Surv Ophthalmol 21:45, 1976.

Biomicroscopy

Berliner ML: Biomicroscopy of the Eye. Volumes I and II. New York, Hoeber, 1949.

Cassin B, Solomon SAB: Dictionary of Eye Terminology, 2nd ed. Gainesville, FL, Triad, 1990.

Coyne SA: Basic slit lamp techniques. J Ophthal Nurs Technol 3:55, 1984.

Ryan GB, Majno F: Inflammation. Kalamazoo, MI, Upjohn Co, 1977.

Sugar J: Corneal examination. In Peyman GA, Sanders DR, Goldberg MF: Principles and Practice of Ophthalmology. Volume I. Philadelphia, WB Saunders, 1980, pp 390.

Tonometry

Boothe WA, Lee DA, Panek WC, et al: The Tono-pen: a manometric and clinical study. Arch Ophthalmol 106:1214, 1988.

Goldmann VH, Schmidt T: Uber Applanationstronometrie. Ophthalmologica 134:221, 1957.

Kao SF, Lichter PR, Terry JB, et al: Clinical comparison of the Oculab Tono-Pen to the Goldmann applanation tonometer. Am J Ophthalmol 94:1541, 1987.

Minckler DS, Buerveldt G, Heuer DK, et al: Clinical evaluation of the Oculab Tono-Pen. Am J Ophthalmol 104:168, 1987.

Refractometry

Corboy JM: The Retinoscopy Book. Thorofare, NJ, Charles B Slack, 1979.

Michaels DD: Visual Optics and Refraction: A Clinical Approach. St Louis, CV Mosby, 1975.

Milder B, Rubin ML: The Fine Art of Prescribing Glasses, 2nd ed. Gainesville, FL, Triad, 1991.

Lensometry

Davis JK: Spectacle lenses. In Duane TD: Clinical Ophthalmology. Volume I. Hagerstown, MD, Harper & Row, 1988.

Humphrey WE: Lensmeters. In Duane TD: Clinical Ophthalmology. Volume I. Hagerstown, MD, Harper & Row, 1988.

Rubin ML: Optics for Clinicians, 2nd ed. Gainesville, FL, Triad, 1974.

Keratometry

Mohrman R: The keratometer. In Duane TR: Clinical Ophthalmology. Volume I. Hagerstown, MD, Harper & Row, 1978.

Rubin ML: Optics for Clinicians, 2nd ed. Gainesville, FL, Triad, 1974.

Interpupillary Distance

Anderson AL: Accurate clinical means of measuring intervisual axis distance. Arch Ophthalmol 52:349, 1954.

Brooks CW, Borish IM: System for Ophthalmic Dispensing. Chicago, Professional Press, 1979.

Exophthalmometry

Keeney AH: Ocular Examination. St Louis, CV Mosby, 1970.

Biometry

Byrne SF: Ultrasound of the Eye and Orbit. St Louis, Mosby-Times Mirror, 1994.

Kendall CJ: Ophthalmic echography. In Wolfe CP, Benes SC (eds): Ophthalmic Technical Skills Series. Thorofare NJ, Slack, 1990.

Introduction to Perimetry

LEARNING OBJECTIVES

- Explain the concept of the hill of vision
- Associate characteristic patterns of visual field defects with abnormalities in specific segments of the afferent visual pathways

- Explain the terms *false positive* and *false negative*

The visual field is a map of the extent of visual space seen without moving the eye. Perimetry is an accurate, noninvasive method of discovering, localizing, and then following abnormalities of the afferent visual pathway by means of their effects on the visual field. Bowl-shaped manual perimeters with standardized, stable, reproducible lighting and target conditions have been the standard since being introduced by Goldmann in 1945. With this instrument, a trained, efficient perimetrist can provide valuable diagnostic information in a reasonable time period. The number of expert perimetrists has not kept pace with demand, however. Many ophthalmologists' offices now use computer-assisted (automated) perimeters that do not require as much technical training for reliable results. The method of recording the field differs, but the concept is the same for both automated and manual perimeters. The testing time is shorter with manual perimetry and the cost is also lower.

● RETINAL SENSITIVITY

Liken the visual field to an island of vision in a sea of darkness. The lowest retinal sensitivity in the peripheral boundaries of the field is the shoreline, the outer limits of poor vision. Even the largest and brightest targets may not be detected here if field loss is advanced. The pointed top of the island represents the fovea, the center of the field with highest retinal sensitivity where the weakest, i.e., the smallest and dim-

mest, targets can be detected in a normal field. Subtle defects are detected first in the central field at the top of the island. Fifteen degrees to the temporal side of the point is a pit (blind spot) with vertical sides down to the "sea." This *"normal"* blind spot represents the optic nerve head, which has no photoreceptors. Without photoreceptors there is no visual perception (Fig. 16–1).

An eye chart measures the fine sharp acuity from the central 5° of field. Most ocular diseases affect the field outside this central 5°. The perimetrist attempts to find and quantify defects that, like craters on the island of vision, have depth, width, and location.

● SPATIAL LOCALIZATION

Our ability to visually localize ourselves and other objects in our environment is related to the particular retinal elements stimulated. A target viewed straight ahead will have its image fall onto the fovea for maximum visual acuity. The brain spatially localizes the fixation target in space along the visual axis at exactly the position that the fixation target occupies. The fovea, the point of reference for the entire retina, carries the principal visual direction, centering the visual space. All other retinal elements carry a retinomotor value related to the fovea. If an image strikes the retina slightly off-center from the fovea, we perceive it in space as being slightly to the side of the fixation object. The fovea divides the retina vertically into temporal

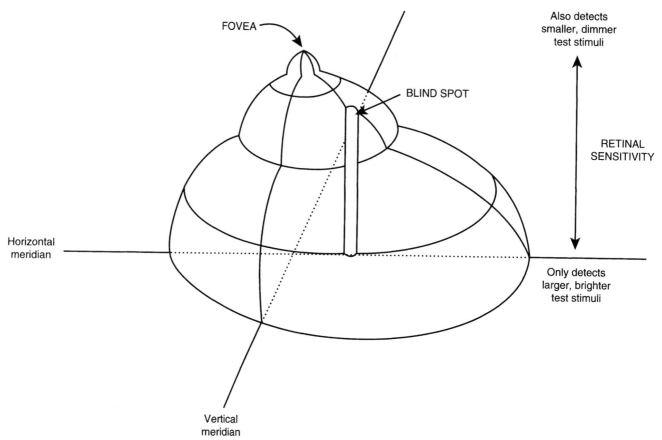

FIGURE 16–1. Island of vision in a sea of darkness.

and nasal halves, and horizontally into upper and lower halves (Fig. 16–2).

The visual field reverses the anatomy of the eye. The retinal receptors organize our visual environment into quadrants exactly opposite those in our retinas. All retinal images are reversed and inverted in the visual field.

• *For example. Nasal photoreceptors stimulated by objects in temporal space spatially localize the images to temporal visual field; inferior photoreceptors stimulated by objects above the fixation target spatially localize the images to the upper visual field, and so forth (Fig. 16–3).*

The optic nerve head is *nasal* to the fovea in the eye. Its corresponding blind spot is *temporal* to the fovea in the visual field. This positions the blind spot on the right side of fixation when testing the right eye and on the left side of fixation when testing the left eye. In the retina, two thirds of the optic nerve head is higher than the fovea. The resulting blind spot is located mostly below the horizontal meridian.

The vertical meridian (90°) of the visual field separates the nasal half of each field from the temporal half.

The temporal field from the right eye and the nasal field from the left eye represent the right half of visual space.

An object appearing to the left of center from us is imaged on temporal retina of the right eye and nasal retina of the left eye. Every two retinal points receiving the image of the same target point, one on the right temporal retina and the other on the left nasal retina, are corresponding points. Both images come from the same object to the *left* of fixation but are on both retinas to the *right* of each fovea. The entire area within the binocular field contains objects imaged on numerous pairs of corresponding points that the brain combines before spatially localizing the object to its correct position in visual space. The two foveas are the most important corresponding points.

• MONOCULAR AND BINOCULAR FIELDS OF VIEW

If an object chosen for fixation is imaged on both foveas simultaneously, such as occurs when both eyes maintain alignment, both foveas aim at the fixation object and both visual fields center on the fixation object. Our central nervous system (CNS) superimposes

A

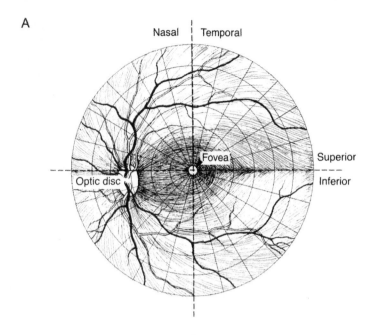

FIGURE 16–2. Quadrants in the retina have reverse representation in the visual field. The fovea centers both the retina and the visual field. *A,* Retina divided into quadrants. (Used with permission from Harrington DO: The Visual Fields. St. Louis, CV Mosby, 1976.) *B,* Peripheral visual field divided into quadrants as recorded by manual perimetry. *C,* Central visual field divided into quadrants as recorded with a 30-2 program by automated perimetry.

B

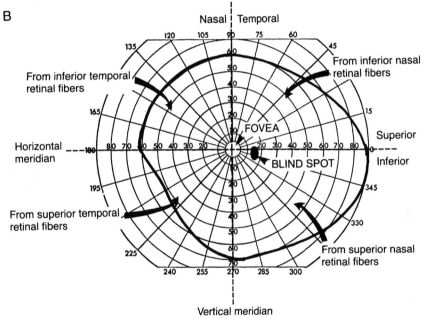

C

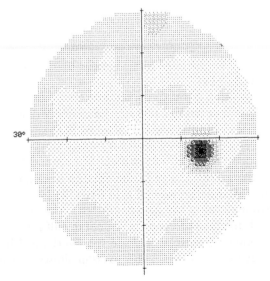

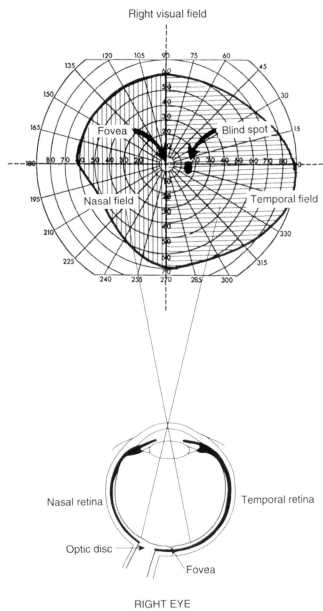

FIGURE 16–3. Right eye spatial localization for its visual field. Nasal retina localizes into temporal field. Temporal retina localizes to nasal field.

both images to form one unified image by producing a binocular overlap.

Because both eyes see simultaneously but singly, each monocular field of 150° (60° nasal and 90° temporal) overlaps to form only 180° of binocular visual field. The binocular field overlaps the 60° of each eye's nasal field, with an extra 30° of temporal field from the right eye on the extreme edge of the field on the right and an extra 30° of left temporal field from the left eye on the extreme edge of the field on the left. When one eye is closed, the field of vision is not cut in half—just the 30° of temporal crescent outside the overlapped field of that eye is "missing." This overlap allows a visual

field defect in one eye to be hidden by the overlap (Fig. 16–4).

Normal peripheral limits of the visual field are 60° nasally, 60° in up gaze, 70° in down gaze, and 90° temporally. Presumably, the nose and brows are responsible for the lower limits perceived nasally and up (Fig. 16–5).

• VISUAL FIELD PATTERNS

Time and energy are saved by knowing what type of defect to look for. Characteristic patterns of visual field defects are associated with abnormalitites in different portions of the sensory visual pathway. The pathway begins in the retina at the level of the photoreceptors and extends back to the visual cortex. With a provisional or known diagnosis, a thorough understanding of the precise architecture of the visual system is essential to reliable perimetry.

The perimetrist must recognize the pattern of different field defects to determine which strategies, targets, or programs to utilize for effective diagnosis and management decisions by the ophthalmologist reading the results of the field test. The perimetrist changes strategy as needed to find enough information to follow change in any defect. Computers need to be programmed to change strategy from detection of defects to quantication and type of defect to look for. Computers still cannot *think* as well as a good perimetrist, especially when dealing with a difficult case, but computerized testing is catching up.

For categorizing most visual field defects, the afferent visual system is partitioned into four distinct anatomic sections. The first two anatomic sections are prechiasmal, affecting only the visual field of the involved eye. The other two are chiasmal and postchiasmal and affect the visual fields of both eyes. Chiasmal defects affect the temporal half of each eye's visual field. Postchiasmal defects affect either both right halves or both left halves of each eye's visual field.

Focal Pathology

Any damage to the outer areas of the retina closer to the choroid from a degenerative process, inflammation, or trauma produces a visual field defect that corresponds in size and location to the area of damage in the involved eye. This portion of the visual pathway includes the choroid, the retinal pigment epithelium (RPE), and the photoreceptor and bipolar cells. The visual field defects produced are of the least specific types. The limit to these defects does not occur at either a vertical or horizontal meridian. These retinal defects are generally visible on funduscopic examina-

A

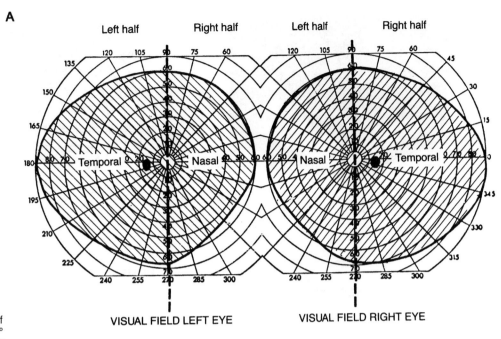

FIGURE 16–4. Binocular overlap of visual field for 120° out of 180° total. Each eye's temporal 30° crescent seen monocularly.

B

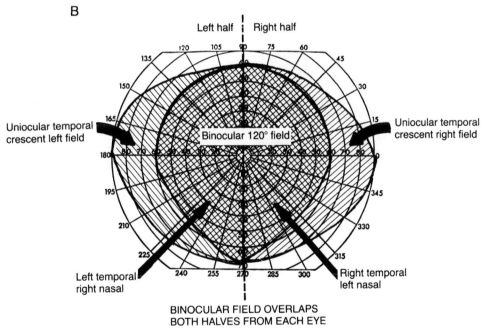

tion; detecting them by perimetry is of little diagnostic value.

Remember spatial reversal. Destruction of tissue in the inferior nasal portion of the fundus produces a corresponding defect in the superior temporal field and so forth. Macular pathology affects the central 10° of field, whereas everything else affects the peripheral field. Examples of focal pathology occur with macular degeneration, retinitis pigmentosa, retinal detachment, cytomegalovirus (CMV) retinitis, or toxoplasmosis scars (Fig 16–6).

Nerve Fiber Layer Pathology

A disease process that affects the ganglion cells, the nerve fiber layer, or the optic nerve on one side produces visual field defects that mirror the architecture of the nerve fiber layer on that side. Nerve fiber bundle defects cause nasal steps and central, centrocecal, wedge, and paracentral scotomas in the visual field of the involved eye only. The limit of the field loss may occur at the nasal horizontal meridian, but will not occur at either the upper or lower vertical meridian.

A

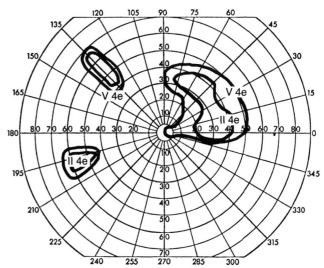

90° Temporal

60° Nasal

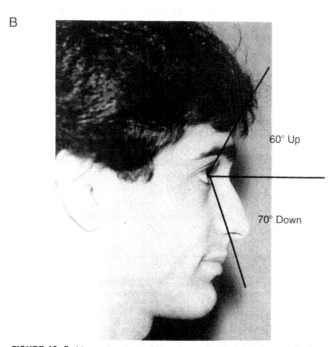

FIGURE 16–6. Visual field by manual perimetry illustrating focal pathology with a few areas of remaining vision from CMV retinitis.

60° Up

70° Down

FIGURE 16–5. Normal extent of the visual field. *A*, Horizontal limits. *B*, Vertical limits.

Because a nerve fiber originates in the retinal ganglion cell layer and terminates in the lateral geniculate body, damage at any location along its length means partial or total loss of visual function at the retinal site that particular nerve fiber subserves. Retinal damage often affects the ganglion cells or the nerve fiber layer in the affected area.

For such abnormalities, central isopters are usually more sensitive than peripheral isopters to subtle paracentral lesions. Because of the pattern of the nerve fiber layer, much more importance is attached to the nasal horizontal meridian and to the area 10 to 20° from fixation. These defects, always monocular, affect nasal fibers, temporal fibers, or both. If both eyes are affected, the defects need not be similar and they are usually not, because bilateral retinal disease is rarely symmetrical (Fig 16–7).

Arcuate nerve fiber bundles flow from the temporal retina, arching above or below the macula to converge into the superior and inferior poles of the optic disc. These nerve fiber bundles surrounding the papillomacular bundle *give way* as they arch out from the disc, enlarging with advancing destruction to form *arcuate,* or Bjerrum, scotomas. These produce paracentral scotomas within 20° of fixation. Paracentral defects either extend from the blind spot or point toward it. They end precisely at the horizontal (180°) meridian on the nasal side and correspond to the anatomic raphe. Partial arcuate scotomata (Seidel scotoma) may appear as an extension of the blind spot adjacent to the disc, either superiorly or inferiorly, or as an ill-defined area of loss somewhere between the physiologic blind spot and the nasal horizontal meridian.

A nasal step is a peripheral decrease in retinal sensitivity with a precise border on the nasal horizontal meridian. The distinct alignment along the horizontal meridian creates a step effect when fibers temporal to the macula are affected. The visual field defect divides into superior or inferior defects precisely along the nasal horizontal meridian. All arcuate nerve fiber bundle defects *respect* the nasal horizontal meridian. Uncommonly, a nerve fiber bundle nasal to the optic disc is destroyed, thus producing a temporal wedge scotoma. These nasal fibers, usually the last to be damaged, are apparently very durable.

Glaucoma is the most common disease producing such nerve fiber bundle defects. In its final stages, temporal islands of poor vision remain when the nerve

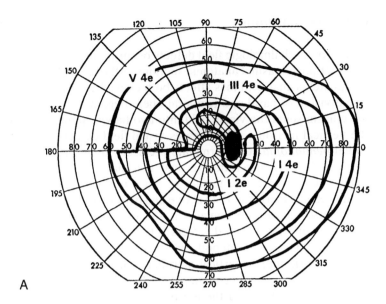

A

FIGURE 16–7. Visual fields with nerve fiber bundle pathology. *A*, Nasal step and incomplete arcuate scotoma from glaucoma by manual perimetry. *B*, Large central scotoma from optic neuritis by automated 60-2 program greyscale.

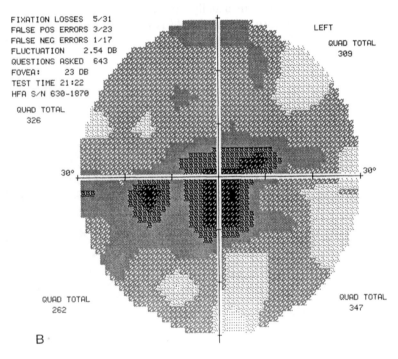

B

fiber layer is destroyed except for some of these nasal fibers.

Optic neuropathies, similar to glaucoma, often affect nerve fiber bundles. Optic neuritis is associated with scotomas of the central 5° of field. Visual acuity usually plummets to 20/200 because the fovea and macula are involved.

If damage occurs in the papillomacular bundle, a centrocecal scotoma connecting the blind spot and central fixation occurs, as in toxic or nutritional amblyopia. The abnormality includes the central 5° out to and including the blind spot (15° temporal). As with central

scotomas, visual acuity usually decreases to 20/200. Progression of these optic neuropathies is often followed clinically by quantifying visual field defects. Toxicity of methyl alcohol, chloroquin, or ethambutol and a deficiency of vitamin B_{12} or folate are examples of possible causes.

Damage to all the optic nerve fibers exiting the superior portion of the optic disc, as with a central retinal vessel occlusion, produces a total loss of the inferior visual field (altitudinal). Conversely, damage to the inferior fibers produces an altitudinal loss of the superior field.

Chiasmal Pathology

Neuro-ophthalmologic field defects occur in the chiasmal or postchiasmal anatomic sections. All chiasmal and postchiasmal field loss affects both eyes. The precise division of nasal and temporal fibers beginning at the chiasm splits the visual field into two halves along the vertical meridian. This creates visual field defects called *hemianopias* that terminate precisely along the vertical. They *respect* the vertical meridian. These fields need comparative testing within a few degrees of the vertical meridian, both above and below fixation.

Because the chiasm contains nasal fibers crossing from both eyes, visual field defects at the chiasm result in temporal field losses in both eyes, most often beginning along the upper vertical meridian. This field cut is called a *bitemporal hemianopsia*. The right half of the right eye's field and the left half of the left eye's field have depressions but usually no temporal fibers are involved; therefore, no nasal field is lost. Central vision may be affected, but often is not.

The most common lesion affecting the nerve fibers in the chiasm is a space-occupying tumor of the pituitary gland. The tumor presses against the chiasm from below, compressing the crossing nasal fibers from both eyes. If the lesion is more anterior and is located toward one side, it may affect the junctional area (von Willebrandt's knee), involving the optic nerve of one eye and the inferior nasal fibers of the other eye. The eye on the side of the lesion will have an optic nerve type defect, most commonly a central scotoma. The opposite eye will have only a superior temporal hemianopsia because only its inferior nasal fibers are affected. This combination is called a junctional visual field defect (Fig 16–8).

Postchiasmal Pathology

This disruption of the visual system involves nerve fibers from both eyes, temporal from one eye, nasal from the other. The resulting bilateral visual field de-

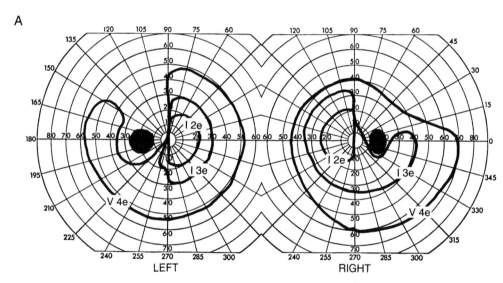

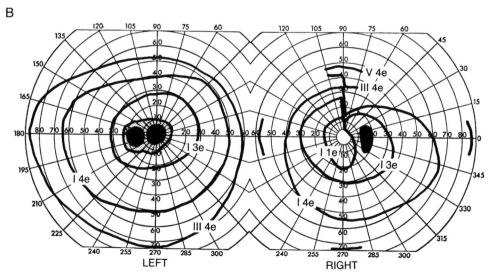

FIGURE 16–8. Visual fields with chiasmal pathology by manual perimetry. *A,* Bitemporal defects OS > OD. Hemianopia complete with I2e target, either eye. Visual field not normal, either eye, even with V4e target. *B,* Junctional defect with upper temporal defect OD respecting vertical meridian except for V4e target. Centrocecal scotoma OS.

fects end with a sharp demarcation along the vertical meridian. Postchiasmal defects are also hemianopic because this rearrangement splits the visual field into two halves. These bilateral defects affect the *same* side of visual space, making them homonymous. The defect in the temporal field of one eye is caused by a defect in the nasal fibers from that eye. The defect in the other eye's nasal field is from a defect in the temporal fibers from that other eye.

Defects in the visual field are opposite to the location of the defect in the postchiasmal pathway, i.e., a right homonymous defect affects the right half of both visual fields, produced by a defect in the left optic tract or radiations. They are described in terms of the affected half of the field (Fig 16–9).

Lesions of the optic tract are often caused by tumor, trauma, or aneurysm of nearby blood vessels (internal carotid artery, posterior communicating artery) or by demyelinating disease, such as multiple sclerosis. Homonymous hemianopias from the lateral geniculate body and optic tract are uncommon.

Fibers in the temporal lobe have their greatest separation from each other. Therefore, lesions in this area often affect the fiber pairs unequally. This results in

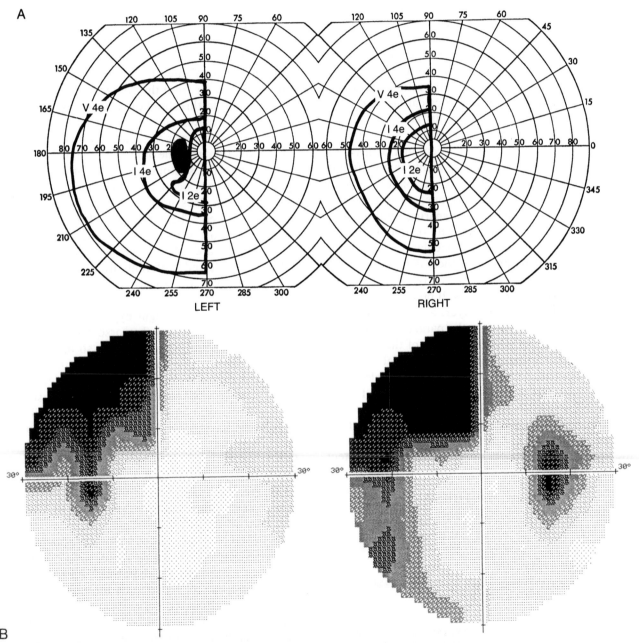

FIGURE 16–9. Visual fields with post-chiasmal pathology. *A*, Congruous right hemianopia splitting fixation from left occipital lobe defect by manual perimetry. *B*, Upper left quadrantanopia (pie-in-the-sky) and OD enlarged blind spot (from papilledema) from right temporal lobe defect by automated 30-2 program greyscale.

variable visual field defects in each eye that may not resemble each other (incongruous) in size, shape, or density, although both defects remain homonymous. Upper quadrantic defects, called *pie-in-the-sky* defects, are localized to the temporal lobe, whereas quadrantic defects in the lower field are localized to the parietal lobe. A left temporal lobe lesion will give a right pie-in-the-sky defect in both eyes, a right superior temporal quadrantic defect in the right eye, and a right superior nasal quadrantic defect in the left eye. The two quadrantanopsias probably will not have similar contours except that they both end along the vertical meridian.

As they travel through the parietal lobe, nerve fibers from corresponding retinal points lie closer together, producing visual field defects in each eye that are more similar (congruous). Eventually, as nerve fibers reach the occipital lobe, visual field defects become identical for each eye. The occipital visual cortex actually has a point-to-point relationship with the retina. Any lesion affecting an area anterior to the calcarine fissure will produce a congruous homonymous hemianopsia that spares central vision. Macular sparing is a 5 to 10° half-moon extending beyond the vertical meridian on the side with the field defect. Visual acuity is not affected when the macula is spared. A left occipital lobe tumor would produce a right homonymous, congruous hemianopia, with or without macular sparing. Without macular sparing, visual acuity may still be unimpaired because each eye still has half its macular function intact.

In summary, a prechiasmal focal defect affects the retinal architecture, but does not respect either the vertical or horizontal meridians. If prechiasmal pathology affects the nerve fiber layer, as in glaucoma, the nasal horizontal meridian or the paracentral areas immediately above or below the limits of the blind spot require special attention, to look for nasal steps and arcuate scotomata. Optic neuropathies may also cause central, centrocecal, and altitudinal defects. The patient with a neuro-ophthalmic defect, either chiasmal or postchiasmal, requires special attention to both upper and lower vertical meridians. The more posterior the lesion, the more congruous the visual field defect.

VISUAL FIELD PATTERNS

Media
  Cornea ⎫
  aqueous ⎬ Defects in the optically clear tissues of
  lens ⎪ the eye cause generalized
  vitreous ⎭ constriction of the visual field

The remainder of the sensory visual pathway is partitioned into four anatomic sections by their relationship to visual field abnormalities.

Focal: monocular defects
  Outer retina
  RPE   Least specific defects correspond to
  Rods and cones   the area of retinal receptors
  Bipolar cells   directly involved by the disease

Nerve fiber bundles: monocular defects
  Ganglion cells—first synapse   Shape of these defects follows the
  Nerve fiber layer   architecture of the nerve fiber
  Optic nerve   layer
Chiasmal: binocular defects
  Optic chiasm   Bitemporal hemianopia
  Von Willebrandt's knee   Junctional defect
Postchiasmal: binocular defects
  Optic tract   Incongruous homonymous
  Lateral geniculate body   hemianopia
  Optic radiations   Homonymous hemianopia that
                                     becomes increasingly congruous
                                     the more posterior the lesion is
  Meyer's Loop   Pie-in-the-sky
  Calcarine Fissure   Congruous

● TESTING STRATEGY

All visual field testing consists of the patient's fixating foveal attention onto an object such as the small mirror in the center of bowl perimeters, then responding to illuminated targets presented from below threshold (too far from the center or too dim or small to be visible) to threshold (just barely visible as it approaches the center, or brighter or larger).

Perimetry is performed separately on each eye. Otherwise, overlap from the other eye's field obscures field loss, as with the scotoma from the physiologic blind spot. The eye not being tested is patched carefully so that the patch does not interfere with the lid of the eye being tested. The central 30° of the visual field is where the most sensitive targets can be detected. Early defects are often found here first. The central field is often tested preferentially over the peripheral field, especially for focal and nerve fiber bundle defects.

By convention, the right eye is tested first. If the vision in one eye is much worse than in the other, however, start with the better eye so that the patient becomes comfortable and successful with the test, especially if this is the patient's first experience with a visual field test. Exceptions to this are those elderly or ill patients with decreased stamina who will be able to tolerate having only one eye tested. Visual fields *can* be obtained in children as young as 5 years, but this is exceptional. Most children can be tested by age 8. When using the Goldmann perimeter, *always* be aware of the patient's position relative to the target arm. If the patient sits back unexpectedly, the target arm may hit the patient's head.

Assessment of the patient's physical and mental status is important for gauging the accuracy of the test. The testing is subjective, requiring both visual perception on the patient's part plus an ability and desire to respond. Often the patient's mental and physical capabilities are already compromised at the beginning of the examination. A patient who is unable to concentrate, to fixate, or to understand will be a poor subject. Fatigue sets in after 40 minutes, and illness and age hasten the time to fatigue. Older patients also take longer to react either because of age or because of slowing caused by certain medications. Efficient use of time is essential to accurate visual field plotting.

Approach a field test as though each patient had a limited attention span, so that you must obtain most of the information in the first 5 minutes. That may be the limit of your useful time. Maximize the production of information. You want to obtain the maximum amount of important data in the shortest period of time for the most accurate field. Expend your energy wisely, i.e., where you anticipate the defect is likely to be, and do not waste time investigating low yield areas.

Despite all this strategy, visual fields cannot be hur-ried. Except for screening techniques there is no such thing as a "quick field" that is both reliable and quanti-tative. The quickest quantitative field test possible is by manual perimetry performed on an intelligent, healthy, young, cooperative adult without visual loss or field defect. In these patients, fields for both eyes can be plotted in 15 minutes by an expert perimetrist. With moderate field loss for any reason, quantitative manual perimetry requires 30 minutes per eye by even an expe-rienced perimetrist. An occasional pause to give the patient a rest is often helpful. The test itself can produce additional anxiety, stress, and frustration in the patient (and sometimes in the perimetrist as well). Increased variation of responses decreases reliability. Increased

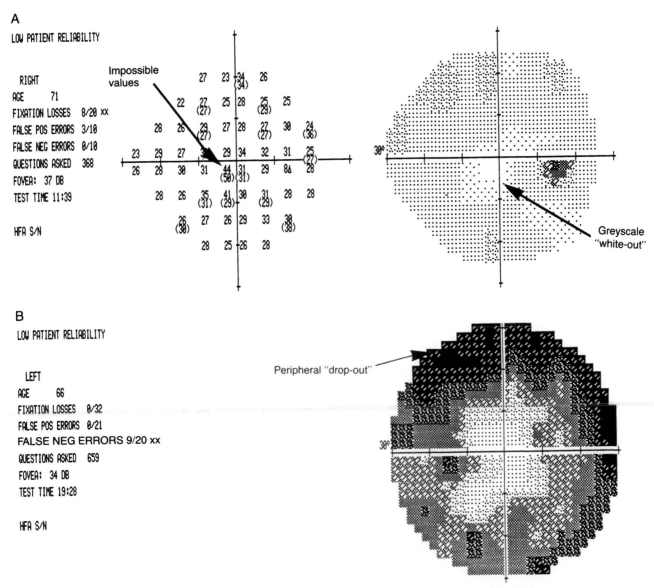

FIGURE 16–10. False responses. *A,* False positive. "Trigger happy" patient may yield impossibly high numeric values and greyscale "white-out." *B,* False negative. Patient fails to respond when target is seen. Most common in the extreme peripheral part of the visual field, it can lead to peripheral drop-out or a false ring scotoma.

reliability occurs as you increase the number of fields evaluated on that patient. The perimetrist's comments can be very helpful. Soothe the patient and remain efficient in completing the task. Sympathy, kindness, and encouragement help.

Expect increasing inconsistent responses with advanced field loss. *A false positive response* is what a patient gives when no stimulus is presented; e.g., when patient buzzes before the stimulus is turned on with manual perimetry. This is difficult to correct, because patients frequently persist in responding to nothing or become overly conservative when cautioned about it and then fail to respond if not absolutely sure. An indication of false positives on automated perimeters is high decibel values disproportionate to what is expected in the numeric grid. Become familiar with the normal range of values on your machine so that you are alert to this type of testing error (Fig. 16–10).

A false negative response occurs when the patient fails to respond to a stimulus greater than the threshold already established for a given point; e.g., when patient doesn't buzz as V 4e stimulus moved toward center past I 4e isopter. Frequently this shows that the patient is not paying attention. Periodically talking with the patient can often avert this error. More than three false positives or negatives means poor cooperation, understanding, or fatigue.

You want to select the right automated program or manual targets for greatest reliability and reproducibility. The perimetrist knows the working diagnosis in order to anticipate probable types of field defects. In any quadrant where the isopter is normal, no suprathreshold static check need be done near the isopter boundary. An exception is straddling the vertical meridian, both at upper and lower limits of the field, in patients in whom the defect may be chiasmal or postchiasmal. You are looking for a hemianopic or quadrantanopic defect.

Straddling the Vertical Meridian for Chiasmal and Post-Chiasmal Defects

1. Four major meridians appear normal. Targets presented farther peripherally than threshold and brought from nonseeing to into seeing areas (Fig. 16–11).

2. Two additional points are plotted in each quadrant for a total of 16 points (Fig. 16–12).

3. When an isopter line is drawn connecting the points, field could still pass for normal although a slight depression is noted at the 60° meridian (Fig. 16–13).

4. If strategy had been placing 24 checkpoints at each meridian, test would have taken longer, but defect now appears at 75° meridian as well as at 60° meridian (Fig. 16–14).

5. When isopter line connects the 24 points, the defect in the upper right quadrant is not much greater (Fig. 16–15).

6. A third strategy straddling meridians could have been

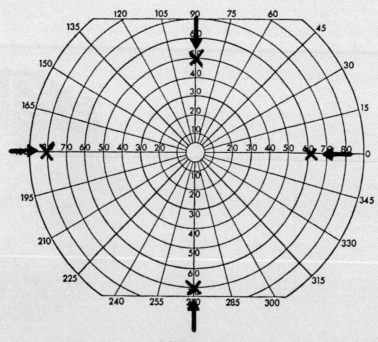

FIGURE 16–11

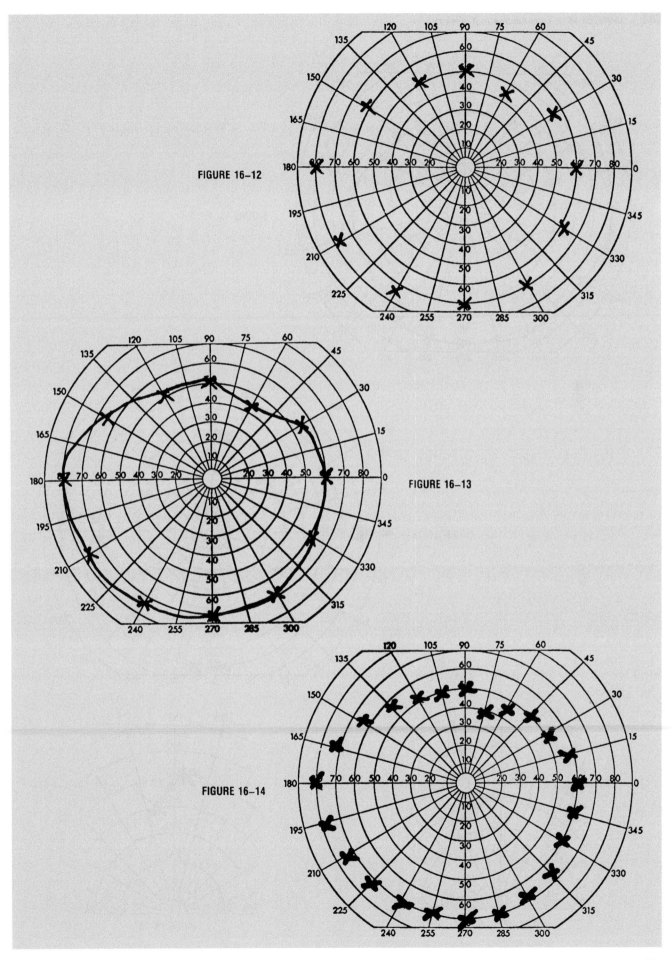

FIGURE 16–12

FIGURE 16–13

FIGURE 16–14

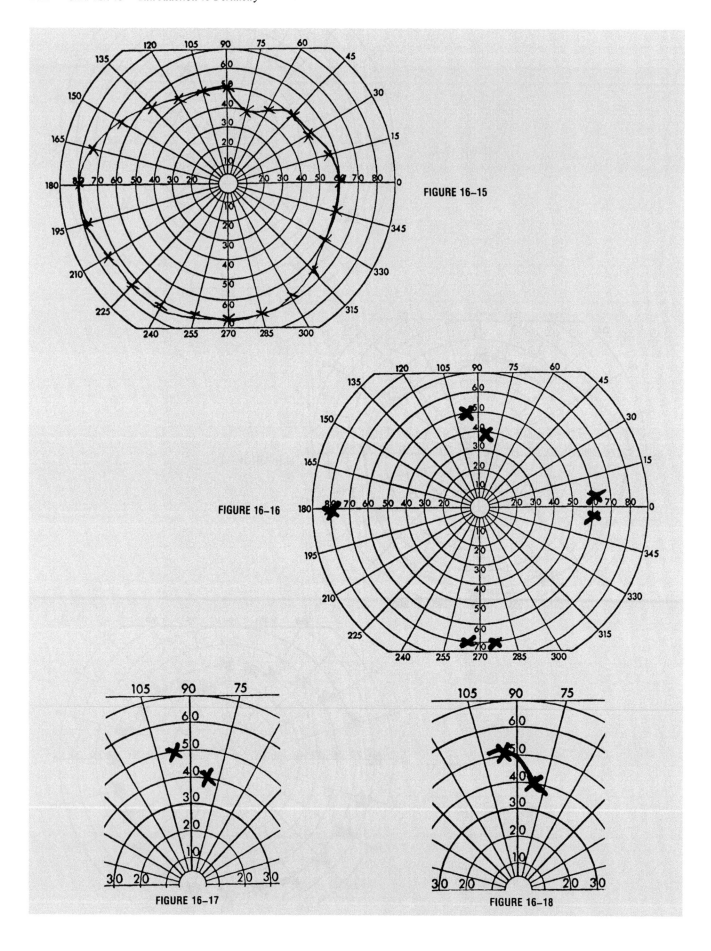

FIGURE 16–15

FIGURE 16–16

FIGURE 16–17

FIGURE 16–18

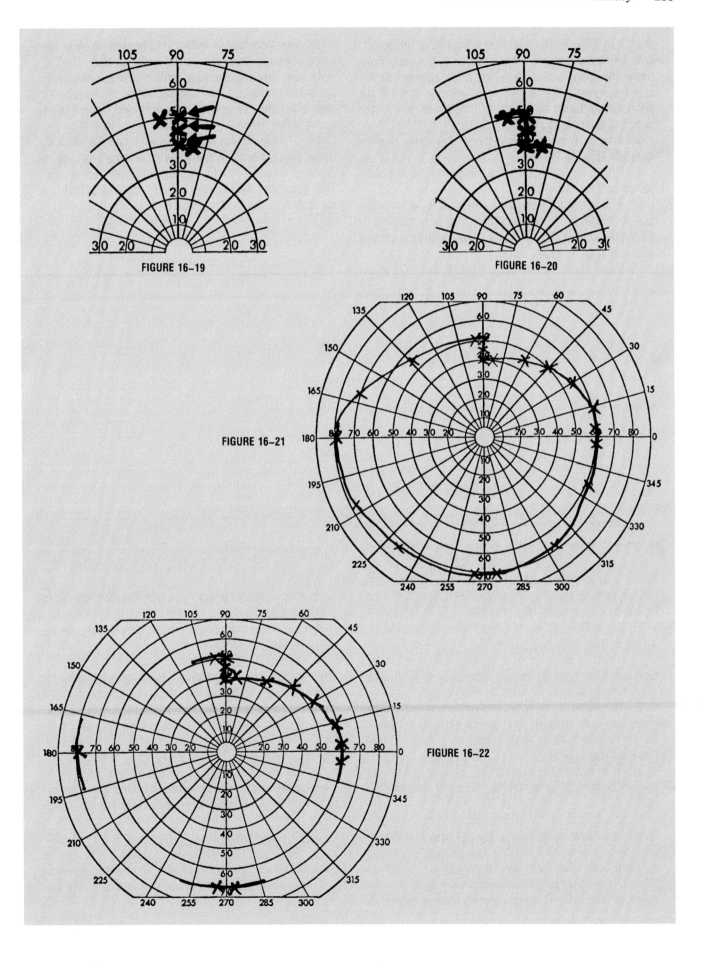

FIGURE 16–19

FIGURE 16–20

FIGURE 16–21

FIGURE 16–22

chosen to show more rapidly the full extent of the defect. With two checks within a few degrees of the nasal horizontal meridian, two each within a few degrees of the upper and lower vertical meridians, and one check at the temporal horizontal for a total of only seven points, the potential defect is found (Fig. 16–16).

7. Area of concern is found near the upper vertical meridian (Fig. 16–17).

8. Isopter line connecting the two points shows potential defect (Fig. 16–18).

9. Exploration for three more checkpoints, moving target perpendicular to potential defect from nonseeing to seeing thus better defines defect as respecting the vertical meridian (Fig. 16–19).

10. Exact contour of defect readily seen when isopter line connecting these five points is drawn (Fig. 16–20).

11. By checking the four remaining meridians in the upper right quadrant, and the two additional meridians in each of the other three quadrants, we have 20 check points and a better definition of the defect (Fig. 16–21).

12. The perimetrist may opt to eliminate the two additional check points in the three quadrants that had no potential defect, so that only 14 points have been plotted. This quickened the test, but without sacrifice of points in the area with the defect (Fig. 16–22).

Straddling the Nasal Horizontal Meridian for Nerve Fiber Bundle Steps

1. Same strategy for nasal horizontal potential defect. Four major meridians appear normal. Targets presented farther peripherally than threshold. Brought from nonseeing to seeing areas (Fig. 16–23).

2. Two additional points plotted in each quadrant for a total of 16 points (Fig. 16–24).

3. When an isopter line is drawn connecting points, field could still pass for normal, although a slight depression is noted at the 30° meridian (Fig. 16–25).

4. If a different strategy had been chosen with 24 checkpoints at each meridian, test would have taken longer, but defect now appears at 15° meridian, as well as at 30° meridian (Fig. 16–26).

5. When isopter line connects the 24 points, the defect in the lower right quadrant is not much greater (Fig. 16–27).

6. A third strategy straddling meridians could have been chosen to reveal more rapidly the full extent of the defect. With two checks within a few degrees of the nasal horizontal meridian, two each within a few degrees of the upper and lower vertical meridians, and one check at the temporal horizontal for a total of only seven

points, and the potential defect could be found (Fig. 16–28).

7. An area of concern is found near the nasal horizontal meridian (Fig. 16–29).

8. Isopter line connecting the two points shows potential defect (Fig. 16–30).

9. Exploration for three more checkpoints, moving the target perpendicular to potential defect from nonseeing to seeing will better define the defect with respect to the nasal horizontal meridian (Fig. 16–31).

10. Exact contour of defect is readily seen when the isopter line connecting these five points is drawn (Fig. 16–32).

11. By checking the four remaining meridians in the lower right quadrant, and two additional meridians in each of the other three quadrants, we have 20 check points and a better defined defect (Fig. 16–33).

12. The perimetrist may opt to eliminate the two additional check points in the three quadrants that had no potential defect. Now we used only 14 points, making the test more rapid, but without sacrifice of points in the area with the defect (Fig. 16–34).

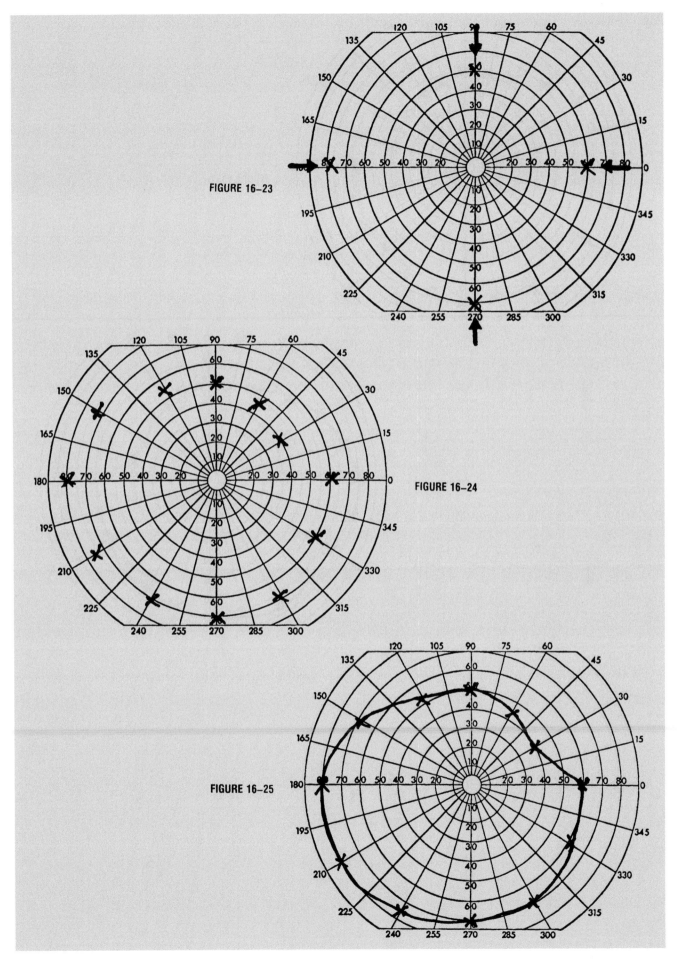

FIGURE 16–23

FIGURE 16–24

FIGURE 16–25

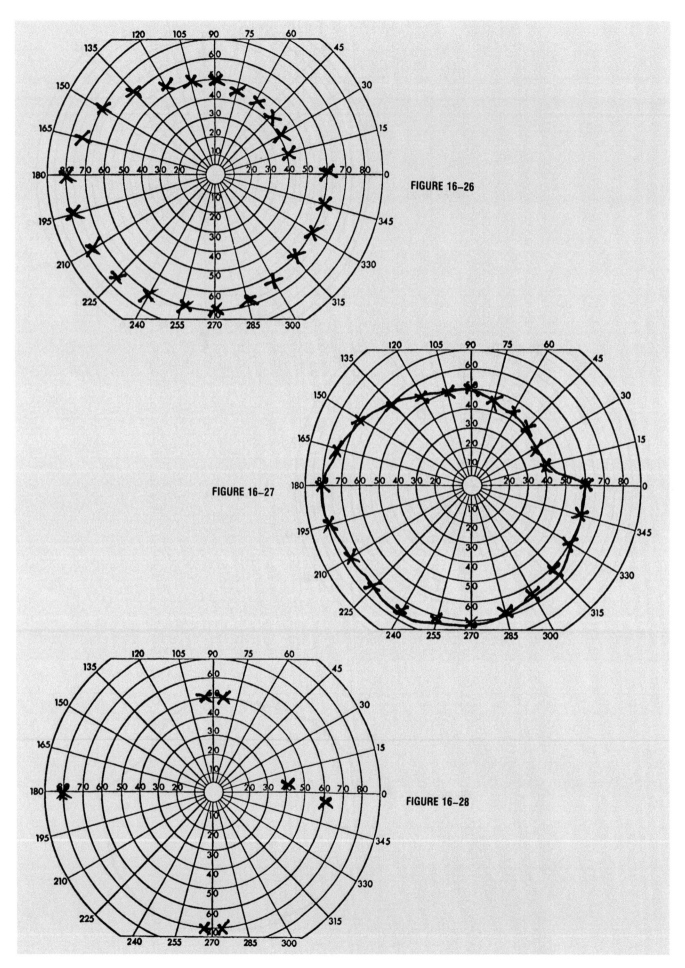

FIGURE 16-26

FIGURE 16-27

FIGURE 16-28

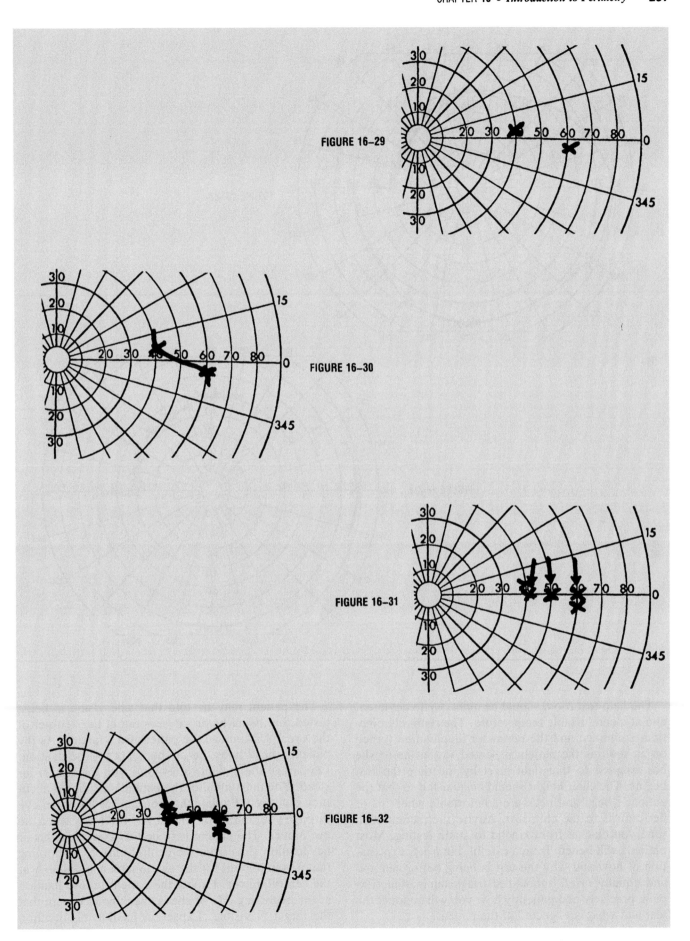

FIGURE 16–29

FIGURE 16–30

FIGURE 16–31

FIGURE 16–32

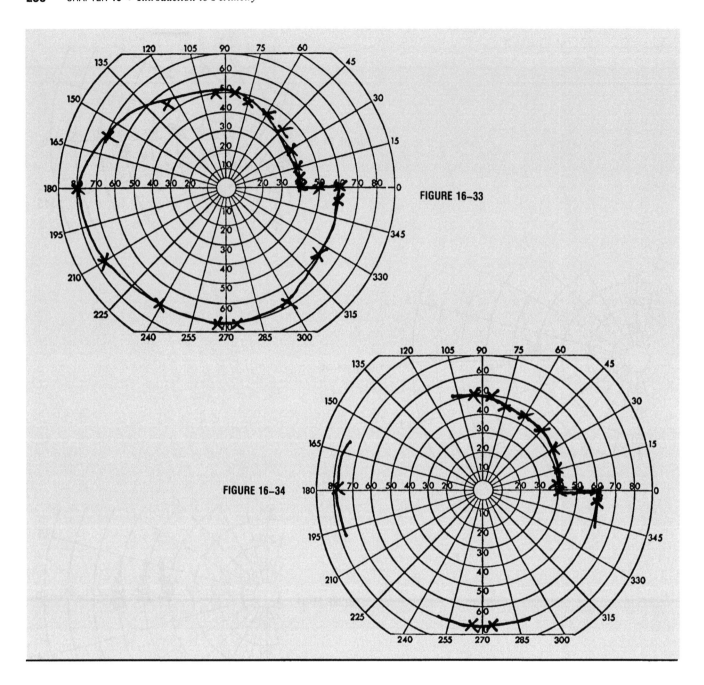

FIGURE 16–33

FIGURE 16–34

The field test room should be quiet, well ventilated, and at a comfortable temperature. The room illumination is dimmed and the perimeter illumination turned on as soon as the patient is seated so that he or she has adapted to that light level by the time the test begins. The chair height should be adjusted so that the patient's head and neck are comfortable when his or her chin is in the chin rest. Advise the patient each time you change from kinetic to static testing. Most patients will benefit from a careful, but *brief,* explanation of how and why the test is being performed and and equally *brief,* announced trial examination. Explain precisely and patiently how you will conduct the test and what is expected of the patient.

The patient may be told that side vision is being tested, i.e., what he or she sees out of the "corner of the eye." Discourage the patient from talking. As the patient's head bobs, he or she is apt to lose fixation. Encourage the patient to respond with the buzzer instead. You must monitor the patient's fixation if accuracy is desired. Explain that you can see his or her eye through your telescope so that you will know when the eye moves. The patient is to be told *every* time his or her fixation slips from the central mirror, reinforcing that it is important for the eye to look *continuously* at the central mirror. Expect the patient to lose fixation at the beginning. He or she is checking to ensure that the target is visible. Lapses in fixation or attention decrease the reliability of the field more than any other factor. Occasionally adjust the patient's head position so that the reticule cross hairs remain centered over the middle of the pupil. This reinforces the idea that the eye can be seen through the telescope.

An apparent field change can be caused by a change in pupil size. If pupil size is smaller than 2 mm, retinal sensitivity decreases. Ptotic lids may be taped up long enough to plot the superior visual field. The patient must still be able to blink normally to keep the cornea lubricated.

No lens is required for testing peripheral fields unless the patient is aphakic and needs a contact lens. The effect of the refractive correction on peripheral retina is minimal. When testing the peripheral field, the patient does not need a central add or any refractive correction worn, unless the error is greater than 6 D. The refractive correction influences the central field because macular function is involved.

On all central isopters, the patient's refractive error *is* corrected. Because most visual field patients are over age 40, most are presbyopic. Because the Goldmann perimeter bowl is only 0.33 m from the eye, the eye needs a near correction, the central plus add, to test vision in the central field. No patient has a visual field test without a refraction on that same day for best visual acuity. If the patient is not wearing the refractive correction that produces best corrected visual acuity, or if you forget to use a central add, there will be an apparent decrease in retinal sensitivity producing a defect that is not there (false positive). Even with a central add, the lens carrier position must be such that the patient looks through the center. A special lens holder is utilized with narrow rim lenses. Otherwise, an artificial scotoma in the shape of the wide rims results.

The spherical equivalent is used for cylinders less than one diopter. Cylinders greater than one diopter are added to the lens holder. All presbyopic patients have the refractive error *plus* the near plus add.

• CALCULATION OF THE CENTRAL ADD

In order to assess the central 30° of the visual field accurately, the central mirror target must be in sharp focus on the fovea of the eye being tested. Because the target in the Goldmann's perimeter bowl is 30 cm from the eye, the maximum accommodative demand is +3.25 D (100 cm/30 cm). Patients with no refractive error need only the amount of add appropriate for their age as their central add. Under the age of 35, none is needed (Table 16–1).

Theoretically, the patient's far point is placed on the fixation target. The spherical equivalent is used only with cylinders less than 1.00 D. For all aphakes and

TABLE 16–1.

Goldmann Table

Age (years)	Add (diopters)
35–40	+1.00
40–50	+1.50
50–55	+2.00
55–60	+2.50
60+	+3.00
Aphakes	+3.25

pseudophakes, use +3.25 D from the Goldmann table. Aphakes should have the distance refractive error worn in a soft contact lens. If a trial lens is used for an aphakic correction, the perimetrist may expect to find a constricted field with the normal blind spot being smaller and closer to fixation than usual, usually near 10°. This is an artifact from the high plus (+) lens, and usually a soft contact lens (around +14 D) is more satisfactory.

For hyperopic patients less than 35 years old, no correction and no central add are necessary unless hyperopia exceeds +5.00 D. For hyperopes with more than +5.00 but younger than 35 years old, employ the refractive correction with no additional add, e.g., for a 30 year old with +6.50 D, employ +6.50. For hyperopes over age 35, take the correction and add the amount listed on Goldmann's table.

For myopic patients younger than 35 years old, no correction and no add are necessary unless the myopia is greater than −3.00 D, e.g., a 25-year-old myope of −2.50, no correction and no add are needed. If the patient is younger than 35 years old but the myopia is greater than −3.00 D, use the excess over −3.00, e.g., a −6.25 D myope would need −3.25. Myopes past age 35 need enough of the myopic correction to put the far point on the Goldmann central mirror, e.g., for a 58-year old myope of −4.00 + 1.00 × 90, calculate the −3.50 D spherical equivalent of the refractive error. Because you use −3.00 to get the far point to the Goldmann mirror (.33 m away), you only need the additional −0.50 for this patient.

The central add is determined for age, then modified by the patient's refractive error. The calculated add is then placed before the patient's eye in a special lensholder as close to the eye as possible without touching the patient's eyelashes.

• RULES FOR RELIABLE FIELD TESTS (SAME FOR MANUAL AND AUTOMATED)

1. Maintain consistent test conditions.
   a. Calibrate the instrument at least on a daily basis.
   b. Keep pupil size the same for subsequent tests.

c. Use the same perimeter type.
d. Use the same test targets or programs.
e. Use the same brightness setting.
f. Use the best corrected visual acuity. Repeat the refraction if measured vision has worsened since previous visit. Aphakic eyes are tested with a contact lens correction.
g. Use a corrective lens, if necessary, for the central 30° of visual field. This is *most important!*
h. Adjust head position slightly as necessary for fixation and for patient to look through the correcting lens.
i. Monitor fixation for steadiness.
j. Move a kinetic target at a steady rate.

2. Move a kinetic target from a nonseeing area to a seeing area, or start with a static target below threshold (too dim to be seen) and brighten it until first perceived.
3. Present targets at randon times and locations.
4. Retest locations where missed targets should have been detected (false negative).
5. Retest locations where defects are found to verify field loss (false positive).
6. Assess patient reliablity. Recognize
a. Illness.
b. Fatigue.
c. Comprehension.
d. Age: Too young? Too old?
e. Cooperation.
7. Provide encouragement. Otherwise, attention and alertness will decrease.
8. Explain the test procedure.

Bibliography

Anderson DR: Perimetry with and without Automation, 2nd ed. St. Louis, CV Mosby, 1987.
Ellenberger C: Perimetry, Principles, Technique, and Interpretation. New York, Raven Press, 1980.
Trobe JD, Glaser JS: The Visual Fields Manual. Gainesville, FL, Triad, 1984.

• CHAPTER 16 INTRODUCTION TO PERIMETRY

1. As the right eye looks straight ahead at a rose bush, a rabbit hops into view to the right and below the rose bush. What is the rabbit imaged on?
a. lower nasal retina
b. fovea
c. lower temporal retina
d. upper nasal retina
e. upper temporal retina.

2. When the right eye is closed, the binocular visual field is decreased by what amount?
a. half
b. 30° on the right side
c. 60° on the right side
d. 60° on the left side
e. 30° on the left side.

3. What does a right homonymous hemianopia affect?
a. chiasm
b. left optic radiations
c. right nerve fiber layer
d. left outer retinal layers
e. right optic radiations.

4. What is a central add used for?
a. aphakes only
b. children
c. central targets
d. all patients
e. presbyopes.

5. A patient does not respond upon presentation of a larger stimulus in an area where a smaller stimulus of the same brightness was perceived. This is known as a
a. suprathreshold
b. false negative
c. sign of field loss
d. false positive
e. threshold.

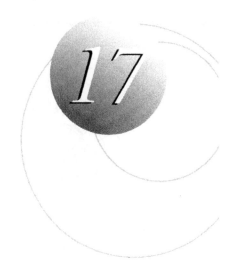

Manual Perimetry

LEARNING OBJECTIVES

- Differentiate static and kinetic perimetry
- Differentiate manual and automated perimetry
- Define isopter, scotoma, depression, contraction, central threshold target, and suprathreshold perimetry

- Describe methods for exploring defects with manual perimetry
- Explain quantification of scotomas and depressions

• TYPES OF PERIMETRY

Kinetic Perimetry

Moving targets are easier to detect than stationary ones. Kinetic perimetry involves *moving* a test stimulus (target) of preselected size and brightness at a constant rate of speed, approxiamtely 5°, or a quarter inch/sec, from a nonseeing to a seeing area, i.e., from within a defect out or from a peripheral point in toward the center (Fig. 17–1). The same stimulus is varied in its location to map its borders. If the test target is moved too fast for the patient's reaction, a falsely contracted field results. If the test target is moved too slowly, the test takes too long, and the patient becomes bored and inattentive.

Kinetic perimetry establishes a boundary of equal retinal sensitivity, an *isopter,* at all points where a specific moving test stimulus is first detected. An isopter is the threshold border between seeing and nonseeing areas for that test target. Similar to contour lines denoting equal elevations on a map, it is the unbroken line drawn by connecting each point where the patient first detects a test target of specific size and brightness as it approaches the central fixation target from the periphery. You are plotting horizontal slices through the island of vision (Fig. 17–2).

From decades of kinetic perimetry, standard defini-

tions about abnormalities in the visual field have been accepted. Cloudiness in the eye's optical media (the cornea, aqueous, lens, and vitreous) causes generalized *contraction* of the visual field. The targets are seen, but the images on the retina are blurred and are not detected by the less sensitive peripheral areas. This produces a symmetrical inward shift to all isopters as though the island of vision partly submerges. The most common example of such cloudiness is a cataract. Corneal opacities, corneal irregularities, and corneal swelling also produce this effect however (Fig. 17–3).

A *depression* is an inward shift of a portion of an isopter from decreased visual sensitivity affecting only some parts of the visual system. Some depressions are shallow, with sloping margins. A shallow defect has markedly different isopters with different size targets. Others are deep, with isopters that pile up from the inability to see in the affected area with brighter, larger targets as well as dimmer, smaller ones. Steeply sloping margins indicate more profound defects. The isopters in these cases will be the same size with many different size test targets (Fig. 17–4).

An area of visual field loss from decreased retinal sensitivity inside an isopter is a *scotoma*. When it disappears with larger, brighter targets, think of it as a *relative* scotoma, a crater in the island of vision. An *absolute scotoma* denotes a blind area of the visual field, even when using the largest, brightest target (Fig. 17–5).

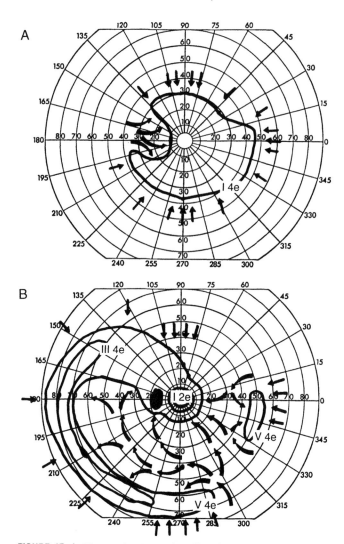

FIGURE 17–1. Non-seeing to seeing. Start by turning the stimulus on in a non-seeing area. The patient signals when the stimulus is first appreciated. Record where the stimulus is perceived moving in from the far periphery at two points per quadrant, two or three points just to either side of the upper and lower vertical meridian, and two points on either side of the nasal horizontal meridian. Ignore the meridian lines. Move the stimulus at right angles toward any defective area to define its borders. Turn the stimulus off before you record to avoid confusing the patient. *A,* Target moved from periphery in. Several additional threshold points are recorded by moving stimulus into defective area at right angles. *B,* Target moved from periphery in. Many additional threshold points are recorded to define both the extensive defect in lower field and the remaining island in right field.

Manual Perimetry

Manual perimetry employs kinetic and static methods with stimuli of variable size and illumination. The goal is detection of the highest normal retinal sensitivity. To do so, you find the smallest, dimmest test stimu-

lus that provides a normal isopter. If a defect is discovered, its boundary is defined with the smallest, dimmest test target that ascertains the defect. You then find the test target having the smallest increment in size and brightness where the defect "disappears." You are now "outside" the pathology. This quantifies the defect for greatest size and depth (Fig. 17–6).

Tangent screen, Goldmann and Goldmann-type perimeters, such as Marco's and Topcon's, are examples of instruments used manually. These instruments are relatively inexpensive and durable. Goldmann perimeters have been the standard for the last 40 years. The validity of the results depend directly on steady fixation by the patient on the central mirror. The telescope has another advantage of permitting constant monitoring of the fixation of the eye under examination. When defects are found, the perimetrist quickly changes strategies and test stimuli for maximum quantitation. Moving targets are utilized to rapidly define isopters and scotomas as recorded by definitive patterns. Most ophthalmologists are familiar with these isopter patterns.

Manual perimetry has the advantages of speed and ability to test the entire visual field. It is useful for peripheral visual fields because of the speed and ease of testing across the vertical midline for hemianopic and quadrantanopic defects.

The main drawback of manual perimetry is that more technical skill is required for reliable results than with automated perimetry. Unskilled technicians have more difficulty finding scotomas other than the blind spot. Unfortunately, kinetic perimetry has not yet been successfully computerized.

Static Perimetry

Static perimetry is the detection of a *stationary* target. Because motionless targets are harder to detect than moving ones, stationary targets are more sensitive. The patient responds to successive lights blinking as they are turned on and off. *Threshold static* perimetry begins with a target too dim to be seen. Target brightness increases until detected. Threshold has been reached. If stimuli are not detected where expected, the field is abnormal. You are plotting vertical slices from above down to the island of vision. Static perimetry tests the visual field within its expected limits.

In 1962 the manual Tubingen perimeter was introduced as a static perimetric method. It never came into wide use, however, because of the inordinate time necessary to test even part of the visual field. Manual static perimetry often takes 2 hours per eye. Automated

A

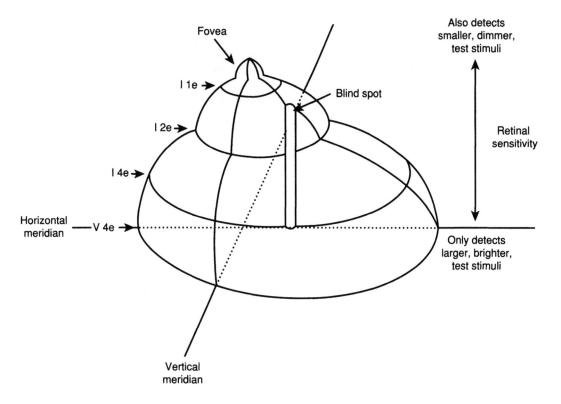

Fovea

Also detects
smaller, dimmer,
test stimuli

I 1e →

Blind spot

I 2e →

Retinal
sensitivity

I 4e →

Horizontal
meridian → V 4e →

Only detects
larger, brighter,
test stimuli

Vertical
meridian

B

Above threshold

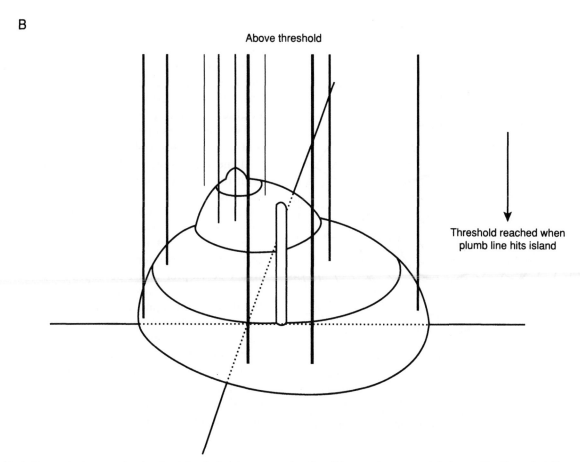

Threshold reached when
plumb line hits island

FIGURE 17–2. Theoretical concept using the island of vision comparing the difference in approach between kinetic and static perimetry. *A,* Horizontal slices through the island of vision with kinetic stimuli. *B,* Vertical plumb lines down to the island of vision with static stimuli. Similar to drilling for oil, the deeper the plumb line, the heavier and stronger it must be. Note that the third plumb line on the left is not strong (intense) enough to reach the island. It remains above threshold.

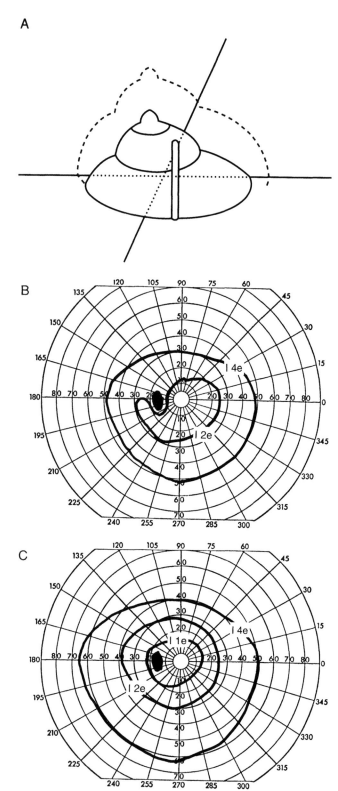

FIGURE 17–3. Contraction of the visual field. *A*, Schematic diagram illustrating a partially sunken island with a contracted field.

B, Media opacity from a moderate cataract in a presbyopic patient contracts the visual field. Without a central add the field contracts more. *C*, Same patient following cataract exraction with an add for central targets.

static perimetry had halved the required time, but it still takes about twice as long as manual kinetic perimetry. Static threshold perimetry is more precise, however, especially for scotomas.

Suprathreshold static perimetry employs a test target of chosen size and brightness to test whether it is seen at preselected locations within the visual field where it should be. On a manual perimeter you test *within* the limits of the isopter boundary at specified locations with the same test target used to map the iospter by kinetic perimetry.

By combining suprathreshold static and kinetic perimetry, the Armaly-Drance method detects an area of potential deficit by static testing within a kinetic isopter. Suprathreshold static screening quickly finds the defects. Kinetic isopters quantify them when smaller, dimmer stimuli are tested. Quantifying will take 30 to 60 minutes and screening less than 10. Screening techniques are especially helpful for patients with no previous visual field examinations. Automated perimetry excels at this technique.

Almost every office has some variation of the Armaly-Drance method as originally described. In all variations, the central threshold test stimulus is determined first, then its isopter and blind spot are plotted. This central isopter with the threshold target is most important for comparisions. It must be mapped using a central add. With adolescents and young adults, often I 1e is the central threshold target. Most patients with good vision in the 20/20 to 20/40 range will see the I 2e. If the I 2e is not seen until the blind spot is passed (around 10°), an I 3e, i.e., the same size but brighter, should be tested.

Two variations are used, one for glaucoma suspects and one for neuro-ophthalmic defects.

If the I 2e isopter and suprathreshold static testing with the I 2e within its isopter are normal, the more sensitive I 1e isopter is plotted and the I 1e suprathreshold static within its isopter is tested. The more sensitive target is used to discover any defect.

If the I 2e isopter or any suprathreshold I 2e static tests within its isopter are abnormal, test the less sensitive I 3e isopter and I 3e suprathreshold static tests within its isopter. Now you want to determine whether the defect you found with the I 2e disappears. If the defect is still found, test with larger, less sensitive targets until it does disappear.

If a test stimulus is first detected at 40° and then is seen on a static check at 45°, either that response is incorrect or the kinetic position is farther out than 40°, certainly beyond the 45° where the suprathreshold static target was seen.

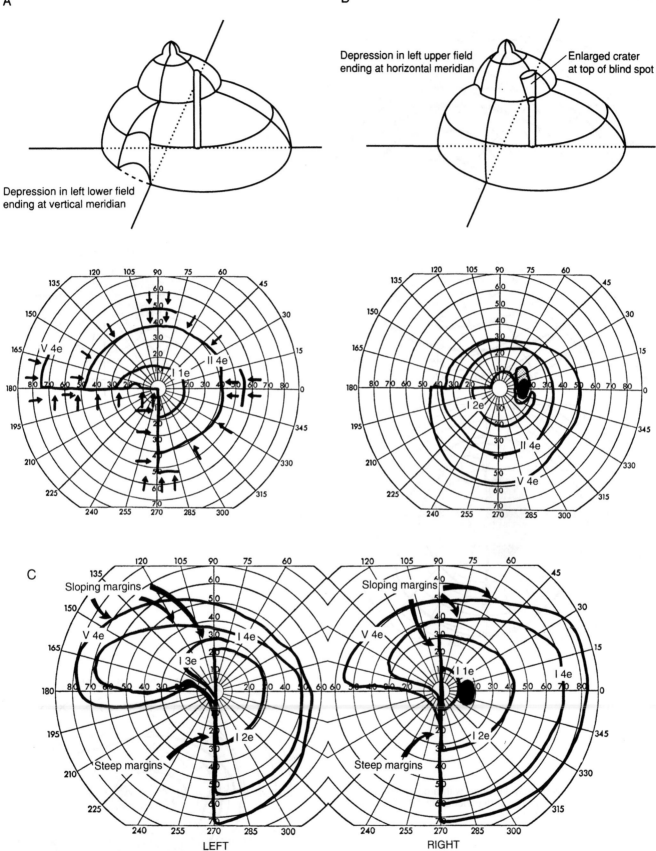

FIGURE 17–4. Craters and depressions in the island of vision. *A,* Schematic diagram illustrating a depression such as occurs with neurological defects respecting a vertical meridian.

B, Schematic diagram illustrating a depression that occurs with a nasal step respecting the nasal horizontal meridian and a crater from an enlarged blind spot. Both often occur with glaucoma.

C, Defects may have isopter margins that slope with fields that enlarge with larger stimuli. Isopter defects with steep margins remain the same with different size stimuli.

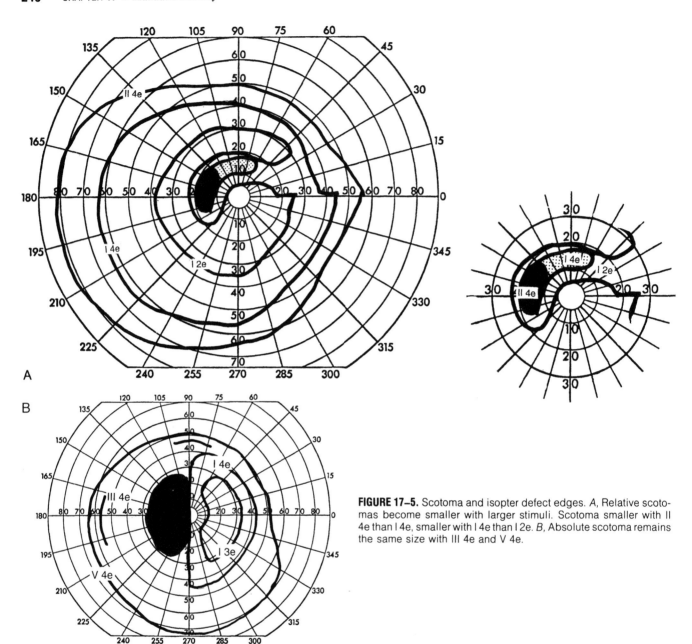

A

B

FIGURE 17–5. Scotoma and isopter defect edges. *A*, Relative scotomas become smaller with larger stimuli. Scotoma smaller with II 4e than I 4e, smaller with I 4e than I 2e. *B*, Absolute scotoma remains the same size with III 4e and V 4e.

FIGURE 17–6. Defects may disappear with larger stimuli as you move outside the pathology. Nasal step found with I 2e, I 3e, I 4e, but III 4e target is outside the defect.

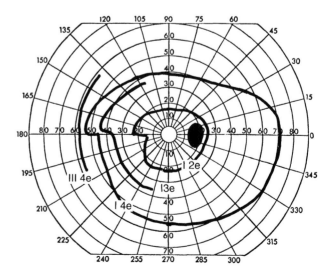

Goldmann's Perimeter Calibration

1. Seat the patient and dim the room illumination to match the testing conditions.

2. Turn the machine on from the back and maintain dim room illumination.

3. Ensure that the patient is well away from the path of the target arm.

4. Place a visual field chart in the rear slot. Center it using bottom center and side center frame notches.

5. Lock the stylus in place at 70° on the right side of the field paper (Fig. 17–7).

6. Turn on the ON/OFF button on the right rear side.

7. Set the target size to V and the illumination level to 4e. Both levers are now pushed to the extreme right position (Fig. 17–8).

8. Remove the barrier (or push up the flag) from the small opening on the left side near the front of the perimeter bowl (Fig. 17–9).

9. With the stimulus button on, hold the light meter at the opening just created. The V 4e light should fall on the light sensitive cell of the light meter, which should read 1400 Lux (lx) (1000 apostilbs [asb]). If a higher reading is noted, adjust the knob on the lower left side of the perimeter. If the light cannot be maximized to 1430 lx, turn the light bulb 180°. If the light meter still does not register 1430 lx, change the bulb in the perimeter bowl (Fig. 17–10).

10. Change the target setting to V le and replace the barrier (or push the flag down) on the left side. This should cover the light sensitive cell (Fig.17–11).

11. Look through the slit in the perimeter bowl from the side opposite the barrier. Using the lever or sleeve at the top of the bowl, adjust the light level so that the brightness of the bowl interior matches that in the barrier opening, usually called the doughnut (Fig. 17–12).

12. Unlock the stylus.

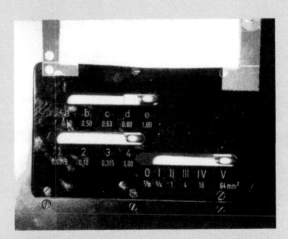

FIGURE 17–8. Push all levers to far right.

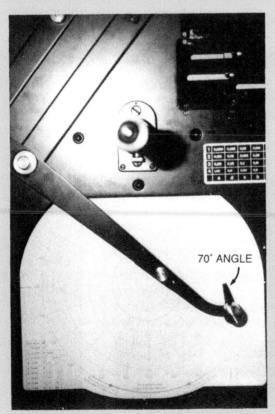

70° ANGLE

FIGURE 17–7. Locking stylus.

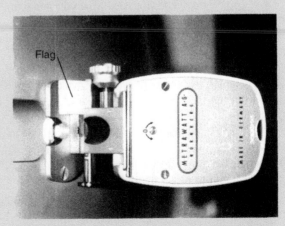

Flag

FIGURE 17–9. Remove the barrier so that light hits meter.

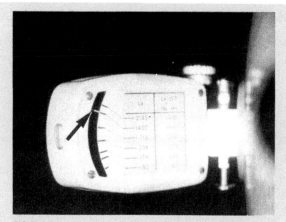

FIGURE 17–10. Reading the light meter.

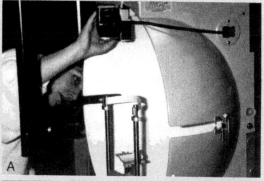

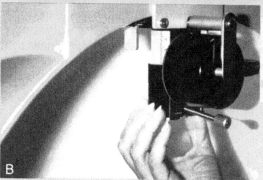

FIGURE 17–12. Lever at top of bowl adjusts light level in the "doughnut."

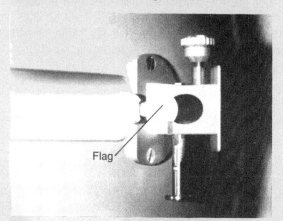

Flag

FIGURE 17–11. Replace the barrier, covering light sensitive cell.

Technique for Manual Perimetry

A. Patient Preparation

1. Adjust the instrument table and the chair for the patient's comfort.

2. Keep the room illumination dim with the perimeter bowl illuminated so that the patient will be appropriately light-adapted for the mesopic conditions of testing.

3. Explain briefly and precisely what you are about to do and what response you expect from the patient.

4. Tell the patient how you will be monitoring fixation and why.

5. Patch the worst eye and test the better eye first. If vision is equal, test the right eye first. Avoid any interference from the patch band to the eyelid of the eye to be tested.

6 Guide the patient's head to rest comfortably in the chin rest with the forehead against the restraining band. Warn that the target arm will strike the patient's head if the chin is not firmly in the rest (Fig. 17–13).

7. Using the horizontal and vertical knobs at the bottom rear of the perimeter, align the eye to be tested so that the pupil is centered in the cross hairs of the reticule when viewed in the telescope at the rear of the instrument (Fig. 17–14).

8. Focus the reticule to measure pupil diameter on the vernier scale of the horizontal cross hair. Make the measurement *without* the central add in front of the eye.

9. Center the visual field paper in the rear slot by using the bottom center and side center frame notches (Fig. 17–15).

10. Set the target levers to I 4e and show the stimulus to the patient. Demonstrate target movement and observe the patient's fixation (Fig. 17–16).

11. Check that the response buzzer is working and that the patient knows how to respond (Fig. 17–17).

12. Adjust the shutter switch on the right rear side of the perimeter so that the illuminated target is seen only when the switch is depressed manually.

13. Place the central add in the lens holder, adjusting it close to the patient's face to touch the brow but not the eyelashes. Utilize a thin-rimmed lens to avoid creating an artificial ring-shaped blind area. If you use a contact lens on the aphakic eye, use the full +3.25 central correction (Fig. 17–18).

14. Always be aware of the patient's position with respect to the target arm. If the patient sits back from the chin rest, he or she may be struck by it.

B. Central Visual Field Exploration

1. Double check to ensure that the eye not being tested is covered.

2. Identify the central threshold target, the smallest, dimmest target the patient can see beyond the blind spot approximately 25° temporal to fixation.

3. Plot the blind spot with the central threshold target by turning the target light on where the patient does *not* see it, then moving the target steadily until the patient *does* see it. About 15° temporal to fixation, 5° below the horizontal meridian, is a good place to begin (Fig. 17–19).

4. Plot the isopter with the threshold target, moving steadily from the nonseeing periphery toward the center, marking each point where the patient first responds. This threshold isopter is an essential part of the examination, providing the major visual field landmark as well as establishing a measure of reliability of the patient's performance.

5. Pay particular attention to the meridians approximately 3° to 5° on either side of the superior and inferior vertical meridians and the nasal horizontal meridian. One seeing point at least 5° closer to fixation than the comparative point on the other side of the meridian defines a *step*. The line connecting these two points aligns exactly along the meridian and does not merely slope across it (Fig. 17–20).

6. Use the same threshold target size for a static check. The target light is turned on without moving it at different points within the isopter. Alert the patient to the change in strategy. The target is now suprathreshold. It should be seen everywhere within the central isopter except the blind spot. If a static point is not seen on two successive trials, that area may contain a scotoma. When using the same target kinetically from the missed points, it should be seen. If not, plot as for any scotoma. If the target is seen, check the same area for a scotoma with the next most sensitive kinetic target.

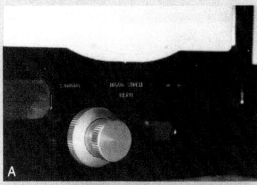

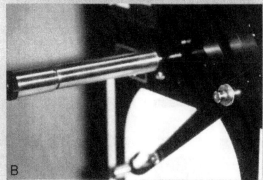

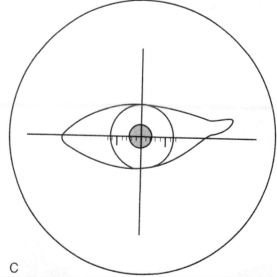

FIGURE 17–14. Pupil centered in cross hairs. *A,* Horizontal and vertical dials move the chin rest. *B,* Telescope allows perimetrist to constantly monitor fixation. *C,* Note that the eye (and the head) appear upside down.

FIGURE 17–13. Patient seated with head in chin rest.

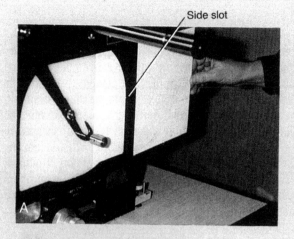

Side slot

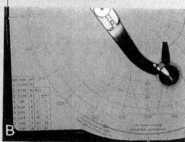

Side center frame notch

Bottom center frame notch

FIGURE 17–15. Centering the visualfield paper in the perimeter frame. *A,* Paper is being slid into place through side slots. *B,* Paper is aligned with side and bottom frame notches.

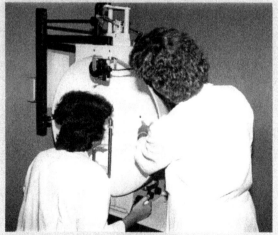

FIGURE 17–16. Show I 4e stimulus on bowl to patient.

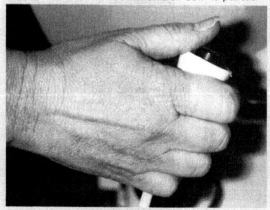

FIGURE 17–17. Response buzzer.

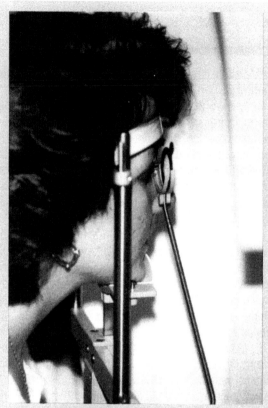

FIGURE 17–18. Central add in lens holder.

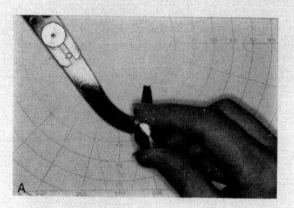

B

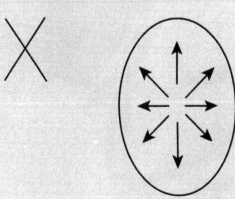

FIGURE 17–19. Plot the blind spot. *A,* Place stimulus "inside" the blind spot before turning the stimulus on. *B,* Always move stimulus from non-seeing to seeing area.

C. Peripheral Visual Field Mapping

1. Remove the central add and give the patient a short rest.

2. Approach the center from the far nasal periphery with a I 4e target until it is seen.

3. Repeat with successively larger targets. As the responses move farther out, the isopters begin to fall very close together. Choose the smallest target where the targets fall close together to plot an entire peripheral isopter (Fig. 17–21).

4. If the I 4e isopter is normal, choose the V 4e stimulus and plot its isopter.

5. Repeat for the other eye.

6. For each eye, record the patient's name and medical record number, the date, whether the patient cooperated, and if reliably, the central add, and the best corrected visual acuity. Comment about the examination to help with interpretation, especially if the test was difficult or inconsistencies were found.

7. Label each isopter.

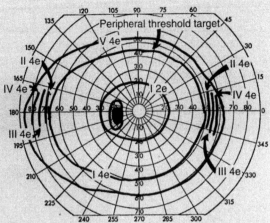

FIGURE 17–21. Plotting the peripheral isopter. Central threshold isopter with the I 2e was plotted first. Peripheral targets I 4e, II 4e, III 4e, IV 4e, and V 4e tested near temporal and nasal horizontal meridians. All five targets fall closely together. I 4e should be chosen as the peripheral isopter and plotted as noted here. The perimetrist had the central I 1e as an option for the third isopter or could have chosen one of the other peripheral targets. She opted for the V 4e.

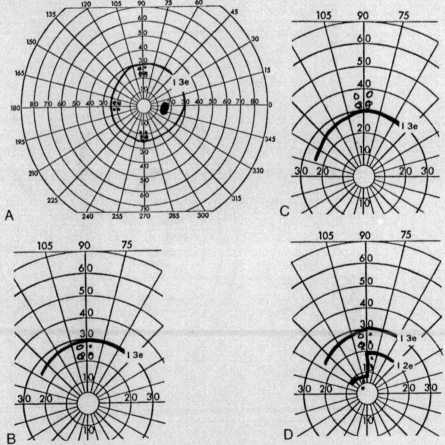

FIGURE 17–20. Suprathreshold static testing with kinetic central threshold target. *A,* Kinetic I 3e is plotted, then used to check static points just within the isopter at both vertical meridians, and at the nasal horizontal meridian. I 3e seen at static positions tested, except at upper vertical meridian where it is not seen on two attempts to the left of the meridian. A dot is used where seen; a small open circle, when not seen. *B,* Static points at upper vertical meridian as seen on repeat test, verifying not seen to the left of the upper vertical meridian. *C,* Checking static points outside the kinetic isopter with the I 3e is not fruitful because static more difficult to see than kinetic. Patient should always, and does here, miss points outside the isopter when inadvertently attempted. *D,* I 2e locates vertical step in area where static check with I 3e was missed. Patient does see I 2e when tested as static target within the I 2e isopter.

Armaly-Drance Technique for Glaucoma Suspect

1. Place the central add in the lens holder.
2. Determine the central threshold stimulus. For example, a central I 2e isopter should ring the field approximately 25° from fixation, just outside the blind spot.
3. Plot the blind spot kinetically with the central threshold stimulus. In this example, the I 2e.
4. Screen the paracentral area statically. Use the central

threshold stimulus as a suprathreshold static stimulus 15° from fixation at every meridian. Check two points at meridians 15° above and 15° below the blind spot.
5. Determine the dimmest stimulus seen kinetically 10° from fixation and map its isopter, which is most often the I 1e.
6. Use this dimmest stimulus as the central supra-

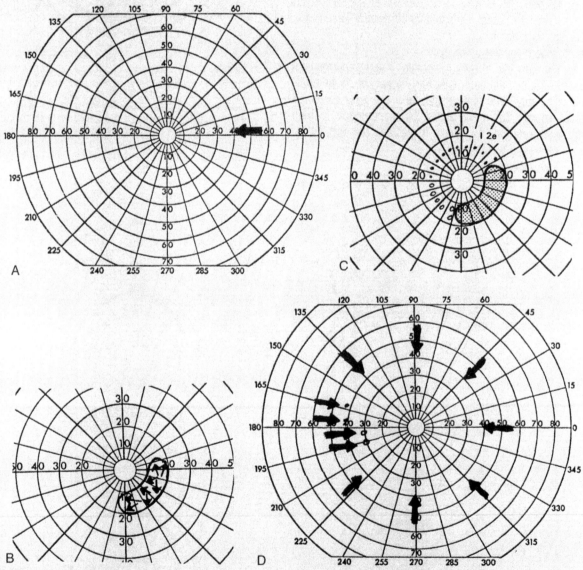

FIGURE 17–22. Armaly-Drance technique for glaucoma. *A,* Central kinetic I 2e moved on temporal horizontal meridian from 50° in towards central mirror. I 2e is perceived at 35°, so I 1e attempted. Because the I 1e was not perceived further out than 10°, the I 2e is chosen as the central threshold isopter. *B,* The blind spot is mapped with the I 2e kinetically, starting within the area where the target is not seen, until the target is seen. *C,* The same I 2e is used as a suprathreshold static target at every meridian 15° from the central mirror, and twice, just above and below the blind spot. I 2e is missed as a static target below the blind spot all the way to the nasal horizontal meridian. *D,* I 2e kinetic isopter tested at the nasal horizontal meridian where two checkpoints just above and two just below are plotted. In this example, a nasal step is found below the nasal horizontal meridian. The I 2e is now used as a suprathreshold static target to test just within the kinetic isopter at the four points found at the nasal horizontal meridian. Note that the two static points just below the nasal horizontal meridian are missed. Only three isopter points about every 45° in the upper field and three isopter points about every 45° in the lower field, including upper and lower vertical meridians, plus the temporal horizontal isopter, are plotted. No pathology is expected in these areas.

threshold static target to test all points 5° from fixation and the four quadrants within 5° of the central fixation mirror.

7. Explore for a central nasal step with the central threshold stimulus. Begin to test kinetically to threshold from 35° nasal of fixation twice above (5° and 10°) and twice below (5° and 10°) the nasal horizontal meridian.

8. Suprathreshold static testing with the same I 2e is performed just within the nasal horizontal isopter, two static checks above (5° and 10°) and below (5° and 10°) the nasal meridian.

9. Complete the central threshold (I 2e) isopter by plotting 3 meridians above (135°, 90°, 45°) and 3 meridians below (225°, 270°, 315°).

10. Remove the central add.

11. Explore for a kinetic peripheral nasal step with a brighter stimulus (usually the I 4e). Begin moving the stimulus in from 70° nasal of fixation twice above (5° and 10°) and twice below (5° and 10°) the nasal horizontal meridian.

12. Use the same peripheral kinetic stimulus to check statically just inside the peripheral isopter twice, two static

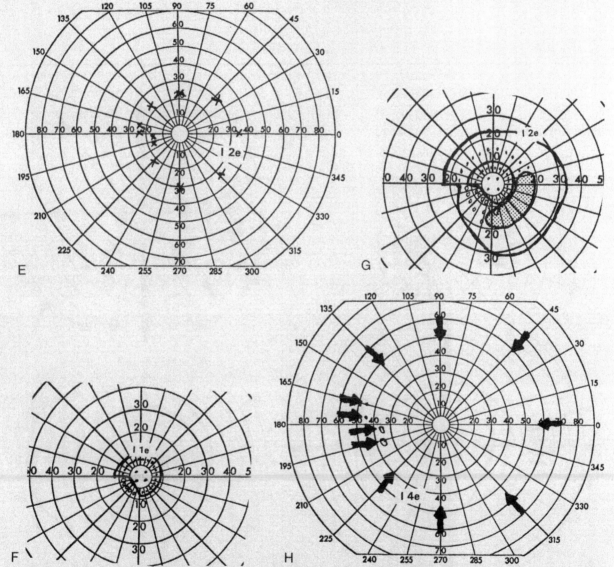

FIGURE 17-22. *Continued E,* Plotted points from figures C and D. We will concentrate our strategy on the nasal horizontal meridian and the blind spot extension below. *F,* The I 1e kinetic isopter is mapped. Then the I 1e is used as a suprathreshold static target in the four quadrants in the central 5°, and in each meridian just outside 5°. As expected, the static I 1e is missed in the lower nasal quadrant outside 5° because the kinetic isopter is closer to fixation here. *G,* The completed central visual field just plotted. *H,* Testing for a peripheral target. The I 4e perceived at 52° on the temporal horizontal meridian is chosen. When the target moved in from 65° toward the central mirror just above and just below the nasal horizontal meridian, the nasal step is still found below. When the I 4e is used as a suprathreshold static target just inside the nasal horizontal isopter, it is seen above but not below. Kinetic isopter points at the upper and lower vertical meridians, the temporal horizontal meridian, and one point per quadrant in between are plotted.

checks above (5° and 10°) and below (5° and 10°) the nasal meridian.

13. Kinetically outline the remaining peripheral isopter at upper (90°) and lower (270°) vertical meridians and the temporal horizontal meridian.

14. Check statically just inside the temporal horizontal meridian isopter and the upper and lower vertical meridian isopters (Fig. 17–22).

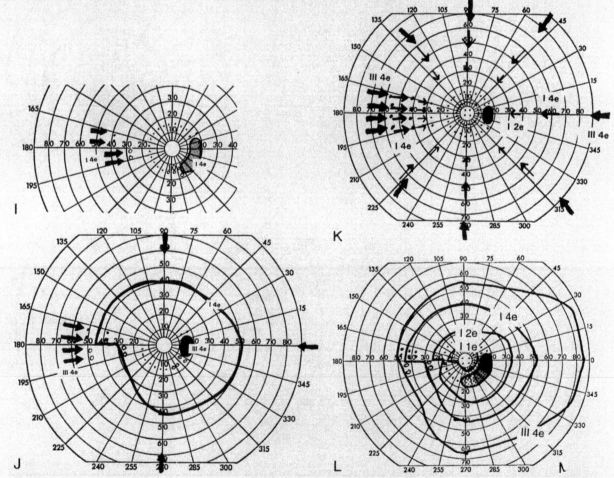

FIGURE 17–22. *Continued I,* Because the blind spot is abnormal with the I 2e, it is replotted with the I 4e. The defect is smaller than with the I 2e, but still not normal. Notice the missing I 4e suprathreshold static points in the lower nasal area 15° from fixation. *J,* Draw the kinetic I 4e isopter. Because the I 4e had an enlarged blind spot and a nasal step, the same procedure was used for the III 4e to determine if it was normal. When target moved in from 75° toward the central mirror just above and just below the nasal horizontal meridian, no nasal step is found. When the blind spot was tested, it was also normal. Because we have gotten outside the pathology, testing any larger peripheral target is unnecessary. *K,* A composite of the Armaly-Drance technique for glaucoma for the peripheral and central visual field. Static checkpoints are marked with a dot if seen. *L,* Entire recorded visual field.

Armaly-Drance Technique for Neuro-ophthalmologic Defects

1. Place the central add in the lens holder.

2. Determine the central threshold stimulus. For example, a central I 2e isopter should ring the field approximately 25° from fixation, just outside the blind spot.

3. Plot the blind spot kinetically with the central threshold stimulus. In this example, it is the I 2e.

4. Screen the paracentral area statically. Use the central threshold stimulus as a suprathreshold static stimulus 15° from fixation at every meridian within the I 2e isopter.

5. Determine the dimmest stimulus seen kinetically 10° from fixation and map its isopter, which is most often the I 1e.

6. Use this dimmest stimulus as the central suprathreshold static target to test all points 5° from fixation and the four quadrants within 5° of the central fixation mirror.

7. Explore for a central vertical step with the same central threshold stimulus (I 2e). Test kinetically to thresh-

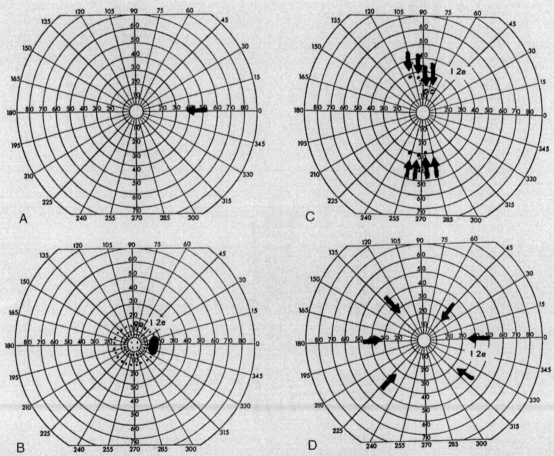

FIGURE 17–23. Armaly-Drance technique for neurological defects. *A,* Central kinetic I 2e moved on temporal horizontal meridian from 50° in towards central mirror. I 2e perceived at 30°, so I 1e attempted. Because the I 1e was not perceived, the I 2e is chosen as the central threshold isopter. *B,* The blind spot is mapped with the I 2e kinetically, starting within where the target is not seen, and moved until the target is seen. The same I 2e is used as a suprathreshold static target at every meridian 15° from the central mirror. Because I 1e target was not seen, the I 2e is used as a suprathreshold static target in the four quadrants in the central 5°, and in each meridian just outside 5°. Static checkpoints are marked with a dot if seen and with a small circle if not seen. The blind spot appears normal as do the central 5° and 15° static points checked at each meridian. Forty-eight suprathreshold static points have now been checked. *C,* I 2e kinetic isopter points are plotted at the upper and lower vertical meridians where two checkpoints just to the right and two just to the left are plotted. In this example, a vertical step is found to the right of the upper vertical meridian. The I 2e is now used as a suprathreshold static target to test points just within the kinetic isopter at the four points found at the upper vertical meridian, and the four points at the lower vertical meridian. Note that the two static points at the upper vertical meridian to the right are missed. *D,* Three kinetic isopter points every 45° in the nasal field, and three every 45° on the temporal field are plotted.

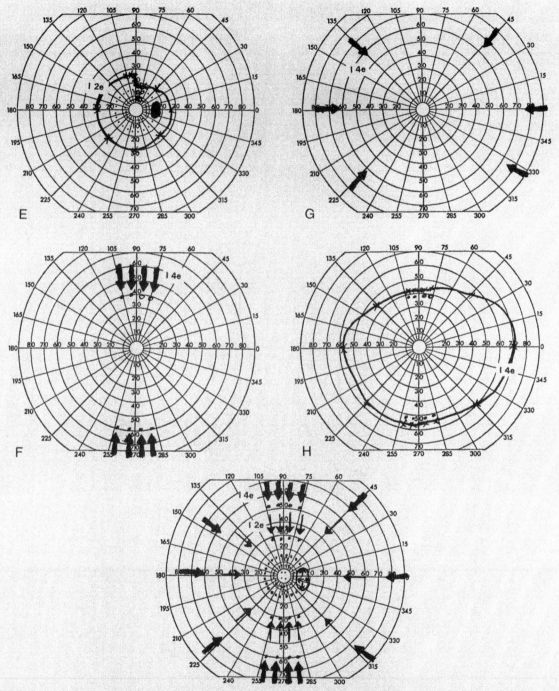

FIGURE 17-23. *Continued E,* The completed central Armaly-Drance isopter as plotted in figures *A* through *D.* Because the defect found is at the upper vertical meridian on the right, we will concentrate our strategy in that area. *F,* Testing for a peripheral target. The I 4e is chosen to test at the upper and lower vertical meridians where two checkpoints just to the right and two just to the left are plotted. No kinetic vertical step is found to the right of the upper vertical meridian. The I 4e is now used as a suprathreshold static target, however, to test just within the kinetic isopter at the four points found at the upper vertical meridian and the four points at the lower vertical meridian. Note that the two static points at the upper vertical meridian are still missed, indicating a probable kinetic defect with smaller, more sensitive targets. *G,* Three isopter points every 45° are plotted in the nasal field and three isopter points every 45° are plotted in the temporal field. No suprathreshold static points are checked because no pathology is expected in these areas. *H,* The I 4e isopter as plotted in figures *F* and *G.* Because there was a normal blind spot and no other defect within 15° to suprathreshold static testing, no further testing in this area is required. *I,* A composite of the completed Armaly-Drance technique for a neurological visual field. Static checkpoints are indicated by a dot.

old from 40° toward fixation twice slightly to the right (5° and 10°) and twice slightly to the left (5° and 10°) of the upper (90°) and lower (270°) vertical meridians.

8. Suprathreshold static testing with the same central threshold stimulus (I 2e) is performed just within the vertical isopter, with a minimum of two static checks to the right (5° and 10°) and left (5° and 10°) of the vertical meridian both upper (90°) and lower (270°).

9. Complete the kinetic central threshold isopter by plotting three meridians (135°, 225°, and the nasal horizontal) on the nasal side and three meridians (45, 315, and temporal horizontal) on the temporal side.

10. Remove the central add.

11. Explore for a kinetic peripheral vertical step with a brighter stimulus (usually the I 4e). Begin moving the stimulus in from 80° above and below fixation twice slightly right (5° and 10°) and twice slightly left (5° and 10°) of the vertical meridian.

12. Use the same peripheral kinetic stimulus to check statically twice just inside the vertical isopters.

13. Kinetically outline the remaining peripheral isopter at three meridians (135°, 225°, and nasal horizontal) on the nasal side and three meridians (45°, 315°, and temporal horizontal) on the temporal side.

14. Check statically just inside the same six meridians (Fig. 17–23).

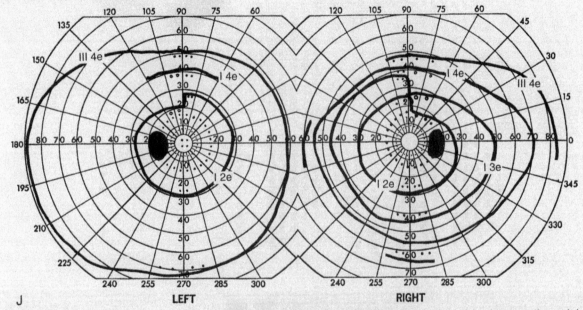

FIGURE 17–23. *Continued J*, Visual field plotted for both eyes. Left eye was plotted first, and the III 4e chosen as the peripheral target. When that target proved normal, the I 4e was tested in the area of concern, i.e., the upper vertical meridian. The right eye was then mapped, using the same targets, adding the I 3e for a possible vertical step, which was found.

Automated

Computerized perimeters utilize static methods in selected programs to record patient responses at grids of predetermined points instead of the familiar isopter contours of manual kinetic perimeters. The Humphrey's Field Analyzer, Digilab, Octopus, and Dicon are examples of automated perimeters.

The perimetrist selects the appropriate screening program. Selection of programs depends on the pattern of points. If unexpected defects are found with a screening program, another program may be selected by the perimetrist to quantify them. Some programs automatically test actual thresholds at each missed point. The perimetrist has to tell the computer when to change strategies by using a new program. Patients become bored and lose concentration more readily with

static testing, thus producing more false positives than with kinetic testing. Almost constant communication between the patient and the perimetrist prevents loss of patient concentration (Fig. 17–24).

● KINETIC TESTING METHODS

Blind Spot

One normal absolute scotoma, the physiological blind spot, reflects the site of the optic disc where the optic nerve exits the eye. Because this area has no photoreceptors, no visual perception takes place when this area is stimulated. In the eye the optic disc is nasal to the macula. In the visual field, this produces a blind spot about 12° to 18° temporal of fixation and from 2°

A Automated central 30-2 program

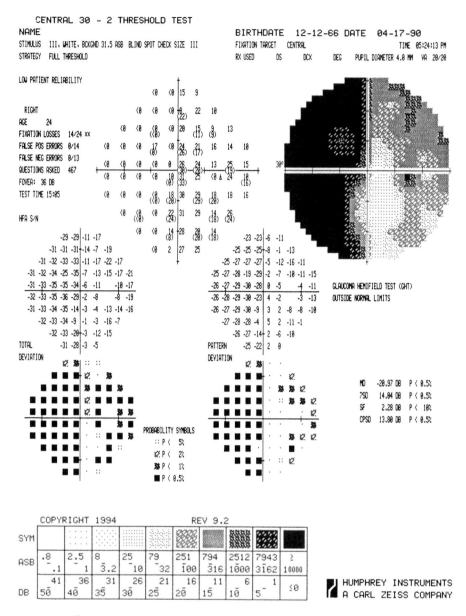

B Same patient, same day as measured on manual perimeter

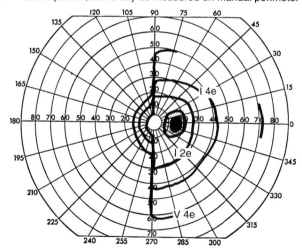

FIGURE 17–24. Perimetrist may have option of either manual or automated perimetry on many patients. *A,* 30-2 detective gray scale on automated perimeter documenting a left hemianopsia. (Courtesy of Humphrey Instruments, San Leandro, CA) *B,* repeat visual field on manual perimeter also documents a left hemianopsia.

above the horizontal meridian to 8° below, making it approximately 6° wide and 10° high.

The patient is advised that everyone has an area where they cannot see, that the blind spot is normal. Otherwise, the patient becomes alarmed when he or she does not see the test stimulus. The technician should keep encouraging patient responses. The blind spot is usually tested with the central threshold target. The blind spot is mapped at the beginning of testing to prove that the patient understands the test procedure and is fixating steadily. If within normal limits, the blind spot is usually not tested with other size targets. Start with the stimulus within the blind spot and move out. It is inadequate to find four points where the test stimulus is first seen. In addition, the four oblique points must also be plotted. If no blind spot is found, verify that you are 15° temporal to fixation, not nasal (you are testing the wrong eye). Verify that the patient is patched and is maintaining steady fixation. If the normal blind spot cannot be plotted, the entire field is suspect because it will be similarly difficult to discover any abnormal blind spots.

Enlarged blind spots are of two different types. With papilledema the blind spot has a concentric enlargement from a swollen optic nerve. With glaucoma, however, damage to the nasal side of the optic disc produces temporal enlargement of the blind spot. This damage to the optic disc first occurs superiorly and inferiorly causing a vertically oval physiological cup and a vertically elongated blind spot (Fig. 17–25).

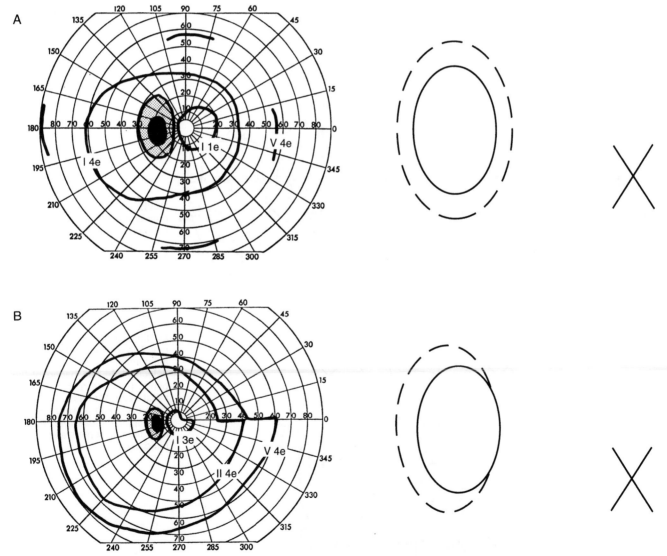

FIGURE 17–25. Enlargement of the blind spot. *A,* Papilledema enlarges blind spot concentrically. *B,* With increased intraocular pressure, nerve fibers at the optic nerve head above, below and nasally are affected elongating the blind spot with enlargement on the temporal side.

Central Field

The fovea, tested where the patient fixes, has the greatest retinal sensitivity, and the retinal periphery the least. The smaller and dimmer the test target, the more sensitive the retina you are testing and the greater the likelihood that a defect will be discovered. If there is no defect to the more sensitive central targets, there usually will not be any to larger, less sensitive peripheral targets. The minimum objectives are to obtain at least one central isopter using a central add with the smallest size target at the lowest illumination possible and to determine the smallest peripheral isopter that is normal.

Central test stimuli may show defects even when peripheral targets have normal isopters. A defect to a particular size target is always found with smaller and dimmer targets, usually with an expanded defect (Fig. 17–26).

Most patients with no field defect will have a peripheral isopter with the I 4e target. Nonmacular retinal pathology (e.g., retinitis pigmentosa, progressive optic neuropathies such as those produced by compressive tumors, and chiasmal and postchiasmal defects) are best followed by peripheral fields. Everything else (e.g., macular pathology and nerve fiber bundle diseases such as glaucoma) is best followed by central perimetry. Central visual field testing remains critical because most visual field loss affects the central 30° either initially or predominantly.

Best corrected vision in the 20/200 range indicates loss of central vision. A patient with such a finding will have difficulty maintaining fixation. Monitoring eye position through the telescope is most important in patients with poor vision. Enhance the patient's fixation with a cross hatch line drawn on two 15-inch strips of paper tape placed around fixation. Never draw a cross hatch on the perimeter bowl. Do not assume that the patient with 20/200 vision will not have an I 2e isopter. With a dense central scotoma there is often an I 2e field just outside the scotoma. There may be a central or centrocecal scotoma with a normal peripheral I 4e

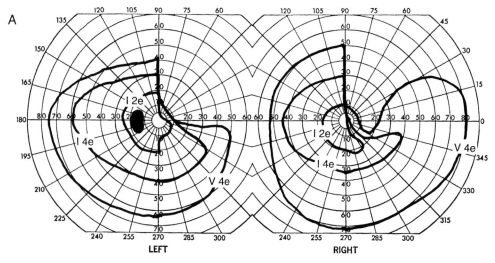

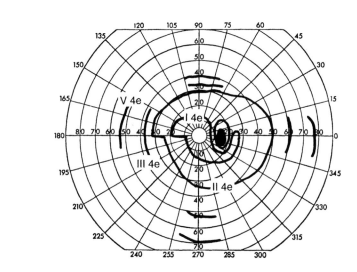

FIGURE 17–26. Defect always greater with smaller stimuli. *A*, Incongruous right hemianopia. The smaller central I 2e stimulus shows an almost complete hemianopic defect. The largest peripheral stimulus, the V 4e, has just an upper right quadrantanopia. Steep margins to all stimuli are found along the upper vertical meridian and sloping margins to all stimuli in the lower right quadrant. The left halves of both fields are normal. B. Nerve fiber bundle defects. I 4e has baring of the blind spot. I 4e and II 4e have nasal steps. II 4e has a Seidel scotoma extending upward from the blind spot, whereas III 4e and V 4e have normal isopters and normal blind spots.

isopter; whereas, if the decrease in visual acuity is from a cataract or some other media opacity, no I 2e field will be found.

A central scotoma always affects the central 5° of the field, sometimes the central 10°, or even 20°. Visual acuity is always decreased, usually to 20/200. With 20/200 vision or less, reverse the usual order and obtain a V 4e field first. The location of the V 4e indicates where the isopter might be to more sensitive targets. Reduce target size from a V 4e to an I 4e.

A paracentral scotoma may show no reduction in vision. Because paracentral scotomas occur with chiasmal lesions or glaucoma, suprathreshold static perimetry in the central area is a must. Generally, three isopters are plotted. The central threshold isopter is one, the most common begin the I 2e. Now record the dimmest central isopter the patient can see. Use the I 1e, if possible, that will be the second. Now record a peripheral isopter as the third one, commonly the I 4e. If the I 4e is abnormal, plot a larger test simulus (e.g., III 4e) as a fourth isopter (Fig. 17–27).

Patient Response

Begin in a nonseeing area. Plot the field where the target first appears and the patient responds by tapping or buzzing with the response object. The starting point should be farther from central fixation than the extent of the visual field could possibly be. Because a normal peripheral field extends 60° nasally and 90° temporally, it is safe to start with a peripheral target 70° nasally. It is not safe unless the target is first presented farther than 90° temporally. Young patients, no matter how poor their central vision, may see a I 4e target 80° to 90° out on the temporal side. Do not anticipate where

the temporal isopter will be by starting at 60° to 70°. An attempt is made to present the target 15° *outside* where it might be seen. If the patient responds when you turn on the stimulus but before you have moved it, you have not started far enough peripherally. The peripheral isopters will be round instead of their normal ovoid shape.

If the field is normal to a I 4e, it will be normal to a V 4e; therefore, only minimal testing need be done with anything larger than I 4e. Having a normal peripheral isopter to the I 4e test stimulus does not mean the central field is normal. If the I 4e peripheral target appears abnormal, however, a second peripheral isopter with a larger size target should be found that produces a normal field. In order to save time, jump to the V 4e target. It can be used to explore key locations. This information is important if the field is abnormal. If the V 4e is normal, the smallest target size that is normal should be determined (the II 4e, III 4e, or IV 4e). It is superfluous to do peripheral isopters with a I 4e, II 4e, III 4e, IV 4e, and V 4e on each patient; it is also not necessary to do a I 1e, I 2e, and I 3e central isopter on each patient. Manual kinetic perimetry allows the perimetrist to adjust the test object sizes according to each patient's ability to see them. The target sizes given are those suggested for starting.

Move the test target perpendicular to the defect you are defining. When a defect is located to any size kinetic stimulus, that defect is fully quantified, not only by recording that size isopter, but with the smallest, dimmest target the patient can perceive. The defect's borders are also tested with smaller, dimmer, test stimuli to define the slope of its margins. Find and record isopters with increasingly larger test targets until an isopter is found with no defect. Either the defect "disappears" (a *relative* scotoma) or you determine that the defect still exists to the largest and brightest test stimulus (V 4e) (an *absolute* scotoma).

The *a, b, c, d,* and *e* log units on the Goldmann perimeter were developed for utilization with static perimetry. For kinetic perimetry, including suprathreshold static perimetry, all isopters are tested with the *e* log unit. The Roman numeral is the test stimulus size. The Arabic numeral designates illumination. With test stimulus sizes II, III, IV, and V, the illumination is always 4e. Only with the size I central target are illumination levels below 4e tested, at I 3e, I 2e, and I 1e, ignoring the a, b, c, and d units.

Both automated and manual perimetry remain subjective. The results are only as good as the patient's ability and willingness to respond. Expend time and effort where you anticipate the defect to be from what you know about that patient and what you know about the sensory visual pathways. Do not neglect to screen, however, for possible unexpected defects. The vertical and nasal horizontal meridians are essential areas to

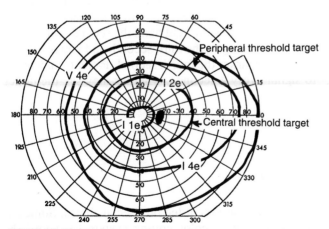

FIGURE 17–27. If 3 isopters are normal with manual perimetry, no additional isopters are necessary. I 2e tested at the temporal horizontal meridian. Because it was seen at 40° beyond the blind spot, it is plotted as the central threshold isopter. I 4e was chosen as the peripheral isopter to plot. I 1e is a good choice for the 3rd isopter. V 4e is superfluous.

test. The minimum number of checkpoints for any one isopter is 14, four (two on either side) straddling the upper vertical meridian, four (two on either side) straddling the lower vertical meridian, four (two above and two below) straddling the nasal horizontal meridian, and two near the temporal horizontal meridian. *Do not test 12 or 15 equally spaced meridians.* The degree lines of the chart paper are landmarks used after the visual field is complete; they need not be used to find kinetic or static points (Fig. 17–28).

Timing

If the nasal horizontal stimulus is seen at 60° as well as the upper vertical meridian at 60°, there is usually

little information to be obtained by testing any of the meridians between these two. Check one or two meridians between so as not to miss a focal depression. If the lower vertical limit is also at 60°, or even 70°, testing radially between the nasal horizontal meridian and the lower vertical meridian will not usually yield much information. If there is also no defect at the vertical meridian, there will usually be no defect at 45° degrees or at 225°. Do not waste time (Fig. 17–29).

From the time the patient sees the stimulus until the patient signals, there is a 1 to 2 second lag, allowing the marker to move an additional few degrees. Record the stimulus threshold location as a few degrees *before* where the pointer is when the patient buzzes. Any response from the patient immediately after turning the stimulus on indicates that the stimulus may have been seen as a static target (suprathreshold). Repeat all such isopter points, starting 15° more peripheral to the first location. *Beware all rapid responses.* These often indicate that the stimulus was not presented initially outside the isopter and beyond detection as it should be, but within the isopter. By the same reasoning, do not assume that a target positioned just below the temporal horizontal meridian at 15° is within the blind spot. When the stimulus is turned on at that location, it is first used as a suprathreshold static target. Otherwise, you incorrectly record a limit of the blind spot if you start to move the target because it takes about 2 seconds for most patients to signal. Check within the blind spot about 5° below the horizontal. If the patient pushes the buzzer 2 seconds later, the stimulus was seen as a static check when it shouldn't have been, thus indicating that the target was not within the blind spot.

When testing a static stimulus in the central area, the timing rhythm with which the target is presented should be varied. It is easy to fall into the trap of grabbing the projector handle with your left hand the first second; depressing the shutter switch to turn the stimulus on with your right hand the second second; the patient signaling on the third second; and you recording with your marker the fourth second. Patients may begin to signal every 4 seconds, whether they see the target or not.

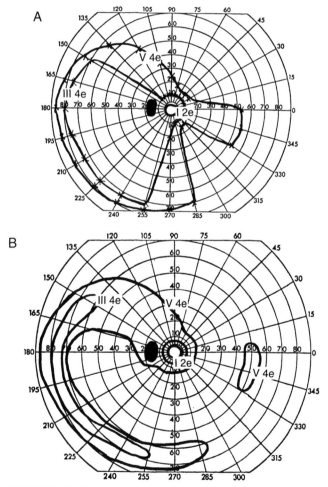

FIGURE 17–28. Change in strategy improves accuracy of definition of defect. *A,* Detection of peripheral kinetic points by moving target along each of the 24 meridians. Huge ring scotoma in lower field was missed. *B,* By spending most of the time moving target perpendicular to defect in lower field, improved definition of the defect occurs.

Recording

Responses are recorded on special charts. Some perimetrists have a color coding system to record the different isopters of a manual field, i.e., a given target is the same designated color on every visual field, but there is no *standard* color code.

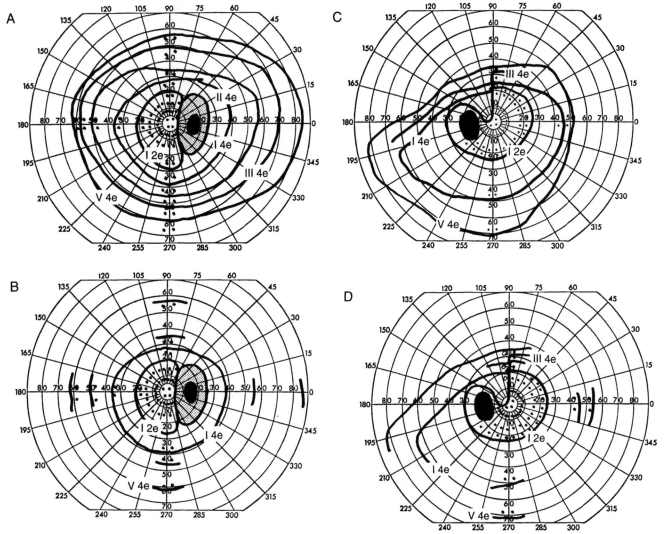

FIGURE 17–29. Two examples of the fastest method to elicit the most information about the defect and adequate information in normal areas. *A,* In the first example, the I 2e has a contracted temporal isopter to 5°. I 4e also has a generally contracted isopter with an enlarged blind spot. II 4e, III 4e, and V 4e have gradually increasing sizes of isopters. III 4e and V 4e have normal blind spots. *B,* The same amount of information is obtained in much less time by plotting fewer points in areas without the defect. I 2e and I 4e are plotted as in *A.* II 4e and III 4e are not tested. Instead, the third isopter chosen is V 4e to determine if the contour has normal limits and the blind spot is of normal size. The only kinetic points obtained were at the two major horizontal and two major vertical meridians. *C,* In the second example, the central I 2e locates defect at upper vertical meridian extending to the left with a slightly enlarged blind spot. I 4e finds much smaller vertical step. III 4e is plotted just sufficiently to know vertical step is still present and that the upper left quadrant isopter remains somewhat contracted. V 4e has no vertical step, but upper left quadrant is still slightly contracted. *D,* Same amount of information can be obtained in much less time by plotting fewer points in areas without the defect. I 2e is plotted same as in *C.* Because I 2e isopter was normal in lower left quadrant and right half of the field, I 4e and V 4e kinetic points are plotted at all 4 major meridians with several points in upper left quadrant. III 4e only is tested at upper vertical meridian to show vertical step is still present.

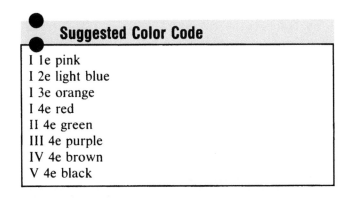

Suggested Color Code

I 1e pink
I 2e light blue
I 3e orange
I 4e red
II 4e green
III 4e purple
IV 4e brown
V 4e black

Another technique will help to avoid confusion while performing the test. The perimetrist chooses different marks for each target (I 2e with a dot (.), I 4e with a check (√), and so forth (Fig. 17–30).

Gathering Patient Information

For both manual and automated perimetry examination, the technician records the patient's identifying

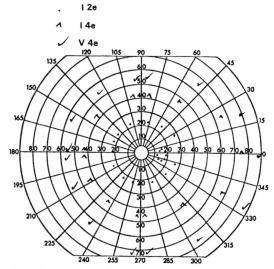

FIGURE 17–30. Use different marks for each isopter.

information on the visual field chart or enters it into the computer (Fig. 17–31).

Name

Most computers identify patients by name and date of birth. This information, including punctuation, must match exactly for each examination or the computer will not recognize the tests as belonging to the same patient. Date of birth is also necessary for computers that employ age-related normals for statistical analysis.

Vision and RX Used

If the vision is not the same as for previous examinations, the results of the examination may be affected. Record the distance refraction plus proper central add for age. Some computers have an option that allows entering the distance prescription and asking the machine to calculate the testing prescription. This is particularly helpful if the perimetrist is not knowledgeable in optics.

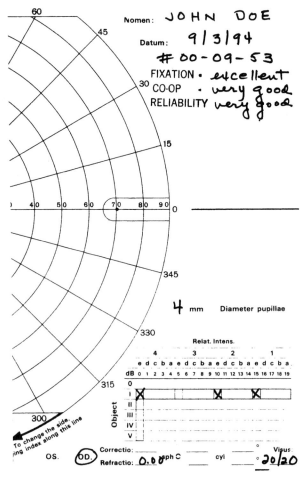

FIGURE 17–31. Enter patient identification.

CENTRAL 30 - 2 THRESHOLD TEST

NAME   JOHN DOE   BIRTHDATE   12-12-66   DATE   04-17-90
STIMULUS   III, WHITE, BCKGND 31.5 ASB BLIND SPOT CHECK SIZE III   FIXATION TARGET   CENTRAL   ID 38-98-35   TIME   05:24:13
B STRATEGY   FULL THRESHOLD   RX USED   DS   DCX   DEG   PUPIL DIAMETER 4.0 MM   YA 20

Pupil Size

A smaller pupil than on previous examinations may affect the field values.

Questions You Want to Answer from Your Plotted Field

I. Is there a defect?
  A. How extensive is it (Fig. 17–32)?
    1. Does it cross the nasal horizontal meridian?
    2. Does it cross the vertical meridian above or below?

3. Is a quadrant out?
4. Is the right or the left half of the field out?
5. Is the blind spot affected?

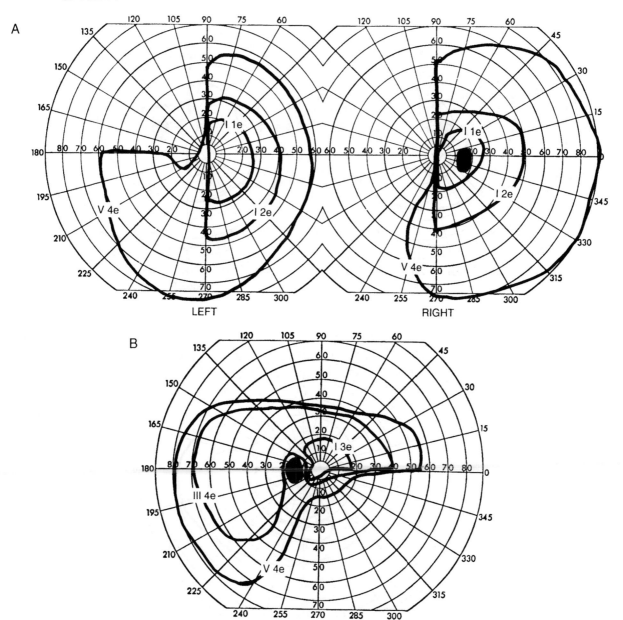

FIGURE 17–32. Determine width and depth of defect, and identify which part of afferent visual pathway is affected. *A,* Postchiasmal left incongruous hemianopic defect in optic radiations. Defect is complete with central targets (I 1e, I 2e) and incomplete with V 4e peripheral target. Right eye field is affected more than left eye field. *B,* Prechiasmal nerve fiber bundle altitudinal defect is present affecting lower field, as often occurs with optic neuropathy. No central field is found with I 1e or I 2e and peripheral field affected almost as much with V 4e as III 4e.

B. How deep is it (Fig. 17–32)?
 1. Does the defect appear with different sized targets?
 2. Just to the dimmest and smallest (I 1e)?
 3. Almost as extensive with the brightest and largest target (V 4e)?
II. Where is it? What part of the sensory visual pathway is affected (Fig. 17–32)?
III. Has it changed since the last field was recorded (Fig. 17–33)?

A. Has the field loss progressed?
 1. Is a previous defect deeper, i.e., found with larger targets than before?
 2. Has a previous defect expanded in size with a particular target size?
B. Is there a new defect? Look for a collapsed isopter in part of the field.
IV. How much quantitation is necessary for later comparison? If you have a baseline program, perhaps a fast thresholding technique can be

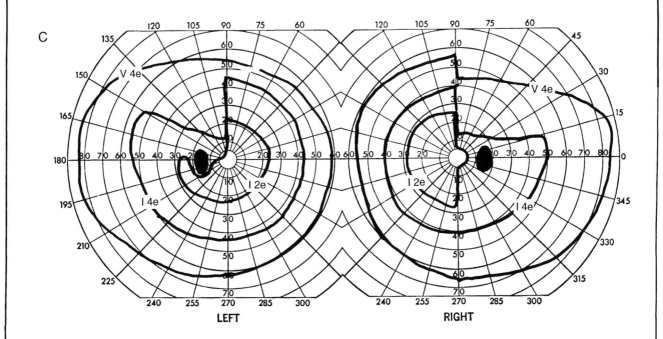

LEFT   RIGHT

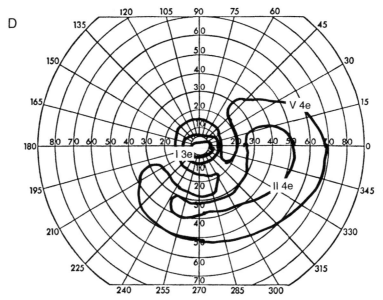

FIGURE 17–32. *Continued C,* Chiasmal bitemporal quadrantanopia. Right eye field is affected more than left eye field. Hemianopia complete in right eye with central I 2e. V 4e stimulus left eye is outside the pathology because it does not have defect at upper vertical meridian. *D,* Advanced nerve fiber bundle defect, right eye, with incomplete arcuate scotoma below pointing to the blind spot, and complete arcuate scotoma above breaking through to the periphery even with V 4e target. This is a typical loss of visual field associated with advanced glaucoma.

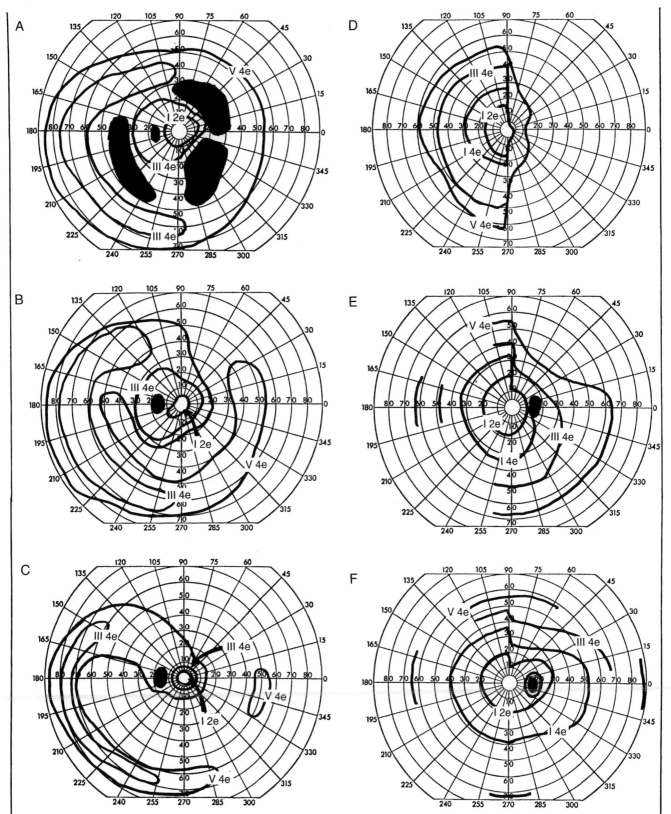

FIGURE 17–33. Comparison with previous fields for documentation of change. Same test targets are used for comparison. *A*, *B*, and *C* document deterioration in patient with retinitis pigmentosa. I 2e seen on all 3 visits, but field gradually contracts. In *A*, V 4e has almost normal isopter with three absolute scotomas in a ring configuration within the isopter. In *B*, absolute scotomas enlarge until they break through to the periphery, markedly contracting V 4e isopter, especially in the upper right quadrant. In *C*, there is continued contraction, both to the III 4e and the V 4e. *D*, *E*, and *F* monitor improvement in the field of vision of patient who had surgery for pituitary adenoma. *D*, Visual field of the right eye on the preoperative visit shows an almost total loss of temporal field to all targets. *E*, Monitors improvement in recovery, especially lower right temporal field to all targets. *F*, Improvement continues. V 4e field no longer has step at upper vertical meridian. Even field of vision to I 2e enlarges to almost normal limits, except for vertical step.

tried on followup tests. In either case, you may add another target or program, but you must have something specific for comparison first. If this is a repeat visit

A. For manual field, use the same size and brightness targets as on the last field.
B. On an automated field, use the same programs and stimulus sizes as the last time.

To summarize, for efficient and reliable perimetry the technician must calibrate the instrument before each day of testing, move the targets from nonseeing to seeing areas, present the targets at random time intervals and locations, retest all missed targets, and test the central field with the correct central add. *And do it all as quickly as possible.*

Bibliography

Anderson DR: Perimetry with and without Automation, 2nd ed. St. Louis, CV Mosby, 1987.

Armaly MF: Selective perimetry for glaucomatous defects in ocular hypertension. Arch Ophthalmol 87:518, 1972.

Cassin B, Solomon SAB: Dictionary of Eye Terminology, 2nd ed. Gainesville, FL, Triad, 1990.

Ellenberger C: Perimetry, Principles, Technique, and Interpretation. New York, Raven Press, 1980.

Lieberman MF, Drake M: A Simplified Guide to Computerized Perimetry. Thorofare, NJ, Slack, 1987.

Trobe JD, Glaser JS: The Visual Fields Manual. Gainesville, FL, Triad, 1984.

Werner EB: Manual of Visual Fields. New York, Churchill Livingstone, 1991.

• CHAPTER 17 MANUAL PERIMETRY

1. What is the threshold border between seeing and nonseeing areas for a particular size and brightness target?
   a. depression
   b. relative scotoma
   c. isopter
   d. step
   e. absolute scotoma

2. Testing begins with a blinking target too dim to be seen. Target brightness is increased until the target is perceived. This is an example of which of the following?
   a. threshold static
   b. central kinetic
   c. screening technique
   d. suprathreshold static
   e. peripheral kinetic

3. What is the central threshold target?
   a. smallest, dimmest target seen within 15° of fixation
   b. always the I 2e
   c. smallest, dimmest target seen 25° temporal to fixation
   d. smallest, dimmest target seen within 10° of fixation
   e. smallest, dimmest target seen 25° nasal to fixation

4. What do we call using the same target size and brightness inside the isopter for a static check?
   a. threshold static
   b. central kinetic
   c. screening technique
   d. suprathreshold static
   e. peripheral kinetic

5. What does the Armaly-Drance technique use in combination?
   a. automated programs
   b. kinetic and threshold static
   c. manual and automated programs
   d. threshold static and suprathreshold static
   e. kinetic and suprathreshold static

Diana J. Shamis

18

Automated Perimetry

LEARNING OBJECTIVES

- Differentiate between threshold static and suprathreshold static perimetry
- Describe automated screening and threshold techniques
- List four advantages to automated perimetry
- Identify which size stimulus on a Goldmann perimeter is equivalent to the usual test stimulus on a Humphrey Field Analyzer

With advances in computer technology, the use of automated perimetry has become widespread. The main advantage of automated static over manual kinetic perimetry is more accurate, reliable, visual field testing within the central 30°. More detailed and subtler defects can be detected and explored than with manual perimetry. Automated perimetry is therefore excellent for retinal macular pathology and for any other small, subtle, central, or paracentral defect.

Although operating an automated perimeter requires less knowledge and expertise on the part of the "perimetrist," an understanding of testing methods, visual field defects, and patient factors that affect reliability can greatly improve the quality of test results obtained with automated perimeters. Communication with the patient is not needed as much as with manual perimetry but is periodically maintained for patient attention.

The main disadvantage to computerized perimetry is the time it consumes and the resulting increased stress on the patient. Patients unsuitable for automated perimetry are those who are

- Too ill for the length of the examination
- Unable to keep their heads still
- Unable or unwilling to cooperate
- Unable to maintain fixation because of nystagmus or poor vision.

The rest of this chapter addresses aspects of automated perimetry that are common to many, but not all, machines. The examples given are from the Humphrey Field Analyzer (HFA). Specific instructions for any machine can be obtained from the manufacturer.

● AUTOMATED PERIMETERS

Differences in background illumination, target stimulus illumination, and software programs in automated perimeters make comparisons among units difficult. Advances in software programs have increased the speed of threshold screening.

Stimulus Type

Automated perimeters can be divided into two types according to the method in which the stimulus is delivered. The more common has a projected light source positioned at different locations in the bowl by a motorized drive controlled by the computer. Filters are used to vary the stimulus intensity. The other type of perimeter has light-emitting diodes (LEDs) or fiberoptics located throughout the bowl to create the stimulus flash.

Stimulus Size and Intensity

In static automated perimetry the size of the stimulus is usually kept constant, whereas the stimulus intensity is varied. Automated visual fields are quantitated by varying stimulus intensity, whereas manual perimetry is quantitated by varying both the stimulus size and intensity. Most standard automated perimeters utilize a 4-mm² round stimulus spot as a standard, which is equivalent to the size III stimulus on a Goldmann manual perimeter. Most projected light automated perimeters have a selection of stimulus sizes that correlate to the Goldmann target sizes I through V. If the patient has significantly decreased vision and difficulty performing the test with the size III target, the target size may be increased to a size V. Other target sizes are not often used in automated perimetry.

White is the standard stimulus color. The HVF also has red, blue, and green stimuli. Red is occasionally chosen to test for macular defects.

Stimulus intensity is measured in apostilbs, which is an absolute measure of light intensity (brightness). A given stimulus, e.g., 400 asb, is the same intensity on all machines; however, maximum stimulus intensity does vary from machine to machine.

Background Illumination

Background illumination is an important factor that varies among machines. With manual perimetry, the background illumination needs to be recalibrated periodically so that the test conditions are the same in all patients for each test. Automated perimeters calibrate themselves. Many, including the Humphrey Field Analyzer (HFA), use a 32-apostilb (asb) brightness background similar to that of the Goldmann manual perimeter, but others, including the Octopus, use a much dimmer, 4-asb background. This dimmer background illumination increases the visibility of the test stimulus.

Comparability of Test Results

Patient results are expressed in decibels (dB), a relative measure of visual as well as auditory sensitivity. The number of decibels is the reduction of light in log units. A reduction of 1 log unit equals 10 dB, so one decibel is one-tenth of a log unit and is also an indication of retinal sensitivity. A measurement of zero decibels and zero log units in perimetry is the maximum target brightness of an instrument. Because a higher number in log units and decibels signifies a dimmer target, this higher number also indicates a greater retinal sensitivity. The decibel changes in value depending on the maximum stimulus intensity (in asb) and the background illumination provided by a given machine. Therefore, a particular decibel reading on one instrument, e.g., the Octopus, does not indicate the same thing as a similar decibel number on another instrument, e.g., HFA. Results from different types of automated perimeters are only comparable if *all* the factors

discussed previously are the same in both machines. Unfortunately, this is frequently not the case.

• PROGRAM SELECTION

Many automated perimeters provide statistical evaluation of visual field loss and progression. Despite this substantial benefit, automated perimetry is not a panacea for the often difficult task of accurately assessing visual fields.

Most automated perimeters use static methods to test the visual field; some also use kinetic targets. Screening techniques are excellent for quickly finding defects, but not defining them. If defects are found, they can be quantified by using automated static threshold perimetry or manual kinetic and static perimetry.

Threshold

Threshold is the sensitivity of any point in the visual field. For testing purposes, it is defined as a test stimulus with a probability of being seen 50% of the time. Threshold value depends on

1. Background illumination and stimulus size
2. Age of the patient (it decreases with age)
3. Location within the field (it decreases away from the fovea).

A numerical value in decibels is assigned to each point tested in the visual field. The values obtained for a patient are compared with the *expected population normals*. Patient values falling outside the range containing 95% of the population values are considered abnormal. Normal threshold values are derived from measurements of many individuals from the *normal population*.

Static Threshold Testing (Quantitative Visual Field)

The strategy is to determine the dimmest light intensity at which the target will be detected. Thresholds are determined by a repetitive up-down bracketing method. The first target should be brighter than threshold, easily seen, and presented at four points (Fig. 18–1). Succeeding targets become dimmer and dimmer until they are not seen by the patient. Threshold confirmation occurs as successively brighter targets are presented until seen again. Testing with stimuli far above or far below threshold wastes time. To further reduce the test duration, the machine tries to select a starting target intensity near threshold level. The closer to threshold at the onset of testing, the shorter the test will be.

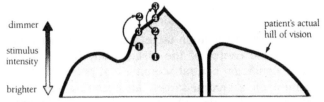

FIGURE 18–1. Static threshold-bracketing technique. Threshold sensitivity at each test point is determined by increasing and decreasing the stimulus intensity in "steps" until the threshold is crossed. (Used with permission from Haley MJ (ed): The Field Analyzer Primer, 2nd ed. San Leandro, CA, Allergan Humphrey, 1987.)

Threshold Strategy

Some automated perimeters, such as the HFA, have several testing strategies available. The major variable is how the machine determines the starting light intensity for each point in the field. Common strategies include

1. Beginning near age-related normal values for all points.

2. Determining the threshold of one point in each quadrant. Those values are used to estimate the starting point for the remainder of the points in that quadrant. This reduces the length of the test as it prevents the machine from beginning from normal in a quadrant that is in fact, actually very abnormal.

3. Choosing previous test results for a given patient for the instrument to begin its thresholding. This can be beneficial when large areas of the field have significant loss. It is not recommended in disease processes, such as optic neuritis, in which the visual fields can rapidly change.

4. Testing the entire field at a level 2 dB brighter than stored values. It then determines "thresholds" at missed points only. As offered on the HFA, this Fast Threshold strategy assumes that the threshold cannot improve. This test should not be given in conditions in which improvement is possible, as is the case with optic neuritis.

Static threshold perimetry is the most accurate automated testing method, but also the most time consuming. Commonly used test programs take 10 to 15 minutes/eye; with setup time and printing the results, this combines to nearly an hour per patient. Some patients lack the attention span or physical endurance to complete the examination. Others have difficulty responding rapidly and reliably enough to static targets, particularly those peripheral to the central 20° of the visual field. If patient responses become inconsistent, the test time lengthens as more stimuli are needed for the program to finish. Although this is also true to some degree of manual perimetry, the manual perimetrist has the option of altering the testing procedure to accommodate the patient's limitations.

Suprathreshold Static Screening (Qualitative Visual Field)

A screening test using a static *suprathreshold* method provides a quick, qualitative assessment of the visual field wherein a problem is suspected. It shows the existence of a defect, but does not define its depth. The instrument determines what a normal threshold level for the patient should be, usually based on age-related data. During the screening test, a single size stimulus slightly brighter than this normal threshold is shown at each point in the array (Fig. 18–2). The idea is to present targets expected to be seen. The patient's answers are recorded simply as points "seen" or "not seen." If the normal stimulus is not seen, it is assumed the point is abnormal. Each program takes 3 to 5 minutes to run.

Long duration screening tests are of limited value for many patients. Instead of screening, some ophthalmologists prefer to perform one full threshold examination as a baseline. Subsequent testing may use a fast bracketing technique to detect changes over the baseline.

Kinetic Threshold

Kinetic thresholding in automated perimetry is similar to the methods used in manual perimetry. The meridians to be tested, target size, and intensity are chosen by the perimetrist. Because most static perimetry involves only the central 30° of the visual field, kinetic testing can provide a relatively quick method to assess the peripheral limits of the visual field. It may also work better with those patients who do not respond reliably to static targets.

Testing Point Array

Many different patterns of testing point arrays are offered by various automated perimeters. Test point locations are selected based on their importance in detecting the types of defects expected. The most commonly used point array measures points located within

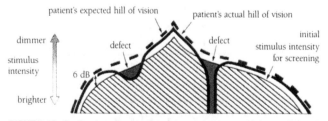

FIGURE 18–2. Static suprathreshold screening technique. Stimuli are presented at an intensity slightly brighter than the patient's visual threshold. Responses are recorded as "seen" or "not seen." (Used with permission from Haley MJ (ed): The Field Analyzer Primer, 2nd ed. San Leandro, CA, Allergan Humphrey, 1987.)

the central 30°, using test points 6° apart. The point array is offset from the vertical and horizontal meridians. This places the first set of points adjacent to the meridians, 3° to either side. Because many visual field defects (Fig. 18–3) are characterized by their relationship to the meridians, this array provides more useful information than arrays that begin with points on the meridians with the next adjacent points 6° away (HFA 30–1 program).

To shorten testing time, some programs have dropped the most peripheral row of points from the superior, inferior, and temporal parts of the 30° field, as in the HFA 24–2 program. The nasal points remain unchanged because of the importance of this area for detection and follow-up of glaucomatous visual field defects. This array is less appropriate in optic nerve disorders other than glaucoma because valuable information may be lost by deleting temporal points.

In patients whose visual field defects approach or include fixation, it may be desirable to test the central 10° with a more tightly compressed array of points spaced only 2° apart, such as the HFA 10–2 program. This provides added detail with which to assess and follow progression.

Test Parameters

Each automated perimeter has a standard set of test parameters, which are utilized unless otherwise specified by the operator. Always check previous parameters for a follow-up patient. If the same test parameters are not used each time, the results cannot be compared, thus wasting your time and the patient's.

Fixation Target

The standard fixation target has the patient fixing a spot in the center of the visual field. If the patient has a significant central scotoma that prevents steady fixation on a central target, an eccentric pattern of targets may be selected, such as the diamond pattern of lights on HFA. The patient is instructed to fixate on the center of the pattern. If an eccentric fixation pattern is selected, the test point array is automatically shifted to correspond to the new fixation point.

Foveal Threshold

Many machines have the ability to test the sensitivity of the center of vision or foveal threshold. Because a target cannot be shown directly on the central fixation target, the patient must fix on an alternate fixation pattern. HFA has a pattern of the four yellow lights. The patient looks for a stimulus to flash in the center of the four lights. Testing the foveal threshold is a useful option because it quickly adds another piece of information by which to verify patient reliability.

Foveal sensitivity can be roughly correlated to patient visual acuity. For example, if the patient has 20/20 vision, the foveal response on an HVF should be in the 30s. Vision decreases proportionately with the foveal threshold. If the response is not within a reasonable range, the patient may not have fully understood the instructions, and this will require reinstruction and retesting.

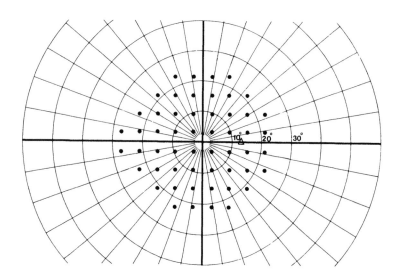

FIGURE 18–3. Point arrays arranged to straddle the horizontal and vertical meridians are most useful for detecting vertical and horizontal "step" defects. (Used with permission from Haley MJ (ed): The Field Analyzer Primer, 2nd ed. San Leandro, CA, Allergan Humphrey, 1987.)

Test Speed

Some machines allow the test speed to be slowed, but because the testing is so lengthy anyway, this is not recommended. If the patient cannot keep up with the usual speed, it is unlikely that slowing it will improve reliability.

Patient Instruction

Patient instruction is important because many unreliable results are caused by an inadequate explanation. Some machines have available on-screen instructions that can be read by the technician, but the perimetrist should feel free to elaborate as necessary to ensure that the patient understands.

Instructions should include the following:

1. Where the patient is to look and especially *not* to look around for the targets.

2. What the stimulus will look like, which is a flashing light that will sometimes be much dimmer than others.

3. The patient should respond even if the light is very faint.

4. The patient will not see all the lights.

5. The patient should blink normally. Patients tend to stare, fearing that they will miss a flash if they blink. This leads to drying of the cornea, blurring, and tearing. Tell the patient to blink immediately *after* a response so as to avoid missing the next target.

6. Suggest that a break is possible if the patient becomes tired. If you intend to leave the room and the machine has a way to pause, tell the patient. A brief pause can often improve the patient's performance significantly.

Performance Assessment

Although it is not necessary to stay in the room for the entire test, always observe the patient for at least the first few minutes of the test and check back every few minutes. Unreliable tests result when patients lose concentration or become misaligned during the test. Reliability typically decreases with the length of the test. The technician can assess patient performance in several ways and take steps to correct unreliable behavior.

Demonstration

If your machine has a demonstration option, use it. It adds only a few seconds to the test and assesses whether the patient is ready and responding properly. If your patient is unclear about what he or she is supposed to be seeing and responding to, the demonstration may spare you from having to restart the test.

Fixation

Fixation monitoring has improved but still remains an important problem. Automated fixation monitoring is done either by continuous photoelectric sensor or periodic blind-spot checks.

The blind-spot method periodically flashes a stimulus in the presumed location of the patient's physiological blind-spot. If the patient is fixing properly, the stimulus should not be seen. If the patient responds, assume he or she is not maintaining adequate fixation. The patient should be reinstructed to keep looking at the central fixation target. If a patient appears to be maintaining fixation but continues to see the blind-spot check stimulus, the machine may not have the blind spot accurately located. Direct the machine to ''relocate the blind spot.'' It may also be helpful to reduce the stimulus size for the fixation check. Periodically communicate with the patient to avoid patient lapses in fixation or attention.

Double Determination Points and Short-Term Fluctuation

Double determination points assess how consistently the patient responded during the test. Threshold responses for several points on the array are determined twice, e.g., the HFA selects ten points in the grid. If the patient gives consistent responses, the two values should be equal. If the patient is inconsistent, the computer increases the number of double determination points. A disadvantage to this strategy is that it lengthens the testing time for the already unreliable patient.

Fluctuation testing compares the threshold values of the double determination points. Short-term fluctuation (SF) is calculated by averaging the amount of fluctuation for all double determination points tested. The greater the SF the more variable and unreliable have been the patient's responses. Short-term fluctuation may increase in patients who have areas of severe visual field loss. It is more difficult for patients to be consistent in and around areas of decreased sensitivity.

• PRINTOUTS

The following types of printouts are common to many automated perimeters.

Screening Examination Printout

Screening examination results are typically presented as a grid of symbols corresponding to the point array tested. The simplest screening tests have only two symbols. One indicates the patient saw the stimulus normal for his or her age at a given point, and the other indicates that he or she did not. More complex screening tests, which carry out a quantitative evaluation of any abnormal points found, may have decibel values for those points or symbols that indicate whether the point represents an absolute or a relative defect.

Numeric Pattern

Static threshold examinations produce decibel values for each point tested. These numbers are displayed on a grid corresponding to the point array. These values represent visual sensitivity. As the sensitivity increases, the number increases. A zero indicates no stimulus was seen (Fig. 18–4).

Grayscale Pattern

The numerical point values are converted to a scale of varying grays ranging from light to dark. The lighter areas correspond to where a dim illumination is seen. The darker areas are where only a brighter illumination is seen. The lighter areas equal better visual fields, and darker areas, worse. This pattern most resembles the isopter patterns recorded with kinetic perimetry. Diagnostic decisions are not based exclusively on the grayscale.

Depth of Defect

This numerical printout, also called total deviation, represents, in decibels, the difference between the patient's test results and the age-related normal values for each point tested. A statistical probability plot may also be provided. This assigns a symbol to each deviation value that indicates the probability of finding such a deviation in the normal reference population. The darker the symbol is, the greater the probability of abnormality.

Comparison

This printout compares the results of two different examinations from the same patient. It also compares the change in each point between the two examinations. The results are stated as positive and negative numbers. This provides a quick, easy means to look for progression of field loss.

• STATISTICAL EVALUATION

Automated perimeters may also provide a statistical evaluation of the progression of visual field loss over the course of multiple examinations. These are extremely useful to the ophthalmologist, because by comparing only the most recent examination results, the clinician may overlook slower, subtle, but significant changes. Specific details of statistical programs can be obtained from their various manufacturers.

Although the following examples of statistical evaluations of static threshold results are from the Humphrey Stat-Pac program, other manufacturers have similar programs (Fig. 18–5).

Pattern Deviation Plots

The statistical program of the HFA attempts to differentiate focal and diffuse visual field loss. With diffuse loss of sensitivity in the visual field, such as that caused by a cataract, the expected values for all points in the field are lowered. Any focal defects will still be included in the pattern deviation plot after the diffuse loss has been eliminated.

Mean Deviation (MD)

Many statistical programs calculate the mean elevation or depression of the patient's overall field compared with the normal reference field. If the MD falls significantly outside the age-matched norms, a probability (P) value will be assigned. The smaller the P value, the higher the probability of an abnormal deviation. For example, for a P value where $P < 5\%$, less than 5% of the normal population obtained a value that low. A significant MD value may indicate either general or localized visual field depression (see Chapter 17).

Pattern Standard Deviation (PSD)

Another approach is to isolate the defect by finding the degree to which the *shape* of the patient's field differs from the shape of a normal age-corrected field. A low PSD indicates a smooth hill of vision, whereas a high PSD indicates an irregular hill with focal visual field defects.

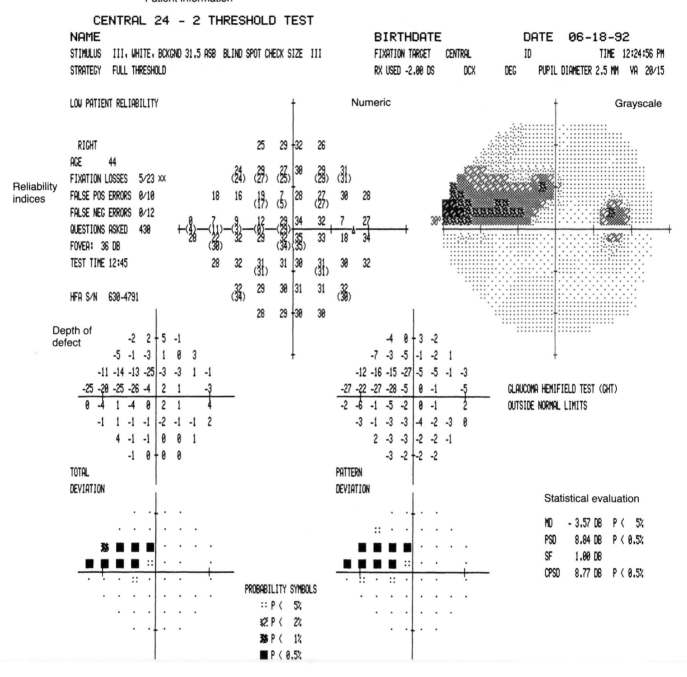

FIGURE 18-4. Humphrey single field analysis includes grayscale, numeric values, depth of defect, evaluation of pattern of vision loss, reliability indices, and statistical evaluation indices.

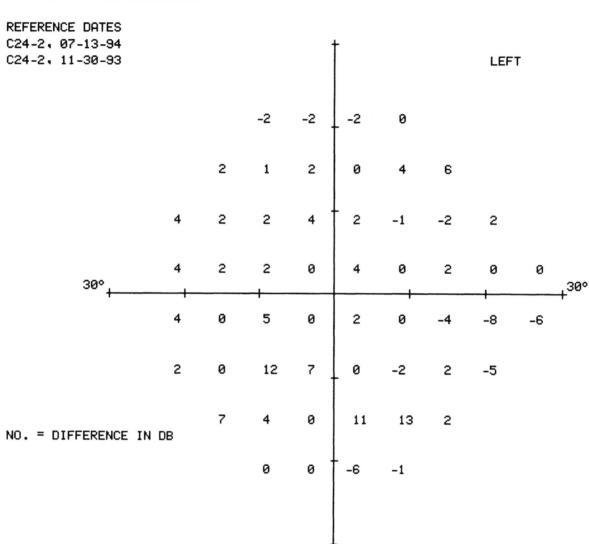

FIGURE 18–5. Comparison printout shows the point-to-point change between two examinations from the same patient.

Corrected Pattern Standard Deviation (CPSD)

This value also compares the total shape of the patient's hill of vision with the shape of the age-corrected hill of vision. In addition, it minimizes the effects of patient variability and isolates the irregularity caused by field loss.

In summary, projection-type automated perimeters have the ability to randomize target presentation. Good manual perimetrists can do this, but unfortunately, not all manual perimetrists are good. Although it takes longer than kinetic perimetry, static threshold and suprathreshold static techniques are best for reliable, accurate fields for the central 30° of the visual field. Many experts consider manual perimetry best for neuroophthalmic defects, e.g., chiasmal and postchiasmal conditions, and consider automated perimetry best for optic nerve or nerve fiber bundle defects, such as optic neuropathies or glaucoma.

Bibliography

Anderson, DR: Perimetry with and without Automation, 2nd ed. St. Louis, CV Mosby, 1987.

Armaly, MF: Selective perimetry for glaucomatous defects in ocular hypertension. Arch Ophthalmol 87: 518, 1972.

Haley MJ (ed): The Field Analyzer Primer, 2nd ed. San Leandro, CA, Allergan Humphrey, 1987.

Lieberman MF, Drake M: A Simplified Guide to Computerized Perimetry. Thorofare, NJ, Slack, 1987.

Silverstone DE, Hirsch J: Automated Visual Field Testing: Techniques of Examination and Interpretation. Norwalk, CT, Appleton-Century-Crofts, 1986.

Werner EB: Manual of Visual Fields. New York, Churchill Livingstone, 1991.

Whalen WR, Spaeth GL: Computerized Visual Fields: What They Are and How to Use Them. Thorofare, NJ, Slack, 1985.

• CHAPTER 18 AUTOMATED PERIMETRY

1. The most common stimulus size used on automated perimeters is equivalent to which one of the Goldmann perimeter sizes?
   a. II
   b. V
   c. I
   d. IV
   e. III

2. What is the maximum target brightness (in decibels) for automated perimetry?
   a. 51
   b. 10
   c. 0
   d. 24
   e. 108

3. What is the most accurate automated testing method?
   a. up-down bracketing
   b. static threshold
   c. suprathreshold static screening
   d. foveal threshold
   e. kinetic threshold

4. Which automated printout most resembles a kinetic isopter map?
   a. grayscale
   b. numeric pattern
   c. double determination point
   d. total deviation
   e. comparison printout

5. Which of the following is a weakness in automated perimetry?
   a. accuracy
   b. perimetrist's skill
   c. detection of subtle defects
   d. reliability
   e. testing time

Ocular Motility: Binocular Function

LEARNING OBJECTIVES
- Explain fixation
- Explain how sensory tests evaluate fusion
- Evaluate fusional amplitudes
- Differentiate types of convergence
- Explain the relationship between accommodation and convergence
- Understand how prisms should be held

● EYE MOVEMENT CONTROL SYSTEMS

Human eyes have a wide range of movement while maintaining coordination with each other. They scan the field of view until an object of interest is found. Once an off-center area of the retina locates the object an "early warning guidance system," activates the complex wiring to the ocular motor system. To change the angle at which the visual stimulus enters the eye, the visual system sends impulses to the extraocular muscles for *saccades,* corrective fast eye movements that function as a homing device, rotating the eye in a predetermined trajectory to steer the desired new image onto the fovea, thus allowing acute examination of the object. Positioning the image onto the fovea is called either *fixation* or refixation because new objects keep attracting attention and supplanting the old. This requires a new eye movement to fixate the new object. The frontal lobes of the brain control the saccades.

Slower following movements, *pursuits,* lock the image of a slow but smooth moving object onto the fovea for tracking. The area around the parieto-occipital lobe junction in the brain controls pursuit.

Although only one eye may be stimulated, both make parallel movements, *versions,* from one gaze position to another. Contraction of one extraocular muscle produces contraction of its *yoke* extraocular muscle in the other eye, according to Hering's law. Both saccades and pursuits use versions to move the eyes into the various gaze positions.

Simultaneously with saccades and pursuits, a feedback mechanism from the *vestibular system* maintains the position of the eyes while the head and body move. As you watch your eyes in a mirror while turning your head to the right, the eyes drive left and appear stationary. If you jump, the eyes appear to remain still, but actually as you go up, they go down. This stabilizing effect keeps the eyes on target. The brain stem, cerebellum, and inner ear coordinate this system.

As a chosen object varies in distance from the eyes, simultaneous inward or outward movements called *vergences* maintain both images on both foveas. The eyes still move equal amounts, but move slowly and in opposite directions. This is the slowest of the slow eye movement systems. The vergence pathways are not well understood but appear to bypass the brain stem gaze centers.

As soon as the newborn human opens its eyes, fixation reflexes begin to develop and reach stability by approximately 6 years of age. Normal development depends on experience for reinforcement. Alertness, the ability to learn, good visual acuity, attention, and interest are all factors in maintaining precise foveal fixation on a target. This finely tuned steering mechanism works synchronously to develop stable fixation even when the eyes, head, and target move.

Fixation

A *fixing,* or *fixating,* eye is one that aims straight at any viewed target. This target is on an imaginary line of direction, the visual axis, that connects the target to its image on the fovea of the retina. The corneal reflex is seen as a reflection when the viewed target is a fixation light. It appears to be located on the cornea where the visual axis crosses the anterior corneal surface. Actually, the corneal reflection is its first Purkinje's image and is located about 4 mm behind the cornea.

Observation of the corneal reflex is one method of corroborating both monocular and binocular foveal fixation. If the corneal reflections match, the image of the target is assumed to be on both foveas. However, a tiny misalignment may be masked. Foveal fixation is also referred to as central fixation, a redundant, but common, term (Fig. 19–1).

The corneal reflex position is seldom centered exactly on the pupil. It is more usually found approximately 0.5 mm nasally. Because the fovea is not at the geometric center of the retina, but *temporal* to it, the corneal reflex comes out *nasal* of center. It can be quite nasal, but still normal, so long as the corneal reflexes are in the *same position in both eyes,* i.e., displaced equidistant from the center of the pupil. Binocular fixation occurs when both visual axes intersect at the fixation object. With an eye misalignment, only one eye deviates at a time. The visual axis of the deviated eye does not intersect the visual axis of the straight eye at the fixation target. The other maintains normal foveal fixation (Fig. 19–2).

When the reflexes match, binocular vision (fusion) may be present or not. The patient may have phoria—a latent deviation. If so, the patient is said to be fusing (simultaneously using both eyes with resulting single binocular vision). Perfect (central) fusion is never found when the corneal reflexes do not match because binocular cooperation requires equal vision and straight eyes.

Sensory Tests

Sensory fusion is the ability of the brain to integrate signals from two similar images, one from each eye, each on a corresponding retinal point, and to unify them into a composite, three dimensional picture. The brain is programmed to see a single binocular image. There is a difference between patients' having the ability to fuse and their demonstrating actual binocular cooperation on examination. The more similar the images are in shape, size, and color, the easier they are to fuse. Confirming motor fusion on examination is proof that the patient can use at least some of his or her sensory fusion capability.

If deviation, i.e., misalignment of the eyes, exists, the patient cannot use his or her sensory fusion capabilities because one image of the target being viewed is on one fovea, and the other is not. The images are not on corresponding retinal points. No fusion is found on sensory testing.

One way to determine the binocular state of a patient is with subjective sensory tests. All subjective tests require some verbal response and decision making on the part of the patient. The examiner has to rely on the patient's honesty, reliability, and comprehension. Later in the text is a discussion of objective tests, such as the cover test, that the examiner conducts with neither verbal response nor decision making from the patient.

When testing children, remember that they do not have the facility with language that adults have. You must interpret what the child is saying. It is easy for the examiner to be misled. Children want to please and are looking for clues. Do not give any, and do not imply that there is a right or a wrong answer. You are only interested in what the patient sees. Be very careful in phrasing your questions. Do not require a yes or no answer; you will get the yes response most of the time. Whenever there is a conflict between objective and subjective results, the objective findings are more likely to be correct.

Worth's 4-dot and stereoacuity tests (e.g., the Titmus test) are examples of subjective sensory tests for single binocular vision. Only patients with aligned foveas demonstrate fusion responses on these tests.

Worth's 4-Dot Test

Worth's 4-dot test is often renamed the Worthless 4-dot test, because it is so poorly done by so many examiners with resulting inaccurate information. Never call it Worth's 4-dot test when the child is lis-

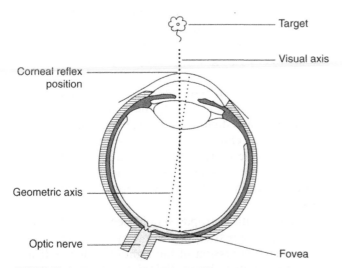

FIGURE 19–1. Fixation target imaged on fovea of right eye.

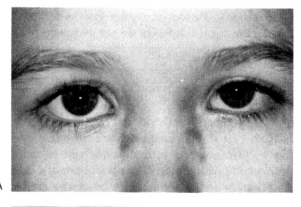

A

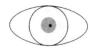

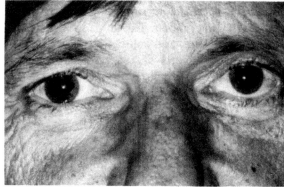

B

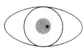

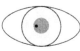

FIGURE 19–2. Variations in position of matching corneal reflexes with straight eyes. *A,* Common slightly nasal corneal reflexes. *B,* Less common very nasal corneal reflexes.

tening, just Worth's test. Avoid giving clues to the right answer. Once you are aware of its pitfalls and limitations, however, this test is easy to explain and quick to perform. It does give important information on whether or not the patient is fusing and the sensory adaptations the patient has developed because of an eye deviation.

Worth's 4-dot test gives information about the patient's current fusion status, i.e., whether there is binocular cooperation. Fusion is only possible with aligned eyes. If there is a misalignment, or *tropia,* the brain acknowledges the visual information it receives from both eyes with diplopia; otherwise, the information from the misaligned eye is ignored, and suppression is found.

Two concepts have to be evaluated on all preschoolers to determine whether they can perform the test. If the patient is too young, e.g., less than 3 years old, to distinguish red from green, the test cannot be done. Can the child identify colors? Red can be described as red, orange, or pink, as long as the child is consistent, just as green can be described as green, blue, or purple. Can the child tell the difference among "two, three, five, or four"? Counting from one to ten is not enough; he or she must be able to reply with the number when fingers are help up. A common problem with this test is the patient with a deviation who unexpectedly answers four dots. This response can be valid and is usually the first clue that this patient has developed anomalous

retinal correspondence (ARC) as an adaptation. The most common explanation, however, is that *the patient has been tested previously* and deduced the correct response from the previous examiner's questions.

To perform the test, a red lens is placed over the right eye and a green one over the left. Then the patient views a modified flashlight with four dots on it, one red, one white, and two green (Fig. 19–3). The right eye looks through the red lens and sees two red lights. The left eye looks through the green lens and sees two green lights and a third light that may be described as either a paler green or yellow. The white dot on the bottom is the only one seen by both eyes. All patients with aligned eyes and binocular control at near (14 inches or 33 cm) should fuse these dots by seeing four simultaneously (Fig. 19–4). They may describe two red and two green dots, one red and three green, or one red with two green and a red-green mixed light. If the patient has a misalignment, the distinction between suppression and diplopia requires explicit questioning, because many children will answer with five dots when they only have four. Some children have difficulty in explaining that the white light is a blend of both colors or that it alternates from red to green to red as they look at it.

Patients with a tropia should see either two red, indicating suppression of the left eye, or three green, indicating suppression of the right eye, or five lights, indicating double vision (diplopia).

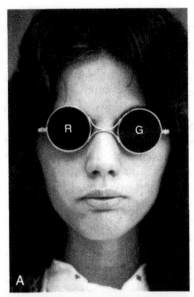

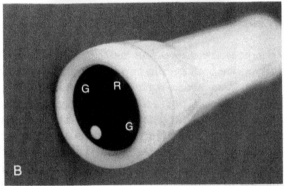

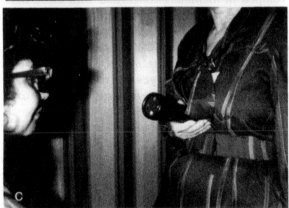

FIGURE 19–3. Testing Worth's 4 Dot. *A*, Patient wearing red-green goggles. *B*, Worth's 4 dot flashlight with 2 green, 1 red, and 1 white lights. C. Patient being tested at near; examiner is holding light 16 inches from patient.

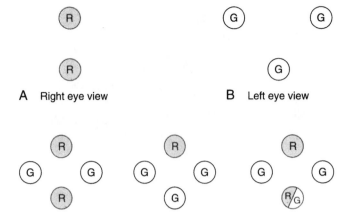

A Right eye view   B Left eye view

C Possible binocular views in straight-eyed patients with fusion

FIGURE 19–4. Dots as they appear to the patient. *A*, Right eye sees 2 red. *B*, Left eye sees 3 green. *C*, Variations of 4 dots as seen by patient fusing with straight eyes.

The patient may have rapidly alternating suppression (two reds for a few seconds, then three greens, then back to the reds). The patient may call this five dots. Ask careful questions. After a response of five dots, ask whether the red and green dots are all there at once, or do two reds appear without green ones, and then change to three greens and no reds. If the patient truly does perceive five dots, the examiner also needs to know whether the reds are to the patient's left or right of the greens. Because children frequently are uncertain about their directions, touch first the right arm, then the left, as you ask which side the reds are on.

When the Worth's flashlight is used at 14 inches, the fusion is peripheral; at 6 feet, central. The closer the flashlight is held, the easier it is to fuse, because the target is imaged over a wider retinal area, thus exceeding the limits of the suppression scotoma.

Stereoacuity

Subjective testing of stereoacuity is also a routine part of the strabismus examination *whenever the patient has a phoria, a deviation less than 10, or an intermittent deviation*. If any stereoacuity is found, it indicates some binocular function, even if no other test has given a fusion response. A positive response on this test is the best indicator of the patient's binocularity.

Stereopsis is the visual appreciation of three dimensionality during binocular vision through fusion of signals from slightly disparate retinal elements. Stereo sensation cannot be learned, even in the presence of fusion, bifoveal fixation, or good visual acuity. It is based on horizontal disparity rather than vertical. Tests for stereoacuity seek to determine the smallest amount of recognizable retinal disparity in seconds of arc, most importantly in judging distance up to 6 feet away. Beyond 20 feet, its influence is considerably diminished (Figs. 19–5 and 19–6).

Currently the most widely employed measure for stereoacuity is probably the Titmus test, which uses the Polaroid principle of two superimposed, nearly identical, vectographic prints, imprinted with polaroid wavelengths 90° to one another. The superimposed prints are viewed at reading distance through Polaroid analyzer filters that have the effect of presenting sepa-

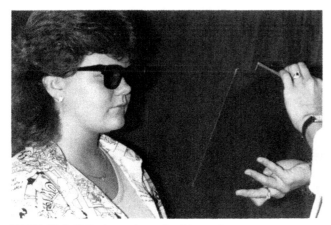

FIGURE 19–5. Patient wearing polaroid goggles.

rate images to each eye. Part of these images are slightly displaced from each other horizontally to stimulate bitemporal retinal elements. This disparate stimulation creates an illusion of nearness, which is seen by the patient as that part of the image coming forward off the page of vectographic prints.

The plate presents a graded series of nine diamonds, each containing four circles, one of which has horizontal retinal disparity. Under the diamonds are three rows of animals, some with greater disparity than the others. On a separate page is a large picture of a fly with raised wings. This is the most peripheral test of stereoacuity. The book is held parallel to the plane of the face. If there is a negative response, it does not mean no stereoacuity, but that none is detectable by *this* test on *this* visit. Granted, stereoacuity can be obtained on some children under age three, looking at the fly, but not consistently. In fact, not until age six do most children without binocular problems give an accurate response.

Although it is more difficult to mislead the examiner on the Titmus test than Worth's 4-dot, this test has pitfalls, as well. In the first three diamonds, patients can frequently guess monocularly which dot is correct, not because they see it in depth as the test is designed, but because it is displaced from a central location. This incorrect response can be verified by using the three rows of animals, which provide no monocular clues. Alternatively, when the page with the diamonds is turned upside down, the disparate pair of circles appears *below* the page. Do *not* ask which circle is now below the page; instead, if anything, ask what is different about the circles. If the sensation of depth is noted, the child will answer correctly.

Central stereopsis operates over a narrow range of spatial disparities. Peripheral stereopsis is much less specific. Corresponding retinal points from the macula and fovea have a point-to-point relationship, whereas more peripheral portions of the retina have a less exact directional value relationship. Instead of point-to-

point, the relationship is area-to-area. This permits *slippage* of corresponding retinal points when dealing with peripheral retina and allows similar visual images in form, contrast, and luminance, but with spatial separation of several degrees to be fusible. This permits peripheral stereopsis to occur with or without central fusion, but central stereopsis never occurs without peripheral fusion.

Central stereopsis is 67 seconds of arc or less, seen by a correct response to at least the 7th set of circles. The Titmus test has its lowest threshold at 40 seconds. The threshold of stereoacuity is approximately 24 seconds of arc at 16 inches. However, the test is graded for a test distance of 15 inches. The seconds of arc disparity changes with testing distance. The 40 seconds on the test booklet become 80 if the test is held at 7 inches, 20 if the test is held at 30 inches.

Vergence

Vergences are disjunctive movements that simultaneously move both eyes in opposite directions in order to obtain, or maintain, single binocular vision. The eyes can move toward one another (convergence), away from each other (divergence), one may move up while the other moves down (vertical vergence), or they can tilt toward (incyclovergence) or away from (excyclovergence) the nose. The ability to converge and diverge developed in mammals concerned with close objects and, coupled with the development of fine motor skills, gradually became refined into excellent eye-hand coordination. Vergences are the motor component of the fusion mechanism that controls horizontal and vertical phorias, which keep the eyes locked in alignment. They are constant corrective movements necessary to continue motor fusion.

The eyes are stimulated to perform these maneuvers as a fixation target changes its distance from the eye. Without such adjustments, the object's image would fall on only one fovea at a time, producing diplopia and eliminating fusion and binocular depth perception. The feedback signal for realigning the eyes is the diplopia (double vision). Within certain limits, our eyes can move in opposite directions through vergences to reunify the images by compensating for the misalignment.

With an eye misalignment, if one image of the target is on the fovea of one eye, the other is not on the fovea of the other eye. The perception is that of two simultaneous but separate images (diplopia). The limit of vergence is exceeded, and the eyes are unable to compensate.

Of the various eye movement systems, the vergences are the slowest, moving only 20° per second. A central nervous system control center for vergence is suspected to be located in the midbrain, but no conclusive

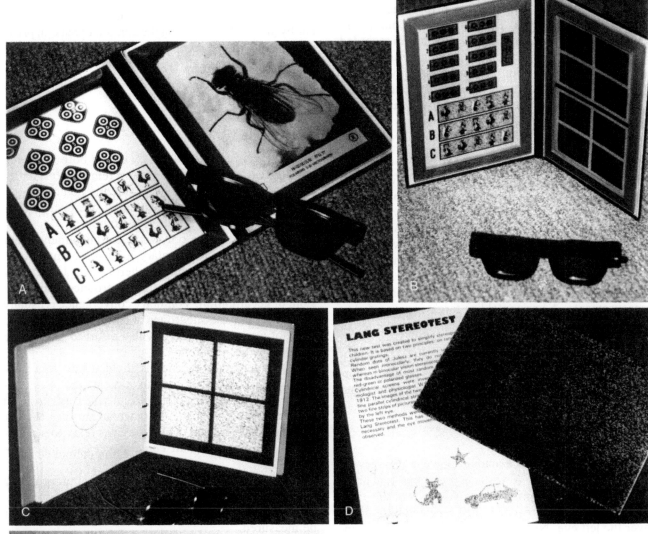

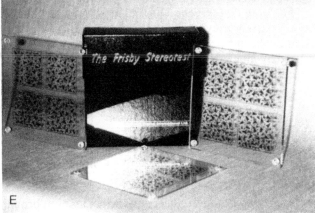

FIGURE 19–6. Various tests for stereoacuity. *A,* Titmus test with polaroid goggles. *B,* Randot's test with polaroid goggles. *C,* TNO test with red-green goggles. *D,* Lang's test without goggles. *E,* Frisby's test without goggles.

evidence yet exists. Eye deviations, especially in childhood, may be caused in part by a faulty vergence mechanism.

The amount the eyes can move to maintain alignment and resist diplopia is the *fusional amplitude*. The unit of vergence measurement, for all except torsional, is the *prism diopter* ($^\Delta$). When fusion reserves are exceeded, diplopia results. The fusion break point (minimum amount of prism that causes diplopia) is recorded as well as the recovery point (maximum amount of prism that allows refusion). Near horizontal vergences are about double the norms for distance, and convergence norms are about double the divergence norms (Table 19–1) (Fig. 19–7).

Cyclovergence (Torsional Vergence)

This is an involuntary rotational reflex movement of both eyes around the anterior-posterior pole. In incyclovergence, both eyes rotate around the visual axis medially relative to the 12 o'clock meridian. In excyclovergence, both eyes rotate around the visual axis temporally relative to the 12 o'clock meridian. Cyclovergence is rarely measured clinically.

Double Maddox rods can be used to make these measurements. A horizontal line target is presented to each eye. For excyclovergence, the temporal ends of the lines are slowly turned down until diplopia is reported. For incyclovergence the temporal ends of each line are turned up slowly until diplopia is reached. Normal values range from 6 to 10° for incyclovergence and 8 to 12° for excyclovergence.

Vertical Vergence

Sursumvergence is the amount one eye can elevate and maintain fusion. A vertical prism bar can place increasingly strong prisms base-down over the right eye until diplopia is reached, then repeated base-down over the left eye. Normal values are 1 to 3 prism diopters in either direction. The eyes involuntarily move in opposite vertical directions to control hyperphorias. In congenital incomitant vertical muscle problems, such as CN IV palsies, or in slowly progressive hyperdeviations, much larger vertical fusional amplitudes may develop over time.

Divergence

Divergence is stimulated by one or both images of the viewed target focused on nasal retina rather than on both foveas. To overcome the homonymous (uncrossed) diplopia caused by this, either or both eyes abduct to return the image of the object of regard onto both foveas. Divergence can be measured with a prism bar by gradually increasing the amount of base-in prism power until the patient reports diplopia. The *break point* has been reached. By slowly decreasing the prism power, a point will be reached where the patient regains single vision, the *recovery point*.

Convergence

Convergence is stimulated by one or both images of the viewed target focused on the temporal retina instead of on both foveas. To overcome the heteronymous (crossed) diplopia this causes, either one or both eyes must adduct to restore bifoveal fixation.

Convergence is the only vergence movement under both involuntary and voluntary control. Voluntary convergence is the mechanism whereby we deliberately cross our eyes to cause laughter, produce double vision, or get attention. Voluntary convergence is usually not included in the subgroups of convergence, because it is not a true reflex but a willed effort to exaggerate the synkinetic near reflex.

Involuntary convergence is divided into four subgroups. In an alert, conscious patient, the eyes converge to a straighter position than when asleep from the tonus present in the extraocular muscles. Under deep anesthesia, or in death, the eyes relax to a divergence position. This *tonic convergence* cannot be measured.

Proximal convergence is the small amount, probably less than 5 prism diopters, induced by psychic awareness of an object's nearness. This awareness cannot be measured.

Fusional convergence, is the fine-tuning mechanism that keeps the eyes aligned and is stimulated by two identical images on disparate retinal points. It is measured by much the same method as fusional divergence, except that increasing amounts of base-out prisms are used until the patient reports diplopia. Just as with divergence, the *break point* and *recovery points* are recorded (Fig. 19–8).

Accommodation/Accommodative Convergence Ratio

Accommodative convergence is that amount brought about by a specific amount of accommodation. At 20 feet, without refractive error, there is no accommodative demand and, therefore no convergence response. The object is seen clearly, and the eyes are parallel.

TABLE 19–1.

Average Fusional Amplitudes

	Convergence	Divergence	Vertical Vergence	Cyclovergence
Distance	$10^\Delta/8^\Delta$ BO	$6^\Delta/4^\Delta$ BI	2^Δ BD OD	10° IN
			2^Δ BU OD	10° EX
Near	$20^\Delta/18^\Delta$ BO	$12^\Delta/10^\Delta$ BI	2^Δ BD OD	10° IN
			2^Δ BU OD	10° EX

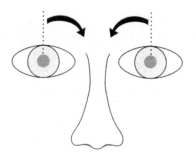
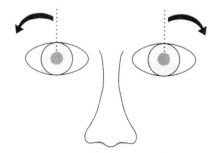

Incyclorotation of both eyes

Excyclorotation of both eyes

A

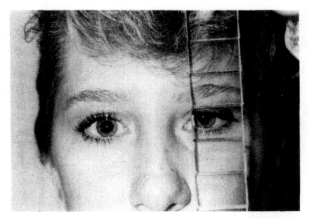

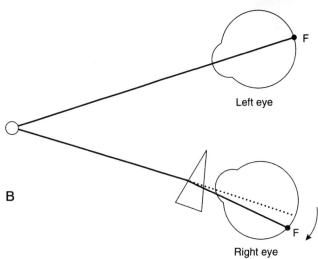

F

Left eye

B

Right eye

F

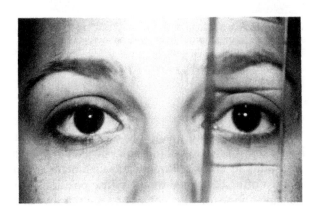

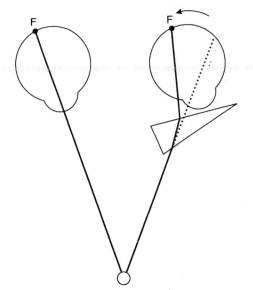

F

F

C

FIGURE 19–7. *A,* Vergences. Cyclovergence. *B,* Vertical vergence testing with base down vertical prism bar. *C,* Divergence testing with base in horizontal prism bar.

Illustration continued on following page

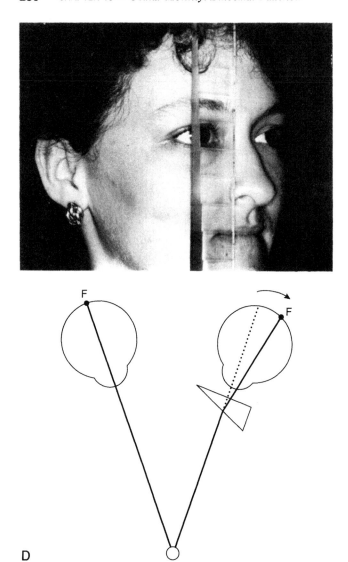

D

FIGURE 19–7. *Continued D,* Convergence testing with base out horizontal prism bar.

Because there is neither accommodative nor convergence demand, any distance deviation will not be influenced by accommodative convergence when the cycloplegic refractive correction is worn.

The eyes must converge in order to keep both foveas aimed at a fixation object as it comes closer than 20 feet. To be seen clearly, the eyes also need to accommodate for the shorter distance. The accommodative demand at a near distance for maintenance of clarity is coupled with the convergence demand for maintenance of single binocular vision. Both depend on how close to the eye the fixation object is, i.e., both mechanisms are distance-dependent. The accommodative convergence/accommodation (AC/A) ratio compares the amount in prism diopters of accommodative convergence generated by each diopter of accommodation. When average, the ratio is about equal to the interpupillary distance measured in centimeters; about 5 : 1 in children and 6 : 1 in adults.

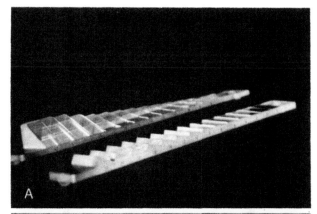

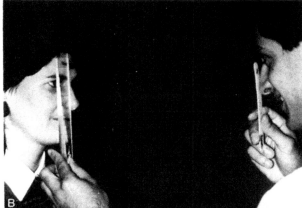

FIGURE 19–8. *A,* Horizontal and vertical prism bars. *B,* Technique. Patient views fixation target held by examiner who is viewing patient's corneal reflexes through horizontal prism bar held base out.

• PRISMS

Prisms are used to quantitate misalignments of the visual axes and are sometimes incorporated in eyeglass corrections to eliminate minor misalignments. Prisms are most often described by their base position, which is usually opposite the deviation, e.g., base-out for inward (eso) deviations, base-down for hyperdeviations (Fig. 19–9).

Prisms should be held so that the rear face is parallel to the plane of the face (frontal plane). Fortunately, small errors in position of the prism produce small errors with weak prisms. Position becomes more critical with prisms above 30^{Δ}. Prisms cannot be stacked

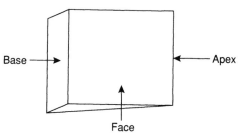

FIGURE 19–9. Prism.

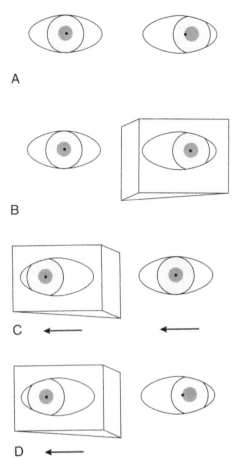

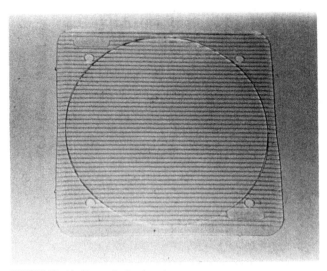

FIGURE 19–11. Fresnel plastic prism.

FIGURE 19–10. Correct and incorrect placement of prisms. *A,* Left eye with uncorrected exotropia. Corneal reflexes do not match. *B,* Exotropic left eye with correcting prism on same eye. Corneal reflexes match. Neither eye moves. Correction occurs whether or not there is a left eye paresis or restriction. *C,* If left eye has no palsy and there is no restriction, corneal reflexes can be made to match with prism on fixing right eye. Right eye moves out to refixate, left eye moves straight by Hering's Law. Right eye is now in exotropic position and left eye is straight. *D,* With palsy or restriction of left eye, corneal reflexes cannot be made to match with prism on right eye. Right eye moves exotropically to refixate with prism, but left eye cannot move when innervated to do so by Hering's Law. Corneal reflex remains uncorrected, left eye.

together in the same direction because the front prism is no longer in the frontal plane and will produce a much greater effect than anticipated. Large deviations are best measured with prisms split before the two eyes. A vertical and a horizontal prism may be stacked together with insignificant error. When measuring incomitant deviations, the prism should be placed before the nonfixing eye to ensure that the fixing eye is in the proper position of gaze. For restrictive syndromes, the restricted eye has the prism before it because that eye cannot properly fix in all cardinal positions. If a prism is held before a fixing eye, the eye moves toward the apex to restore fixation (Fig. 19–10).

Two types of eyeglass prism are available. Prisms can be incorporated into spectacles by being ground in, up to 10^Δ each lens. Weight and expense cause

limitations. The reduction in visual acuity is negligible. Ground-in prisms are usually preferred for long-term use. Press-on, plastic Fresnel prisms are much cheaper, and can range up to 30^Δ, but they reduce visual acuity and are easily scratched. Still they are excellent for short-term use (Fig. 19–11).

Fresnels are much more easily tolerated when applied to the lens of the non-preferred eye. With the smooth side of the press-on facing the inner surface of the eyeglass lens, trace the shape of the lens just inside the frame with a felt tip pen. Be sure that the base is in the right direction. Remove the press-on from the spectacle lens and cut out the Fresnel prism just inside the marked line with scissors. Wash the eyeglasses and the cut Fresnel with contact lens cleaning solution, rinse them thoroughly, and position the Fresnel with the smooth side against the inner surface of the eyeglass lens. Adjust the position of the Fresnel by gently sliding it. Press out air bubbles with the ball of your thumb. Once applied, the press-on should neither overlap the lens bevel nor contact the eyeglass frame. It will be dry enough for wear in 20 minutes.

Bibliography

Cassin B, Solomon SAB: Dictionary of Eye Terminology, 2nd ed. Gainesville, FL, Triad Publishing Co., 1990.

Flom MC, Addams AJ: Fresnel optics. In Duane TD (ed): Clinical Ophthalmology, vol 1. Hagerstown MD, Harper & Row, 1987.

Nelson LB, Catalano RA: Atlas of Ocular Motility. Philadelphia, WB Saunders, 1989.

Thompson JT, Guyton DL: Ophthalmic prisms: Measurement errors and how to minimize them. Ophthalmology 90:204, 1983.

von Noorden GK (ed): Burian-von Noorden's Binocular Vision and Ocular Motility, 4th ed. St Louis, Mosby-Year Book, 1990.

● CHAPTER 19 OCULAR MOTILITY: BINOCULAR FUNCTION

1. Where does fixation move the image of an object of interest on to?
   a. corneal reflex
   b. pupil
   c. visual axis
   d. fovea
   e. cornea

2. What must you have in order to have fusion?
   a. phoria
   b. matching corneal reflexes
   c. one eye fixating
   d. tropia
   e. misalignment

3. What is the response for proof of fusion on the Worth test?
   a. 2 dots
   b. 3 dots
   c. 4 dots
   d. 5 dots
   e. 6 dots

4. How is binocular depth perception tested?
   a. Worth test
   b. prism diopters
   c. prism bar
   d. fusional amplitudes
   e. Titmus test

5. To correct a horizontal deviation larger than 45^Δ, the base of a prism is held in which direction?
   a. same direction as the deviation with two prisms stacked together on one eye
   b. direction opposite the deviation with two prisms, one on each eye
   c. same direction as the deviation with two prisms, one on each eye
   d. direction opposite the deviation with two prisms stacked together on one eye
   e. direction opposite the deviation with one prism on one eye, and in the same direction with one prism on the other eye.

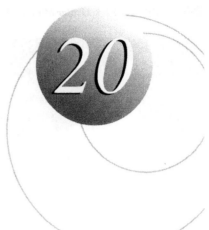

Ocular Motility: Strabismus Evaluation

LEARNING OBJECTIVES

- Assess fixation in both eyes simultaneously
- Differentiate a phoria from a tropia
- Perform a cover-uncover test
- Measure deviation by prism and alternate cover test
- Measure deviation by Krimsky's method
- Estimate deviation by Hirschberg's method
- Understand the strabismus notations used to record the amount and direction of deviation

There are two ways to detect a misalignment of the eyes. One is by shining a fixation light into the eyes of a patient who is looking at the light to determine where the light is reflected on the cornea. The other is to use some form of cover test. Because cover tests give more information, the light reflection is used as a basic screening test, and this is followed by the cover test whenever feasible.

Before performing either of the tests, the cooperation of the patient must be assessed. Strabismus evaluations are most commonly performed on children who often present specific difficulties. They do not recognize their eye problem, are not interested in being examined, have short attention spans, and are frequently apprehensive in a medical surrounding.

To ensure a reliable evaluation, the child *must* be looking at an accommodative target of some type, usually a toy on or around a fixation light (Fig. 20–1). The child's attention *must* be kept on the toy. The rule one toy–one look is a good one. After a short time, even the most interesting toy becomes boring, so have a pocketful ready. Besides producing a steady stream of new toys, ask the child questions about each toy. If it is a toy dog, ask what color the collar is, or what is the dog standing on, and so forth. You can ask if there is a fly on the dog's nose. You know there is not, but expect the child to look longer and harder to make sure. One ploy is to ask the child to touch your light. He must look at it to touch it, although some children

are more apt to touch the light if you ask them not to. Another ploy is to give the child a small toy to hold, but only if the child touches the toy to your light.

Only assess corneal reflexes when the patient is *looking at* the light, not just *seeing* it. Note whether the corneal reflexes are in exactly the same position in both eyes (Fig. 20–2). If not, which corneal reflex is too far nasal, or too far temporal? Or is the misplaced corneal reflex too far up, or too far down? If the patient did as instructed, i.e., fixed on the light or toy, at least one corneal reflex *is* correctly positioned. You must learn to identify which one. If both eyes appear to be misaligned simultaneously, the patient is *seeing,* but not *looking at* the light.

Before taking another toy for another look, assess what you have observed. If the corneal reflexes matched, the patient has straight eyes or an extremely small deviation. If so, sensory tests should be evaluated next, before the cover test. If the corneal reflexes are asymmetric when the patient looks at the target around the fixation light, there is a misalignment (deviation, tropia, strabismus). Determine which eye is straight, i.e., has its corneal reflex in the correct position. The misaligned eye turns in the direction opposite from its incorrect corneal reflex, e.g., when the corneal reflex is too far *in* (toward the nose) from mid-position, the eye is turned out. If the corneal reflex is too high, the eye is deviated downward. By this manuever, you decide whether there is a misalignment, in which eye

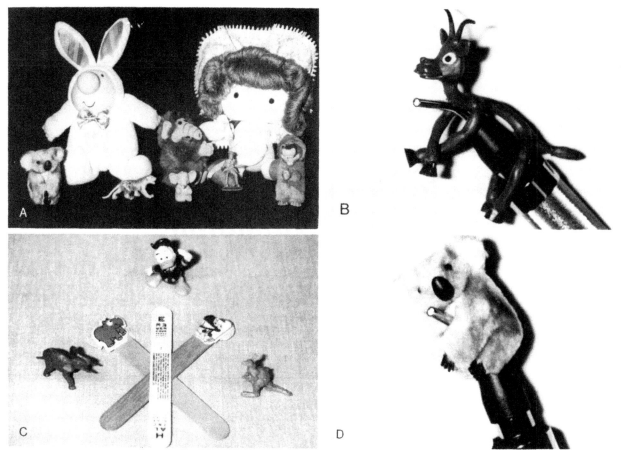

FIGURE 20–1. *A to D,* Accommodative Targets.

and in which direction. Further assessment requires the ability of the examiner to perform the cover test (Fig. 20–3).

● COVER TEST

There are many variations of the cover test. We are concerned only with the cover-uncover test, the cross-cover test (also called alternate cover), and the prism and alternate cover test (PACT).

Cover tests are used to determine whether a deviation is a phoria or a tropia, and whether constant, intermittent, or alternating. The presumption is that both eyes want to maintain foveal (central) fixation on a target, so that the brain can fuse the two images into one. *Central fusion,* fusion of the images on both foveas, cannot occur without simultaneous, almost iden-

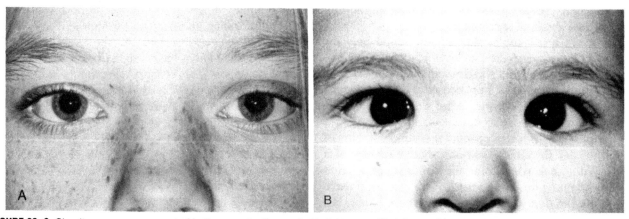

FIGURE 20–2. Simultaneous assessment of both corneal reflexes. *A,* Straight eyes. Slightly nasal but equal corneal reflexes. No epicanthal folds. *B,* Thirty prism diopters right esotropia. Normal left corneal reflex. Temporal position right corneal reflex. Deviation appears cosmetically worse because of large epicanthal folds.

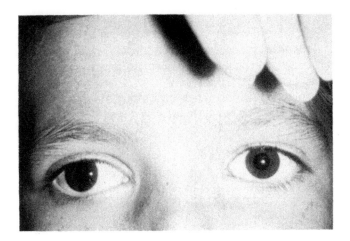

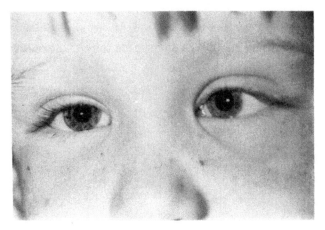

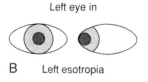

Right eye out

A   Right exotropia

Left eye in

B   Left esotropia

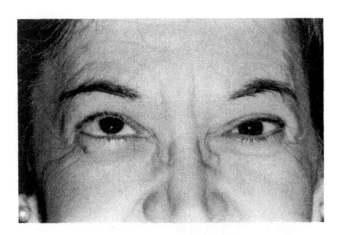

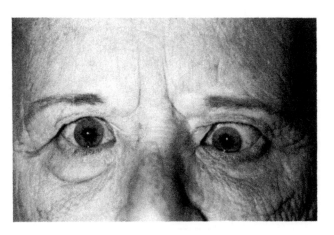

Right eye up

C   Right hypertropia

Left eye down

D   Left hypotropia

FIGURE 20–3. *A* to *D*, Types of tropia.

tical images positioned on both foveas. Even when this correct positioning occurs, central fusion may not exist. *Peripheral fusion,* the fusion of images on the retina surrounding the fovea, is possible when simultaneous images are positioned on only one fovea but must be near the fovea of the other eye. With fusion our brain unifies the two simultaneous images, one from each eye, into one composite image, usually with some binocular depth perception.

A deviation may be seen as a phoria or a tropia. A phoria is locked in control by the fusion mechanism.

When both eyes are able to fix a target onto the fovea correctly, they do so. A phoria can be revealed only when fusion is disrupted, as occurs when an eye is covered (occluded). A patient with a phoria sees double momentarily as the eye is uncovered, then straightens that eye to regain fusion, eliminating the double vision. Phorias that measure more than 2^Δ (about 1°) can be detected by the cover-uncover test. If no movement is seen of either eye on a cover-uncover test, however, whether the cover is being put on an eye or being removed from an eye, the patient might still have a tiny

Cover-Uncover Test: Exophoria

1. In normal bifixation, there are correct position corneal reflexes in both eyes (Fig. 20–4A).

2. With right eye covered, right eye deviates outward under cover, left eye does not move because it is already fixating correctly (Fig. 20–4B).

3. With right eye uncovered, right eye moves to straighten, the left eye does not move because it is still straight (Fig. 20–4C).

4. With left eye covered, left eye deviates outward under cover, although right eye does not move because it is now fixating correctly (Fig. 20–4D).

5. With left eye uncovered, left eye moves to straighten, but right eye does not move because it is already straight (Fig. 20–4E).

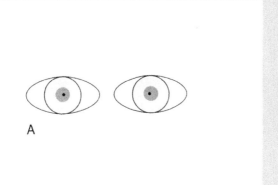

A

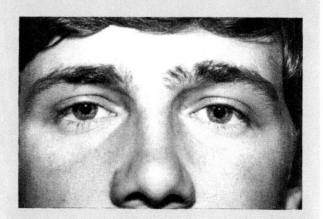

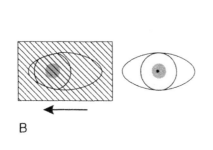

B

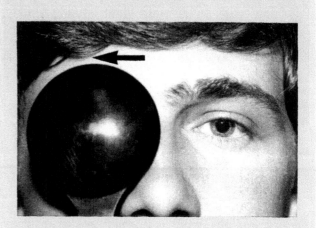

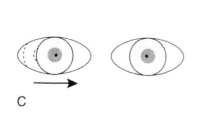

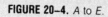

C

FIGURE 20–4. *A* to *E.*

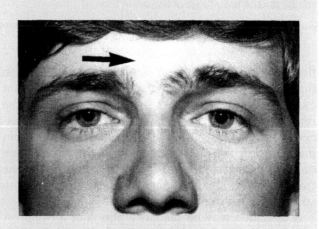

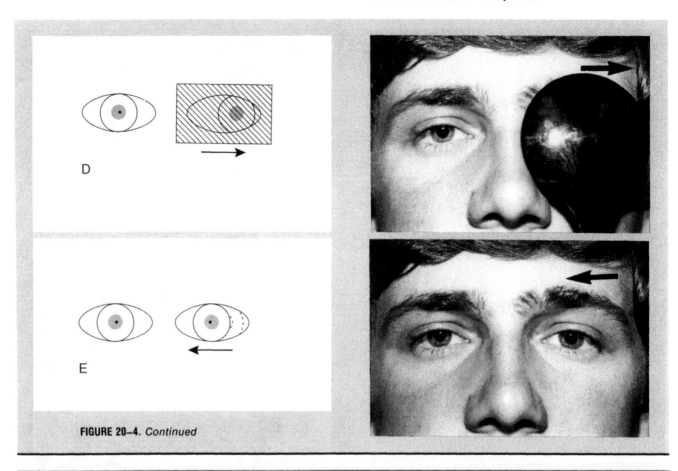

D

E

FIGURE 20–4. *Continued*

Cover-Uncover Test: Left Esotropia

1. Right eye fixates. Left eye deviates inwards with its corneal reflex temporal (out), compared with correct position of corneal reflex of right eye (Fig. 20–5*A*).

2. Left eye is covered, but neither eye moves. Right eye stays straight. Left eye under cover remains deviated (Fig. 20–5*B*).

3. Left eye is uncovered and neither eye moves. Right eye is still straight; left eye is still misaligned (Fig. 20–5*C*).

4. When the straight right eye is covered, left eye moves outward to *pick up* central fixation. Its corneal reflex assumes a correct position, but right eye now deviates under the cover (Fig. 20–5*D*).

5. When cover is removed, there are two possibilities. Both eyes may shift to the right so that eyes return to original position with right eye fixating and left eye deviating. This misalignment is neither intermittent nor alternating (Fig. 20–5*E*).

6. Alternatively, neither eye moves, but patient's corneal reflex is now temporal in right eye, which is deviating, but left eye is straight with its corneal reflex in the correct position. This misalignment is alternating, but not intermittent (Fig. 20–5*F*).

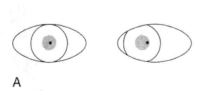

A

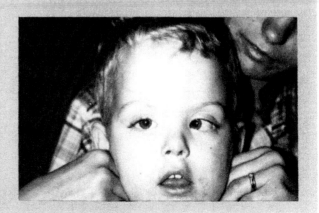

FIGURE 20–5. *A to F. Illustration continued on following page*

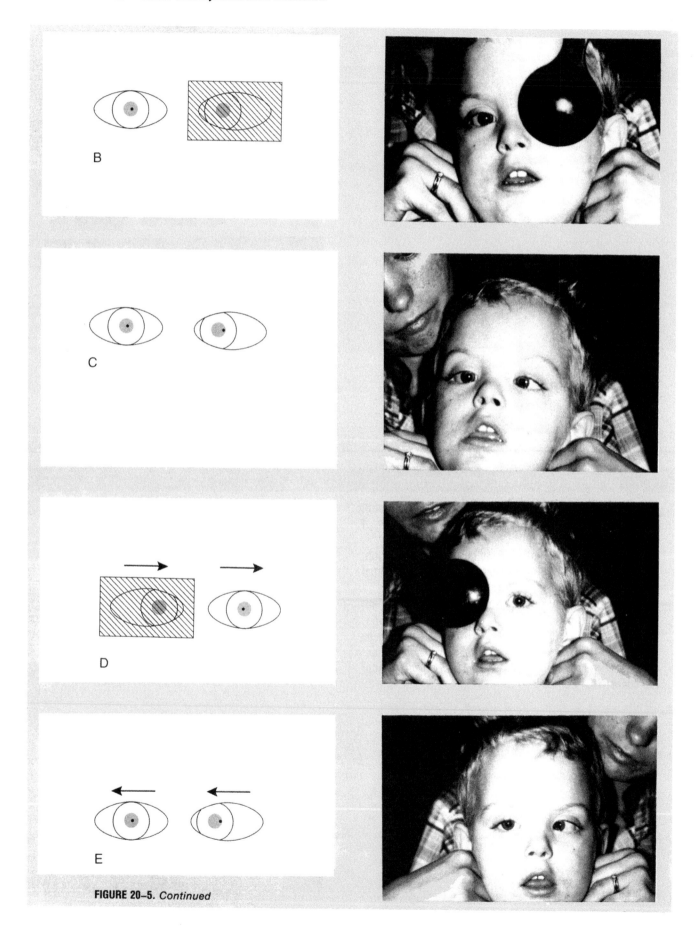

FIGURE 20–5. *Continued*

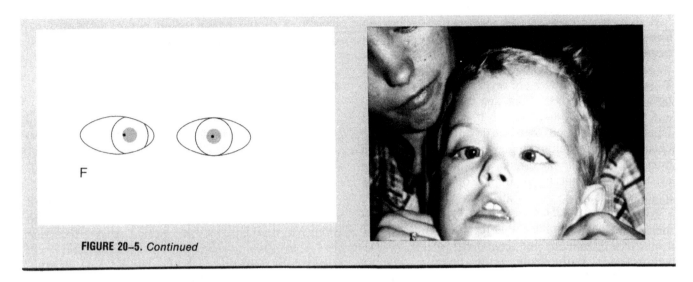

FIGURE 20–5. *Continued*

phoria, detected only on alternate cover test. Direction (eso, exo, hyper, hypo)* as well as magnitude, can be detected by the alternate cover test, but this test does not differentiate whether the misalignment is controlled by fusion, a *phoria,* or not, a *tropia.* The cover-uncover test does.

● COVER-UNCOVER TEST

The patient's corneal reflexes and eye movements are observed as you cover one eye, then uncover it, cover the other eye, then uncover it. With each maneuver, eye movements or changes in corneal reflex position are noted. If the patient is not able to centrally fixate with each fovea in turn, becomes distracted, or shifts fixation from the light, the test is invalid.

If the corneal reflections match, the cover-uncover test verifies that the eyes are straight, and possibly phoric, but signifying probable binocular function. Equal corneal reflex positions before covering either eye do not distinguish whether the patient is orthophoric, orthotropic, esophoric, exophoric, hyperphoric, or hypophoric. All patients with phoria, as well as patients with no phoria, will have identical corneal reflections when fixating a target light because they are fusing and their eyes are straight. The patient may even have a very small tropia. When there is a manifest misalignment (tropia) the nonaligned eye does not have its visual axis aimed at the fixation target. Its corneal reflex does not match the corneal reflex position on the fixating eye. The cover-uncover test verifies the deviation.

If the patient has a phoria, there will be a movement noted only as the eye is *uncovered.* The patient begins the test fusing, with straight eyes (corneal reflexes match) and ends up the same way. When the examiner

covers an eye, he notes no movement of the eye he did not cover. It does not need to move because it was already straight, but the covered eye may have moved under the occluder. As this covered eye is uncovered, it may move back into alignment and return both corneal reflexes to the same position. The test must then be repeated, covering and uncovering the other eye. The only movement noted will be of this covered eye as it is *un*covered. The occluded eye deviates to its natural, slightly misaligned position under the cover. When the cover is removed, the eye returns to exact alignment by the fusion mechanism.

To summarize; with a phoria, every time we cover an eye, no movement is seen in the eye left uncovered. When the covered eye is uncovered, it moves to straighten from its misaligned position under the cover.

A tropic patient on the cover-uncover test will have asymmetric corneal reflexes at the beginning and at the end of the test, but he or she may change which eye is misaligned. Tropic patients do not fuse when both eyes are uncovered, even if they have ability to do so. Because the patient is tested while fixing a desired target, one eye will always be straight, whereas the other is misaligned. This misalignment remains constant between the two eyes, no matter which one fixates. If the patient has a tropia, a corrective eye movement will be seen as the fixing eye is *covered.* The eye not being covered is the one that moves. The idea is to pick the straight, fixing eye to cover. This forces the misaligned eye to move to straighten itself, and you notice the shift. Because the eyes move in tandem, the eye under the cover moves in the same direction and amount as the eye you forced to straighten itself. You shifted the misalignment to the eye under the cover. If you mistakenly cover the misaligned eye, no movement is seen of the other eye not covered because it is already straight, and no movement is seen when the misaligned eye is uncovered, because it stays misaligned.

---

* Eso deviation (turned in); exo deviation (turned out); hyper deviation (turned up); hypo deviation (turned down).

A movement made by the nonfixing eye when the fixing eye is *covered* tells you that the patient has a tropia. The nonfixing eye that was deviating has straightened to fixate. If both eyes move when that eye is uncovered, both eyes are reverting to their position before the cover. The nonfixing eye deviates again, and the fixing eye fixes again. If neither eye moves when that eye is uncovered, the deviation is alternating because the originally fixing eye is now nonfixing and deviating, whereas the previously nonfixing, deviated eye is now straight and fixating. You shifted the misalignment from one eye to the other.

To summarize; whenever both eyes are uncovered, such as at the beginning and at the end of the test, the tropia is apparent by the asymmetry of the corneal light reflexes. With a tropia, every time we cover, or uncover, the deviated eye, neither eye moves. Every time we cover the straight eye, the other eye moves from its misaligned position to straighten and fixate properly. The straight eye, under the cover, deviates, however. When we uncover what had been the straight fixing eye, either both eyes shift, and we end as we

began, or no movement occurs and we have reversed which eye is misaligned (Fig. 20–6).

● ALTERNATE COVER TEST

The examiner covers the right eye, pauses, quickly moves the cover to the left eye, pauses, then quickly recovers the right eye and pauses. The pause allows time for the eye just uncovered to fixate. The movement of the cover must be rapid when it is moved from one eye to another. This maneuver may be repeated several times, as long as the patient's attention is held on the fixation target. As the cover is crossed from one eye to the other, each eye as it is being uncovered will make a movement to pick up fixation if there is *either* a phoria *or* a tropia. An outward movement of the eye being uncovered will be noted if that eye is in toward the nose from straight ahead. An inward movement will be noted if that eye is deviated outward from straight ahead, a downward movement if misaligned up, and an upward movement if down. The correcting

COVER-UNCOVER TEST

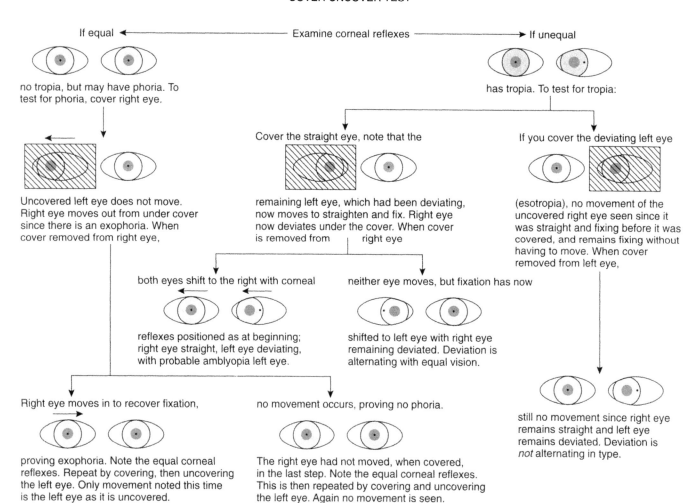

If equal ←———— Examine corneal reflexes ————→ If unequal

no tropia, but may have phoria. To test for phoria, cover right eye.

has tropia. To test for tropia:

Uncovered left eye does not move. Right eye moves out from under cover since there is an exophoria. When cover removed from right eye,

Cover the straight eye, note that the

remaining left eye, which had been deviating, now moves to straighten and fix. Right eye now deviates under the cover. When cover is removed from right eye

If you cover the deviating left eye

(esotropia), no movement of the uncovered right eye seen since it was straight and fixing before it was covered, and remains fixing without having to move. When cover removed from left eye,

both eyes shift to the right with corneal

reflexes positioned as at beginning; right eye straight, left eye deviating, with probable amblyopia left eye.

neither eye moves, but fixation has now

shifted to left eye with right eye remaining deviated. Deviation is alternating with equal vision.

Right eye moves in to recover fixation,

proving exophoria. Note the equal corneal reflexes. Repeat by covering, then uncovering the left eye. Only movement noted this time is the left eye as it is uncovered.

no movement occurs, proving no phoria.

The right eye had not moved, when covered, in the last step. Note the equal corneal reflexes. This is then repeated by covering and uncovering the left eye. Again no movement is seen.

still no movement since right eye remains straight and left eye remains deviated. Deviation is *not* alternating in type.

FIGURE 20–6. Algorithm for cover-uncover test.

eye movement is in the direction opposite to the eye misalignment. Tiny phorias as small as 2^Δ can be detected. Only if no movement is detected by cross covering, can the patient be considered to be orthophoric, if sensory tests (e.g., Worth's test, Titmus test) prove fusion. If there is no subjective proof of fusion, he or she is considered to be orthotropic—no deviation but no proof of fusion, either. This test disrupts fusion. It uncovers all the phoria and tropia (Fig. 20–7).

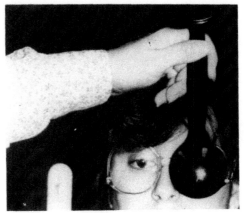

FIGURE 20–7. Technique for covering (occluding) one eye as other eye continues to look at, i.e., fixate on light.

Cover-Uncover Test Determines Alternation of Misalignment

1. Right esotropia present. Left eye is fixating (Fig. 20–8A).

2. Left eye is occluded and this forces right eye fixation (Fig. 20–8B).

3. Right eye fixation is maintained. There is now left esotropia (Fig. 20–8C).

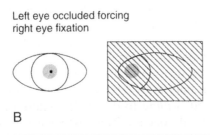

Right esotropia, left eye fixating

A

Left eye occluded forcing right eye fixation

B

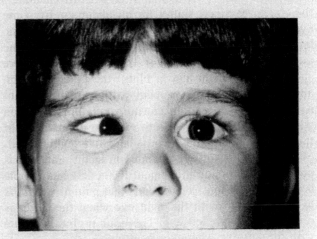

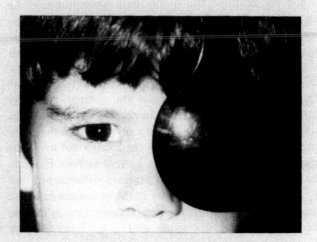

FIGURE 20–8. *A to C. Illustration continued on following page*

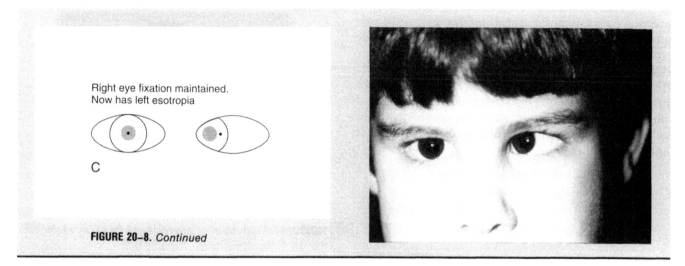

Right eye fixation maintained.
Now has left esotropia

C

FIGURE 20–8. *Continued*

• COMPLETING THE STRABISMUS EVALUATION

If on the first look at the corneal reflexes you determine that the patient has a problem with the right eye turning in (corneal reflex is out), on the second look you determine whether the patient can hold the right eye straight with the left one turned in (see cover-uncover test). Cover the straight left eye so that the misaligned right eye straightens (left eye turns in under-the-cover). We have shifted the misalignment from one eye to the other. The cover is then removed from the left eye while the patient continues to fixate on the target. If the right eye stays straight and the left eye stays turned in (through a blink) the patient has an alternating strabismus, probably with equal visual acuity. This means the patient can *hold* or *maintain* fixation with the right eye when both eyes are uncovered. If the patient immediately reverts back to fix with the left eye while the right eye deviates in again, and this is noticed as a version movement to the left, amblyopia is probably present. This means that patient is *unable* to hold fixation with the right eye when the cover is removed from the left eye. The brain prefers to fixate with the left eye whenever possible.

Do not confuse alternation with intermittency: An *intermittent tropia* is one where the deviation is sometimes present, sometimes absent. For example, on inspection of a patient's corneal reflexes the right eye is the straight, fixing eye and the left is exotropic (Fig. 20–9). The left eye's corneal reflex is too nasal or too far "in." During examination the patient suddenly straightens the left eye, and the corneal reflex from the left eye moves from a nasal to a more central position, matching the corneal reflex in the fixing right eye. The right eye stays straight. This patient is now foveally fixating with both eyes and appears orthotropic, but is actually exophoric. Intermittent misalignments are sometimes straight and phoric and controlled by fusion, but at other times are tropic and so not controlled by the fusion mechanism.

• MEASUREMENT OF THE MISALIGNMENT

Prism and Alternate Cover Test

The alternate cover test will not distinguish a tropia from a phoria. It simply shows the direction of the misalignment, not whether it is controlled by fusion. When combined with a prism (clear calibrated wedge type), the alternate cover test becomes the prism and alternate cover test (PACT) (Fig. 20–10). Phorias and tropias are measured the same way. Assuming a patient is cooperative, this produces the most accurate measurement of the amount of deviation. The shift needed to fixate the target first with one fovea, then the other, is measured. If there is an eso misalignment, an *outward* movement will be seen. It will stop (be neutralized) when the base-out prism that corrects the misalignment is placed in front of the eye. If the amount of base-out prism is insufficient, the outward movement of each eye as it is uncovered will be dampened but still present. If too large a base-out prism is placed before an eye with an eso deviation, a reverse or *inward* movement of either eye as it is uncovered, will be noted. The patient now is overcorrected. If the examiner inadvertently puts the prism base-in instead of base-out, the amount of outward movement of the eye on cross-cover will increase rather than decrease (Fig. 20–11).

It does not matter which eye has the prism in front of it. The total amount of prism may even be split before each eye. It is important to continue to increase the size of the prism until a reversal is seen. The most precise measurement is the largest prism that stops the movement *before* reversal. A horizontal prism bar is preferred by many examiners over loose prisms. The patient not only must be *able* to fixate normally with each eye but *willing* to do so. In children under age two, this rarely occurs. This test measures the entire deviation, phoria, and tropia.

Precise measurements are not possible if a prism is positioned in front of one eye with the fellow eye first

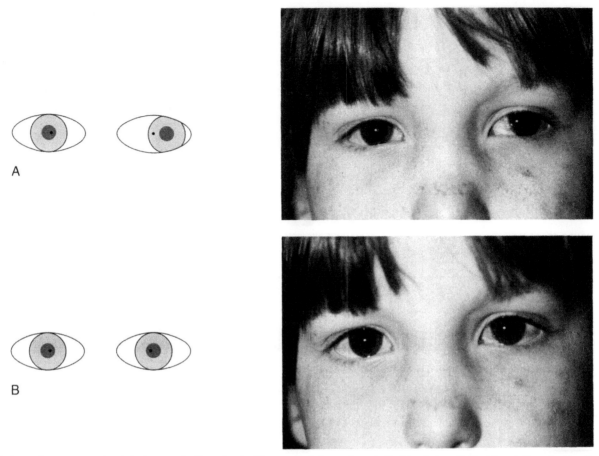

FIGURE 20–9. Intermittent exotropia. *A*, Left eye misaligned out with exo deviation not controlled by fusion. Patient has left exotropia. *B*, Both eyes straight with exo deviation controlled by fusion. Patient now has exophoria.

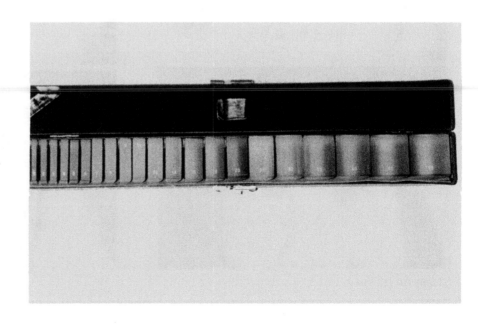

FIGURE 20–10. Set of loose prisms.

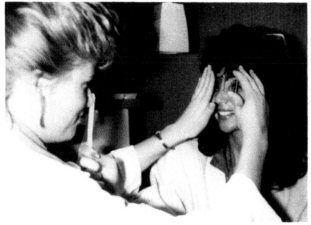

FIGURE 20–11. Measuring misalignment with prism and alternate cover test while viewing accommodative target.

covered, then uncovered. Every time the fellow eye is uncovered, fusional movements may be made which will influence the movement of the eye under the prism. This will not permit accurate assessment of the amount of deviation, whether phoria or tropia, but especially phoria. Neutralization with prisms must be evaluated by *alternate* cover, never by cover-uncover.

Krimsky's Test

The cover test is not possible if there is poor vision in one eye or if the patient lacks the desire to continuously fix on the target. In these cases, the deviation is measured by the next most accurate method, Krimsky's corneal reflex test. First, the position of the corneal reflex in the straight fixing eye is carefully noted. Then the prism is placed in front of the straight eye with the base in the same direction that the corneal reflex in the misaligned eye is off-set, e.g., if the corneal

Krimsky's Method for Measuring Misalignments

1. Neutralizing the prism base-out produces equal position of corneal reflexes (Fig. 20–12A).

2. Prism base-out is too small for full correction (Fig. 20–12B).

3. Prism base-in increases the deviation (Fig. 20–12C).

4. Two smaller prisms, both base out, can neutralize deviation (Fig. 20–12D).

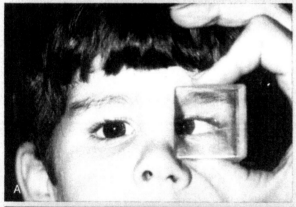

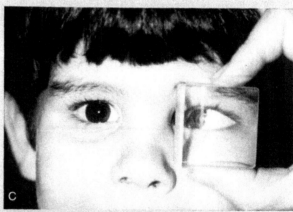

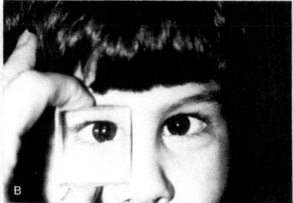

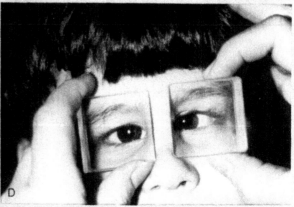

FIGURE 20–12. *A to D.*

Krimsky Corneal Reflex Test: Right Exotropia

1. Right eye is out, its corneal reflex is in. Image strikes right eye temporal retina (Fig. 20–13A).

2. Correcting base-in prism normalizes right eye corneal reflex position. Neither eye moves. Right eye stays out under prism. Left eye stays straight. Image strikes right eye fovea from light rays bent by prism. Both corneal reflexes match (Fig. 20–13B).

3. Alternatively, correcting base-in prism over fixing left eye shifts corneal reflex toward prism apex onto temporal cornea. Image shifts off the left fovea of the straight left

eye. In less than a second, however, there is a resulting version movement of both eyes to the left that repositions the left corneal reflex to its correct position as left fovea regains fixation. This shift also corrects right corneal reflex position. Right eye is now straight however, and the left eye is now out under the prism. Prisms bend light rays from target so that image strikes left fovea as light rays from same target simultaneously produce image on right fovea. Both corneal reflexes match (Fig. 20–13C).

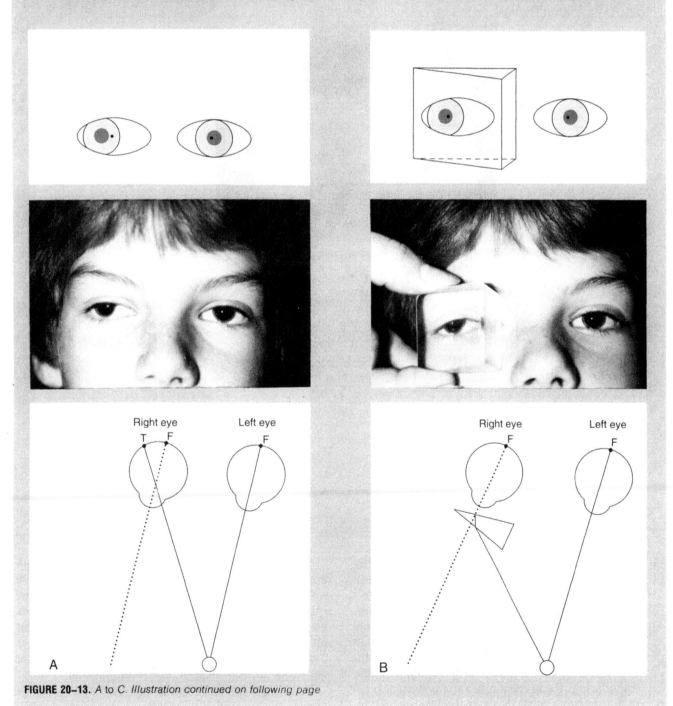

FIGURE 20–13. *A to C. Illustration continued on following page*

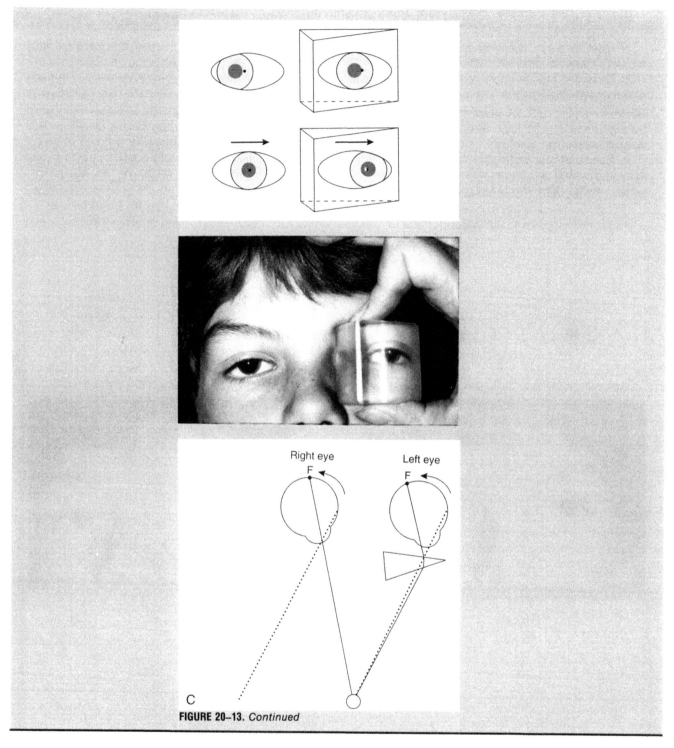

FIGURE 20–13. *Continued*

reflex is *out* away from the center, then the base of the prism is held on the out or temporal side. If the deviated eye has its corneal reflex offset *in* toward the nose, then the base of the prism is held in toward the nose. The correcting prism in front of *either* eye will bring symmetry to both corneal reflex positions. Observation of the corneal reflex on the deviated eye is easier without looking through the prism. The strength of the prism that brings the corneal reflex to the correct position in the deviating eye is the most crucial observation.

As with the alternate cover, *too small* a base-out prism will partly correct the corneal reflexes with an eso deviation. Too *large* a prism will overcorrect and reverse the deviation of the off corneal reflex; the prism placed the wrong way (base-in) will increase how far off the corneal reflex is. If a deviation (over 40^Δ) is present, it is best to split the prism into two smaller ones, one in front of each eye, both base-out.

If the right eye is 30^Δ exotropic, and a 30^Δ prism is placed in front of the fixing left eye, the corneal reflex image shifts toward the apex of the prism to a more temporal position on the left eye. The image is deflected off the fovea, forcing both eyes to shift in a version movement. The straight left eye shifts temporally to refixate, and the deviated right eye shifts nasally to straighten, thereby correcting its corneal reflex. At the end of this version movement to the left, both corneal reflexes match.

If the prism is placed before the misaligned right eye, however, the 30$^\Delta$ prism shifts the corneal reflex toward the apex of the prism, which moves it nasally on the cornea. Neither eye moves. The right eye does not straighten under the prism. The corneal reflex, which had been nasal on the right eye before the prism was introduced, now matches the corneal reflex position of the fixing left eye.

Hirschberg's Estimation

To perform Krimsky's test, the patient must allow the examiner to put a prism in front of one eye. Not all patients are willing to do so, especially youngsters under age two. Fortunately, another way to quantitate the amount of deviation exists, although it is less accurate than Krimsky's test. Hirschberg's method estimates the number of millimeters the corneal reflex is off in the misaligned eye compared with the position that reflex should be to match the straight eye. With experience, it should take only a few seconds to perform. The ease and speed of performing the test provide its distinct advantage.

How do we estimate in millimeters? The most important guideline is that the average cornea is 12 mm in diameter (Fig. 20–14). In average room illumination the average pupil is 4 mm. This breaks the average cornea into three segments of 4 mm. For each millimeter of deviation there is 7° or 15$^\Delta$ deviation.

The examiner, on the first look, estimates how many millimeters the corneal reflex is off in the misaligned eye and notes which direction. By cheating a little, it can be assumed that the corneal reflex is dead center. An eso misalignment at the temporal edge of the pupil would compute to be approximately 2 mm off, or 30$^\Delta$.

If the misaligned eye has its corneal reflex halfway onto the iris, there is an approximate 4 mm displacement and therefore 60$^\Delta$ of deviation. If the misaligned eye has its corneal reflex at the limbus, there is a 6 mm displacement of the corneal reflex and therefore 90$^\Delta$ of deviation. This 30$^\Delta$, 60$^\Delta$, 90$^\Delta$ rule helps guide Hirschberg's estimations (Fig. 20–15).

To develop proficiency in measuring misalignments, evaluate each patient by estimation of the corneal reflex malposition in millimeters first. Then attempt a Krimsky's test measurement with prisms. If the patient continues to cooperate, try a PACT. It takes the longest to do and requires the greatest cooperation from the patient. The first two are faster and easier to perform, but less accurate. After several attempts, measurements from the three tests should begin to agree. Then whenever the alternate prism and cover cannot be performed on a patient, Krimsky's measurement and Hirschberg's estimation will have more validity. Krimsky's test often agrees within 5$^\Delta$ of the PACT measurement and Hirschberg's within 10$^\Delta$. Hirschberg's and Krimsky's methods measure only tropias. The PACT measures tropias and phorias (Fig. 20–16).

Hirschberg's test is done at near. In order to estimate as accurately as possible, draw an imaginary vertical line and an imaginary horizontal line through the corneal reflexes of both eyes. The horizontal lines in both eyes are then compared to see whether one is higher or lower than the other for any vertical misalignment. The vertical lines are compared to see whether one is closer or farther to the center of the pupil then the other for any horizontal misalignment. This aids in

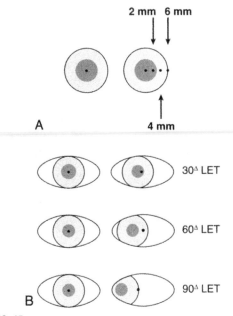

FIGURE 20–15. Hirschberg's estimations from millimeter displacements. *A,* Millimeter displacements for eso deviations. *B,* Prism diopter equivalents for eso deviations.

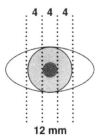

FIGURE 20–14. Average pupil size indoors and its relationship to corneal diameter.

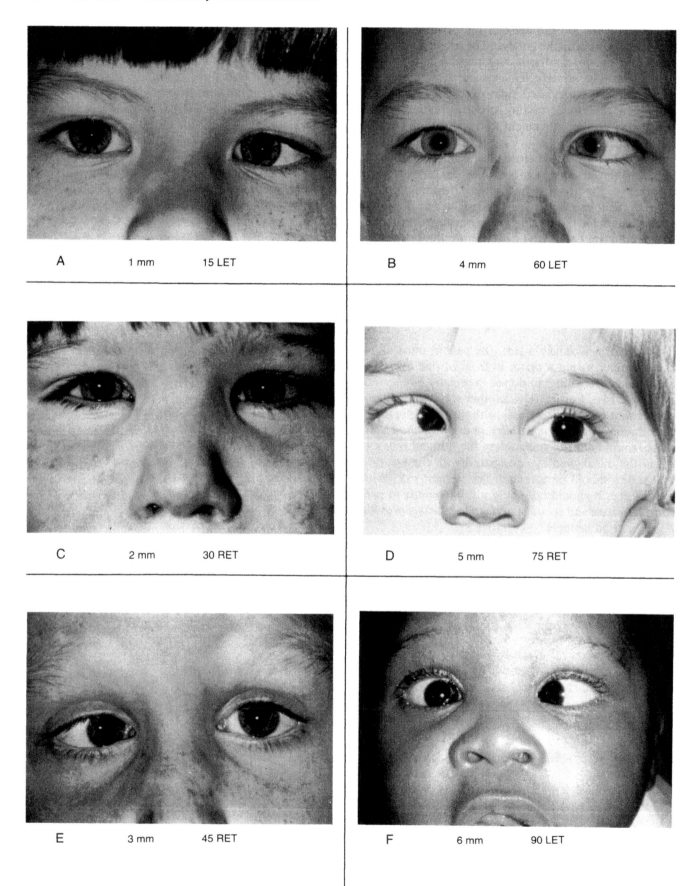

A	1 mm	15 LET
B	4 mm	60 LET
C	2 mm	30 RET
D	5 mm	75 RET
E	3 mm	45 RET
F	6 mm	90 LET

FIGURE 20–16. *A* to *F*, Hirschberg's estimations.

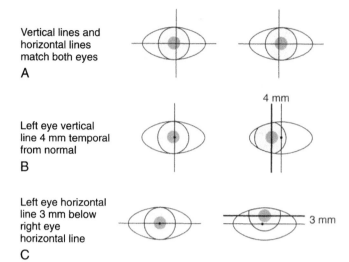

Vertical lines and horizontal lines match both eyes

A

Left eye vertical line 4 mm temporal from normal

B

4 mm

Left eye horizontal line 3 mm below right eye horizontal line

C

3 mm

FIGURE 20–17. Comparing abnormal to normal corneal reflex positions using horizontal and vertical lines. *A,* Vertical lines and horizontal lines match both eyes. *B,* Left eye vertical line 4 mm temporal from normal. *C,* Left eye horizontal line 3 mm below right eye horizontal line.

deciding how many millimeters off the corneal reflex is in the deviated eye (Fig. 20–17).

In the following example, the corneal reflex of the left eye is 3 mm more nasal than the one in the right eye and 1 mm higher than in the right eye, giving this patient 45^Δ of left exotropia and 15^Δ of left hypotropia (right hypertropia) (Fig. 20–18).

● PROCEDURE

Whenever eyeglasses are worn, measurements are done both with and without correction using 20/30 targets, both distance and near, to ascertain the accommodative component. If there is one, the eso deviation will increase when the eyeglasses are removed. Special attention is paid to the distance measurement with cycloplegic refraction worn. This measurement is the

basic deviation showing the amount of misalignment that needs surgical correction.

Most patients with intermittent exo deviations have good fusion control, often starting with a comparatively small exo-shift (less than 5^Δ). When measuring with small base-in prisms, neutrality occurs after one or two alternate covers. As one continues to alternately cover, however, the exo shift increases and the small prism is not enough. Keep one eye occluded and change to a larger prism, then resume alternating the cover. Do not uncover both eyes until the patient is neutralized for a minimum of six cross-cover maneuvers. A larger base-in prism than the neutralizing one must be tested until continuous reversal movements are seen. The largest base-in prism that stops the eye movements without reversal is the measure of the exo deviation.

● RECORDING

How do we record these strabismus measurements? It is really quite simple, if not entirely logical. E stands for eso (misaligned in), X for exo (misaligned out), H is for hyper (misaligned up), and h is for hypo (misaligned down). Vertical deviations are usually designated by the higher eye. Nothing is added with a phoria, but T is added if there is a tropia. A prime sign (′) after the designation means the measurement was done at near (14″), so the absence of ′ after the designation means the measurement was done at distance (20′). Frequently, D for distance and N for near are added for further clarification. CC (con correction) means with glasses on, SC (sine correction) glasses not worn. If the deviation is alternating, there is no symbol, but if there is a definite eye preference, R or L is added before the E, X, or H. The numbers preceding all these letters are the measurements of the phoria or tropia in prism diopters, which uses the symbol delta ($^\Delta$) in the superscript position. If the T is bracketed, X (T), it means the deviation is intermittent.

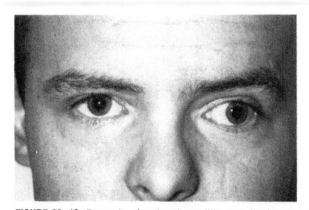

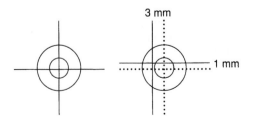

3 mm

1 mm

FIGURE 20–18. Example of estimating millimeter displacement for patient with both exo and hypo deviations.

• *Here are several examples:*

$20^{\Delta}X(T)'$ = 20 prism diopters (about 10°) of intermittent exotropia measured at 14 inches (near)

$75^{\Delta}RET$ = 75 prism diopters (about 40°) of right esotropia measured at a distance of 20 feet

$45^{\Delta}ET'10^{\Delta}LHT'$ = 45 prism diopters (about 25°) of esotropia with 10 prism diopters (about 5°) of left hypertropia measured at near

PACT: $\quad$ cc $3^{\Delta}E + 5^{\Delta}E'$
$\quad\quad\quad\quad\quad$ sc $30^{\Delta}ET + 35^{\Delta}ET'$

• *These are measurements done with eyeglasses on (cc) by prism and alternate cover test showing 3 prism diopters of esophoria at distance and 5 prism diopters (about 3°) of esophoria at near. With eyeglasses removed (sc), the patient measured 30 prism diopters (about 15°) of esotropia at distance and 35 prism diopters (about 18°) of esotropia at near.*

Bibliography

Nelson LB, Catalano RA: Atlas of Ocular Motility. Philadelphia, WB Saunders, 1989.

von Noorden GK: Atlas of Strabismus, 4th ed. St Louis, CV Mosby, 1983.

von Noorden GK (ed): Burian-von Noorden's Binocular Vision and Ocular Motility, 4th ed. St Louis, Mosby-Year Book, 1990.

• CHAPTER 20 OCULAR MOTILITY: STRABISMUS EVALUATION

1. You inspect this patient's corneal reflexes. If you cover the patient's right eye, you see no movement of the left eye. When you uncover the right eye, it moves out. You then cover the left eye, but see no movement of the right eye. You uncover the left eye, and it moves out. What does this patient have?

   a. alternating esotropia
   b. intermittent esotropia
   c. exophoria
   d. intermittent exotropia
   e. esophoria

2. You cover the patient's right eye and the left eye doesn't move. You uncover the right eye, which still does not move. You cover the patient's left eye. The right eye moves in. What happens to the left eye under the cover?

   a. It moves up.
   b. Nothing.
   c. It moves in.
   d. It moves out.
   e. It moves down.

3. You cover the right eye and the left eye moves out. You then uncover the right eye and neither eye moves. What has happened?

   a. The patient has fused.
   b. You shifted the deviation from the left eye to the right eye.
   c. The patient has retained left esotropia.
   d. Intermittent deviation disappeared.
   e. The patient cannot hold fixation with the right eye.

4. Estimate the following deviation using Hirschberg's method.

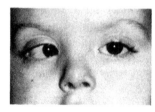

   a. 30^{Δ} RET
   b. 90^{Δ} RET
   c. 30^{Δ} RET 30^{Δ} LHT
   d. 60^{Δ} RXT
   e. 60^{Δ} RET 20^{Δ} RHT

5. Estimate the following deviation using Hirschberg's method.

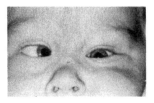

   a. 45^{Δ} RET 20^{Δ} RHT
   b. 75^{Δ} RET
   c. 60^{Δ} RET 15^{Δ} RHT
   d. 45^{Δ} RET
   e. 60^{Δ} RET 10^{Δ} LHT

Ocular Motility: Extraocular Muscle Function

The eye is the only sense organ that can move independently. The coordinated actions of the extraocular muscles provide precise guidance, allow the eyes to have a large range of view, and provide single binocular vision for both distance and near.

● EXTRAOCULAR MUSCLES

Six extraocular muscles attached to each eye move the eyes with great speed and accuracy. The muscles are long and thin, giving them a favorable mechanical advantage to move a small sphere with tremendous power. This is especially effective if the muscle pulls from behind and attaches far forward, as it does with the rectus muscles (Fig. 21–1).

Both orbits have medial walls that are approximately parallel to one another. The lateral walls of the orbit form an angle approximately 90° to one another, making the angle between the medial and lateral orbital wall 45°. Every muscle *except* the inferior oblique originates at Zinn's annulus. This annulus surrounds the apex at the rear of the orbit near the medial wall (Fig. 21–2).

The muscles originating at the Zinn's annulus travel forward as a muscle cone to attach to the eyeball *forward* of the center of rotation, approximately 0.25 inch from the limbus. All except the superior oblique run from Zinn's annulus to attach onto the eyeball anterior

to the center of rotation, at approximately 22°, or half the 45° angle. In contrast, the inferior oblique (IO) originates on the orbital floor near the front medial wall and the superior oblique (SO) functions as though it originates at the trochlea near the medial orbital roof. The obliques insert on the eyeball at an approximate 50° angle from the anteroposterior axis when the eye is in the straight-ahead position. The obliques insert onto the eyeball on the *temporal* side *behind* the center of rotation. Therefore, all four rectus muscles pull from the rear of the orbit near the nasal wall, but the oblique muscles pull from the front of the orbit near the nasal wall. The rectus muscles exert a backward pull on the eyeball. The oblique muscles exert a forward pull. The angle between the orientation of the obliques and the orientation of the vertical recti is approximately 73°. The direction of the muscle pull produces different vertical movements of the eyeball, depending on whether or not the eye is looking straight ahead (primary position) (Fig. 21–3).

The medial rectus (MR) runs alongside the nasal wall of the orbit. When it contracts, the eye moves from straight-ahead (primary position) *in* toward the nose. The lateral rectus (LR) attaches to the lateral side of the eye. When it contracts, it pulls the eye *out* toward the ear (Fig. 21–4).

When the eyes look straight ahead, they are parallel to the medial wall of the orbit. From the primary position, each eye is pulled up by a combination of its SR

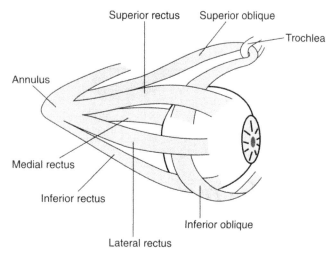

FIGURE 21–1. Six extraocular muscles.

and IO. Neither muscle pulls as effectively as when the eye position is in the same direction as the muscle plane, however.

The SR and IO contract to pull the eye up to provide *elevation*. The IR and SO contract to pull the eye down in *depression*.

The vertical recti move the eye up and down best when the eye is in the out (abducted) position. The obliques move the eye vertically best when the eye is in the *in* (adducted) position. The explanation lies with the differences in the direction of contraction and the orientation of muscle planes.

The direction of the muscle plane of the SR and IR is about half the 45° angle of the *temporal* wall. Therefore, if the eye is in the out (abducted) position, it is in the same orientation as the SR and IR, increasing their efficiency at pulling the eye up (SR) or down (IR). When the eye is in this out position, the obliques are ineffective at pulling the eye up or down (Fig. 21–5).

If the eye looks in toward the nose (adducted) however, then the eye is in the same direction as the plane of the obliques. They become most efficient at moving the eye up (IO) or down (SO). In this *in* position (adducted) the SR and IR are ineffective at moving the eyeball up or down. Because the superior oblique pulls from the trochlea and is attached toward the back of the eye it tips the front of the eye down, whereas the inferior oblique under the eye pulls the back of the eye down and flips the front of the eye up. The obliques are contrary. They do everything opposite to what you expect until you understand the mechanics of the line of pull.

The 12 extraocular muscles interrelate to one another in several different ways. Any one muscle in one eye relates in some fashion to every other muscle in that same eye, but also to every muscle in the opposite eye. Whenever the relationship is such that one muscle, the *agonist*, has another muscle either in that eye or the other eye to help it move the eye, the helping muscle

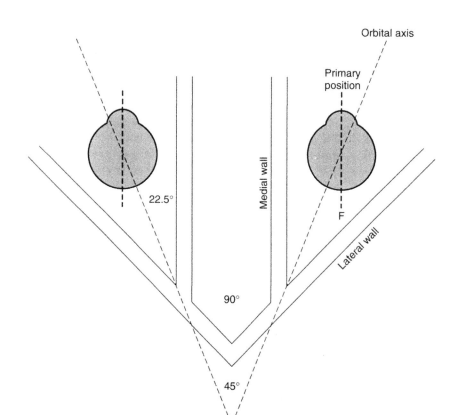

FIGURE 21–2. Schematic diagram of the orbital walls.

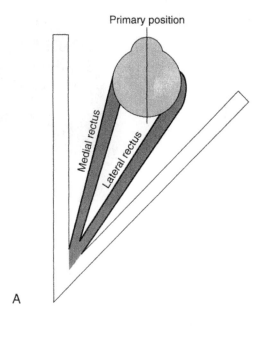

Primary position

Medial rectus

Lateral rectus

A

Medial wall

Vertical recti

Obliques

Lateral wall

B

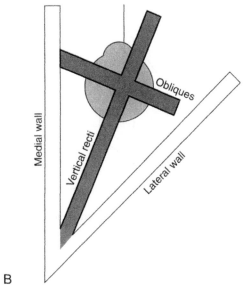

FIGURE 21–3. Schematic diagram of the extraocular muscles in primary position. *A,* Muscles that act horizontally. *B,* Muscles that act vertically.

is called a *synergist.* On the other hand, when another muscle contracts to perform the opposite function, it is called an *antagonist.*

When a muscle contracts to pull the eye in its direction of action, its task is made easier if the muscle that pulls in the opposite direction relaxes. That combination is Sherrington's law of reciprocal innervation, which states that when an agonist muscle contracts, an equal and opposite innervation to relax is received by its direct antagonist.

● **For example.** *If the left medial rectus (LMR) contracts to pull the left eye in, the left lateral rectus (LLR) is the direct antagonist trying to pull the left eye out. The LMR can only pull the left eye in if the LLR allows it to do so by relaxing.*

● **Types of Eye Muscles**

Agonist	Muscle that moves the eye by contracting
Antagonist	Muscle that moves the eye by relaxing as the agonist contracts
Ipsilateral	Same side or same eye
Contralateral	Opposite side or opposite eye
Synergist	Muscle that contracts to help another muscle (the agonist)
Direct Antagonist	Ipsilateral antagonist directly opposite the agonist
Yoke Muscle	Contralateral synergist
Contralateral Antagonist	Yoke muscle of the direct antagonist

For example, the right superior rectus moves the right eye up when it contracts. Because it is the agonist, its ipsilateral synergist is the right inferior oblique (RIO), which also moves the right eye up. The right inferior rectus (RIR) is an ipsilateral antagonist. It opposes the action of the agonist right superior rectus (RSR). The left inferior oblique (LIO) is a muscle in the left eye that is a contralateral synergist, a yoke muscle that moves the *left eye up* in right gaze, matching the RSR which moves the *right eye up* in right gaze. The contralateral antagonist moves the other eye in the opposite direction in the same gaze. In this case, the left superior oblique (LSO) is the contralateral antagonist of the RSR. It moves the *left eye down* in right gaze (Fig. 21–6).

A one-eye movement is a *duction* movement. An eye *abducts* when its LR, attached to the outside of the eye on its temporal side, contracts. The eye moves out toward the ear. An eye *adducts* when its MR, attached to the outside of the eye on its nasal side, contracts. The eye moves in toward the nose. *Supraduction,* or elevation, occurs when the eye looks up. Looking down is *infraduction,* or depression. *Incycloduction,* or intorsion, is when the top of the eye tilts in toward the nose. *Excycloduction,* or extorsion, is when the top of the eye tilts away from the nose (Fig. 21–7) (Table 21–1).

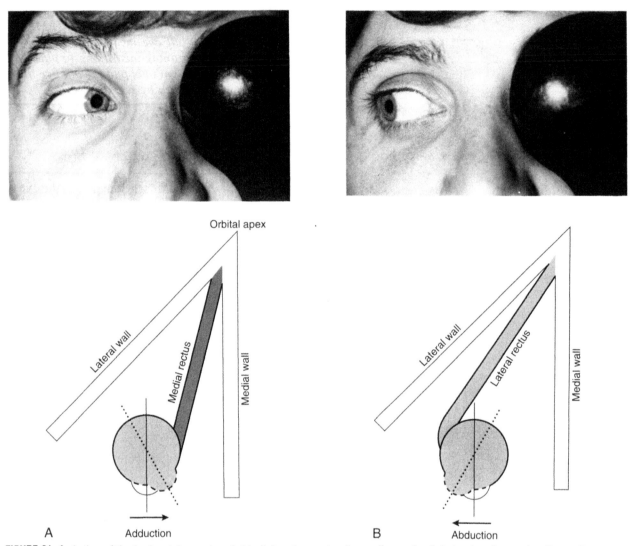

FIGURE 21-4. Action of the horizontal muscles. *A,* Medial rectus contraction pulls eye in. *B,* Lateral rectus contraction pulls eye out.

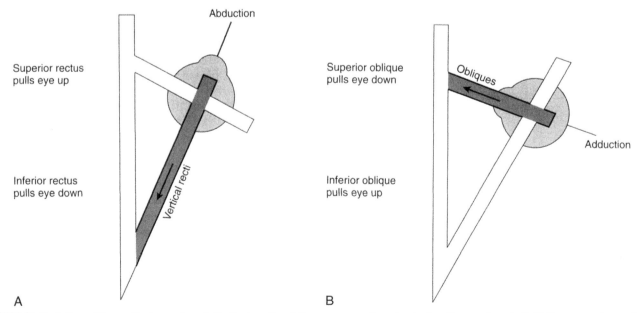

FIGURE 21-5. Action of the vertical muscles. *A,* Vertical recti pull the eye up or down best when the eye is out. *B,* Oblique muscles pull the eye up or down best when the eye is in.

Agonist   Ipsilateral synergist

RSR   RIO   LIO Contralateral synergist (yoke)

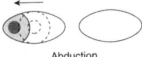

RIR ⟶ **LSO**

Direct antagonist   **Contralateral antagonist**

FIGURE 21–6. Steps in finding the contralateral antagonist of the RSR. *First,* at the vertical arrow, find its direct antagonist (RIR). *Second,* at the horizontal arrow, find the yoke of the direct antagonist (LSO), which is the contralateral antagonist of the RSR.

TABLE 21–1.

Characteristics of Eye Movements

EOM	Contralateral Synergist = Yoke	Ipsilateral Antagonist	Contralateral Antagonist = Yoke of Ipsilateral Antagonist	Ipsilateral Synergist	Function
RMR	LLR	RLR	LMR	RSR RIR	Adduction
RLR	LMR	RMR	LLR	RSO RIO	Abduction
RSR	LIO	RIR	LSO	RIO	Elevation
RIR	LSO	RSR	LIO	RSO	Depression
RSO	LIR	RIO	LSR	RSR	Intorsion
RIO	LSR	RSO	LIR	RIR	Extorsion

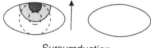

Abduction

A

Sursumduction

B

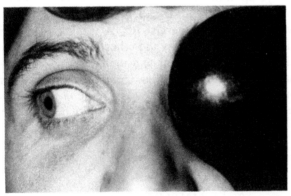

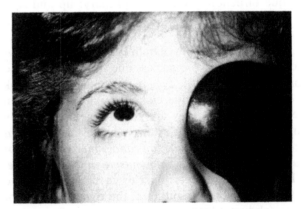

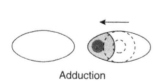

Adduction

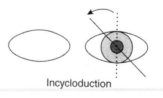

Incycloduction

C

D

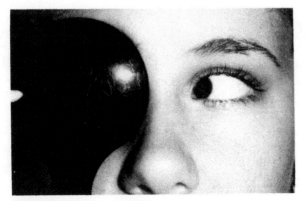

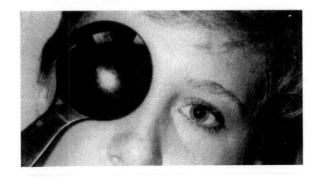

FIGURE 21–7. Types of ductions.

Types of Single Eye Movements

Abduction	Eye moves from straight ahead out towards the ear
Adduction	Eye moves from straight ahead in towards the nose
Elevation (Supraduction)	Eye moves from straight ahead up
Depression (Infraduction)	Eye moves from straight ahead down
Intorsion (Incycloduction)	Top of eye tilts towards the nose
Extorsion (Excycloduction)	Top of eye tilts away from the nose

When the eyes look straight ahead, they are in primary position. Secondary positions are gazes directed up, down, right, or left. Tertiary positions are the four oblique directions away from primary: up and right, down and right, up and left, and down and left (Fig. 21–8).

A parallel movement of both eyes is a version movement. We have two muscles, one in each eye, which contract to guide both eyes in the same direction, like two car wheels on either end of an axle. The two muscles act as though they are yoked together. That eye function obeys Hering's law, which states *when an agonist muscle contracts, an equal innervation to contract is received by its yoke muscle in the other eye.*

Hering's law affects muscles in both eyes. When both eyes look into right gaze, the right eye turns out away (abducts) from the nose, and the left eye turns in toward (adducts) the nose. The LMR contracts to pull the left eye in, the right lateral rectus (RLR) contracts to pull the right eye out (Fig. 21–9). Sherrington's law affects muscles in one eye. The chemical formula for hydrogen sulfide, H_2S (which smells like rotten eggs) is often used as a mnemonic to remember which law affects both eyes, H_2 (Hering's), and which law affects one eye, S (Sherrington's).

When the eyes make version movements, they can be directed into six positions, three on each side, the cardinal directions, where the 12 extraocular muscles pair off. In these positions, only one muscle for each eye can maneuver the eyeball to that location. For right and left gaze, the two pairs of MR and LR are tested. Notice that for right gaze the RLR pairs with the LMR to move the eyes in parallel. For left gaze the LLR pairs with the right medial rectus (RMR). That leaves the four pairs of vertical muscles to be tested in the four tertiary positions of gaze (Fig. 21–10).

When extraocular muscles are tested for their functions, the obliques and the vertical recti are only tested for their vertical function, i.e., how well they move the eye up or down. When an eye moves from primary position straight up, the superior rectus (SR) is helped by its ipsilateral synergist IO. A weakness of either one could be masked by the other. Both muscles have other functions, torsion and abduction or adduction that are not being evaluated. Oblique function is therefore tested only when the eye is in the *in* position and vertical rectus function is tested only when the eye is in the *out* position.

Types of Eye Movements

Duction	Movement of one eye into a cardinal position
Version	Movement of both eyes into a cardinal position
Right Gaze (Dextroversion)	Both eyes move to the right
Left Gaze (Levoversion)	Both eyes move to the left
Elevation (Sursumversion) (Supraversion)	Both eyes move up
Depression (Deosumversion) (Supraversion)	Both eyes move down

A. PRIMARY POSITION OF GAZE

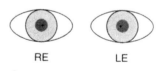

RE   LE

A

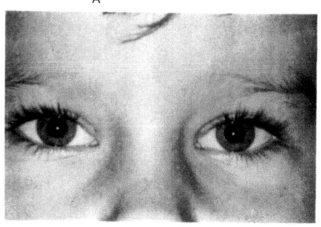

FIGURE 21–8. *A* to *C.* Positions of gaze.

B. SECONDARY
POSITIONS
OF GAZE

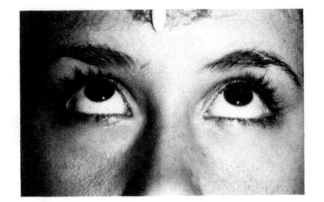

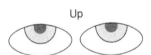

Up

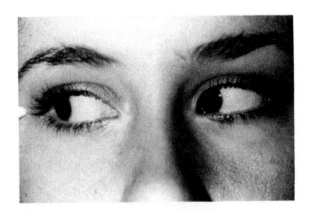

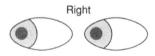

Right

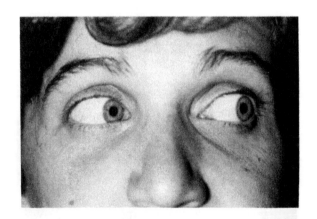

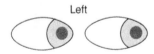

Left

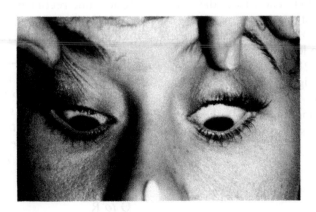

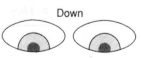

Down

FIGURE 21–8. *Continued*   B

Illustration continued on following page

C. TERTIARY POSITIONS OF GAZE

Up + right

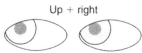

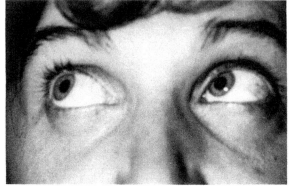

Down + right

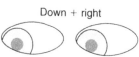

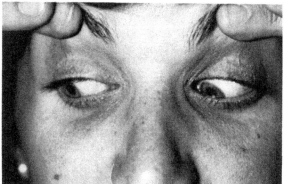

Up + left

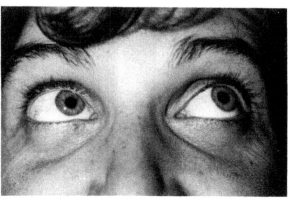

Down + left

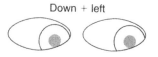

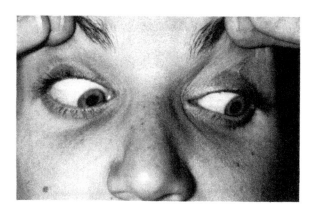

FIGURE 21–8. *Continued*

For example, if we look into left gaze, the left eye is in the *abducted* (out) position. The LIR is the only muscle in the left eye capable of moving it down. When the right eye looks into left gaze, however, it is in the *adducted* (in) position and so looks down by contraction only of the RSO (Fig. 21–11). Note the lower corneal reflex in the higher right eye with the weak right superior oblique muscle.

In muscles with vertical function pairs (yoke muscles), there is always one muscle from the right eye

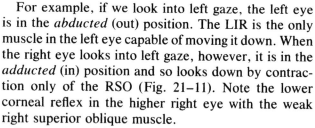

RLR   LMR

RE   LE

FIGURE 21–9. Example of Hering's Law that when the RLR conracts to pull the right eye out, the LMR contracts to pull the left eye in. Both eyes move to the right.

and one from the left, one superior muscle and one inferior, one rectus and one oblique. If you know one muscle from one eye, by transposing you can find its yoke in the opposite eye.

• **For Example.** *Start with the* RSR. *To find its yoke:*
  R *(right) changes to* L *(left)*
  S *(superior) changes to* I *(inferior)*
  R *(rectus) changes to* O *(oblique)*
  Thus, the LIO *is the yoke of the* RSR.
• *Start with the* RIO. *To find its yoke, we transpose:*
  R *to* L
  I *to* S
  O *to* R
• *Therefore, its yoke is the* LSR.

See Figure 21–12.

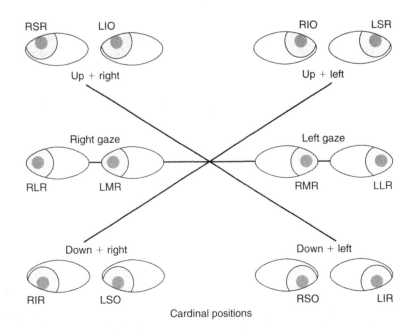

RSR   LIO   RIO   LSR

Up + right   Up + left

Right gaze   Left gaze

RLR   LMR   RMR   LLR

Down + right   Down + left

RIR   LSO   RSO   LIR

Cardinal positions

FIGURE 21–10. When the extraocular muscles are tested for their functions, the obliques and the vertical recti are only tested for their vertical function. Therefore, oblique function is only tested with the eye in the *in* position and vertical rectus function is tested with the eye in the *out* position.

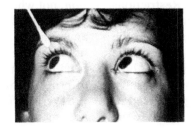
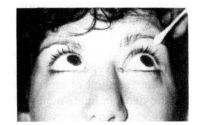
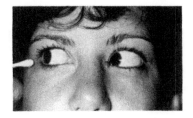
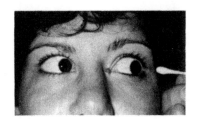
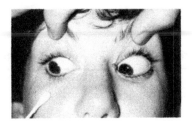
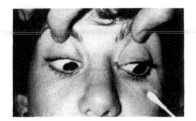

● EVALUATION OF EYE MOVEMENTS

Versions and ductions are tested in the six cardinal positions (up and right, right gaze, down and right, up and left, left gaze, down and left) in which the six pairs of yoke muscles are evaluated.

Analysis of deviations to find any underactive muscle relies on comparing yoke muscles, because the two receive equal innervation. If neither muscle nor its nerve is dysfunctional, both yoke muscles will respond equally, no overaction or underaction will be noted when their movements are compared. If versions are

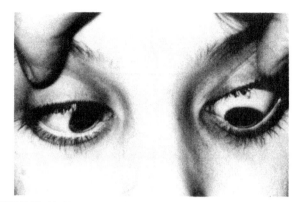

FIGURE 21–11. Up and right (U + R) is the only tertiary position that tests the RSR and the LIO. RSR is the only muscle in the right eye that can elevate in abduction. LIO is the only muscle in the left eye that can elevate in adduction.

abnormal, ductions may be normal or abnormal, but if versions are normal, ductions will *always* be normal. Therefore, ductions do not need to be tested unless there is an abnormal version movement. Restrictions show abnormal versions with no improvement on ductions. Most palsies have improved ductions when the versions are abnormal. Most of the time more can be learned from versions than ductions. Versions test how the same amount of innervation moves both eyes.

The fixation light, with its fixation target around it, is brought from primary position (straight ahead) to the other fields of gaze, as the observer notes any limitation of movement. Only the patient's eyes must move, not the patient's head (Fig. 21–13).

The observer's eyes should be about 2 feet away from the patient, with the fixation light about 15 inches away, in whatever direction the observer wishes to test. The fixation target is brought from primary position to up gaze, then down gaze. By this maneuver, the patient is examined for an A or a V pattern, defined as a difference in the eso or exo measurement in up gaze compared with down gaze. Then the fixation light is moved from right gaze to left gaze, to detect a medial rectus or lateral rectus defect. If there is a defect, a difference in eso or exo measurement is seen in right gaze compared with left gaze. Apparent limitations of any eye movement in any of the six cardinal poistions when versions are evaluated must be retested using ductions (one eye movements).

In schematic diagrams of the extraocular muscles, note that the obliques are positioned where they *function,* not where they are located anatomically, e.g., the RSO appears in the *down and in* position, even though, anatomically, it is found above the eye. The SO does not bring the eye to the in position. When the eye has been brought in, mostly by the MR, the SO contracts to bring it down (or the IO contracts to pull it up).

Several different schemes are utilized to record overactions and underactions of the extraocular muscles

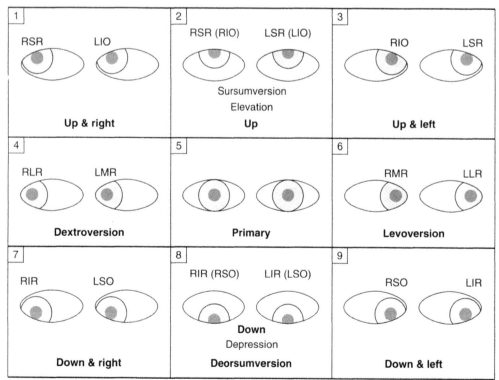

FIGURE 21–12. Nine diagnostic positions of gaze.

Secondary positions of gaze 2, 4, 6, 8
Tertiary positions of gaze 1, 3, 7, 9

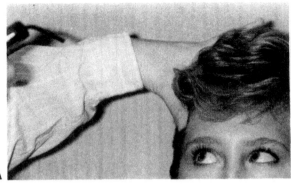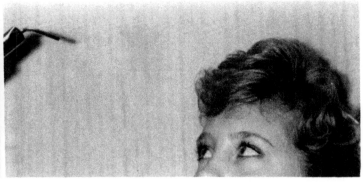

FIGURE 21–13. Technique for testing versions. *A,* Right. Patient's head straight, eyes up and right. *B,* Wrong. Patient's head up and right, eyes in primary position.

found on versions. My preferred method is shown in the following series of diagrams (Fig. 21–14). A horizontal line is used to represent the medial and lateral rectus fields of action, and two crossed lines at 45° and 135° are used to represent the fields of action of the vertical movers of the eye, both elevators and depressors.

For example, if we look up and to the right we are testing the RSR and the LIO. According to Hering's law, if both muscles have normal function, then the same amount of innervation to the RSR to elevate the right eye in abduction is received by the LIO to elevate the left eye in adduction. If one of those two muscles is weak, any given amount of innervation will not ele-

vate the involved eye to the same extent as the normal eye (Fig. 21–15). If the RSR is weak, as in this case, on up and right gaze the right eye will be lower. Therefore, the right corneal reflex will ride higher than on the normal left eye. The patient will have a left hyper (right hypo) in that field of gaze. The underaction of the RSR is recorded on a scale of −1 to −4. An alternative way of recording this shows the left inferior oblique as overactive, using a scale of +1 to +4.

Whenever yoke muscles are compared, it is only necessary to record one. Recording one muscle as underactive is the same as saying its yoke is overactive, e.g., +2 overaction of the LIO is the same as saying a −2 underaction of the RSR. It is not necessary to

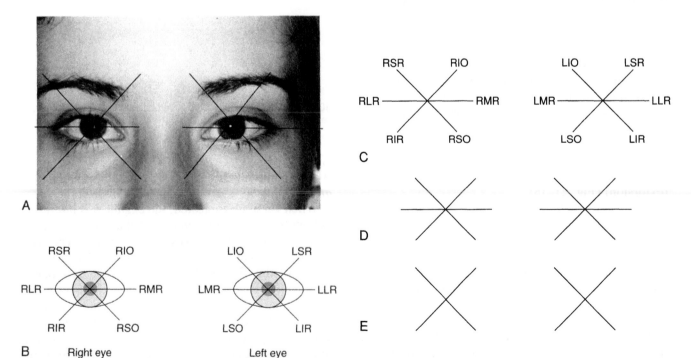

FIGURE 21–14. Variations on one scheme for recording versions. *A,* Lines for muscle function superimposed on eyes of patient. *B,* Diagram of lines for muscle function superimposed on eyes with muscles labelled. *C,* Diagram of lines for muscle function with muscles labelled. No eyes shown. *D,* Diagram of lines for muscle function. Muscles not labelled. *E,* Diagram of lines for muscles with vertical action only. Horizontal lines removed.

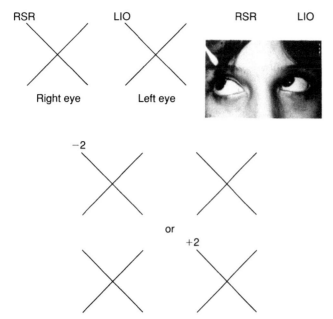

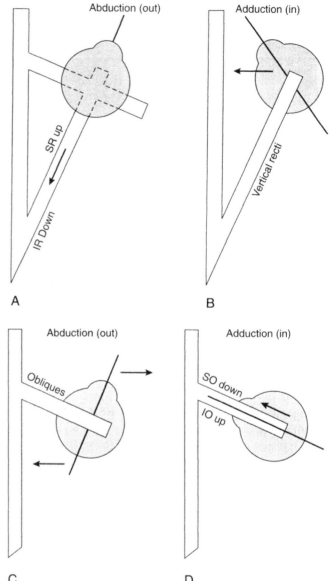

FIGURE 21–15. Example of recording vertical extraocular muscle dysfunction. Patient has left hypertropia in up and right gaze.

designate both minus for the RSR as well as plus for the LIO. The most common muscle imbalance recorded as overactive is for an oblique muscle. Pairs of overactive obliques are common, usually with an A or a V pattern.

• NONVERTICAL FUNCTION OF THE VERTICAL EXTRAOCULAR MUSCLES

The vertical rectus muscles do not move the eye out (abduct). Once the eye is in the out position, these muscles move the eye up or down. In fact, when the eye is in the in position (adducted), both vertical recti help the MR keep the eye adducted. They pull the front of the eye toward the medial wall. In addition, the SR tilts the top of the eye in toward the nose (intorsion). The IR tilts the bottom of the eye toward the nose, which tilts the top of the eye out away from the nose (extorsion) (Fig. 21–16).

The oblique muscles pull from the *front* of the orbit near the nasal side. The obliques do not move the eye in (adduct). They move the eye up or down once the eye is already in (adducted). See Table 21–2.

When the eye is abducted (out), the obliques help the LR in keeping the eye out by pulling the back of the eye towards the medial wall of the orbit, which moves the front of the eye toward the lateral wall into abduction. The SO also tilts the top of the eye toward the nose (intorsion). The IO tilts the bottom of the eye toward the nose, which tilts the top of the eye away from the nose (extorsion). In primary position, the obliques are the primary torters of the eye (Fig. 21–17).

FIGURE 21–16. Functions of the vertical extraocular muscles. *A,* Vertical recti in abduction. *B,* Vertical recti in adduction. *C,* Obliques in abduction. *D,* Obliques in adduction.

A mnemonic for this function is as follows: *superiors are in* (intorters); *inferiors are out* (extorters).

When versions are tested, the examiner is interested only in the vertical movements of the obliques and the vertical recti. To move an eye up or down from primary position, a combination of the IR and SO is used for down, or the SR and IO for up. If all the extraocular muscles have normal function, when the eye moves from primary position to any other, the amount of intorsion by the SR and SO is balanced by the amount of extorsion by the IR and IO. No torsion occurs unless one of these four muscles is out of balance by being overactive or underactive. The torting ability of the vertical muscles becomes apparent only when one of the four is defective or when pairs of obliques are over-

TABLE 21–2.

Changes in Extraocular Muscle (EOM) Function with Changes in Position

EOM		
Abducted Position	**Primary Position**	**Adducted Position**
Superior rectus		
Elevation	Elevation	Adduction
	Adduction	Intorsion
	Intorsion	
Inferior rectus		
Depression	Depression	Adduction
	Adduction	Extorsion
	Extorsion	
Superior oblique		
Intorsion	Intorsion	Depression
Abduction	Depression	
	Abduction	
Inferior oblique		
Extorsion	Extorsion	Elevation
Abduction	Elevation	
	Abduction	
Medial rectus		
Adduction	Adduction	Adduction
Lateral rectus		
Abduction	Abduction	Abduction

active with an A or a V pattern. The SR and IR are the primary vertical movers of the eye, but with some assistance from the obliques. The recti primarily move the eye vertically with some adduction and some torsion. The obliques primarily turn the eye with some abduction and vertical movement.

In summary, a muscle that moves the eye is called an agonist. All those muscles in the same (ipsilateral) eye that help move the eye in that direction are synergists. When the MR pulls the eye in, it is helped by the SR and IR. When the LR pulls the eye out, it is helped by the obliques. Therefore, the obliques are ipsilateral synergists of the lateral rectus for abduction. The vertical recti are ipsilateral synergists of the medial rectus for adduction. Because both superior muscles

(SR and SO) intort the eye, they are ipsilateral synergists for intorsion. Because both inferior muscles extort the eye, they are ipsilateral synergists for extorsion.

Bibliography

Nelson LB, Catalano RA: Atlas of Ocular Motility. Philadelphia, WB Saunders, 1989.
von Noorden GK: Atlas of Strabismus, 4th ed. St Louis, CV Mosby, 1983.

• CHAPTER 21 OCULAR MOTILITY: EXTRAOCULAR MUSCLE FUNCTION

1. What are the yoke muscles in this diagram, and what is this version movement called?

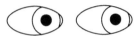

   a. LMR and RMR, dextroversion
   b. RMR and LLR, levoversion
   c. RMR and RLR, levoversion
   d. RMR and LLR, dextroversion
   e. LMR and RMR, levoversion

2. What are the yoke muscles in this diagram, and what is this position of gaze?

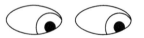

   a. RSO and LIR, down and left
   b. RIR and LSO, down and right
   c. RIO and LIR, down and left
   d. LIO and RIR, down and right
   e. RIR and LSO, down and left

3. A 20-year old male was examined for vertical diplopia, which he has had ever since he fell off his motorcycle 2 months ago. What is wrong with the extraocular muscles if his versions look like the following?

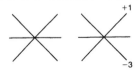

   a. Underaction of LSO is more marked than the overaction of LIO.
   b. Overaction of RIO is more marked than the underaction of RSO.
   c. Underaction of LIR is more marked than the overaction of LSR.
   d. Overaction of RSR is more marked than the underaction of RIR.
   e. Underaction of RIR is more marked than the overaction of RSR.

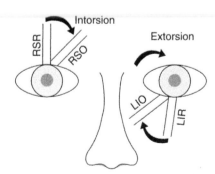

Incyclorotation of both eyes

FIGURE 21–17. Torsion. Intorsion mostly from the superior oblique with help from the superior rectus. Extorsion mostly from the inferior oblique with help from the inferior rectus.

4. The primary function of the RSR is to pull the right eye up when that eye is in the *out* (abducted) position. What is its ipsilateral synergist for its primary function?
   a. RIR
   b. RLR
   c. RSO
   d. LSR
   e. RIO

5. What extraocular muscle appears to be underactive?

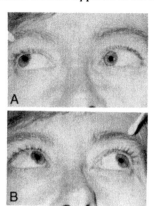

   a. RSR
   b. RIO
   c. LSO
   d. LIO
   e. LSR

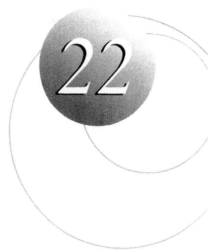

Ocular Motility: Incomitant Deviations

LEARNING OBJECTIVES

- Differentiate comitant from incomitant deviations
- Perform and evaluate the results of Bielschowsky's head tilt test
- Perform and evaluate the results of a three-step test to find the paretic extraocular muscle
- Evaluate A and V patterns
- Understand the how and why of abnormal head postures

Comitant eye misalignments measure the same in different directions of gaze. The most common examples are childhood eso and exo deviations. An incomitant deviation has different measurements of the misalignment in different fields of gaze. By testing extraocular muscle function, the examiner determines which muscle is defective. Incomitant deviations can be caused by a malfunction of one of the extraocular muscles, a defect of the nerve supplying the muscle, an A or a V pattern, or a mechanical restriction of the muscle or its surrounding tissues (Fig. 22–1). Eye misalignments occurring before age four are usually comitant, and after age 20 they are usually incomitant.

Weakened muscles cannot move the eye into their field of action by the anticipated amount, resulting in increased deviation in the field of action of the weak muscle. The opposite field of action has the least amount of deviation. When partially weakened, however, the muscles have the remarkable ability to retain good function whenever they receive more than the normal amount of innervation, e.g., on ductions. A weakness of the nerve supply to a muscle is *paresis*. Most nerve defects are partial, not total. On ductions, such partial nerve defects appear to have normal movement. Only when both eyes receive equal amounts of innervation (such as occurs with versions) do the two eyes move in different amounts, one less than the other. The eye's paretic (weakened) muscle does not move as well as the yoke muscle in the other eye. Therefore, versions are a better test for pareses than ductions. If versions are normal, ductions will always be normal. Ductions are tested only when versions are abnormal.

One example is a right lateral rectus (RLR) palsy. If the palsy is total, the right eye will not come out past midline when looking to the right (abduction). The right eye goes no farther than midline whether or not the left eye is covered. In most incomitant deviations however, there is still *some* function of the defective nerve.

If the left eye is the fixing eye, there will be normal innervation going to the left medial rectus (LMR) to move to the right (adduct). Normal innervation will go to the weak RLR, but this amount of innervation will be ineffective for a full version movement. On ductions, the RLR receives excessive innervation. It comes out past midline. On versions with the paretic right eye fixing, the LMR also receives excessive innervation which it does not need. It overacts and adducts past where it should go.

● RESTRICTIONS

An incomitant deviation caused by a mechanical restriction around the eyeball is as common as one caused by a weakness of the nerve supply to a muscle. A restricted muscle cannot relax when its direct antagonist contracts. When this occurs, the incomitant deviation is still analyzed as though the examiner expects to find a weak muscle. Once the apparently paretic muscle is diagnosed, a mechanical restriction must be ruled out. The mechanical restriction occurs in or around the direct antagonist of the apparently weak muscle. What appears to be an RLR palsy may actually be a bound-down right medial rectus (RMR) muscle.

With a paresis, the involved eye can usually move better on ductions than versions. With restrictions, the

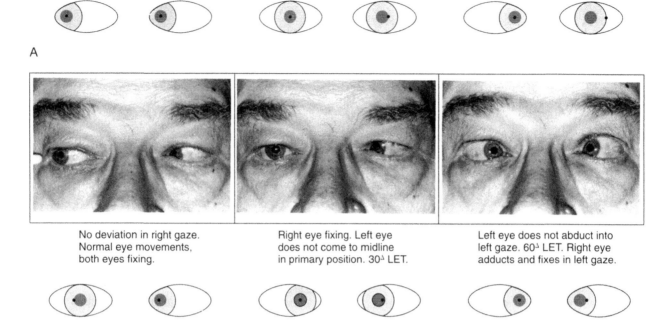

A

| No deviation in right gaze. Normal eye movements, both eyes fixing. | Right eye fixing. Left eye does not come to midline in primary position. 30$^\Delta$ LET. | Left eye does not abduct into left gaze. 60$^\Delta$ LET. Right eye adducts and fixes in left gaze. |

B

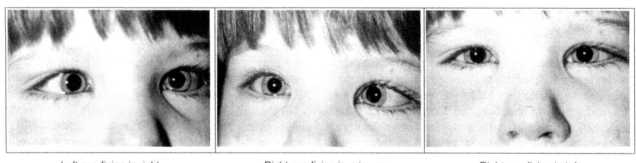

| Left eye fixing in right gaze. 30$^\Delta$ RET. | Right eye fixing in primary position. 30$^\Delta$ LET. | Right eye fixing in left gaze. 30$^\Delta$ LET. |

FIGURE 22–1. *A,* Incomitant left esotropia. Incomitant horizontal deviations change in amount from primary position to right and left gazes. The fixing eye usually remains the same. *B,* Comitant esotropia. Comitant horizontal deviations do not change in amount from primary position to right and left gazes. However, the fixing eye may change.

duction movement does not improve over the version movement. An eye with a paretic RLR would move more into right gaze on ductions than on versions. An eye with a restricted RMR would not move any better into right gaze on ductions than on versions. Instead of a weak RLR, it becomes a restriction of its direct antagonist, the RMR.

For another example, a thyroid patient with fibrosis of the inferior rectus (IR) muscle depresses the involved eye normally, but cannot elevate it. It looks as though the superior rectus (SR) of the involved eye is paretic instead of the IR being restricted. The largest deviation is not found in the field of action of the restricted muscle, but in the field of action of its direct antagonist, the muscle that seems paretic (Fig. 22–2).

● BIELSCHOWSKY HEAD TILT TEST

The Bielschowsky head tilt test is based on input from the vestibular system that then attempts to return the eyes to an upright position despite head tilt. On right head tilt, the right eye intorts while the left eye extorts; on left head tilt, the right eye extorts while the left eye intorts. The extorters are the inferior muscles; the intorters are the superior muscles (Fig. 22–3*A* and *B*).

The patient's head is tilted first to the right shoulder—the hypertropia is measured—and then to the left shoulder—the hypertropia is remeasured.

● THREE STEP TEST

The three step test is commonly used diagnostically to determine which extraocular muscle is paretic in an incomitant vertical deviation. This method for finding which paretic muscle is at fault eliminates half the vertical muscles with each step.

FIGURE 22–2. Thyroid ophthalmopathy. *A,* No vertical deviation in primary position. *B,* Left hypotropia in up gaze since LIR restriction prevents left eye from elevating, simulating RSR paresis.

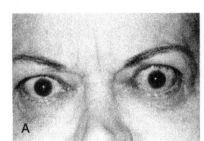
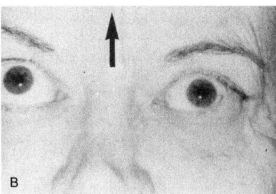

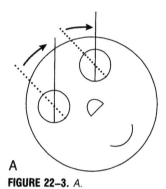

Right eye intorters
RSR + RSO
Left eye extorters
LIO + LIR

A
FIGURE 22–3. *A.*

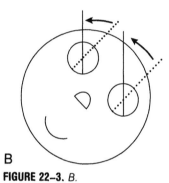

Left eye intorters
LSR + LSO
Right eye extorters
RIO + RIR

B
FIGURE 22–3. *B.*

Bielschowsky Head Tilt Test

If all the extraocular muscles that move the eye vertically have normal function, no vertical imbalance (hypertropia) is found on head tilt to either shoulder.

1. Head tilts to right shoulder (Fig. 22–3*C*).
2. Head tilts to left shoulder.

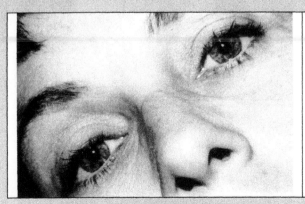
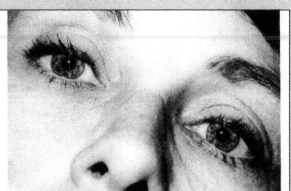

C   OD intorters and OS extorters in balance. No hyper on right head tilt.

OD extorters and OS intorters in balance. No hyper on left head tilt.

FIGURE 22–3. *C,* No vertical muscle imbalance on cover test and head tilt test.

Three Step Test

Step One—Is There a Right Hyper or a Left Hyper? The first step determines whether the deviation is a right or a left hypertropia, i.e., which eye is higher (Fig. 22–4A). In our example, the first step eliminates four of the eight muscles with vertical action—leaving only those four that, if weak, would cause a right hypertropia. The paretic muscle could be one of the two muscles of the right eye that pull that eye down, right inferior rectus (RIR) or right superior oblique (RSO), or one of the two muscles of the left eye that pull that eye up, left inferior oblique (LIO) or left superior rectus (LSR).

RIO̶   LIO
RSO   L̶S̶O̶
RIR   L̶I̶R̶
R̶S̶R̶   LSR

The cross outs show the muscles circled that could cause a *right* hypertropia.

Step Two—To Which Side Gaze Is the Hyper Larger? The second step eliminates two of the remaining four muscles that have their vertical function in the gaze in which the hyperdeviation is less. Our patient has a marked increase in right hyperdeviation in left gaze (Fig. 22–4B). Only the vertical extraocular muscles that can function in left gaze are implicated. The right inferior rectus and the left inferior oblique are deleted since they are right gaze vertical muscles.

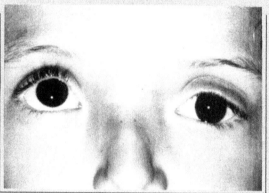

FIGURE 22–4. *A.*

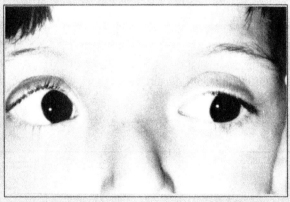

Right hypertropia

Right eye depressors
RIR
RSO

Left eye elevators
LIO
LSR

A

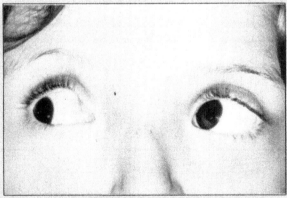

RSO   L̶I̶O̶
R̶I̶R̶   LSR

FIGURE 22–4. *B.*

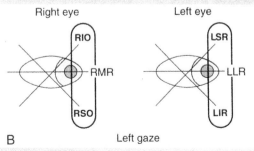

B   Left gaze

By combining the two diagrams we see that we have only two muscles circled both times: the right superior oblique and the left superior rectus. We have remaining only the contralateral antagonists: two muscles, one in each eye, either two intorters or two extorters, that move the eyes in the *opposite* direction but in the same gaze (Fig. 22–4C). The two superior muscles remaining are both intorters.

Step Three—Which Head Tilt Increases the Hyderdeviation? Of the two muscles remaining, the Bielschowsky head tilt tests one on right head tilt, the other on left head tilt (Fig. 22–4D). The test implicates one of the two muscles by which head tilt produces the larger hyperdeviation.

An increased right hyperdeviation is found on right head tilt. The intorters also have vertical function. The SR ele-

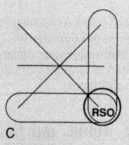
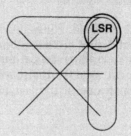

C

FIGURE 22–4. *C.*

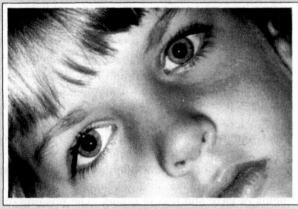
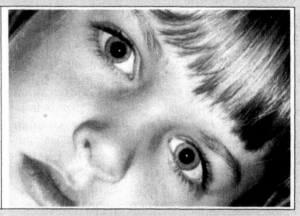

FIGURE 22–4. *D.* OD intorters out of balance. OS extorters in balance. Large RHT on right head tilt.

OD extorters in balance. OS intorters in balance. No RHT on left head tilt.

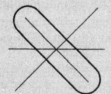

FIGURE 22–4. *E,* RHT worse on right head tilt.

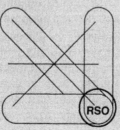
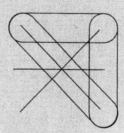

FIGURE 22–4. *F.*

vates the eye; the SO depresses it. When the head tilt is to the side where the paretic muscle (RSO) torts, its ipsilateral synergist (RSR) for torsion outperforms the paretic muscle. Because the RSR is also an elevator, it pulls the eye up more out of alignment, increasing the right hyperdeviation.

On left head tilt, the right extorters and the left intorters are tested. In this example, the right hyperdeviation is less since the left superior rectus is normal. It opposes the normal left superior oblique as it should, resulting in only intorsion of the left eye, with less vertical imbalance.

If we return to our crossed-out technique and circle those muscles tested in right head tilt and then combine all three steps, the RSO is the only muscle circled all three times (Fig. 22–4*E, F*).

In this example, we chose an RHT worse in left gaze and worse on right head tilt. For any incomitant deviation, the first step eliminates four vertical muscles; the second step, another two; and the Bielschowsky head tilt helps decide which one of the last two muscles is at fault.

• A AND V PATTERNS

Although childhood eso and exo misalignments are usually horizontally comitant, they may be vertically incomitant because of an A or a V pattern. The eso measurement in right gaze will be the same as in primary position and in left gaze. However, the deviation will be more in up gaze and less in down gaze than in primary, or the reverse. Any incomitance, such as an A or a V pattern, always complicates the management of childhood eye misalignments (Fig 22–5).

A and V patterns are caused by pairs of overactive oblique muscles. V patterns most often have overaction of both IO and A patterns most often have overaction of both SO. The up and right and up and left positions, or the down and right and down and left positions, will have a vertical deviation in addition to the horizontal deviation because of the overaction of oblique muscles (Fig. 22–6).

The following case illustrates this point. The patient has a V eso, similar to that shown in Figure 22–5*A*, measuring 25$^\Delta$ ET in primary position, as well as right and left gaze. The down gaze measurement is 35$^\Delta$ esotropia as is the down and right and down and left measurement. The up gaze measurement decreases to 15$^\Delta$ ET, which is also measured up and right and up and left. However, up and right there is also 10$^\Delta$ of left hyper caused by the overactive left inferior oblique. Up and left there is 10$^\Delta$ of right hypertropia caused by the overaction of the right inferior oblique. This patient is horizontally comitant for his eso deviation. He is vertically incomitant on two counts. He has a vertical that changes in up and right from up and left, and he has an up gaze horizontal measurement and a down gaze horizontal measurement that differ from the primary position measurement (Fig. 22–7).

If we illustrate a V exo, similar to Figure 22–5*B*, the deviation is now worse in up gaze, but both the inferior obliques remain overactive. In Figure 22–7*C* we have the typical appearance and measurements found with A exo patterns, similar to Figure 22–5*D*, with overactive superior obliques.

• TIPS, TURNS, AND TILTS

Patients with incomitant deviations frequently retain single binocular vision in one or several fields of gaze where the deviation is not present or is so small that it can be controlled. In order to utilize the fields of gaze in which fusion is still available, the patient adopts an abnormal head posture that puts the eyes into the position of least deviation. It may be quite marked or hardly noticeable. The *head* turns *toward* the field of gaze where the weak muscle usually functions. The *eyes* look in the field of gaze directly *opposite* where the greatest deviation is found.

Another cause of abnormal head posture is *nystagmus*. Some patients have nystagmus greater in some fields of gaze and less in others. The position of least nystagmus is the patient's null position where visual acuity is often best. The abnormal head position places the null straight ahead (Fig. 22–8).

Tips of the chin either up or down are usually adopted when there is an A or V pattern. A esos and V exos may fuse in down gaze; V esos and A exos may fuse in up gaze.

Face *turns* to the right or left are adopted whenever the incomitancy is due to an MR or LR problem. A patient with a CN VI palsy will turn their face to the side where the eye can't move. For example, an LLR palsy causes a deviation in left gaze. The face turns to the left so that the patient's eyes are in right gaze, where he retains fusion (Fig. 22–9).

Head *tilts* are adopted when there is an oblique muscle problem. IO palsies are much less common than SO palsies. Patients with SO palsies adopt a head tilt to the opposite shoulder. Because the right superior oblique functions in down and left gaze the head tilts down and to the left, allowing patients to utilize gaze up and to the right. *Right* superior oblique palsies maintain fusion with a *left* head tilt. They are worse in right head tilt. If a patient with a vertical eye misalignment walks

Text continued on page 333

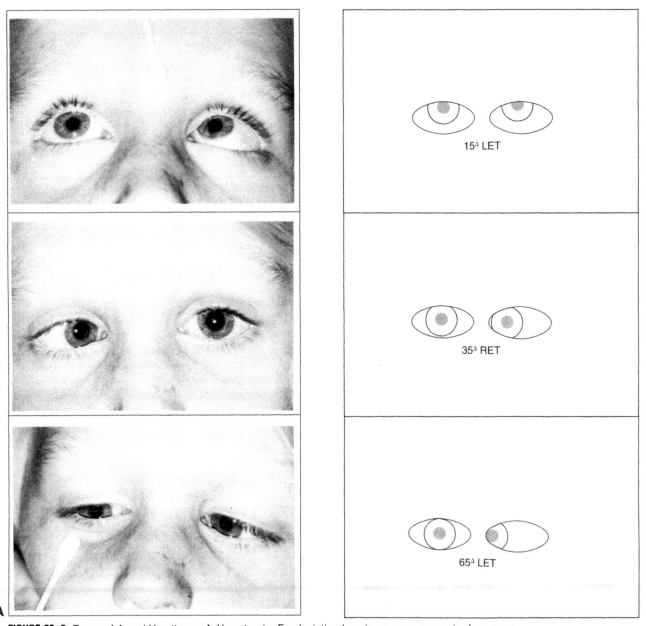

FIGURE 22–5. Types of A and V patterns. *A,* V esotropia. Esodeviation less in up gaze, worse in down gaze.

Illustration continued on following page

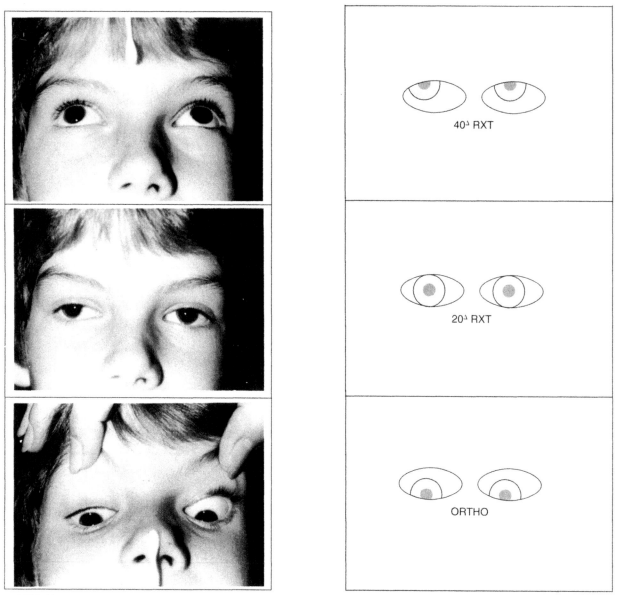

B

FIGURE 22–5. *Continued B*, V exotropia. Exodeviation worse in up gaze, less in down gaze.

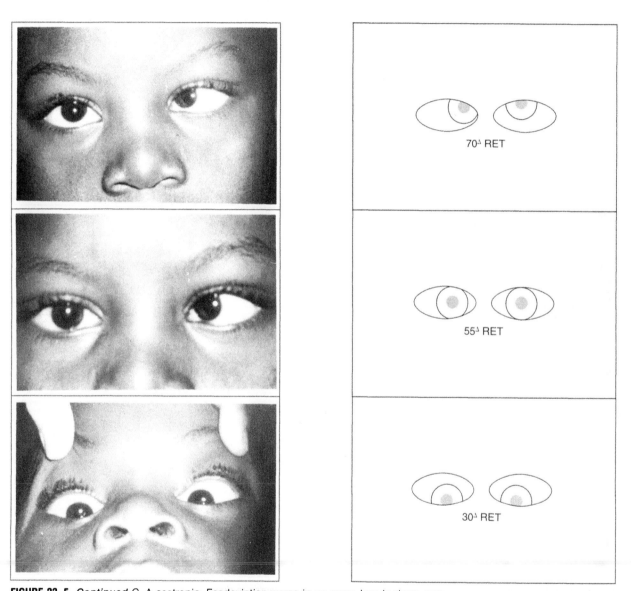

C

FIGURE 22–5. *Continued* C, A esotropia. Esodeviation worse in up gaze, less in down gaze.

Illustration continued on following page

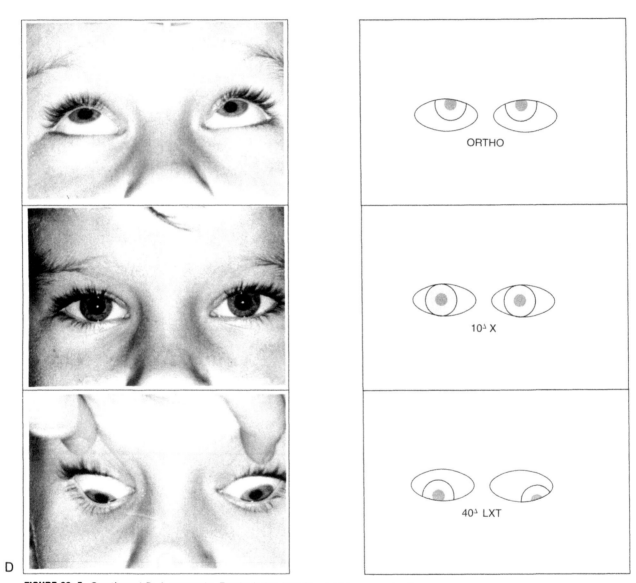

D

FIGURE 22–5. *Continued D*, A exotropia. Exodeviation less in up gaze, worse in down gaze.

Marked overaction   LIO

Marked overaction   RIO

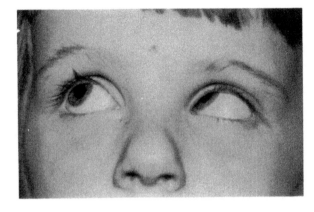

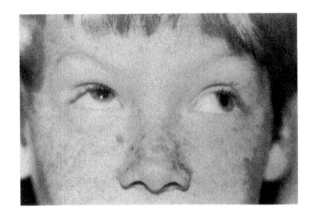

A

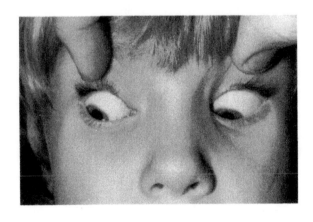

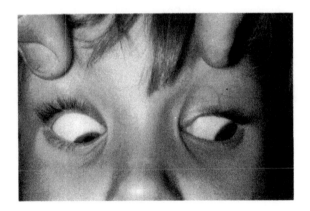

B

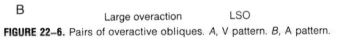

Large overaction   LSO

Large overaction   RSO

FIGURE 22–6. Pairs of overactive obliques. *A,* V pattern. *B,* A pattern.

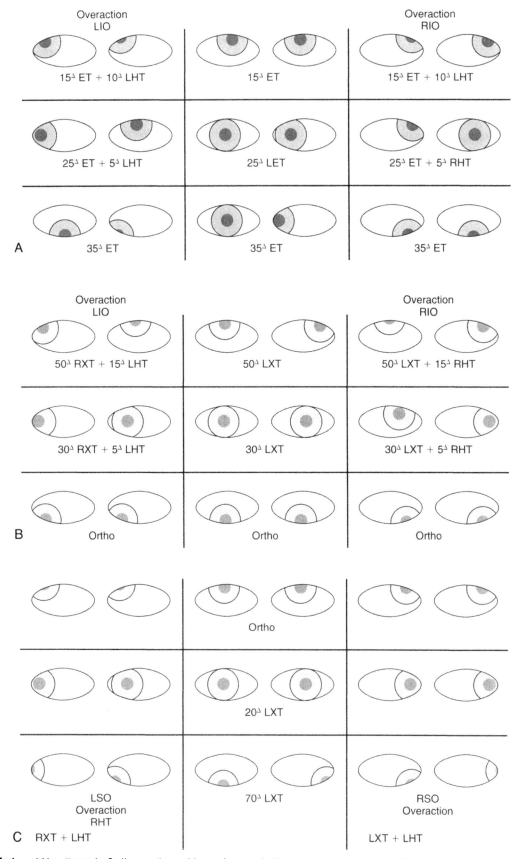

FIGURE 22–7. A and V patterns in 9 diagnostic positions of gaze. *A*, V esodeviation with overactive inferior obliques. *B*, V exodeviation with overactive inferior obliques. *C*, A exodeviation with overactive superior obliques.

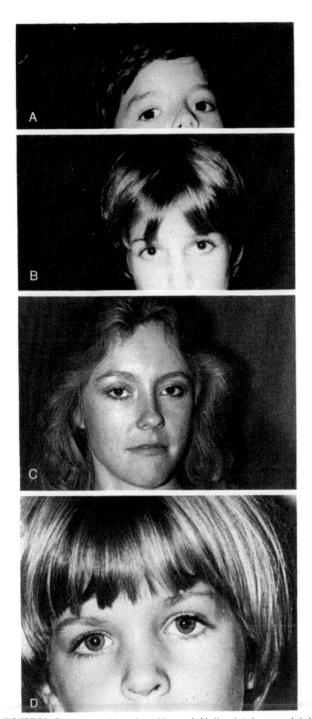

FIGURE 22–8. Abnormal head positions. *A,* Null point down and right with nystagmus. Head up and in left gaze. *B,* V eso has small deviation in up gaze where he fuses with chin in down position. *C,* Left head turn to fuse in right gaze in patient with weak LLR. *D,* Moderate right head tilt producing fusion in patient with left superior oblique palsy.

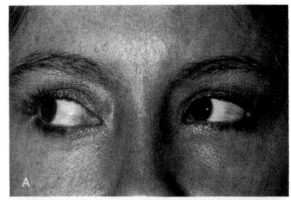

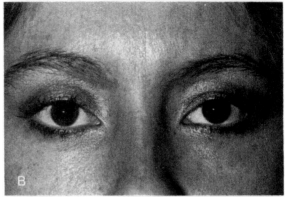

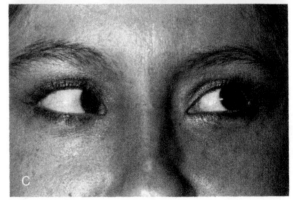

FIGURE 22–9. Mild paresis of left lateral rectus. *A,* Normal right gaze with fusion. *B,* Small esodeviation in primary position with diplopia. *C,* Incomplete abduction of the left eye with diplopia in left gaze from left esodeviation.

is in the field of gaze where the head is aimed. All tests for binocularity should be done with the patient using the abnormal head position.

Bibliography

Koch P: An aid for the diagnosis of a vertical muscle paresis. J Pediatr Ophthalmol Strabismus 17:272, 1980.

Nelson LB, Catalano RA: Atlas of Ocular Motility. Philadelphia, WB Saunders, 1989.

Parks MM: Ocular Motility and Strabismus. Hagerstown, MD, Harper & Row, 1975.

von Noorden GK: Atlas of Strabismus, 4th ed. St Louis, CV Mosby, 1983.

von Noorden GK (ed): Burian-von Noorden's Binocular Vision and Ocular Motility, 3rd ed. St Louis, CV Mosby, 1985.

into a room with a left head tilt, an RSO palsy is suspected until proven otherwise.

Often, abnormal head postures have a combination of turns, tilts, and tips. The basic rule usually holds. Notice in which fields of gaze the eyes are placed by the abnormal head posture. This is where fusion is retained, or nystagmus is least. The maximum problem

● CHAPTER 22 OCULAR MOTILITY: INCOMITANT DEVIATIONS

1. In this patient, choose the pattern that applies.
   a. V esotropia
   b. V exotropia
   c. No pattern
   d. A esotropia
   e. A exotropia

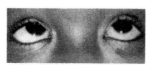
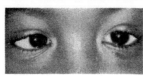
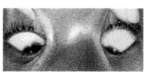

2. What is the most likely underaction?
   a. LLR
   b. LMR
   c. RLR
   d. LSO
   e. RMR

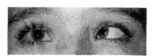
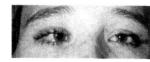
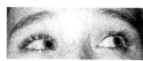

3. This patient has hypertropia in right gaze only as shown. Which *diagram* of the underactive muscles is most correct?

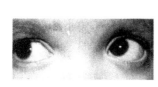

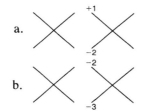

a.

b.

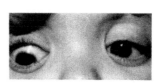

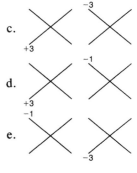

c.

d.

e.

4. The up and right and up and left gaze positions shown are the only abnormalities in versions. What does this patient most likely have?

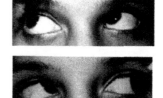

   a. V esotropia
   b. overactive superior obliques
   c. A exotropia
   d. A esotropia
   e. underactive inferior obliques

5. Which extraocular muscle would be implicated if the third step shows an increased hypertropia on head tilt to the left shoulder?
   a. RSR
   b. LIO
   c. LIR
   d. LSO
   e. RSO

Eileen Harrell

Contact Lenses

LEARNING OBJECTIVES

- Discuss differences among hard, gas permeable, and soft contact lenses
- Explain base curve, diameter, optical zone, and Dk (i.e., oxygen permeability) level
- Explain the use of keratometry and refractometry results in choosing contact lenses
- Explain centration, movement, and fluorescein patterns in the assessment of contact lens fit

- Explain the calculations in steepening and flattening a lens
- Understand the difference between corneal and lenticular astigmatism and how each affects choice of contact lens
- Explain how the cornea acquires its oxygen with and without wearing contact lenses
- List signs of corneal irregularity
- List five contact lens complications

Contact lenses are a popular method of optical correction for refractive errors such as myopia, hyperopia, and astigmatism. The use of contact lenses has expanded over the decades to include alternative functions for improved visual acuity, enhanced cosmetic appearance, and recuperation of the cornea.

In a normally healthy eye, optimal visual acuity can be achieved with either glasses or contact lenses. The eye with an abnormal corneal surface may reach visual acuity levels with a contact lens unobtainable by glasses. A rigid contact lens can be made to create a new, smooth refractive surface for an eye with corneal irregularity secondary to ocular trauma, corneal transplant, keratoconus, or a corneal dystrophy.

Contact lenses are the ideal correction when cataract surgery is required and an intraocular lens implant may be inadvisable, as with congenital cataracts or ocular trauma. Because the dioptric power of a contact lens has less effect on the image size than eyeglasses, a contact lens becomes essential to preserve binocularity with monocular aphakia due to the image size difference induced by the anisometropia, that is, the difference in refractive power of the two eyes.

Extended-wear soft contact lenses can be worn as a protective bandage to promote healing of the corneal epithelium in eyes with anterior corneal dystrophy, post-penetrating keratoplasty surgery with delayed re-epithelialization, and aphakic or pseudophakic bullous keratopathy. Their use requires frequent return examinations because a de-epithelialized cornea is prone to infection and so must be monitored closely. Following corneal evaluation, the lens is removed, surfactant cleaned, rinsed, disinfected in the clinical setting, and if necessary, reinserted.

Rigid and soft contact lenses can also be used to mask the appearance of a disfigured eye. The lenses are beneficial with corneal scars, opaque corneas, leukocoria, and iridodialysis. Masking lenses can provide partial occlusion to diminish photophobia in patients with ocular albinism, aniridia, or loss of iris tissue following ocular trauma. Refractive power can be cut into the lenses for sighted eyes. Black occluder pupils are frequently used for nonsighted eyes (Fig. 23–1).

Occlusion therapy using masking lenses can treat amblyopia and diplopia. Patch therapy is the most common treatment for amblyopia. Because of the limited cooperation of the children in which amblyopia is treatable (approximately birth to age 7 years), patch treatment may be unsuccessful. A contact lens is, in some cases, more tolerable for the pediatric patient and, therefore, more successful. Cooperation is required for the insertion and removal of the contact lens. The use and care of the lens is the responsibility of the child's parents or caregivers. They need to be aware of potential complications, including occlusion amblyopia of

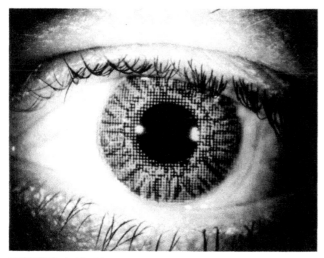

FIGURE 23–1. Masking contact lens with black occluder pupil.

the normal eye and contact lens–related problems, including solution and lens-related allergies, corneal abrasions, and corneal infections.

Occluder contact lenses are utilized to treat diplopia when methods to restore fusion, such as prisms, eye exercises, and surgery have been unsuccessful. When binocular vision cannot be achieved and double vision is intolerable, an occluder contact lens blocks the second image.

• CONTACT LENS CATEGORIES

Contact lens polymers are of three basic varieties. Two are rigid plastics: polymethylmethacrylate (PMMA) or "hard" contact lenses and gas-permeable lenses. The third variety is soft hydrogel contact lenses. Although all three can be worn interchangeably in many diagnoses, each has its own advantages and disadvantages. Understanding these differences greatly enhances the ability of the contact lens fitter to match the needs of the patient with the most appropriate lens.

Hard Contact Lenses

Hard contact lenses are cut from the PMMA polymer. The dioptric curve on the concave (back) side reflects the curvature of the cornea. The dioptric curve on its front surface is cut to summate the dioptric power necessary to correct the refractive error of the eye. Because it maintains its own curvature and thus resists warpage, PMMA lenses are excellent for correcting toric corneas and irregular astigmatism, and for providing a smooth, stable refractive surface for the cornea. The plastic is durable and reproducible. It is moderately resistant to coating with tear film products and can be mechanically or chemically polished to diminish surface scratches and deposits. These properties

lengthen the life of the lens considerably and decrease the overall expense.

PMMA lenses have several disadvantages. Because the cornea has no blood supply, it derives its oxygen from the atmosphere and the tear film. The plastic does not allow transmission of oxygen, and a PMMA lens can thereby induce an anoxic environment. To help counteract this, the lens is usually cut small, approximately 8.0 to 8.7 mm. With the blink motion, the excursion of the lens allows the tear film, carrying the oxygen, to be exchanged under the lens (tear pump). At the onset, these lenses are generally uncomfortable. Adaptation to the sensation of the eyelid striking the surface of the hard contact lens takes approximately 2 to 4 weeks. The lens is initially worn for limited periods, gradually increasing wear each day. Once a comfortable level of wearing time is reached, it must be maintained by daily wearing of the lenses. Maximum wear time should be kept under 15 hours per day.

Long-term wearing of PMMA contact lenses may induce corneal warpage. Treatment is difficult because corneal curvature can fluctuate, changing the amount and axis of corneal astigmatism. The warpage results in an irregular astigmatism that eyeglasses cannot fully correct optically.

Rigid Gas-Permeable Lenses

Rigid gas-permeable lenses offer good visual acuity for spherical refractive errors and moderate amounts of corneal astigmatism. Rigid gas-permeable lenses offer many advantages characteristic of PMMA lenses while having the additional benefit of transmitting considerable oxygen to the cornea. The permeability of the plastic, the ease with which oxygen passes through it, is called the Dk level of the material.

The oxygen permeability of rigid lenses was improved by adding silicone to PMMA. Silicone is extremely permeable to oxygen. The disadvantage of silicone is its poor wettability and lack of resistance to coating with tear film deposits. Fluorosilicone acrylates have been developed that maintain the oxygen permeability while they decrease the tendency toward deposit accumulation on the lens surface. Increased oxygen permeability allows these lenses to be cut with a larger diameter, approximately 9.0 to 9.6 mm. Lenses of this diameter commonly fit under the upper eyelid, lessening the eyelid hitting the lens during a blink, thereby improving comfort and adaptation to the lens (i.e., alignment fit).

The disadvantage of gas-permeable lenses is the greater fragility of the material compared with PMMA lenses. The tendency to become coated with components of the tear film, to scratch on the surface, and to crack along the edge of the lens requires more frequent replacement than that of a PMMA lens. The usable longevity of rigid gas-permeable lenses is approximately 18 to 24 months. Warpage of the lens (i.e., lens flexure) can also occur, especially with high Dk materials. Assessment of warpage is made with a radius gauge by measuring the base curve of rigid contact lenses (Fig. 23–2).

Rigid gas-permeable contact lenses should be considered for the following situations:

1. Past success with rigid gas-permeable lenses
2. Moderate corneal astigmatism
3. Corneal irregularity e.g., from scars, corneal transplants, and early to moderate keratoconus
4. Overwear syndrome with PMMA or soft contact lenses
5. Poor success with soft contact lenses, e.g., decreased visual acuity, neovascularization, solution toxicity, and hypoxia (lack of oxygen)
6. History of giant papillary conjunctivitis (GPC)
7. Occupation; i.e., use in an environment with gaseous air contaminants
8. Prominent allergy history.

Soft Contact Lenses

Most soft contact lenses are hydroxyethylmethacrylate (HEMA) polymers comprising a variety of hydrated polymers cut by a multitude of soft lens manufacturers. Water content varies from 38 to 79%, and this is one determinant of oxygen transmission through the soft plastic lens. The higher the water content, the greater the amount of oxygen transmitted. Lens thickness, along with water content, contributes to the effective Dk of any material. Soft contact lenses are

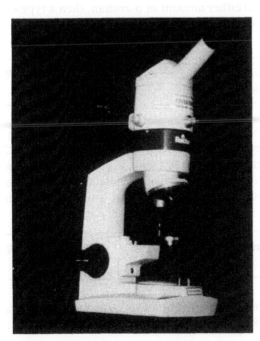

FIGURE 23–2. Radius gauge.

fitted with diameters that extend beyond the limbus (scleral lenses) and tuck under the upper eyelid. The large diameter, along with the lens hydration, contributes to the comfort of soft contact lenses, allowing them to be worn on a flexible schedule. Soft contact lenses can be worn intermittently without requiring a readaptation to the lens. Some soft lens polymers are approved by the Food and Drug Administration (FDA) for extended wear, referring to lens wear 24 hours per day during both waking and sleeping. The FDA has a current limit of 7 days of continuous wear. Because of the increased rate of contact lens–related infections with extended wear lenses compared with daily wear lenses, it is advisable to discuss the risks of extended wear with a contact lens candidate. An informed consent form is advisable for extended wear.

Soft contact lenses have several disadvantages for the contact lens wearer. Contrast may decrease particularly when compared with RGF lenses with less deformable surfaces. Mild amounts of refractive cylinder, although not significant enough to use an astigmatic soft lens, may be enough to lessen visual perception. The hydration of the lens can fluctuate depending on tear production. Dehydration of the soft lens induces a steepening effect, changing both the fit and the optics.

Soft lens polymers are capable of absorbing water-soluble chemicals, which may potentially be toxic to corneal tissue. Soft lenses are prone to tear film deposits, particularly protein and calcium. Increased lens filming decreases the ease with which oxygen can permeate the lens. The film also acts as a site for bacterial accumulation. As a result, it is advisable to replace soft contact lenses more frequently than PMMA or gas-permeable contact lenses. At least an annual replacement schedule, combined with an eye examination, is advisable. Replacement can take place more frequently, depending on the rate of depositing on or deterioration of the lens.

Alternative lens choices are available for the contact lens wearer. Lenses with water content of 55% and above, and those requiring heat for lens disinfection, are generally more prone to deposits. Lenses with water content under 45% and with chemical or peroxide disinfection systems can be beneficial. Other options include wearing disposable contact lenses on a daily basis for 2 weeks, replacing conventional soft lenses more frequently with a fresh lens or changing to a rigid gas permeable lens.

Disposable Contact Lenses

Disposable contact lenses are dispensed as multipack units. The lenses are approved by the FDA for extended wear on a 7-day limit time basis. The soft lens may then be disposed of or disinfected with an appropriate lens disinfection system and reinserted for one additional 7-day period. Two weeks is the general limitation for wear of disposable contact lenses. (Always check the manufacturer's guidelines.) The lenses may also be used on a flexible wear schedule with removal more frequent than weekly. Day wear use of these lenses is recommended for those who have a history of giant papillary conjunctivitis or who are moderate-to-heavy lens depositors.

Frequent Replacement Contact Lenses

Multipackaged lenses are available from a limited number of companies. These are available in spherical, toric, tinted, and multifocal lens types. Utilization is on a 1- to 3-month basis, depending on the manufacturer's specifications.

Soft contact lenses should be especially considered for the following situations:

1. Past success with soft contact lenses
2. Spherical refractive error
3. Past discomfort with rigid contact lenses
4. Request for tinted lenses, whether cosmetic, masking, or occluder
5. Occupation with an environment with particulate debris
6. Bandage lens for epithelial healing—recurrent corneal erosion or postoperative corneal transplant healing.

Silicone Contact Lenses

Contact lenses made of pure silicone are also available, primarily for aphakia in infants and young children. The high DK, or oxygen permeability, of the material allows adequate oxygen transmission through a high-powered contact lens.

• CONTACT LENS FITTING

Fitting depends on the type of contact lens. The results of keratometry and refractometry tests are used to choose the initial trial lens. Keratometry measures the curvature of the anterior surface of the cornea. Accuracy is critical as the curvature readings will be reflected in the curvature of the chosen contact lens. Recordings are most commonly listed with the flattest meridian first, the steepest meridian second, along with the location, in degrees, of the steepest meridian. The curvature readings are listed both in diopters and in millimeters of radius. These numbers have a direct relationship with one another, e.g., 43.00 diopters (*D*) = 7.84 mm of radius. Normal corneal curvature readings range from approximately 41.00 to 46.00 D. These numbers indicate the amount of power of the cornea to focus light. The difference between the two

meridians indicates the amount of corneal astigmatism present.

• ***Example:*** *42.50/44.25 at 90° 42.50 is the flattest corneal meridian. 44.25 is the steepest corneal meridian at 90°. The amount of astigmatism is 1.75 diopters.*

Other information from keratometry that benefits the fitter includes the regularity of the corneal astigmatism. The axes of the two corneal meridians are usually 90° apart. Any irregularity of the keratometer mires, i. e., a condition with corneal warpage, must be determined. Keratometry is employed to select the appropriate diameter of a contact lens, the base curve of the lens, and to assess the long-term tolerance of the cornea to the contact lens.

Refractometry is necessary to determine the power of the contact lens. Both rigid and soft toric lenses require the minus cylinder form of refractometry, so transposition may be necessary. In minus cylinder, the power of the sphere corrects the flatter of the two corneal meridians. The combined power of the sphere and cylinder corrects the steeper corneal meridian.

• ***Example:*** *Keratometry: 43.00/44.75 at 90° Refractometry: − 4.00 − 1.75 × 180°. The flattest corneal meridian is 43.00 D with a corrective power of − 4.00 D. The steepest corneal meridian is 44.75 D with a corrective power of − 5.75 D.*

When the amount of corneal astigmatism as seen with keratometry differs from the refractive astigmatism in either amount or meridian, then a type of astigmatism, lenticular, is present in the natural lens.

• ***Example:*** *Keratometry: 43.00/43.50 at 90° Refractometry: − 3.50 − 2.00 × 180°*

There is 0.50 D corneal astigmatism at 90° by keratometry. Refractometry in minus cylinder has 2.00 D astigmatism axis 180° (90° in plus cylinder). An additional 1.50 D of lenticular astigmatism is in the same meridian as the steep corneal astigmatic meridian.

• ***Example:*** *Keratometry: 43.00/44.00 at 90° Refractometry: − 3.00 − 1.00 × 90°*

This cornea has 1.00 D of astigmatism by keratometry. Refractometry in minus cylinder should be at axis

180°. Here it is at axis 90°. There must be 2.00 D of lenticular astigmatism at the 180° meridian. Refractometry results only in a 1.00 D cylinder because the second diopter of lenticular astigmatism is neutralized by the 1.00 D of corneal astigmatism 90° away.

Recognizing these numbers and the source of the astigmatism is important to the potential success of a rigid contact lens because rigid lenses correct corneal astigmatism by providing a new spherical optical surface. When significant lenticular astigmatism is present, either specially designed toric rigid lenses or soft toric lenses must be worn.

Rigid Contact Lens Fitting Technique

Base Curve

Determination of the base, or posterior central, curve of a trial rigid contact lens is obtained from the keratometer readings. Fitting philosophies vary. In general, with less than 1.50 D of corneal astigmatism, the lens is fit between the flattest corneal curvature and 0.50 D steeper.

• **Example:** *43.00/44.25 at 90° Base curve: 43.00 D, 43.25 D, or 43.50 D*

With astigmatism greater than 1.50 D, the base curve is chosen by splitting the difference between the two curvatures. Selection of base curve is also determined by the lens diameter.

• **Example:** *43.00/46.00 at 90° Base curve: 44.00 D, 44.50 D*

Diameter

Initial estimation of the diameter of the rigid contact lens follows the general rule that a cornea with a curvature flatter than 43.00 tends to be large, whereas a cornea with a curvature steeper than 44.00 tends to be small. Average diameters for large (flat) corneas range from 9.0 to 9.6 mm, and smaller (steep) corneas range from 8.5 to 8.8 mm. With larger diameter lenses (e.g., 9.6 mm) lenses are fit more toward the flattest corneal curvature as the lens bears on the flatter part of the cornea.

Changing the diameter of the lens alters its fit. As the diameter increases, the sagittal depth also increases, thus steepening the lens. Sagittal depth is the length of a line extending perpendicular from the central apex of the posterior curve of a lens to the line

formed by the chord diameter. The chord (Fig. 23–3) diameter is the distance from one edge of the lens to the other edge. As the diameter decreases, the sagittal depth decreases and flattens the lens. In general, a 0.50-D change in base curve, or a 0.50 mm change in diameter, is necessary to alter the fitting characteristics. When both parameters are adjusted, smaller amounts may be effective.

Lens Steepening

	Base curve	Diameter			Base curve	Diameter
Change base curve	43.00 D	9.0 mm	→	→	43.50 D	9.0 mm
Change diameter	43.00 D	9.0 mm	→	→	43.00 D	9.5 mm
Change base curve and diameter	43.00 D	9.0 mm	→	→	43.25 D	9.3 mm

Lens Flattening

	Base curve	Diameter			Base curve	Diameter
Change base curve	43.00 D	9.0 mm	→	→	42.50 D	9.0 mm
Change diameter	43.00 D	9.0 mm	→	→	43.00 D	8.5 mm
Change base curve and diameter	43.00 D	9.0 mm	→	→	42.75 D	8.8 mm

In summary, to steepen the fit of a contact lens, increase the dioptric curve (decrease the millimeters of radius of curve), make the lens larger in diameter, or both. To flatten the fit of a contact lens, decrease the dioptric curve (increase the millimeters of radius of curve), make the lens smaller in diameter, or both.

Power

The power of a rigid contact lens in diopters is derived from refractometry in minus cylinder and the base curve from keratometry readings. The sphere of the minus cylinder from refractometry is the power of the flattest corneal meridian. The power of the cornea is modified by the resurfacing from the contact lens. The change in the anterior curvature of the eye by

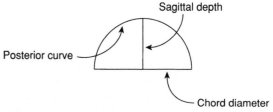

FIGURE 23–3. Lens parameters.

placing the contact lens over its surface requires a corresponding change in the power needed to focus light on the retina. Steepening the base curve of the contact lens increases the dioptric power induced by that curve. Flattening the base curve decreases the dioptric power. To maintain the appropriate power to focus light on the retina, the power of the lens is adjusted corresponding to the dioptric difference between the flattest corneal meridian and the base curve of the contact lens.

- *Example: Keratometry: 43.00/44.50 at 90°*
  Refractometry: −3.00 − 1.50 × 180°
  Base curve: 43.50
  Power: −3.50 D

The chosen base curve of 43.50 is 0.50 D steeper than the flattest corneal meridian of 43.00. The increased lens curvature will add +0.50 D, which must be adjusted for by adding −0.50 D to the sphere: −3.00 + (−0.50) = −3.50 D.

- *Example: Keratometry: 44.00/44.75 at 170°*
  Refractometry: −3.00 − 0.75 × 80°
  Base curve: 44.00
  Power: −3.00 D

No change in base curve is needed from the flattest corneal meridian of 44.00, so the power remains unchanged. Trial lenses are adjusted in the same manner. The dioptric change in base curve is equivalent to the dioptric change in power.

- *Example: Base curve: 43.50*
  Power: −4.00 D
  To steepen the base curve to 44.00 the power is adjusted to −4.50 D.
  To flatten the base curve to 43.00, the power is adjusted to −3.50 D.

Change in the diameter of the rigid lens affects the fitting characteristics of the lens without requiring a change in the power of the lens. A change in the dioptric power of the lens can be made without altering the base curve.

Assessment of the fit of the rigid contact lens is done with a slit lamp. Characteristics of a good fit include appropriate centration, movement, and fluorescein pattern. Centration of the lens keeps the optical zone over the visual axis. The optical zone of the contact lens is the central area containing the full refractive correc-

tion. Decentration of the optical zone can induce visual symptoms such as ghosting of images and glare from lights.

Movement of the contact lens, essential for appropriate tear exchange, is induced by blinking and ocular movement. The blink should induce decentration of the lens superiorly followed by a rapid repositioning. Lateral gaze results in a lagging decentration of the lens, an excursion that should remain within the corneal limbus. Fluorescein dye turns the tear film yellow, thereby allowing the fitter to determine how well the lens fits. Steep lenses do not move well and capture the fluorescein dye underneath the center of the lens with absence of fluorescein at the peripheral edge of the lens. Flat lenses move excessively and bear on the central cornea with an absence of dye centrally and with fluorescein pooling around the peripheral edge of the lens. A good fit shows a thin layer of fluorescein under the lens with a mild peripheral pooling (Fig. 23–4). (See Color Plates 25 and 26.)

Modifications

The following lens modifications can help improve fit and comfort:

Lenticular Carrier. Plus lenticular carriers added to the anterior edge of a high minus lens decrease the

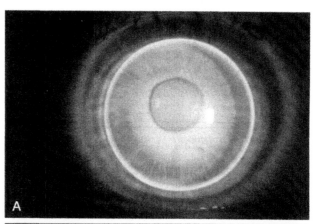

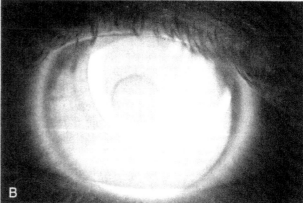

FIGURE 23–4. Fluorescein patterns in contact lens fitting. *A,* Normal appearance. *B,* Flat fit.

edge thickness and decrease the effect of the eyelid which can cause the lens to ride high following a blink. Minus lenticular carriers thicken the edge of high plus lenses to enhance eyelid pickup of the lens for better movement and centration. Plus and minus lenticular carriers should be considered for lens powers greater than ± 4.00 D.

Aspheric Curve. Increasing flattening of the base curve toward the periphery reflects more closely the aspheric curve of the cornea. This can improve centration and improve alignment fitting, particularly if the cornea has an irregular surface and high astigmatism.

Conlesh (CN) Bevel. Manufacturing procedure to thin the outer edge of the contact lens.

• SOFT CONTACT LENS FITTING TECHNIQUE

Base curve

Soft lenses rest outside the corneal limbus and are really scleral lenses. Given the aspheric shape of the cornea, the curvature is considerably flatter in the corneal periphery and sclera than in the central cornea. As a result, the base curve chosen for these lenses is 3 to 4 D flatter than the flattest corneal meridian measured by central keratometry.

The unit of measurement for the base curve is expressed in millimeters of radius. The millimeters of radius refers to the circle created by the dioptric curvature. The greater the power of the dioptric curve, the smaller/shorter the radius in millimeters (Fig. 23–5).

• **Example:** *K: 44.00 D = 7.67 mm radius*
or
K: 46.00 D = 7.33 mm radius

Soft contact lens fitting begins with refractometry and keratometry. Selection of the base curve is an estimation taken from keratometry results. Average corneal curvatures range from 42.00 to 44.00 D and use base curves ranging from 8.4 mm (40.12) to 8.6 mm (39.25 D). Corneal curvature greater than 44.00 D (7.67-mm radius) is considered steep. Typically, the base curve range for a steep cornea is 8.1 mm (41.75 D), 8.2 mm (41.12 D), and 8.3 mm (40.62 D). Corneal curvature less than 42.00 D (8.03-mm radius) is considered flat. Common base curves for flat corneas are 8.8 mm (38.25 D), 8.9 mm (37.87 D), and 9.0 mm (37.50 D).

Diameter

The diameter of soft contact lenses varies by manufacturer, most frequently ranging from 13.5 to 15.0 mm. A modified diameter can alter the fitting characteristic of the soft lens with the base curve held constant. Increasing the diameter steepens the fit of the lens; decreasing it flattens the lens fit (Fig. 23–6).

Power

The power of a soft contact lens derives from the spherical equivalent determined by refractometry. In contrast to rigid lenses, a soft lens rests on the anterior corneal surface without influencing curvature. As a result, the base curve of the soft lens, as it varies from the corneal curvature, does not change the refractive power of the eye. Changing the base curve during fitting does not require a change in power. Base curve and power are independent factors.

• **Example:** *Keratometry: 41.50/42.00 at 90°*
Refractometry: −3.25 + 0.50 × 90°
Base curve: 8.8 mm radius
Diameter: 14.0 mm
Power: −3.25 + (+0.25) = −3.00 D sphere equivalent.

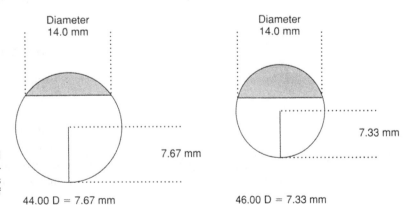

FIGURE 23–5. Relationship between the sagittal depth of a lens and its dioptric curve. If the diameter remains constant, the sagittal depth deepens when the dioptric curve increases (millimeters of radius smaller).

Diameter 14.0 mm

7.67 mm

44.00 D = 7.67 mm

Diameter 14.0 mm

7.33 mm

46.00 D = 7.33 mm

• *Example:* *Keratometry: 43.00/43.25 at 90°*
Refractometry: −5.00 Sph
Base curve: 8.6 mm radius
Diameter: 13.8 mm
Power: −4.75 D (adjusted for vertex distance)

Unlike rigid contact lenses, in which the lens is cut to the fitter's specifications, soft contact lenses are cut with a limited number of parameters within specified guidelines. Availability of various base curves, diameter, and power depends on the lens manufacturers. In general, one to three base curves, one or two different diameters, and a power range within ± 20.00 D are available. Any need for a parameter outside those available with a particular lens type requires a different lens from another manufacturer. Custom lens designs are, however, supplied by some manufacturers.

Vertex distance is that between the corneal surface and the eyeglasses' correction. As the power of the prescription increases to > ± 4.00 D, an adjustment must be made when determining the power of the contact lens. The vertex distance of a contact lens power is zero. Minus lenses require less power, and plus lenses more, when brought to the plane of the cornea.

Assessment of the fit of a soft contact lens includes appropriate movement and centration with stability of vision and comfort. Requirements for movement include 0.50- to 1.5-mm shift following a blink with minimal observable lag in lateral gaze. The optical zone should remain over the visual axis with excursions into all fields of gaze. Steep lenses tend to ride low; flat lenses tend to ride high and to de-center.

Visual acuity can be influenced by an inappropriate fit. Steep lenses flatten with a blink and briefly allow clearer vision. Flat lenses induce a blur immediately following a blink caused by excessive displacement of the optical zone.

The fit of soft contact lenses can be modified by changing either base curve or diameter. Increasing the base curve in millimeters of radius or decreasing the diameter flattens the lens. Decreasing the base curve or increasing the diameter steepens the lens.

• *Example:* *Base curve: 8.6*
Diameter: 13.8 mm
Power: −4.00 D
Steepen the lens by decreasing the base curve to 8.3 or by increasing the diameter to 14.5 mm.
Flatten the lens by increasing the base curve to 8.9. (Decreasing the diameter is another option, although not applicable in this situation due to such a lens' unavailability.)
The power remains at −4.00 D.

• CONTACT LENSES FOR ASTIGMATISM

Several factors determine the best contact lens choice. Determining the type of astigmatism is critical. Corneal astigmatism can be corrected by both rigid and soft toric lenses. Significant lenticular astigmatism usually requires a toric rigid lens or a soft toric lens. When both types of astigmatism are present, a toric soft lens is generally the best option.

An additional factor is the amount of astigmatism. Soft toric lens manufacturers cut lenses that correct approximately 0.75 to 2.50 D of cylinder. Custom lenses can be made with additional correction, however. Rigid lenses can mask significant amounts of corneal cylinder by creating a new spherical optical surface for the eye. When the amount of astigmatic correction exceeds 4.00 D, success with a rigid contact lens with a spherical base curve becomes more limited and a bitoric lens is often required. Two curves 90° apart are cut in the lens, reflecting the curvature of the cornea.

Final considerations in choosing the most appropriate lens for astigmatism are the same as with spherical contact lenses: visual acuity expectations, preferred wearing schedule, and history of success with rigid or toric soft contact lenses.

Toric Soft Contact Lens Fitting

The fitting technique for toric soft contact lenses uses the same guidelines as those for spherical soft lenses for choice of base curve and diameter. Power is determined by the refractometry results in minus cylinder, adjusted for vertex distance. Soft toric lenses incorporate the full refractive correction, sphere, cylinder, and axis, into the lens. Because of the anatomical

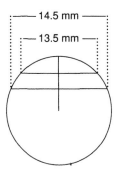

FIGURE 23–6. Relationship between the sagittal depth of a lens and its diameter. If the base curve remains constant, the sagittal depth increases as the diameter increases.

features of the anterior segment of the eye, the lens may shift nasally or temporally rather than rest at the preferred six o'clock position. Assessment of the orientation of the lens on the eye is essential for determination of the cylindrical axis to be ordered. Displacement of the lens marking away from the six o'clock position on the cornea requires adjustment of the axis of the refraction to coordinate the refractive axis with the resting position of the lens. Each clock hour corresponds to a 30° change of axis. The positioning of the axis is determined from the examiner's point of view. As the lens shifts to the left, the change, in degrees, must be added to the refractive axis. As the lens shifts to the right, the change, in degrees, is subtracted from the refractive axis. The mnemonic used for lens axis adjustment is

LARS: Left Add, Right Subtract
The adjustment is made to the axis of the refraction, not to the axis of the trial lens for fitting.

● ***Example:*** *Refraction:* $-3.00 - 1.50 \times 85°$
Trial lens: $2.00 - 1.25 \times 90°$
Position: Axis rests at the 5:30 position on the right eye.
Half a clock hour corresponds to 15°.
The shift is to the right, requiring subtraction from the refractive axis ($85° - 15° = 70°$).
Cylinder power: Set astigmatic powers are available from toric lens manufacturers. Decreasing the amount of cylinder is occasionally tolerated, in part due to the power of the steeper meridian requiring adjustment for vertex distance. The power of the steepest meridian is obtained by adding the power of the sphere to the cylinder in the minus cylinder form of the refraction.
Here: $-3.00 \ D + [-1.50 \ D] \rightarrow -4.50 \ D$
Final lens prescription: $-3.00 - 1.25 \times 70°$.

Success with these lenses depends on the lens's maintaining the same orientation so that of the axis ordered is properly lined up. Stabilization is achieved by employing the following lens designs.

Prism ballast. 1 to 2^Δ base down prism to enhance gravitational pull.

Double slab off. Superior and inferior thin zones to position the lens within the palpebral fissure.

Back surface toric: Optics cut on the posterior lens surface, reflecting the toric curve found with corneal astigmatism.

Eccentric lenticulation. Circumferential lens design to achieve uniform edge thickness.

Truncation. Linear cut along the inferior border of the lens designed for alignment with the lower lid.

● CONTACT LENSES FOR APHAKIA

Contact lenses for aphakia are used most frequently when intraocular lenses are undesirable or contraindicated. Following penetrating ocular trauma, it may be impossible to position and secure an implant. Cataract removal in infants and young children usually requires an aphakic contact lens; an implant often cannot be used because of the changing size of the developing eye in a child.

The type of contact lens for correcting aphakia, whether rigid or soft, depends on the status of the cornea, amount of the tear film, and overall health of the eye. Corneal scarring, whether caused by ocular disease or trauma, results in an irregular corneal surface, and frequently requires a rigid contact lens. Because the plus power necessary to correct aphakia (generally $+10.00$ to $+16.00$ D) is high, the resulting heavy rigid lenses tend to ride low on the cornea. Centration often improves by utilizing an aspheric curvature design which matches the cornea's aspheric surface. An aspheric contact lens will have a greater tendency to remain centered, thus positioning the optical zone of the contact lens over the visual axis. The addition of a minus lenticular carrier (i.e., myoflange) to the rigid lens also enhances lens pick-up by the upper eyelid.

A cornea with a smooth regular surface is generally successful with a soft aphakic contact lens. These lenses are particularly beneficial for comfort. Along with the contact lens, correction for regular corneal astigmatism can be ground into eyeglasses to be worn for distance vision with the necessary bifocal lens for near vision.

When monocular aphakia is present, the prescription for the other eye is taken into consideration to reduce the disparity of image size between the two eyes. The dioptric correction in eyeglasses induces a greater effect on image size than that in a contact lens of the same power. The aphakic eye requires a high plus lens correction. When the phakic eye is myopic, requiring a minus lens for the eyeglasses' prescription, the image size difference from the anisometropia is commonly intolerable, disrupting binocularity. By applying additional plus power in the aphakic contact lens, which is neutralized by applying an equivalent amount of minus power in the eyeglasses' prescription for the aphakic eye, the image size difference is minimized, enhancing binocularity. The following example has a prescription for an aphakic right eye and a myopic left eye:

● ***Example:*** *Right eye (OD):* $+12.00$ *Sph (adjusted for vertex distance)*
Left eye (OS): -2.00 *Sph*
Contact lens: $+14.00$

Eyeglasses' prescription: OD:−2.00 Sph
OS: −2.00 Sph
The focal point is now equal with and without the eyeglasses' correction in place. An increase in the contact lens power to +16.00 D would require an overcorrection of −4.00 D, increasing the minification effect on the image size.

The prescription of the eyeglass lenses should remain within 2.50 D of the disparity, as greater amounts can induce significant prismatic effect (Prentice's rule), when viewing binocularly outside the optical centers of the spectacle correction.

Because of the high power necessary to correct aphakia, the soft contact lens is substantially thicker, ranging from approximately 0.4 to 0.6 mm. As a result, the cornea may receive insufficient oxygen, producing complications such as central superficial punctate keratopathy (SPK), corneal edema, peripheral neovascularization of the cornea, contact lens intolerance, and corneal infections (Fig. 23–7). Contact lenses approved for extended wear but utilized on a daily wear basis improve oxygen delivery, whereas they omit the corneal stress induced by overnight wear.

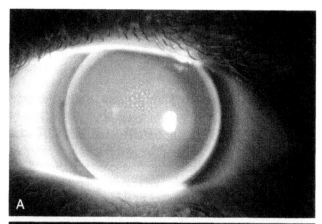

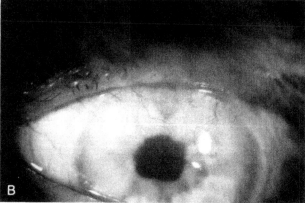

FIGURE 23–7. Complications from contact lens wear. *A,* Superficial punctate keratitis. *B,* Neovascularization.

Pediatric Aphakia

Approximately one week after the removal of an infantile cataract, an aphakic contact lens can be fitted. The steep corneal curvature in infants necessitates a steep base curve for the contact lens (e.g., 7.5 − 7.9 mm). Because of the short axial length of the eye, approximately 17 mm, the power required is high, in the range of +25.00 to +35.00 D. The rapid growth of a child's eye requires changes in power and curvature of the lens and frequent replacement.

Contact lenses composed of 100% silicone are excellent for aphakic correction in infants. The breathability of the material is superior to all other contact lens plastics. Silicone is prone to film—coating with protein from the tear material. This requires replacement approximately every six months.

Soft (HEMA) contact lenses are available for pediatric aphakia. A limited number of companies manufacture lenses with the characteristics of steep base curve and high plus power.

Rigid gas-permeable lenses can be used for aphakic correction in infants. Whereas these lenses transmit oxygen less readily than those of pure silicone, there is less tendency for them to coat with tear film products and the oxygen delivery is adequate.

Both silicone and rigid gas-permeable lenses can be fitted by trial and error with fluorescein to examine fit and tear film exchange (Fig. 23–8). (See Color Plate 39.) Retinoscopy utilizing hand-held trial lenses or a skiascopy bar is performed over a trial contact lens of the appropriate base curve to determine the correct power. Vertex distance of an over-refraction ≥ ± 4.00 D and the working distance of the examiner must be calculated. The distance power, normally corrected for infinity in adults, is overcorrected by +3.00 D to focus the infant at .33 m, the child's primary area of vision. This overcorrection is decreased as the child develops, moving the focal point toward infinity. Amblyopia

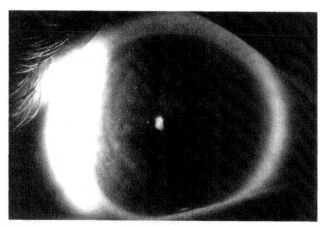

FIGURE 23–8. Subepithelial infiltrates.

treatment is necessary for monocular aphakia in children, requiring patching of the normal phakic eye.

● KERATOCONUS

Keratoconus is a progressive steepening of the anterior cornea accompanied by an increase in myopic correction, astigmatism, and surface irregularity. In its early stages, glasses or soft contact lenses, spherical or toric, may be successful for visual correction. As corneal irregularity worsens, the need for a rigid contact lens becomes necessary to provide the eye with a smooth refractive surface.

Fitting rigid contact lenses for keratoconus begins with estimation of the curvature by keratometry. Corneal curvature, along with myopia, astigmatism, and corneal irregularity, increases as the keratoconus progresses. Keratometry is beneficial for documentation of corneal progression. For early to moderate keratoconus (K of 45.00–50.00 D), rigid gas-permeable lenses are generally successful. As the cone progressively steepens, thinly cut PMMA lenses are often better suited. PMMA lenses have greater resistance to flexure than do gas-permeable lenses, resulting in improved optical clarity. They are thinner than gas-permeable lenses of the same diameter and power. Their decreased mass improves lens performance.

Selection of a base curve that adequately vaults the apex of the cone often results in a lens with a curvature too steep for the peripheral cornea. A small lens diameter (8.0–8.5 mm) allows the steeper lens curvature with the preservation of adequate lens movement and tear exchange. Minimal apical touch can be acceptable provided the lens movement allows tear exchange (see Fig. 24–7).

If a lens curvature steep enough to provide sufficient apical clearance while maintaining appropriate movement cannot be achieved, special design lenses can be used. These include the following:

Soper. Bicurve design with a central curve cut steeper than the peripheral curve to reflect the corneal curvature.

McGuire or "Nipple" Cone. Contour design with a 5.5-mm optical zone, an 8.1-mm diameter, and four peripheral curves reflecting the peripheral cornea.

"Globus" Cone. Similar design using a 6.5-mm optical zone and a 9.1-mm diameter (manufacturer suggested).

● PRESBYOPIA

Correction of presbyopia by contact lenses can be achieved in the following ways:

1. Eyeglasses for reading can be worn over distance powered contact lenses. The advantage is preservation of binocular vision at both distance and near. One disadvantage is the inconvenient and intermittent necessity of eyeglasses.

2. Monovision can be achieved by correcting the dominant eye with a contact lens powered for distance, and correcting the nondominant eye with a contact lens powered for near. The focal point is no longer equal in the two eyes, resulting in decreased stereopsis. An eyeglass prescription which significantly corrects the near reading eye for distance is required for driving purposes. With higher reading powers (e.g., +2.25 D, +2.50 D), this distance correction can result in an anisometropic prescription. Subjective comfort is enhanced by limiting the distance prescription to the minimal power necessary to achieve a visual acuity level that is legal for driving purposes. The advantage of this approach is the clarity of visual acuity achieved with single vision lenses in each eye. The disadvantage is compromised stereopsis.

3. Monobivision involves correcting the dominant eye for distance with a single vision lens, and fitting the nondominant eye with a bifocal contact lens. The advantage is the maintenance of binocularity for distance vision. Disadvantages include decreased stereopsis at near and possible distortion induced by the transitional power zones in the bifocal lens, particularly with a dilated pupil in dim lighting.

4. Bifocal contact lenses correct each eye for both distance and near, maintaining binocularity and stereopsis. Success with bifocal lenses improves when the candidate tolerates potential compromises in visual acuity, accepting optical aberrations including glare, image ghosting, and decreased contrast sensitivity. The presence of a significant distance and near prescription along with an uncomplicated history with contact lenses also improves the rate of success with bifocal contact lenses.

Bifocal lenses can be divided into two basic designs: alternating and simultaneous. Alternating vision lenses provide specific distance and near zones. Translation of the lens is necessary to position the correct zone over the visual axis at the appropriate time. Alternating vision lenses can be categorized as follows:

Segmental. Distance correction centrally with a segment for near correction inferiorly. This design requires stabilization (e.g., prism ballast, truncation).

Annular. A concentric design generally with the distance correction centrally surrounded by a near zone. Alternatively, the central zone can correct for near with the distance zone peripherally.

Simultaneous vision lenses focus for both the distance and near at the same time. The viewer must select which image to focus on. Simultaneous vision lenses can be categorized as follows:

Annular. A concentric design with a small zone for distance or near power with the alternative power in the intermediate peripheral zone.

Aspheric. The central zone is corrected for distance or near with a progressive change in power toward the periphery of the lens.

Diffractive. Concentric echellettes are designed to deflect light, separating it into distance and near components.

Soft and rigid (gas permeable and PMMA) materials are available in both alternating and simultaneous vision designs. Choice of the most appropriate lens material rests on the past experience of the bifocal candidate, visual acuity requirements, and general ocular conditions.

Success with the presbyopic contact lens wearer requires selection of motivated participants who fully understand and are tolerant of the limits of the chosen method of correction.

• CONTACT LENS EXAMINATION TECHNIQUES

New Patient

The contact lens fitting examination begins with a discussion concerning expectations of the lens wearer about contact lenses, and past experiences with contact lenses, so that the fitter understands which type of lens will be most appropriate. Determining the desired wearing schedule (daily, extended, intermittent), visual acuity requirements, and occupational environment is important. Contact lens history including the type of lens worn, the disinfection system used, and any related complications experienced will guide the fitter toward the optimal lens and lens care system. Getting an ocular history is also imperative. Questions are essential concerning ocular surgery, including cataract extraction, glaucoma procedures, corneal transplant, retinal surgery, or blepharoplasty. Strabismus, amblyopia, retinal disease, glaucoma, and trauma may decrease visual acuity potential. In some cases, contact lenses will provide better visual acuity than eyeglasses. This is especially true in anterior corneal dystrophy, corneal scarring, and keratoconus.

A complete medical history, when pertinent for potential ocular involvement, should be documented. Ocular and systemic medications may influence the toleration of contact lenses (e.g., antihistamines).

Following the discussion of ocular and contact lens history, the eye examination begins by testing visual acuity with the patient wearing his or her present correction, either eyeglasses or contact lenses. Refraction over the contact lenses may be necessary, particularly when the chief complaint relates to vision with lenses. Before removal, the lenses should be examined for problems related to fit, including centration, movement with a blink and with lateral gaze, surface deposits, and lens integrity.

Following lens removal, refractometry is performed. Vertex distance is measured in a trial frame for refractive powers of ≥ 4.00 D. Keratometry documents the corneal curvature, indicating its amount and regularity.

A slit-lamp examination of the eye precedes insertion of the trial lens. Corneal clarity, thickness, epithelial integrity, scars, neovascularization, conjunctival injection, tear film amount and integrity, and the eyelid margin and palpebral conjunctiva are examined to provide a baseline status of the eye from which future changes can be assessed. Careful examination can show evidence of complications incurred from previous lens wear. This is of particular concern in follow-up visits for patients with extended wear contact lenses and those who have had corneal trauma. Under these circumstances, ophthalmic technical personnel work closely with the ophthalmologist, because contact lenses induce a greater level of stress to the corneal tissue, and changes are important for assessment and treatment.

Trial lenses (soft, gas-permeable, or hard) with the estimated base curve, diameter, and power are inserted. These lenses are adjusted as necessary, initially by providing the optimal fit, and then with another refraction *over* the lenses to achieve the best power for optimal vision.

Success with contact lenses may rely on appropriate instruction. Before dispensing the lenses, instruction on correct insertion and removal techniques is necessary, including

1. Washing hands prior to handling the lenses
2. Avoiding soaps with (lotions or) moisturizers
3. Inserting the lens before applying hand/facial cream, make-up, hair spray, or the like
4. Being certain the area for placement is clean and free of airborne contaminants
5. Beginning with the same eye each time
6. Understanding a dropped lens requires thorough surfactant cleaning, rinsing, and disinfection
7. Disinfecting immediately following lens removal when surface deposits are still at body temperature.

Thorough discussion concerning contact lens disinfection must be completed to avoid unnecessary complications. It is advisable to have the disinfection procedure verbally repeated by the wearer in a sequential manner to avoid any misunderstandings. Every lens care kit contains instructions. Attention should be brought to this fact.

Scheduled wearing time is given in writing to all new lens wearers as follows:

Rigid gas-permeable and hard lenses

Days 1 to 3—Wear 3 hours, remove for 1 hour, wear 3 hours

Days 4 to 6—Wear 4 hours, remove for 1 hour, wear 4 hours

Days 7 to 10—Wear for 5 to 6 hours.

Increase 1 additional hour every other day

Maximum advised wearing time: 15 hours/day

The cornea benefits from an hour (prior to sleeping) without the contact lens every night

Soft contact lenses

Days 1 to 3—Wear 8 to 10 hours

Days 4 to 6—Wear 10 to 12 hours

After the first week, wear the lenses up to 15 hours/ day. Allow a minimum hour without the contact lens each night.

A final note of caution ought to accompany dispensing the lenses. Should the patient's eye become red or painful, should they experience a decrease in visual acuity, or should they produce *any* discharge, remove the lenses immediately. In most cases, the incident is nothing more than a torn contact lens or foreign matter in the eye. If the symptoms do not resolve within an hour after removal contact an emergency care physician.

Planned follow-up examinations are essential for subjective complaints, difficulties, questions, and reassessment of lens fit. The first follow-up with daily wear lenses occurs 1 to 2 weeks after dispensing. Changes in the base curve or power may be required at that time. Signs of allergies to solutions (itchiness) or toxicity (redness, punctate epitheliopathy) will necessitate a change in the lens care system. Transient complaints with lenses often include foreign body sensation (FBS), tearing, photophobia, and slight visual acuity fluctuations. These are generally adaptive and diminish with time.

At the final follow-up examination a month later, toleration by the eye to the contact lens is assessed, while examining for signs of corneal edema, SPK, and limbal injection. Subjective comfort, wear time, and visual stability are key indicators of toleration.

Regular annual checkups are necessary for daily lens wearers. Lens replacement for conventional daily soft lenses should be expected at least annually. Gas-permeable lenses need replacement every 18 to 24 months. Frequent replacement lenses are replaced according to manufacturer's guidelines.

Extended-Wear Lenses

Extended-wear lenses should be used with substantial caution. These are fitted if their wearing is justified, if the eye is healthy, if there is no history of contact lens complications, and if the patient is aware of the increased risk of infection. They are not usually pre-scribed for the novice contact lens wearer. Following the dispensing of extended-wear lenses, it is advisable for the patient to wear them during waking hours for a few days to assess comfort and tolerance prior to overnight use. The lenses can thereafter be kept in during sleep. Lubrication is advised prior to sleeping and upon awakening. Visual acuity should be normal within 15 minutes of awakening. A follow-up visit is usually scheduled for early the morning after beginning extended wear. Examination should show a freely moving lens without adherence to the ocular tissue, and no signs of corneal edema or conjunctival injection.

Following the overnight examination, the lens may be kept in for a maximum of 7 days with a return visit prior to removal, when increasing stress is placed on the ocular tissue, so that signs of intolerance may be seen. A repeat examination is scheduled about a month later, near the end of a 7-day wearing period.

A consent form must be read, discussed, and signed, for all extended-wear lens patients because there is an increased risk of complication and infection. Responsibility rests with the contact lens fitter to ensure that the risks are understood. Because of the extended wear time and increased stress on ocular tissues, follow-up examinations and lens replacements are usually scheduled at least every 6 months.

Regular Follow-up Examination

When the contact lens wearer is seen for regular follow-up, the fitter inquires about (1) present lens comfort, (2) average daily wearing time, (3) stability and clarity of visual acuity both with the contact lenses and with the present eyeglasses, and (4) excessive blurred vision with eyeglasses after contact lens removal. This spectacle blur is induced by a cornea with a curvature that has transiently been modified by the wearing of a contact lens. Compliance and knowledge of the lens cleaning and disinfection system and frequency of enzyme cleaning should be discussed.

The examination includes testing visual acuity with present contact lenses and eyeglasses. An over-refraction may be necessary, but because of increased accommodation brought on by subnormal vision through filmed, aged lenses, accuracy may be improved by refraction without the contact lens followed by an over-refraction with the new trial lenses in place. Expect to reach the same visual acuity level as on the initial examination. If subnormal vision persists, pay close attention to signs of corneal warpage. Both soft and rigid lenses can induce corneal irregularities, signs of which include irregular retinoscopic reflex, irregular keratometric mires, increased astigmatism and/or change in astigmatic axis, and improvement of vision by a spherical rigid lens to resurface the cornea.

Achieving normal vision by refraction does not negate the necessity for assessment of keratometry on a regular basis. Keratometry often provides the earliest indication of potential corneal warpage. This is followed by a slit-lamp examination for a close view of both the ocular tissues and the contact lens. Key elements of ocular examination include

Bulbar conjunctiva, lining the eye, should be quiet. Injection, particularly in the limbal region, is evidence of hypoxia or solution allergies.

Palpebral conjunctiva, lining the upper eyelids, is viewed for signs of papillary or follicular reactions, i.e., giant papillary conjunctivitis

Corneal examination for clarity of the tissue, overall thickness, epithelial integrity, subepithelial infiltrates, and peripheral neovascularization (see Fig. 23–8).

All can indicate poor contact lens tolerance and must be treated accordingly. Lens wear must be discontinued until the tissue returns to normal.

The avascular cornea gets its oxygen from direct exposure to the air and tear film. Long-term covering with a contact lens can induce a low grade "suffoca-tion" of the cornea. Peripheral neovascularization extending from the limbus onto the cornea is evidence of hypoxia. Treatment may not require discontinuing lens wear, but rather improvement may follow a reduction of lens wear time, a change in lens plastic to one with a higher water content, thinner design, or an extended-wear lens but on a daily wear basis. With success, the blood will recede from the vessels, leaving "ghost" vessels.

Along with examination of the eye, a close evaluation of the contact lenses must be made. Tear film deposits, such as protein, calcium, and mucin, layer out on both soft and gas-permeable lenses. They decrease the wettability by the tear film over the surface of the lens, reduce oxygen transmission, decrease visual acuity, lessen comfortable wear time, and cause increased bacterial coverage over the lens surface. The integrity of the lens must be examined for surface scratches, cracks within the body of the lens, and chips along the lens edge. The presence of such defects requires lens replacement (Fig. 23–9).

Follow-up examinations provide an excellent opportunity to recheck intraocular pressure for glaucoma screening and to complete a dilated fundus examination by the ophthalmologist.

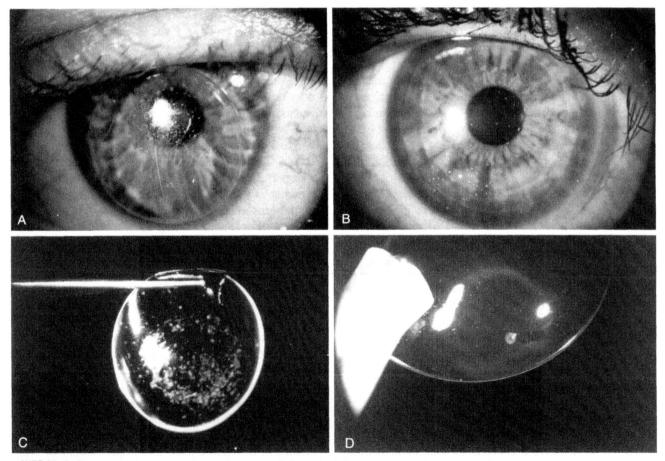

FIGURE 23–9. Old contact lenses needing replacement. *A,* Scratched rigid gas-permeable lens with film. *B,* Lens with calcium deposits. *C,* Tear along lens edge, and deposits. *D,* Fungus growing on lens.

CONTACT LENS COMPLICATIONS

Successful contact lens wear can be enhanced when relative contraindications to lens wear are addressed. These include

Dry eye

Blepharitis

Ocular/systemic allergies

Corneal dystrophy

History of lack of success in wearing contact lenses

Occupation

Cleanliness

Comprehension of contact lens care and handling

Recognition of these situations may require a change in the contact lens or the lens care system dispensed, or it may ultimately rule out the use of contact lenses. The following is a list of common contact lens problems and their potential causes. (See Color Plates 18, 19, 23, and 24.)

1. Poor visual acuity
   Change in prescription
   Aged lens
   Lens deposits
   Lens switch
   Poorly fitted lens
   Lens manufacturing
2. Red eye
   Adapting to new lenses
   Contamination of the lens by foreign matter
   Lens too tight
   Poor blink
   Contact lens overwear
   Conjunctivitis
   Ocular infection
3. Contact lens discomfort
   Adaptation to new lenses
   Lens deposits
   Inverted lens
   Foreign body
   Corneal abrasion
   Allergy related to lens or solutions
   Contact lens overwear
   Ocular infection
4. Giant papillary conjunctivitis
   Generalized allergies
   Allergy to lens plastic
   Reaction to lens film
5. Contact lens overwear
   Tight lens fit
   Aged contact lens
   Excessive lens wear time either daily or over years
   Inadequate oxygen transmission for corneal needs
   Inadequate lens care
   Corneal intolerance to contact lenses
6. Contact lens–related sterile corneal infiltrates
   Toxic reaction to solutions
   Corneal hypoxia
   Lens-related allergies

Contact Lens Disinfection

General rules for contact lens disinfection
- Lenses should be disinfected every time they are removed from the eye.
- Only sterile contact lens solution should be used. Tap water, distilled water, or homemade saline solutions should *never* be used.
- A 4-hour minimum time period is generally required for chemical disinfection of both soft and rigid contact lenses.
- Lenses can be stored for up to 48 hours following disinfection. Longer periods require redisinfection prior to insertion.
- Contact lens cases should be replaced every 2 to 3 months. This greatly diminishes the accumulation that builds up from daily contamination. (Fig. 23–10).
- Open containers of any ocular or contact lens solutions should be discarded after 1 month. The pre-servative in the solution can become over-whelmed by microbial growth.

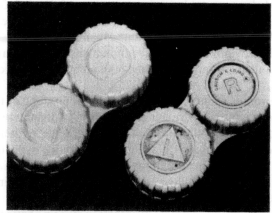

FIGURE 23–10. Lens cases. Case on left is new. Soiled case on right is 6 months old.

7. Contact lens–related infections

Organism (bacterial, fungal, or acanthamoebic), derived from contamination of lens, cleaning solutions, case, or corneal hypoxia

Awareness of the effects of these potential complications is important. Educating the contact lens wearer about them is essential. Contact lens–related problems can most often be avoided with planned follow-up care, appropriate lens replacement, and adequate lens care.

Rigid Contact Lenses

Surfactant cleaners work to remove surface debris, microbial biofilm, and tear film deposits. The cleaning process should be maintained for 30 seconds. Advise the patient to rinse the lens thoroughly with sterile contact lens saline solution. Immerse the lens in a soaking and disinfection solution. Disinfection takes place as the preservative acts in the solution, and a 4 hour minimum soak is required.

Weekly use of an enzymatic cleaner is strongly advised with gas-permeable lenses. The suggested soak time is 2 hours. Surfactant cleaning, rinsing, and disinfection should follow this procedure. Prior to insertion, a gentle massage with a wetting, soaking, or conditioning solution is beneficial. The purpose of this solution is to lower the wetting angle of the plastic, thus allowing the tear film to spread evenly over the lens surface following the blink.

Soft Contact Lenses

There are three basic disinfection procedures for soft contact lenses, including peroxide, other chemicals, and heat. All systems require the initial surfactant cleaner for 30 seconds, followed by a sterile saline rinse. The surfactant allows greater lens surface exposure for the disinfectant. Enzymatic cleaning is recommended on a weekly basis, regardless of the disinfection system. All soft contact lenses can utilize a peroxide or chemical system. Heat systems can be employed only for most soft contact lenses with a water content less than 55% (check manufacturer's guidelines).

Peroxide disinfection systems are consistent in the presence of 3% hydrogen peroxide as the disinfectant, but they vary in the duration of the peroxide soak and in the method of neutralization. The peroxide exposure time ranges from 10 minutes to overnight. Neutralization of peroxide follows, leaving the lens soaking in a buffered saline solution and ready for insertion.

Nonperoxide chemical disinfection systems have the action of a preservative in the solution as the antimicrobial agent. A 4-hour minimum soak is mandatory. Ocular sensitivities to the preservative may occur, necessitating changing lens care systems.

Heat disinfection requires a minimum 10-minute soak at a temperature of $\geq 80°C$. Whereas heat is very effective as a disinfectant, it has several disadvantages. First of all, heat frequently shortens the life span of the soft lens. Second, if tear film deposits are not adequately removed during use of the surfactant cleaner, they can be heated onto the surface. Electricity is needed, which can be inconvenient.

Compliance and comprehension are the key factors to be stressed when giving instruction concerning contact lens care. Complete understanding of the cleaning and disinfection procedure and the potential complications of improper use should be known.

Finally, relay to the patient the importance of continuing with the lens care system dispensed. A change to a different brand can lead to misuse, or incomplete disinfection. Patients wanting to change should be requested to discuss this with qualified personnel.

Bibliography

Crews MJ, Driebe WT, Stern GA: The Clinical Management of Keratoconus: A Six-Year Retrospective Study. CLAO J 20:194–197, 1994.
Hales RH: Contact Lenses: A Clinical Approach to Fitting, 2nd ed. Baltimore, Williams & Wilkins, 1982.
Key JE: CLAO Pocket Guide to Contact Lens Fitting. New York, Kellner/McCaffery Assoc. Inc., 1994.

• CHAPTER 23 CONTACT LENSES

1. What defines the ease with which oxygen passes through a contact lens?
   a. Dk level
   b. water content
   c. acrylate content
   d. fragility factor
   e. sagittal depth.

2. Average corneal curvatures use soft contact lenses with base curves of which value (mm)?
   a. 8.1–8.3
   b. 8.8–9.0
   c. 7.6–7.8
   d. 8.4–8.6
   e. 7.8–8.0.

3. If a patient has keratometry readings of 43.00/44.50 @ 90° and refractometry of $-4.00 -1.50 \times 180°$, which astigmatism is described?
   a. 1.50 D corneal astigmatism and 3.00 D lenticular astigmatism
   b. 1.50 D corneal astigmatism
   c. 1.50 D corneal astigmatism and 1.50 D lenticular astigmatism
   d. 1.50 D lenticular astigmatism
   e. no astigmatism.

4. How do you steepen the fit of a rigid contact lens?
    a. increase the diameter of the radius of curvature
    b. decrease the base curve in diopters
    c. decrease the lens diameter
    d. decrease base curve and decrease lens diameter
    e. increase the base curve in diopters.

5. What is the power of the flattest corneal meridian equal to?
    a. spherical equivalent
    b. sphere of the refraction in minus cylinder form
    c. sphere of the refraction in plus cylinder form plus +0.50 D
    d. sphere of the refraction in plus cylinder form
    e. sphere of the refraction in minus cylinder form plus −0.50 D.

Donald Enkerud

Ophthalmic Photography

LEARNING OBJECTIVES

- Describe the relationships among shutter speed, aperture number, and film speed
- Define the relationship between ISO film rating and film sensitivity
- Describe the benefit of an electronic flash unit
- Differentiate among telephoto, normal, and wide-angle lenses
- Differentiate digital, fluorescein, and indocyanine green angiograms
- List three contraindications to angiography
- List four mild reactions to fluorescein injection
- List three major reactions to fluorescein injection

Ophthalmic photography improves patient care by providing documentary and diagnostic photographic evidence. *Documentary photographs* provide the viewer with a rapid factual record of the eye as it was seen on a particular visit. Some examples of documentary photography include

1. Fundus photography
2. Endothelial photography
3. Slit-lamp biomicrography
4. External photography

Diagnostic photographs allow the physician to see things normally hidden. Examples of diagnostic photography include

1. Fluorescein angiography
2. Digital angiography
3. Indocyanine green (ICG) angiography.

To many ophthalmic technical personnel, learning to do ophthalmic photography may be intimidating. Ophthalmic technical personnel should understand two general photographic guidelines. The fundamental principles of photography must first be understood, and then this knowledge is adapted to the specific needs of ophthalmic photography. We explore the basics of photographic theory here only as necessary to accomplish our task.

● PHOTOGRAPHIC BASICS

Photography uses a camera body (light-proof box) with an imaging mechanism (lens) to place an image on light-sensitive material (film). The light passes through a small opening (aperture), which opens and closes (shutter), briefly to allow light to strike the film.

Camera Body

Basic, important components in the capture and control of the photographic image involve the camera, which keeps film in the dark, until we are ready to take a picture. In contemporary photography, the most basic part is the camera body. This term refers to a camera without a lens or accessories. The camera body is frequently modified by adding tools to make our tasks easier.

Shutter

The shutter is an opaque window that opens and closes rapidly to allow the film to be briefly exposed to light. This shutter stays open for a finite, but variable, length of time, controlled by a dial usually located somewhere on the camera body. The shutter is most often located just in front of the light-sensitive film. Many common focal plane shutters are not one piece, but two. One opaque window moves out of the way and then a second opaque window races across the film aperture to stop the exposure. The width of the gap between the two opaque windows controls the length of the time the film is exposed to light, measured in fractions of a second, i.e, 1/15, 1/30, or 1/60. The gaps are arranged so that each speed halves the next speed, so, thereby if you increase shutter speed from 1/60 to 1/125, you halve the exposure time. This variable can be controlled manually or automatically, depending on the camera (Fig. 24–1).

Camera shutters usually work reliably but may occasionally fail. Ophthalmic photographers usually recognize the characteristic images created by a camera with a malfunctioning shutter. Typically, this type of failure needs to be corrected by a qualified camera repair technician.

Film Transport

So far, we have described a box that holds our film and a shutter to regulate how long the light strikes the film. Film is bought in long rolls so that we can take numerous pictures before reloading. The film transport within the camera body moves the film from one picture to the next after an exposure is made. Many cameras use a manual film transport. Typically, there is a winding lever on top of the camera body which you advance with your thumb to pull the film through the camera. Other cameras use a motorized system to pull the film through automatically. Besides being convenient, this automatic system allows the ophthalmic photographer to move quickly from picture to picture without pausing to advance the film. Because the film transport is a mechanical device, it is prone to failure.

Once we have taken all the desired pictures, the film has to be removed from the camera. Most 35mm cameras use a *rewind knob* to roll the film backward through the camera into the cassette from which it came. On manual-wind cameras, this rewind is also manual. On most motor-driven film transports, there is a motor-driven rewind. With both systems, there is usually a locking device or switch that must be disengaged before the camera will allow the film to be rewound. This switch allows the camera to be temporarily "put in reverse" as we recover the film (Fig. 24–2).

Lens

A lens is attached to the camera body to take pictures, and is used either as a freestanding device, which we could hold in our hands, or on a tripod, e.g., to photograph a face. Frequently, however, we take pictures of the inside of the eye or highly magnified pictures of the external eye. In this case, we remove the lens from the body and attach the body to special optical systems to take the required pictures. These devices, such as fundus cameras or photo-slit lamps, are specialized optical tools that effectively replace the lens.

A simple lens is similar to those on most 35mm cameras. Although a camera body can be simple in design, a quality lens is generally complex. That complexity is usually not considered by photographers, but a few variables should be known. The first is *focal length*. The focal length of a lens is the distance from its optical center to the point where the rays of light being imaged pop into focus. Focal length is usually measured in millimeters (mm).

Photographers categorize lenses by focal length into three broad categories (Fig. 24–3).

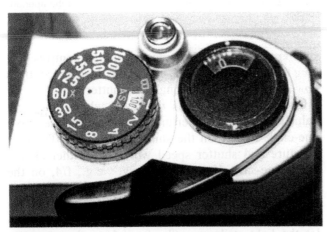

FIGURE 24–1. Shutter speed dial (on the left). (Copyright owned by Donald Enkerud.)

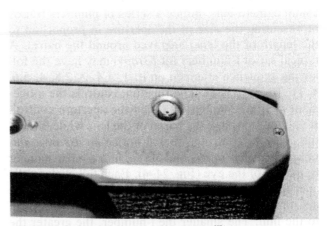

FIGURE 24–2. This push button, similar to the clutch in a car, allows the film transport to turn to reverse, so that the film can rewind. (Copyright owned by Donald Enkerud.)

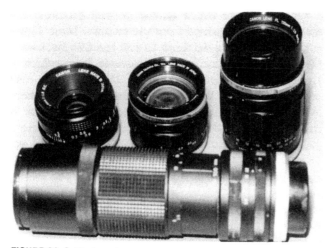

FIGURE 24–3. Various lenses.

1. Telephoto—This lens has a long focal length. The optics of a telephoto lens make the image appear to be larger, or closer, than when viewed with the naked eye.

2. Normal—The normal lens renders an image with the perspective approximately equivalent to what we see with our own eyes, i.e., the image looks neither bigger nor smaller than we would perceive it.

3. Wide-angle—A wide-angle lens has a very short focal length; this has the opposite effect of a telephoto lens. This lens pushes things farther away, but increases the angle of view. As a consequence, it enables a photographer to incorporate a greater area into a photographic space.

This classification of lenses as telephoto, normal, or wide-angle is somewhat subjective. For our purposes, wide-angle lenses are smaller than 45mm, normal lenses range from 45mm to 70mm, and telephoto lenses are larger than 75mm. Thus, a 35mm lens is considered moderately wide-angle. A 50–55mm lens is the most common normal lens. A 200mm lens is a moderately powerful telephoto.

A lens offers aperture control. Looking at a typical 35mm camera lens, notice a series of numbers (ratios representing the size of the aperture in proportion to the length of the lens) engraved around the barrel. A typical set of f-numbers (or *f-stops*) may have the following sequence stamped on it: 1, 1.4, 2, 2.8, 4, 5.6, 8, 11, 16, 22, 32, 45. The ring that controls the movement of these numbers is called the aperture control. If you look through the barrel of the lens while turning the aperture control, you will notice an *iris* or a *diaphragm,* which opens and closes in a similar manner to the iris of the eye (Fig. 24–4). Each full click on the aperture dial either doubles or halves the size of the aperture and the amount of light that we allow through to the film. The smaller the f-number, the greater the amount of light admitted. The larger the f-number, the

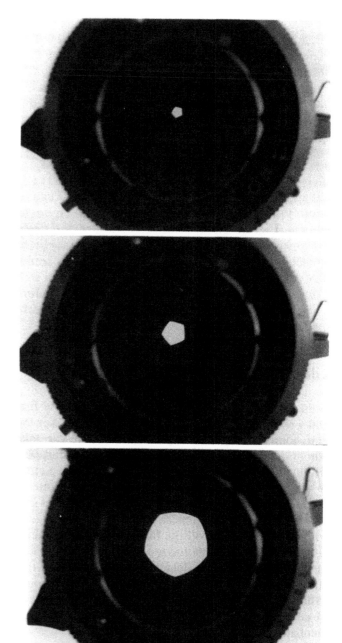

FIGURE 24–4. Changes in aperture size by adjusting the aperture control.

smaller the aperture. Whereas the *shutter* controls *how long* light hits our film, the size of the *aperture* controls *how much* light gets through the shutter.

The next key point is that each whole numerical value change of the aperture control is equivalent to a one-click change on the shutter speed dial. Think of aperture and shutter speed working together almost like a see-saw. If we go ''heavy,'' e.g., f/4, on the amount of light we are letting into our camera, we can compensate by allowing the light to strike the film for a shorter duration time. Alternatively, if we desire to let the light strike our film for a long time, we can balance the effect by making the hole, or aperture, very small, e.g., f/8.

Depth of Field

Depth of field may dictate whether our photographs are sharp or fuzzy. For any given subject, there is exactly one spot where the rays of light falling on the film are exactly in focus. The location of that spot is infinitesimally thin. Rays of light focusing in front of or behind that spot are unfocused in a photograph. The term *depth of field* refers to the amount of distance that can be induced into the focusing system and still render an image of acceptable sharpness. The depth of field is the distance between the nearest object and farthest object in a scene that are both acceptably in focus.

Depth of field can be regulated by two controls. Aperture is the most common way. A smaller aperture (higher f-number) generally yields greater depth of field. Larger apertures (lower f-number) restrict the depth of acceptable focus. Focal length can also alter depth of field. A wide angle lens with its shorter focal length gives greater apparent depth of field for a given aperture than a telephoto lens does. Increasing the f-number and using a brighter light source can also compensate. The high levels of magnification so critical to ophthalmic photographers are not forgiving because the closer to the lens the photographic object lies, the shallower the depth of focus. Accurate focus is critical for the ophthalmic photographer.

Film

Film may be the most important link in the entire chain. It is the last general photographic component to understand before we concentrate on specific ophthalmic-related details. Although there are hundreds of types of film available, we need be concerned with only a few choices. Ophthalmic photographers usually either take color slides of patient pathology or perform fluorescein angiograms with black-and-white film.

Color slide film creates a positive image on the film, which can be developed and viewed immediately. The film itself is processed, turning into a usable color image, cut, and then mounted into plastic or cardboard slide mounts. Because there are neither negatives nor prints made from them, the images are sharper and more faithful to the original subject. There is usually little interpretation of the colors or brightness that would ordinarily be introduced in the printing process. Color slide film is employed most often in ophthalmic photography. Almost all major film manufacturers make acceptable color slide film. Kodachrome, Fujichrome, and Ektachrome are three such slide films. Although photographers tend to be biased toward the brand of film they prefer, most high quality slide films work well for ophthalmic photography.

Quality aside, however, all films are not the same. The variable is *film speed,* the sensitivity of film to light. A film that is very sensitive is called "fast" film. Conversely, a film that requires more light to take the same picture is "slow." There exists a relative film speed scale that is uniform from film to film, manufacturer to manufacturer, and nation to nation. This *film speed rating* is regulated by the International Standards Organization (ISO). (It was previously measured as an ASA number.) Every roll of film has an ISO rating. The smaller the number, the slower (or less light sensitive) the film is, and the higher the number, the greater the film's light sensitivity. If we were to take samples of film and place them on a table in increasing order or sensitivity, we might read the following ISO numbers on the film boxes: 25, 50, 64, 100, 160, 200, 400, 800, 1600, and 3200. The highest number, 3200, is the most sensitive (fastest) film listed; ISO 25 film is the slowest listed.

There are many reasons to choose one film over another based on relative film speed. The most significant reason is image quality. In general, the faster (more light sensitive) the film, the poorer the image quality. Faster film must incorporate larger pieces of light-sensitive compound in its make-up, which allow more rays of light to strike and activate it. The film, when developed, will show a "graininess" that may be disturbing. Slow film, by comparison, has an almost imperceptible grain structure. This very high quality image requires a greater amount of light to form the image because there are many elements of an image-forming, light-sensitive compound. Their great number gives the image incredible detail. Because they are small, however, it takes more light to activate them. Ophthalmic photographers typically use color slide film with an ISO ranging from 25 to 200. Both Kodak Ektachrome 100 and Fuji Fujichrome 100 are excellent general purpose films (Fig. 24–5).

Color adds no usable information to the fluorescein angiographic process. It would be a waste of time, money, and effort to use it. Black-and-white negative films for angiography come in similar speed-rated categories. Because we are taking rapid sequence pictures with many filters on the lens, which impair the passage of light, ophthalmic photographers almost always use a fairly fast black-and-white film. Some popular black-and-white films include Kodak Tri-X, Kodak T-MAX, and Ilford HP5. All these films have an ISO rating of 400, which makes them relatively fast.

If the ISO rating of a film is doubled, the sensitivity of that film is increased by a factor of two, i.e., ISO

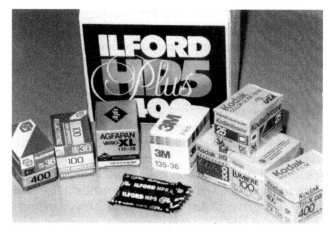

FIGURE 24–5. Examples of color film of various light sensitivities.

200 film is twice as sensitive to light as ISO 100. There is a 1 to 1 correlation among film speed, aperture, and shutter speed. A one unit change in any one of these variables is exactly equivalent to a corresponding one unit change in one of the other variables in the opposite direction.

Exposure

So far, we have discussed the camera hardware. With the addition of film, we are ready to take a picture. For any given "scene" that we would like to photograph, whether a beach, a party, or the inside of an eye, a certain amount of light is required to generate the proper exposure. Many cameras available today solve this problem with on-board computer chips or indicators to determine the optimal exposure.

The amount of light coming through a lens can be monitored by a light meter, which is calibrated to a medium level of color brightness and mounted inside the camera. The standard visual reference point is a medium (18%) gray. The light meter forces you to set the controls on the camera in such a way that standardized reference brightness is reproduced. Most of the time, this works readily enough.

Assume you have chosen a fast shutter speed that allows light to expose the film for only a short period of time because you want to stop the action. The light meter then tells you that you need more light to reach the film in order to compensate for the short exposure. You either open the aperture to a larger diameter (smaller f-stop) or have a higher speed film (higher ISO number) in the camera. By manipulating aperture, shutter speed, and film speed, we can almost always arrive at a correct exposure.

When performing fluorescein angiography or color photography of the retina, we use a very bright, but also very brief (<1/1000 sec), light burst from an electronic

flash unit to illuminate the inside of the eye. The intensity of the electronic flash is so strong that it becomes the exposure setting tool in a flash photograph. With flash photography we either run tests by trial and error or rely on the on-board computer chips to determine the correct exposure.

Filters

Filters serve many purposes in photography. Some change colors; some lighten or darken a subject; some eliminate reflections. All modify light in some way.

There are two broad classes of filters. *Absorption filters* absorb every color of light except the color of the filter, e.g., a green filter appears green because it is absorbing every color of light except green. Green passes through and is perceived by your visual system. Absorption filters are very common and easy to produce. For scientific work, however, we can obtain much more precision with the interference filters of ophthalmic photography. *Interference filters* consist of a precision coating evaporated onto an optical glass surface. This coating reflects every color of the spectrum *except* the color to be passed through the filter. Looking at these filters, they may appear silvery or mirrored. They are much more precise and much more costly then absorption filters.

External Photography

The simplest application of ophthalmic photography is external photography, which uses a camera that most closely resembles a standard 35mm camera. The only additions are a *macro lens* and an *electronic flash unit*. A macro lens is a conventional lens that has been designed to allow focusing very close up. The ability to focus closely allows the image recorded on the film to be much larger than normal. An electronic flash unit is added to the camera body to provide sufficient light to enhance the clarity and detail of the photograph. Current computerized electronic flash units make calculating exposures extremely easy.

External photography records clinical details at a level generally observable by the human eye. The photographer may photograph both eyes, one eye, the entire head or face of a patient, or other anatomic structures. The following types are the most common:

1. *Full-face photography* images the entire head and face of a patient. The patient should be facing in the direction that offers the best view of the pathologic condition under consideration, but generally with the patient looking straight ahead at the photographer. A plain, unpatterned, nondistracting background in a neutral color, such as a medium gray, is desirable.

When framing the subject in the viewfinder, try to compose tightly without excessive background visible around the patient, but do not compose so tightly that the top of the head, chin, or ears are cropped off.

2. *Mask photography* is done by moving the camera close enough to the patient so that both eyes and the bridge of the nose can be imaged within the 35mm frame. The ears and the background should not be visible. These mask-like photographs are taken for many diagnostic purposes. The most common is to document ocular alignment, sometimes called "strabismus series," or the "nine diagnostic positions of gaze." In this series, the patient's head is looking straight ahead at all times. The patient then shifts the gaze from straight ahead to up, up and toward the patient's left, left, down and toward the left, down, down and toward the patient's right, right, up and toward the right, and then straight ahead once again. It is similar to going around a clock, with the patient's nose at the center of the dial: up is the 12-o'clock position, left is the 3-o'clock position, and right is 9 o'clock.

Special Considerations in External Photography

Although while relatively straightforward, the photographer may avoid some pitfalls by attending to basic techniques, including

1. Holding the camera steady. Because we work at higher than normal magnifications, the camera must be braced tightly between your face, arms, and body to provide a stable platform to ensure clear and sharp photographs. Photographers hold their breath and squeeze (not press) the shutter release button at the exact moment of exposure. Competent camera handling and accurate focusing are essential to limit the lack of sharpness within any photograph.

2. Depth of field. Maximize depth of field by using an electronic flash to allow working with small apertures. Even so, the range of depth of field in macrophotography is very limited.

3. Unusual pathology. Knowing exactly what to photograph and how to do it come with experience. Certain photographic tricks help illustrate a diagnostic entity. For example, proptosis (protrusion of the eyes) can be best shown by photographing the eyes from above the patient's head looking down toward the chin. To do so, have the patient recline in an examination chair and stand behind the patient's head. When photographing lesions, use a simple paper or nonreflective plastic scale to document size.

Special Equipment for External Photography

We have mentioned macro lenses that focus at closer working distances than normal, thus allowing the image size to be considerably larger than one obtained with a conventional lens. Macro lenses are probably best suited for this task, but it *is* possible to take very high quality close-up photographs without a macro lens. A simple device for close focusing capability is the extension tube, which is a spacer placed between the camera lens and the camera body. Another alternative is a close-up lens set, which can be screwed in front of a conventional lens much as a magnifying glass is held in front of your eye (Fig. 24–6).

Electronic Flash Units

An electronic flash unit is almost essential with external photography. First, the brief flash illumination is brilliant, thus allowing the use of a smaller aperture to create greater depth of field. Moreover, the direct nature of the light tends to show imperfections extremely well. Many electronic flash units couple electronically with the camera to provide automatic exposure calculation. This is generally very reliable and is an excellent way to deal with the subtle variables encountered in macro photography. Automated electronic flash units reading from the automatic light meters in cameras, however, can be fooled. Remember that an extremely bright or extremely dark subject can confuse the meter into calculating exposures that can result in substandard photographs. Remember that your light meter will probably not work with a dark black background or an overly bright background. Similarly, a camera-mounted electronic flash unit can completely miss the subject when brought within a few inches of the patient. Even a patient's complexion will be factored into the exposure equation. Heavily pigmented individuals may have their images somewhat overexposed as the built-in light meter tries to adjust the light to illuminate the subject. Many photographers utilize a more sensitive film, for example ISO 200, for external photography in an effort to maximize depth of field.

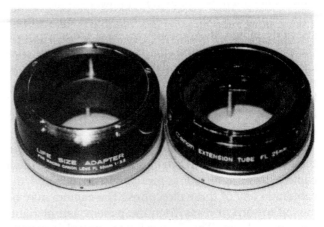

FIGURE 24–6. A close-up lens with an extension tube.

● COLOR FUNDUS PHOTOGRAPHY

Fundus photography is relatively easy despite the unusual equipment necessary.

Equipment

The fundus camera has an incredibly complex lens and an electronic flash unit that combine to produce a camera with a modified ophthalmoscope. Think of the fundus camera as a low-powered microscope lying on its side. We attach a camera body to the optics of a system that images the inside of the eye. The term fundus camera describes the assembly of the optics, flash unit, and 35mm camera body required to photograph the human retina. Whereas the optics of a fundus camera are fairly complex, the important points are few and easily remembered.

1. The illumination system of a fundus camera projects a "doughnut" of light, a circular ring of illumination, onto the retina. By the time the light reaches the retina, it has diffused. The light reflected from the retina passes back through the "doughnut hole" to be recorded on 35mm film.

2. There are two built-in illumination systems. First is a *viewing illumination system* which is powered by a continuous light source such as an incandescent lamp or halogen lamp inside the optical head assembly. Normally, this is coupled to a brightness control regulated by the photographer. A balance must be struck between illuminating the fundus with sufficient brightness to focus the camera and maintaining a comfortable environment for the patient. Trial and error is the only way to establish that balance.

The second illumination system is an *electronic flash source*. The electronic flash of light allows a sharp image to be reflected back to the film. The brief duration of an electronic flash also helps to stop motion from the patient's eye. The electronic flash unit inside the camera head will be coupled to a power supply. Some of these power supplies are floor mounted while others are table mounted. Some newer cameras incorporate the power supply within the camera body itself. Regardless, controls are available to the photographer to regulate the brightness or intensity of the flash. The brightness may be regulated for patient comfort, but it is primarily to adjust the flash levels for the various film sensitivities (speed) chosen.

3. The ophthalmic photographer should think in three dimensions when handling a fundus camera. Each camera has a controlling mechanism to position the camera in any of three directions. The camera may be moved toward or away from the patient, left or right, and up or down. This 3-coordinate control is usually present in the form of a handgrip, or joystick, located on the table surface that supports the fundus camera (Fig. 24–7). Some joysticks are coaxial. The stick that controls forward/backward, and left/right functions also controls up/down using a rotary motion. Other cameras have two controls, one for forward/backward, and the other for up/down. By necessity, the tables that support the fundus camera move easily, to allow positioning of the camera in front of the patient's eye.

4. The camera body and film are attached to the optical and electronic components. The camera body may or may not look like the camera we take on vacation. Nevertheless, it is still a box in which the film is kept dark until the moment of exposure. Some fundus cameras are coupled to their 35mm camera bodies by myriad wires and cables. Others have internal coupling pins to link the two systems (Fig. 24–8). The three circuits that must be controlled are power to the camera body, a trigger to release the shutter, and a cable to synchronize the shutter with the flash. On newer camera systems, the wires controlling these functions are replaced by electrical contacts recessed in the camera body.

Procedures

Color fundus photography is flash photography of the patient's eye. The basic procedures follow.

1. Educate the patient. Because we are not photographing inanimate objects, we have an obligation to help the patient understand the purpose and nature of the procedure. Color fundus photographs document the evolution of the patient's condition from visit to visit. Sequential fundus photography is one of the best tools available to the ophthalmologist to monitor a given condition.

2. Dilate the patient's eyes. Ophthalmic photogra-

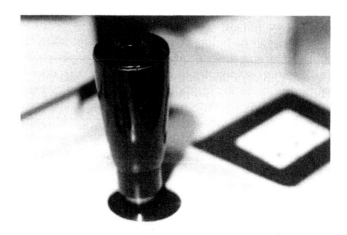

FIGURE 24–7. Joystick on the fundus camera allows control of position for back and forth, side to side, and up and down.

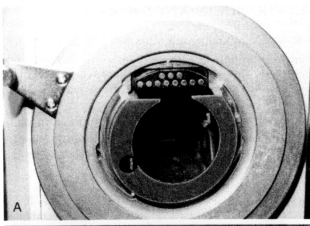

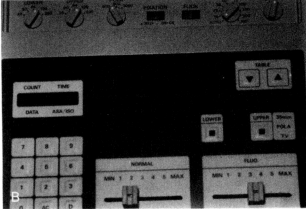

FIGURE 24–8. *A,* Modern fundus cameras connect to camera bodies with pin connectors rather than cables. *B,* An example of a fundus camera control panel. Note the controls for flash, viewing illumination, and timer.

phers typically do this in a two-step fashion. Most often, 1/2% Mydriacyl (tropicamide) and 2 1/2% Neo-Synephrine (phenylephrine) are administered. Drops should always be administered under the direction and supervision of a physician. The amount of dilation necessary is somewhat relative. For some cameras, particularly those with a narrow angle of view, 3 to 4 mm of pupillary dilation will be adequate for simple fundus photography. For other cameras, especially those with wider fields of view, more than 6 mm of dilation will be essential. Maximum dilation is even more critical when performing stereo/photography.

3. Adjust the camera to the patient. Each camera has adjustments that allow it to best "fit" your patient for reasonable comfort and support. Set the seat so that the patient is able to place the head in the chin rest without excessive hunching of the shoulders or straining of the neck. The forehead should be against the forehead rest, ensuring that focus is maintained. Fix the chin rest so that the beam of light from the camera illuminates the ocular area while still providing ample adjustment with the camera controls up and down. A comfortable chair is helpful. Removing the casters from the chair base ensures that the patient will not slip off the stool during the procedure.

4. Verify that the camera is turned on and ready to operate. Load the camera with an appropriate film, which may be either 35mm color film, such as Kodak Ektachrome 100, or a Polaroid color print film back.

5. Adjust camera controls and illumination system. Adjust the brightness of the viewing system so that you have adequate illumination to see fundus detail. Focus the camera. There is a threshold beyond which the patient will be unable to tolerate the intensity of the light. Sacrifice a bit of brightness so that the patient is comfortable and more cooperative.

6. Set the ocular on the camera viewfinder to match the patient's refractive error. Place a plain white paper or card in the viewing path. Sit behind the camera, viewing through the ocular. Notice the reticle with engraved lines designed to appear at optical infinity. Determine your eyepiece setting by turning the ocular to the farthest "plus" setting available. Your visual system is "fogged." Dial the ocular *slowly* toward the "minus" until the reticle lines appear crisp and sharp. Stop exactly at that point. **Do not oscillate or hunt for the best focus.** The human eye can accommodate, which allows the photographer to focus on the reticle at many different points. Avoid this temptation by stopping rotation of the ocular as soon as the reticle lines become sharp. Repeat this procedure several times until a comfortable and repeatable stopping point is found. This will generally be your setting for each session. It is possible that there will be some changes based on your patient's age, fatigue, or other metabolic functions. Similar cameras often have totally different ocular settings.

7. Position the light beam over the patient's iris before you look into the camera. If you move the camera forward and backward with the joystick, you will notice that at some point, the doughnut of light projected onto the iris and cornea becomes sharper and more distinct. When this doughnut is at its sharpest point, you are at the correct working distance. Move the camera left and right, or up and down, until the doughnut of light is centered squarely over the dilated pupil. If you look through the camera's ocular at this point, you may be surprised to find a nearly correctly aligned image of the patient's retina. Fine tune this image while looking through the ocular by moving the joystick in any of your three axes of control.

8. Select an angle of view from the variable angles of view found in many modern fundus cameras. They are able to take a photograph that encompasses a great, broad view of the patient's fundus, or they can take a narrow, magnified view. Use the view which best suits the condition you are photographing. If in doubt, check with your ophthalmologist.

9. No filters are added during color photography.

10. Maneuver the patient into looking in the correct position for optimum photography. This may be other

than just straight ahead into the light. Most fundus cameras have a fixation target located either inside the light path, next to the light path, or both. Most often, the external fixation target is used to move the patient's eye from point to point (Fig. 24–9). This is done by positioning the external fixation light in front of the eye *not* being photographed. As the patient tracks the fixation light with the nonstudy eye, the study eye follows along.

11. Compose your picture for optimal clarity, ask your patient to blink in order to wet the cornea, and then take your photograph.

12. At the conclusion of color photography, remove the film from the camera unless sufficient film remains to photograph another patient. In any case, identify the contents of the roll of film before you send it to the processor. A good strategy is to make a photograph of the patient's name on a piece of paper before you begin photographing the eye. This step ensures that a name record is on the film before the imaging begins.

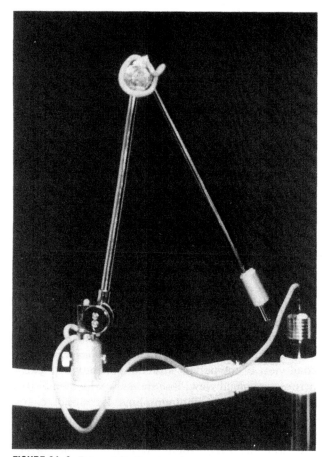

FIGURE 24–9. External fixation target.

FLUORESCEIN ANGIOGRAPHY

Fluorescein angiography involves an injection of a contrast solution into the patient's arm. Timing and coordination are of paramount importance. The realization that the patient may become ill, or perhaps even die, does nothing to lessen the anxiety of beginning ophthalmic photographers. In reality, fluorescein angiography is similar to driving a car, in that it consists of many small steps linked together to make a whole.

Background

The concept of stereophotography is important in understanding various photographic techniques, including fundus photography and fluorescein angiography. With stereophotography, the resulting image is similar to that seen in the Viewmaster you may have played with as a child. When viewed through special binocular magnifiers, the resulting fundus image has an apparent depth. This is achieved by taking two nearly simultaneous images of approximately the same view which are separated by a small amount of lateral distance. When these two slightly dissimilar images are put side by side and viewed by our binocular visual system, the resulting fused image appears three dimensional. Why should we go through the trouble of doing that? Many physicians do not avail themselves of this kind of photography, but the retina is made of several layers, some of which are transparent. Other physicians believe that it is extremely important to localize retinal lesions in the third dimension. They want to know not only where the third bifurcation of the superior arcade is but also whether it is above, underneath, or within the retinal structure.

While viewing the retinal image through the fundus camera, notice the margin of error within which you can maneuver the camera's controls and still perceive a reasonably good quality image. This is done in the left to right direction only. Stereophotography exploits that spatial tolerance by requiring that you take two photographs of almost the same view of the patient's retina. The first is taken with the camera positioned slightly to the right of the clear central image, and the second is taken with the camera positioned slightly to the left of the clear central image. The two resulting images look very much alike, but they are slightly shifted in space. The quality of both images should be very good. Some photographers like to take one of the two stereoimages right through the center of the optical axis, thereby ensuring that one of the two is of optimum quality. This strategy slightly diminishes the amount of stereo separation and, therefore, perceived depth. Trial and error with a few patients will yield a technique with which you will be comfortable. At first, your images may have numerous artifacts and other unwanted photographic flaws, but these will diminish with perseverance and practice. Stereophotography during angiography is frequently advocated even if the results are not used. If you take stereophotographs and your physician chooses not to use them, the physician can still get valuable information from the "flat" photographs. If you do not photograph the patient in stereo, however, you cannot create stereoimages after the fact.

A major consideration is the choice of photographic media for the angiography process. Traditionally, film-based products were utilized to acquire the photographic image. Today, however, it is possible to perform fluorescein angiography digitally, using a slightly modified fundus camera, coupled with a fairly powerful personal computer, (a "filmless" solution). Rather than the image being recorded on film, it is electronically transmitted to a computer that captures the image on a storage medium, usually the hard drive. Software on the computer converts the digital information to an image that very closely resembles one obtained by conventional film. These systems have many advantages. The angiographic results are available almost immediately after the procedure. The images can be manipulated and enhanced to best demonstrate the area a physician may wish to treat. Because we are not dealing with slides and negatives, storage and retrieval of a particular patient's images are rapid.

At present, debate exists over which is the better methodology, conventional or digital angiography. Conventional film still offers high resolution and is cost-effective. Conventional film angiograms can be produced, generally, at less expense than digital angiograms because the cost of the equipment and film is lower than the cost of the storage media and computers required by the digital alternative. The high film resolution is also not subject to digital manipulation, which could bias or obscure objective findings. It is likely that digital angiography will be preferred after further refinement.

Steps in Angiography

Fluorescein angiography refers to the specific part of a photographic study wherein a bolus of fluorescein dye is injected into a patient intravenously and sequential black-and-white photographs are taken as the dye progresses through retinal blood vessels. From a procedural basis, however, this is somewhat incomplete. Angiographic steps might be listed as

1. Documentation
2. Evaluation
3. Patient education
4. Color fundus photography
5. Fluorescein angiography.

The fluorescein *process* is like a continuum from initially greeting the patient to finishing the paperwork at the end.

Documentation

The extent of written documentation varies from practice to practice. Current Medicare guidelines, for instance, dictate that certain minimum levels of patient record keeping be maintained to qualify for reimbursement. Irrespective of the amount of documentation, it is crucial that it is correct. You should have a diagnosis from the physician, information about the exact clinical entity to be photographed, and know which eye is of primary interest, because fundus cameras can photograph only one eye at a time. The early, or transit, phases of the angiogram occur so quickly, with so much information, that you cannot shuttle between eyes. Documentation should also include some basic patient information, such as medical record number, name, and address, for record-keeping purposes. Good clerical skills and labeling habits are important to avoid confusion.

Examination

Most ophthalmic photographers are not physicians. The examination portion of the fluorescein angiogram allows the photographer to rule out the obvious and to look for the few contraindications to fluorescein angiography. Before dilating a patient's eyes, you may want to perform the flashlight test to see if the anterior chamber is narrow. This is done by shining the beam of a penlight tangentially across the plane of the iris. If the far side of the beam appears markedly in shadow, you may want to reconsider dilating the patient's eyes before a more thorough examination is done by the ophthalmologist. Inquire about known allergies. Whereas there is no documented link between other specific allergies and sodium fluorescein, you should be alert for the patient who has strong allergies to many substances. Inquire if the patient is pregnant. Although sodium fluorescein is generally a safe compound, angiography during pregnancy is normally not recommended. Ask if a patient is diabetic, which may cause a change in the way you administer the dye. If the patient is a child, or has a physical handicap, you may need to reposition the patient's chair or the camera to provide a more comfortable position.

Your initial meeting with the patient may reveal other interesting findings. For example, you may find that you do not speak the language your patient speaks. You may discover that your patient is hearing impaired. Any number of surprising details can make performing the angiogram more challenging. The time to determine these problems is before, not during, the angiogram.

Education

This phase begins when you greet the patient and ends when the patient leaves your care at the end of the procedure. Some believe that most fluorescein reactions are not caused by a chemical reaction with the fluorescein dye, but rather by apprehension over the procedure itself. By educating the patient about what you are about to do, how you will do it, and what you expect to find, more cooperation and better pictures can be obtained. Patient education does not mean that you should discuss diagnostic or therapeutic details. Leave that task to the ophthalmologist.

Fluorescein Angiography Procedure

All our skills (photographic principles, basic ophthalmic pathology, fundus camera handling technique, and patient management) culminate during fluorescein angiography. Not that fluorescein angiography is difficult, but it does require integrating skills previously learned individually.

Fluorescein angiography works because of a basic principle called fluorescence. Nontoxic sodium fluorescein dye is administered into a patient's bloodstream and is carried by the blood throughout the circulatory system. The dye rapidly diffuses throughout the body, then clears the system. We pay attention to this dye-treated blood flow only when it passes through the retinal and choroidal blood vessels. The vasculature of the retina is transparent. It appears red because you see the blood column flow through the clear vessel walls.

When we shine white light from the camera flash through a blue exciter filter that only allows blue light of 465 to 490 nm wavelength to reach the retina, we cause molecules of the fluorescein dye in the blood to become temporarily excited by picking up light energy. This extra energy causes the molecules to become unstable. In an effort to stabilize themselves, the molecules release some of this energy in the form of green-yellow light that has a higher wavelength (about 520 nm) than the blue light that stimulated the molecules. The photographer illuminates the retina with a bluish light, and the fluorescein returns a bright, glowing, green-yellow light. A barrier filter built into the camera excludes all light except the green-yellow light to pass back to the film. Only light of that particular color is imaged on our negatives.

The only portions of the eye that are imaged on film are those areas that contain the fluorescent dye at that point in time when the picture is taken. If there is no disease, fluorescein dye does not leak out of retinal blood vessels. Abnormalities may fluoresce less (*hypo*fluoresence) from interruptions and blockages in blood vessels, or more (*hyper*fluorescence) if blood leaks out of blood vessels.

Fluorescein Preparation

The contraindications for angiography are pregnancy, history of previous reaction to angiography, and strong history of general allergic reactions. With these in mind, angiography is still safe for almost every patient. It is not, however, uncommon to see some kind of adverse, usually mild, reaction. Some common reactions are nausea (sometimes progressing to vomiting), itching (sometimes accompanied by hives), numbness of the lips or tongue, sneezing, and injection-related problems, such as bleeding around the venipuncture site. All these are considered minor reactions to fluorescein, and almost all are self-limiting.

Every photographer worries about more serious complications, including fainting, respiratory arrest, cardiac arrest, and pulmonary edema (lung swelling). Although this list may sound daunting, the chances of a serious, life-threatening reaction are very slim ($<0.5\%$). Still, it is important to have an understanding of the basic treatments for each of the complications. Table 24–1 summarizes those reactions. In order to respond appropriately to a potentially serious adverse reaction, the photographer should have a basic emergency kit. There are many commercial kits available for cardiac and respiratory arrest. Consult with your physician, or the physician's nurse manager to determine how your area should be equipped. The ophthalmic photographer should be certified in cardiopulmonary resuscitation (CPR) as it may be necessary to intervene in a life-threatening situation.

Fluorescein Sequence

Check your equipment to determine that it is functioning properly. Clean the lenses and load black-and-white film into the fluorescein camera. Typically, Kodak Tri-X, T-Max, Ilford HP-5, or some similar film, is chosen for fluorescein angiography. Each of these films will yield a good quality angiogram, although they should not be interchanged without experimentation.

We are ready to begin the angiogram sequence, but not ready to call our nurse (or physician) to begin the injection. We record on film the preliminary information which, together with the angiogram proper, provides a complete photographic survey. For the sake of this discussion, we will assume that you will have a standard 36-exposure roll of photographic film. Whereas there is no set limit on how many frames a complete angiogram should have, we will attempt to expose all 36 available frames in the series about to be

TABLE 24–1.

Fluorescein Reactions and Management

Local Effects	Manifestation	Management	Comments
Leakage of fluorescein at site of injection	Complaints of burning or dull ache around site of injection for 1/2–1 hour	Reassure patient that dye inadvertently leaked. Cold soaks	*Not* recommended to give a local anesthetic at site of injection
Chemical thrombophlebitis	Cord-like tender line running along antecubital vein which drains the site of injection	Self-limited process. No treatment	Duration: 7–10 days
Direct intra-arterial puncture	Immediate severe pain and extreme discoloration of distal end of extremity	Submerge arm in cold water. Systemic analgesic (e.g., aspirin and codeine)	Discolorations will disappear in 24 hours

Systemic Effects			
Nausea and/or vomiting	Transient—usual onset 1–2 min. post-injection	Reassurance. If strong prior history of nausea and vomiting, consider 25 mg promethazine HCl intramuscularly (IM) 30 min preinjection	Approximately 10% of fluorescein patients suffer nausea. About 2% proceed to vomiting.
Flushing of skin. Pruritus. Paresthesia. Dull metallic taste	Itching. Local or systemic numbness of lips or tongue	Antihistamines administered by physician, e.g., diphenhydramine (Benadryl) 50 mg oral or IM	Monitor patient for 1 hour
Hives	Localized thickening and elevation with red weal can be mild or dramatic	50 mg diphenhydramine (Benadryl)	<1% occurrence
Profuse angioedema	Swelling of skin, lips, and other soft tissues	Antihistamines oral or intravenously (IV)	<1% occurrence
Fainting		Patient supine. Monitor blood pressure	Result of systemic hypotension or shock, more often among women. Sometimes vagal response
Bronchospasm or asthma		Epinephrine 1:1000 0.2–0.4 ml subcutaneously, as necessary. Aminophylline 250 mg IV slowly over 5 min	Administered only by physician
Anaphylactic shock		Epinephrine 1:1000 0.3–0.5 ml subcutaneously. Repeat 15–30 min as needed. Intravenous fluids to replenish intravascular volume. Maintain airway and administer O$_2$ as needed. Antihistamines, e.g., diphenhydramine (Benadryl) 10–20 mg IV	Severe bronchospasm and variations in blood pressure are likely complications

These are general guidelines. All patient care is under the direct supervision of the ophthalmologist. © 1995. Donald Enkerud.

described. You may need a second roll to complete an angiogram, or you may end early and still have film remaining. You want to have all the correct pictures rather than many pictures of the wrong thing.

After the camera is loaded, identify the patient by photographing a slip of paper, or name tag, directly on film with the fundus camera. Because paper is white and highly reflective, it may be necessary to lower flash intensity to avoid overexposing the film. It is advisable to shoot three name tags in a row to avoid photographing a name tag on the exposed leader of the film which was struck by light when being loaded into the camera. Three exposures of the name tags will ensure that at least one will survive to identify the angiogram.

When we review the processed film, only one name tag will be retained, which becomes the first frame of the angiographic sequence.

"Red-free" Photographs

The next four photographs in the preangiographic sequence are the "red-free" photographs obtained by turning the power of the fundus camera to its lowest setting and exposing the retinal image to the film under green light. Most fundus cameras have a green filter, which can be switched on, built into the optical system. The green filter absorbs much of the red illumination returning from blood-filled vessels, thus resulting in a dark image wherever red occurs on the film. Be sure to remove this filter when you finish with this series. The red-free photographs provide an ophthalmoscopic view, i.e., an image that most closely represents a color image, even though the pictures are black-and-white. Vascular architecture and major landmarks should be readily apparent.

A stereo pair of the nonstudy eye is followed by a stereo pair of the study eye. Stereo pairs are done by taking two photographs in rapid succession of nearly the same area, displaced by moving the joystick only a few millimeters. Make sure that both images are of good optical quality. Reset the power to normal fluorescein levels at this point.

Control Photo

The control photo is the one photograph of the study eye taken exactly as if the angiogram were being performed, but without the dye. All camera controls, filters, and light controls are placed on the same settings as those during the angiographic series. Ironically, on a processed angiogram, a good control photograph should show almost nothing because it is a record of flaws in the filter system of the fundus camera. If the camera system has an imperfectly matched set of retinal filters, the control photograph would show faint, ghost-like images of the retinal vasculature and architecture. If the filters are perfectly matched, as they should be, the control photo will show almost nothing because the *only* light that will reach the film is the green-yellow light from the stimulated fluorescein molecules. Perhaps there will be a circle outlining the field of view of the retinal image.

Note that the fluorescein exciter and barrier filters are not permanent devices. They may be damaged by age, improper maintenance, humidity, and other factors. By regularly taking control photographs for each angiogram, a photographer can be alert to any indications of deterioration of the fluorescein filters.

This set of images, the preangiographic sequence, becomes our first angiographic building block. That this sequence required six frames is no accident. It is not uncommon for photographers to store their film negatives in plastic negative sleeves available from many photographic suppliers. Commonly, these negative preservers allow you to cut your finished film into six pieces of six frames each (36 exposures). Conveniently, our six frame preangiographic sequence neatly fills the first row of a six frame angiographic preserver. This may sound excessive, but its regular use provides the photographer with an unchanging platform with which to evaluate performance. Similarly, the physi-

cian will become accustomed to this standardized format.

In summary, our first building block, the preangiographic sequence, consists of three subpieces—the name tag, the red-free photographs, and the control photograph.

Dye Administration

Sodium fluorescein is available from many vendors in various formulations. Most commonly, it is available as either 5 ml of 10% sodium fluorescein or as 2.5% ml of 25% sodium fluorescein. Although each photographer has his or her own personal bias, both are acceptable. Similarly, fluorescein is available in both light- and dark-colored formulations, which are chemically identical. Physicians and nurses tend to prefer lighter formulations because they allow differentiation of the fluorescein from the blood in the intravenous tubing prior to injection.

In addition to fluorescein, your physician or nurse manager may help determine other items necessary to administer the fluorescein. Typically, these consist of butterfly injection sets, in either 21 or 25 gauge, syringes for drawing up and pushing fluorescein, alcohol wipes or other germicidals, tourniquets, gauze, adhesive strips and bandaids. (Fig. 24–10).

Actual administration of the fluorescein is critical to the entire angiographic process, requiring the greatest coordination among photographer, patient, and injection provider. It is strongly recommended that ophthalmic photographers lead during this crucial time and direct when the injection should begin. The injection process is synchronized by a timer to the rapid, sequential, photographic analysis of the fluorescein as it travels through the ocular circulation. A miscue here biases the entire sequence of events. A typical injection sequence is as follows.

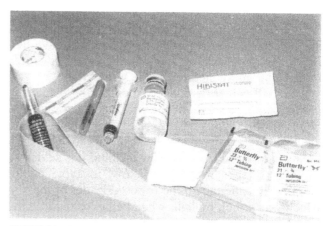

FIGURE 24–10. Items necessary to instill fluorescein dye.

1. After fundus photography, the patient is briefed on what to expect during the angiographic process and is given the opportunity to ask questions.

2. The injection provider is introduced and he or she may or may not answer additional questions.

3. Position the patient's arm comfortably, such that the antecubital vein is accessible to the injector. A tourniquet is applied to the upper arm, and the patient is verbally prepared for the injection.

4. The patient is asked to place his or her head against the forehead rest and the chin into the chin rest. Using the fixation target, orient the patient's eye to the specific area to be photographed during the early phases of the angiogram. This serves two purposes. First, if the patient is following your directions, he or she will be less preoccupied with the idea of the needle about to be received. Second, once the needle is introduced, you are ready to photograph the study, even if the injection is premature.

5. Immediately before the injection, disinfect the injection site with an antibiotic wipe or alcohol swab.

6. The needle is introduced into the antecubital vein, and the nurse or physician verifies that there is blood return into the butterfly tubing, thus signifying that the needle is in the vein and not in the extravascular space.

7. The nurse or physician signals readiness to administer fluorescein and awaits the photographer's cue to begin because the photographer must synchronize the injection with the first photographs and the resetting of the timer to zero. A timer is almost always utilized because it helps to quantify the rate of blood flow through the vascular system. These data also provide valuable clues to a physician, particularly in occlusive vascular diseases. The timer is usually reset and activated with the touch of a button exactly at the moment the injection begins.

Early Phase Photography

We are now ready to administer the injection and to take the most crucial photographs of the entire angiographic sequence. These are the early, or transit, images that document the arterial filling phase of the angiogram. The nurse or physician begins the injection process. When the photographer signals that the injection is to begin, the timer is reset to zero, and this begins its film recording. Each time the shutter is depressed, an accurate elapsed time figure will be recorded with each frame. The first image is made as the nurse or physician injects the dye at the moment the photographer says, "Go." The next image is taken the moment the physician completes the injection. These first two pictures document the elapsed time of injection. This helps answer many questions about the speed of injection and its resultant effect on the quality of the angiogram.

The photographer will be viewing the patient's retina through a filtered system, either with exciter filter alone or with exciter and barrier filters together. The resulting viewed image is very dim. After the injection, there may be a period of 8 to 10 seconds when no image is visible. Most photographers wait this period before taking any more photographs. With practice, it is possible to visualize the arrival of the fluorescein-laden blood into the choriocapillaris during what is commonly called choroidal flush. This has been likened by some photographers to "watching lightning bolts" spread across a "dark night sky." A good angiogram includes a few frames of this phenomenon before moving on.

At this point, rapid sequence photography begins at one frame per second or faster. The goal is to record accurately choroidal and arterial filling during the 30 seconds before venous return begins. This is a good point for the photographer to pause. Unfortunately, it is also the point at which most patients might become ill. (Be aware that some patients [about 1 in 20] feel some nausea and a few vomit.)

This completes the second building block of a fluorescein angiogram, i.e., the early, or transit, phase. This sequence also has landmark images: the beginning of the fluorescein injection, with the timer set to zero, and the documentation of the end of injection. From that point on, the early phase is "free-form," encompassing another 8 to 12 images until venous return begins.

Midphase Photography

More correctly called venous phase, photographs taken in this sequence document the flow of blood returning from the eye to the venous side of the heart. The overall intensity of the viewed field increases as the concentration of fluorescein dye in the venous blood increases. Because the liver and kidneys are constantly working to remove the fluorescein, recirculation of the blood results in decreased intensity. As time goes by, the arteries and capillaries show less fluorescence whereas the veins still show great fluorescence.

As angiographers, we strive to document this transition from arterial to venous circulation, and the slow diminishment of arterial flow, by taking a few stereo photographs of both eyes. After photographing the eye of primary interest, the photographer, for the first time, can direct attention to the other eye and document its retinal appearance. Many photographers are tempted to try to move the camera to the companion eye earlier in the angiographic sequence in hopes of obtaining early high quality photographs of both eyes. These efforts are usually futile. Because the dynamics of early phase angiography are so brisk, it is unusual to obtain meaningful data on both eyes within such a short time frame. Mid-phase venous angiography is the first time that the photographer can pause and move the camera to the opposite eye without compromising the essential information from the eye of primary interest.

It is common to make another three or four pairs of photographic images of both eyes. At this point, the patient can have a brief rest because several minutes usually elapse before the next angiographic phase. This gives the photographer time to complete the necessary paperwork and to remind the patient of the effects that they may observe after angiography. Most patients will have very bright yellow urine for the next 24 to 48 hours, and their skin may be tinted yellow for the next few hours. These observations are normal and resolve completely by themselves.

With mid-phase, or venous, angiography, we have completed the third building block of our angiographic sequence. Three or four stereo pairs were taken (six or eight individual pictures), occupying all of the third row of our six frame angiographic strip and part of the fourth. This leaves us with six to ten blank frames with which to conclude the angiogram.

Late Phase Angiography

The final phase consists of taking late photos. Late is an indefinite term and in different institutions can range from 10 to 20 minutes. The exact amount should be arrived at through consultation between the photographer and the physician. Abnormalities, such as cystoid macular edema, may dictate that a longer than normal amount of time be allowed to elapse before concluding the late phase photographs. Other abnormalities, e.g., proliferative diabetic retinopathy, may force the photographer to conclude the late phase relatively early because of profuse fluorescein leakage into the vitreous cavity, which will totally obscure the retina from further view. The remaining 10 or so frames should document late photographs of both the companion eye and the eye of primary interest. Use this time, also, to look about the fundus and document other areas of interest. It is not unusual for the ophthalmic photographer to notice abnormalities that were undocumented by the physician during indirect examination.

Our last phase, late photographs, is the simplest. Both the photographer and patient are under little pressure, and both can concentrate on creating the best possible photographs. Late photographs are the last building block of the complete angiographic sequence.

Angiographic Sequence Summary (Figure 24–11)

1. The preangiographic sequence begins with photographs of the name tag, red-free photographs of each eye, and a control photograph.

2. Early (arterial) phase photographs document the injection sequence and the earliest phases of retinal circulation.

3. Mid-phase (venous) circulation photographs document the increase of venous blood flow in both the primary eye and the companion eye. They can also show other areas of interest for possible treatment by the ophthalmologist.

4. Late phase photographs complete the angiogram by documenting the now nearly depleted venous and arterial fluorescent circulation. What remains at this point may be pooling of fluorescein in intraretinal spaces or staining of tissue. Table 24–2 provides a step by step guide to this technique.

● PHOTOGRAPHIC ANGIOGRAPHIC PROCESSING

Learning to photograph may well become a requirement in your duties. Taking the photograph is only half the process—processing the film delivers a meaningful product into the hands of the physician.

Color Processing

Don't do it. At the low volumes of use encountered in most ophthalmic practices without a dedicated photographer, in-house color processing is unnecessary. Working with a local laboratory to process color film is usually more cost-effective at low volume and almost always delivers a consistent product.

Some photographers choose not to have a local laboratory but to purchase *prepaid mailers*. These envelopes can be purchased from many laboratories at competitive prices. Purchase of the envelope includes processing of the film. The film is placed in the envelope and mailed to the laboratory. Within a few days completed film will be mailed back.

Black-and-White Processing

Whereas color processing is best left to color laboratories, black-and-white processing is within reach of most technicians. Usually the first obstacle is not the processing itself, but rather the lack of a darkroom. A darkroom is not necessary, however. It is possible to

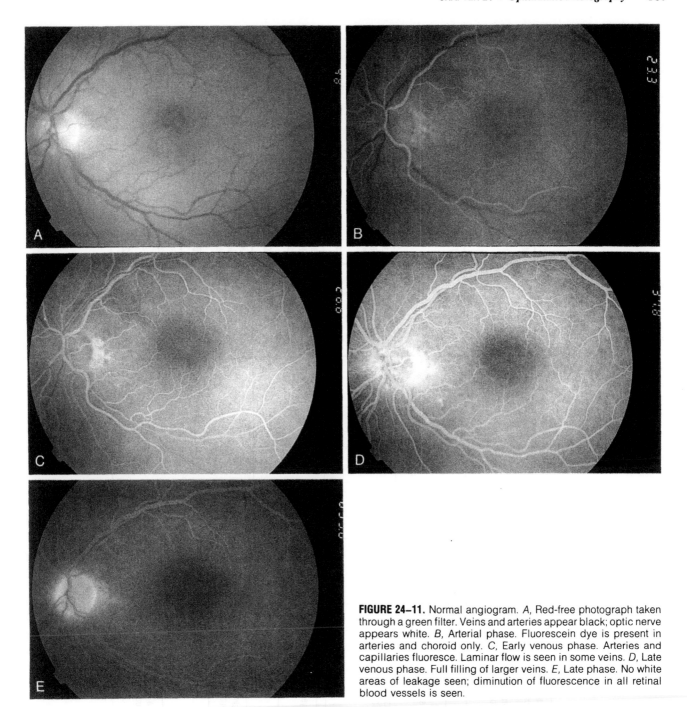

FIGURE 24–11. Normal angiogram. *A,* Red-free photograph taken through a green filter. Veins and arteries appear black; optic nerve appears white. *B,* Arterial phase. Fluorescein dye is present in arteries and choroid only. *C,* Early venous phase. Arteries and capillaries fluoresce. Laminar flow is seen in some veins. *D,* Late venous phase. Full filling of larger veins. *E,* Late phase. No white areas of leakage seen; diminution of fluorescence in all retinal blood vessels is seen.

assemble the equipment necessary to process fluorescein angiograms for less than $100.

An Instant Darkroom (Figure 24–12)

Even the smallest practice doing fluorescein angiography can process film with the addition of a few basic pieces of equipment, which would readily fit into a filing cabinet. A dedicated darkroom is not required.

The following equipment allows a technician to completely process a fluorescein angiogram.

1. Changing bag. This light-tight sack looks like a sweater with no neck opening. Instead, it has a zipper at the "waist" and is really a double-lined bag. This changing bag serves as a portable darkroom. You lay the changing bag on a table, place the necessary tools and film inside, insert your arms into the sleeves, and manipulate the light sensitive components in the dark

TABLE 24–2.

Ready Reference for Flawless Fluorescein

Name tag	Stereo red-free (Pt 1)	Stereo red-free (Pt 2)	Stereo red-free (Pt 1)	Stereo red-free (Pt 2)	Control photo
1	**2**	**3**	**4**	**5**	**6**
Start injection **7**	End injection **8**	First angio Photo after pause **9**	Choroidal Flush 1° Eye **10**	Early phase Stereo half 1° Eye **11**	Early phase Stereo half 1° Eye **12**
Early phase Stereo half 1° Eye **13**	Early phase Stereo half 1° Eye **14**	Early phase Stereo half 1° Eye **15**	Early phase Stereo half 1° Eye **16**	Early phase Stereo half 1° Eye **17**	Early phase Stereo half 1° Eye **18**
Early phase Stereo half Fellow eye **19**	Early phase Stereo half Fellow eye **20**	Early phase Stereo half Fellow eye **21**	Early phase Stereo half Fellow eye **22**	Early phase Stereo half Fellow eye **23**	Early phase Stereo half Fellow eye **24**
Late photos Stereo half Fellow Eye **25**	Late photos Stereo half Fellow Eye **26**	Late photos Stereo half Fellow Eye **27**	Late photos Stereo half Fellow Eye **28**	Late photos Stereo half 1° Eye **29**	Late photos Stereo half 1° Eye **30**
Late photos Stereo half 1° Eye **31**	Late photos Stereo half 1° Eye **32**	Late photos Stereo half 1° Eye **33**	Late photos Stereo half 1° Eye **34**	Late photos Stereo half 1° Eye **35**	Late photos Stereo half 1° Eye **36**

© 1995. Donald Enkerud.

Name tag and red-free photos at low power; green filter (optional)

Control photo with all fluorescent filters and at regular fluorescent power settings.

Injection photos document speed of injection; start timer at start of injection.

Move quickly in early phase. Most critical; first dye visible 8–10 secs (average).

Always photograph both eyes if possible.

Patient and photographer take a break here until about 10 minute mark.

Start late photos with fellow eye because that is where you last left off

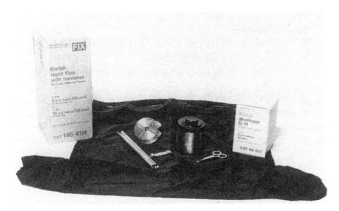

FIGURE 24–12. Darkroom equipment for black and white photographs: changing bag, reels, tanks, scissors, can opener, and chemicals.

center of the bag. The few parts of the developing process that have to be conducted in absolute darkness can be accommodated by the changing bag.

2. Film tanks and reels. Tanks and reels are light-proof containers that hold the film and chemicals while the film is being processed. Within the changing bag, the film is wound onto reels. The reels are then placed in the tanks that have tight-fitting, light-proof lids. The lids generally have a second light-proof opening that allows chemicals to be freely poured in and out without light's striking the film. Plastic and metal developer reels are available and both are equally effective. The photographer should choose the developer reel to suit temperament, skill, and budget.

3. Scissors and a can opener. The rounded end of the can opener will pry open the light-proof film cassette, and the scissors will trim the tongue-shaped leader from the edge of the film. The film can then be wound around the spiral reel.

4. Chemicals. Most photographers use one of two developing chemicals. The first is Kodak D-11, a powder that makes one gallon of solution, which is used at full strength to process the angiographic negative. Some trial and error may be necessary to determine the correct film processing time, but 8 or 9 minutes is typical. Some photographers prefer HC-110, a more versatile developer that is widely available in most camera shops. The "B" dilution is preferred by many photographers to process angiographic negatives. A development duration of 8 to 10 minutes is a good starting point.

5. Rapid fix. Fixer removes the undeveloped light sensitive compounds in the film and fixes the image on the film. Kodak Rapid Fix is a timesaver by concluding the developing process in 5 to 8 minutes.

6. Running water. Plain tap water can be used to wash the film thoroughly before drying. Specialized film washers can be purchased inexpensively to improve the washing action tremendously. Wash the film

thoroughly for at least 30 minutes to 1 hour under running water. The washed film can be air dried or gently force dried with any number of commercial film dryers.

As easy as this procedure can be, some photographers elect not to process their own negatives, selecting one of the many angiographic processing services located throughout the country. For a nominal fee, these services will process your exposed film in a timely manner.

It is likely that health care reform will result in more ophthalmic technical personnel acting as ophthalmic photographers. The skills required are not out of reach, but mastery of the techniques takes time. Basic steps to success are a fundamental understanding of the photographic processes, a knowledge of basic camera mechanics, and a grasp of the building blocks that make a fluorescein angiograph. All of these skills are acquired with simple practice.

References

Berkow JW, Orth DH, Kelley JS: Fluorescein Angiography: Technique and Interpretation. San Francisco, American Academy of Ophthalmology, 1991.
Cassin B, Solomon SAB: Dictionary of Eye Terminology, 2nd ed. Gainesville, FL, Triad, 1990.
Coppinger JM, Maio M, Miller K: Ophthalmic photography. In Ophthalmic Technical Skills Series. Wolfe CP, Benes SC, eds.: Thorofare, NJ, Slack, 1990.
Jalkh AE, Celorio JM: Atlas of Fluorescein Angiography. Philadelphia, WB Saunders, 1993.
Justice J (ed:) Ophthalmic Photography. Boston, Little, Brown, 1982.
Wong D: Textbook of Ophthalmic Photography. New York, Don Wong, 1990.

● CHAPTER 24 OPHTHALMIC PHOTOGRAPHY

1. How do you compensate when you increase shutter speed?
   a. changing to a faster ISO rated film
   b. decreasing aperture size
   c. changing to a larger F number
   d. enlarging aperture size
   e. changing to a slower film speed.

2. Ophthalmic photography usually magnifies the area of interest. What is one way to also increase the depth of field?
   a. decreasing aperture size
   b. using a telephoto lens
   c. using slower film
   d. increasing the focal length
   e. using a smaller F number.

3. Which of the following adverse reactions to fluorescein is the most serious?
   a. nausea
   b. fainting
   c. itching

d. sneezing

e. vomiting

4. What is mid-phase fluorescein angiography more commonly known as?

a. arterial phase

b. red-free photos

c. fluorescein leakage

d. choroidal flush

e. venous phase.

5. When is the correct working distance reached with the fundus camera?

a. light intensity is just above the patient's threshold

b. patient looks straight ahead

c. doughnut of light is focused most distinctly on the cornea

d. patient fixes with the study eye

e. joystick is used to "fine tune" the image.

Patricia T. Lamell
Charisse Barcelo Hines

Surgical Assisting

LEARNING OBJECTIVES

- List the members of the surgical team and explain the duties of each
- Discuss aseptic technique
- Explain the reason for and technique of the surgical scrub
- Explain gowning and gloving procedures
- Define a sterile field
- Describe how to apply an eye patch
- Explain the use of a Fox shield
- Describe the care of ophthalmic surgical instruments
- Explain the differences between the three methods of sterilization
- Identify 12 common instruments for ophthalmic surgery
- Name six common ophthalmic surgical procedures

Once the decision to perform surgery is made, preoperative preparations begin. A physical examination, including taking a medical history and a general physical assessment (H&P), and laboratory tests, including a complete blood count (CBC) and urinalysis (U/A), are performed to ensure that the state of health of the patient permits the operation. The ophthalmologic history and examination is included in the preoperative report.

Pre- and postoperative instructions are explained to the patient and family by the ophthalmologist, who often provides written instructions if needed. Most patients become anxious—some become terrified—before surgery, especially eye surgery with its potential threat of blindness. The surgical ophthalmic assistant can help allay some of the fears by reiterating to the patient and family a brief description of the procedure and what to expect before and after surgery and by answering questions. Be relaxed, cheerful, and optimistic in your interactions with patients.

Instruct patients to bring personal identification, and medical insurance information, and a minimum of personal items with them to the surgical facility. Jewelry, money, and excess clothing should be left at home. Nail polish and make-up should be removed.

● INFORMED CONSENT

Before surgery, written permission is obtained from the patient or legal guardian. A legal guardian signs the permit if the patient is under age or incapable of understanding the procedure. The preoperative permit is a legal document disclosing all potential risks and benefits, is written without abbreviations and with as little "medicalese" as possible. This form should be discussed before any preoperative medication is administered. The physician, patient (or legal guardian), and a witness sign this document. Ideally, someone other than a member of the surgical team witnesses the signature.

● THE OPERATING ROOM

The surgical suite is an isolated room kept as free as possible of micro-organisms. Each facility follows strict procedures as dictated by hospital accreditation and infection control. The operating room staff includes people who manage the front desk, who maintain sterile supplies, and those who do housekeeping, as well as radiologists, pathologists, and the surgical team itself. Professional behavior, following standard medical ethics, must be observed.

Upon entering the surgical area, personnel change into special clothing known as scrub suits or "greens." Scrub clothing fabric, as well as any linen in surgery, is made from nonconductive cotton to avoid generating static electricity. Although laundered after each wearing, it is not sterile. Some type of leg and foot covering, usually socks, is worn under scrub clothing, and shoe covers are worn over street shoes. All hair on the head and face should be confined by a covering. Beards are enclosed with special hoods. A disposable surgical mask covers the nose and mouth. Jewelry in the operating room is kept to a minimum, if worn at all. Fingernails are trimmed short and round, without nail polish. Although operating room procedures do not vary greatly from one facility to another, each person entering the surgical area must adhere to the rules and regulations particular to that institution.

• THE SURGICAL TEAM

The drama and seriousness associated with operating rooms intimidate student surgical assistants as well as most patients. Learn the standard steps of all surgical procedures one by one so that you can anticipate the surgeon's requirements and desires.

All members of the operating room staff directly involved in the surgical procedures have specific duties and work together to perform an efficient safe procedure. The surgical team of health care personnel is divided into scrubbed and nonscrubbed. The scrubbed members are surgically sterile, the nonscrubbed, circulating personnel are not. In ophthalmology, this closely knit unit includes the surgeon, the surgical assistant, the scrub nurse or technician, the circulator, and the anesthesiologist.

Scrubbed Personnel

Surgeon. The leader of the surgical team has ultimate responsibility for the welfare of the patient and directs the operating room activities.

Surgical Assistant. As a direct assistant to the surgeon, this is often another surgeon, but it may be a scrub nurse, an ophthalmic technical person, or a surgical technologist. The assistant follows the directions of the surgeon, anticipating the sequence of the surgical procedures. The assistant provides exposure of the surgical field, cuts sutures, and assists in hemostasis.

Scrub Nurse or Scrub Technician. Responsible for preparing and maintaining a sterile field, the scrub person selects all necessary sterile supplies, instruments, and garments, and assists the circulator in opening them. During the case, the scrub person hands the surgeon instruments and supplies in the anticipated sequence. Instruments are placed firmly in the surgeon's hand with tips in the position the surgeon will use them. As instruments are passed to the surgeon, the surgeon will pass others back to the scrub person. All supplies such as drugs and solutions must be clearly and accurately labelled. The scrub person may be a nurse, an ophthalmic technical person, or a surgical technologist. In some instances, the scrub person also acts as the surgical assistant (Fig. 25–1).

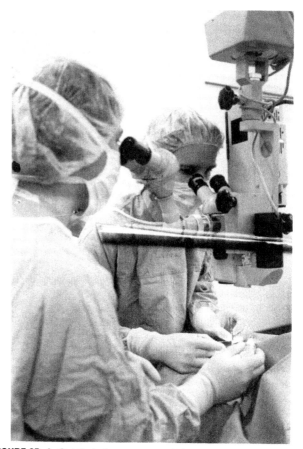

FIGURE 25–1. Ophthalmic surgeon and the surgical assistant viewing through operating microscope.

Circulating Personnel

Circulator. By legal mandate, either an RN (registered nurse), a surgical technologist, or ophthalmic technical person supervised by an RN who is the patient's advocate during the operative period, is present to guard the patient's safety. The circulator has knowledge of the temperature and humidity guidelines, patient care and comfort measures, and positioning techniques for surgical wound exposure. The circulator is the go-between in the operating room, communicating between the scrubbed and nonscrubbed members of the operating room staff; assisting the anesthetist during induction and extubation; delivering necessary supplies to the scrub technician as needed; and connecting, placing, and adjusting nonsterile equipment during surgery. The circulator may assist with the patient's skin preparation. It is also the circulator's task to request a stretcher to transport the patient from the operating room, to help the patient move from the OR table, and to transport the patient until relieved by other health care personnel. In addition, the circulator is responsible for completing legal documentation of the surgical procedure.

Anesthetist. A physician (anesthesiologist) or a nonphysician (certified registered nurse anesthetist) who acts under the direct supervision of a physician to induce general anesthesia (putting the patient "to sleep") if required, to provide patient comfort, and to monitor the patient's vital signs (blood pressure, pulse, respiration). In many institutions, the anesthesiologist also performs the local block (retrobulbar/peribulbar).

• ANESTHESIA

The ophthalmic surgeon and the anesthetist, guided by the patient's wishes, recommend the type of anesthesia depending on the type and duration of the surgical procedure along with the physical and emotional state of the patient. Systemic medications, such as analgesics, sedatives, and anti-anxiety drugs, are commonly administered to relax the patient. The patient's physical health and the surgeon's preference dictate which medications are selected. Needles and syringes of various sizes are prepared for injection with strengths and amounts of anesthetic drugs ordered by the ophthalmic surgeon. Epinephrine solution is often added to prolong the duration of anesthesia. When general anesthesia is chosen, the patient is anesthetized prior to the surgical preparations. Much eye surgery is, however, done using local anesthesia to minimize systemic risks and to avoid postoperative nausea and vomiting.

Topical Anesthesia

Anesthetic drops, such as tetracaine (Pontocaine), proparacaine (Ophthaine, Ophthetic), and cocaine, are all that is required for minor procedures on the conjunctiva, removal of superficial foreign bodies, and removal of corneoscleral sutures postoperatively. Tetracaine, unlike proparacaine, penetrates deeply. Both are fast-acting, producing topical anesthesia within 1 minute and lasting approximately 10 to 20 minutes. Superficial punctate keratitis may develop after instillation, but systemic reactions are extremely rare. Cocaine is not often used because it damages the corneal epithelium and produces pupillary dilation. Topical anesthetic drops may be added to supplement the effects of the local anesthetic.

Local Anesthesia

Removal of skin and conjunctival lesions and repair of eyelid lacerations require tissue infiltration by an injected anesthetic such as 1% lidocaine (Xylocaine) and 0.75% bupivacaine (Marcaine). Lidocaine is popu-

lar because of rapid penetration of tissue, taking 4 to 6 minutes to act and lasting 40 to 60 minutes. When combined with epinephrine, anesthesia lasts 2 hours. Bupivacaine lasts longest, approximately 8 to 12 hours when combined with epinephrine, but takes 5 to 11 mintues for a slower onset of action. Lidocaine is often combined with bupivacaine, producing both fast onset of action and long duration.

Regional Anesthesia

A nerve block, such as a facial or retrobulbar block, is chosen when a larger area of anesthesia is required. The facial nerve is sometimes blocked before the retrobulbar injection. A facial nerve block is essential to immobilize the orbicularis muscle, thus preventing squeezing of the eyelid during surgery. Injection of an anesthetic agent along the course of the seventh (facial) cranial nerve (CN VII) is achieved by one of the following methods:

1. Nad-bath's method blocks the seventh nerve as it emerges from the skull behind the ear.
2. O'Brien's method blocks the nerve at its proximal trunk at the jaw angle in front of the ear.
3. Van Lint's method blocks the nerve at its terminal branches along the superior and inferior orbital rims near the lateral canthus.

Retrobulbar Block

Injection of an anesthetic agent into the muscle cone behind the globe abolishes all movement and sensation of the globe except for the fourth (trochlear) cranial nerve (CN IV), which enters the orbit above the muscle cone and therefore is unaffected. In most cases, a single injection, often a mixture ("cocktail") of xylocaine (with or without epinephrine), bupivacaine (Marcaine), and hyaluronidase (Wydase), temporarily paralyzes the second, third, fifth, and sixth cranial nerves (CN II, III, V, VI). Wydase is an enzyme that helps increase diffusion of the anesthetic.

The retrobulbar injection is given through the skin of the lower lid with the needle then guided slightly superiorly into the muscle cone. The injection is carefully administered to reduce the possibility of complications such as a retrobulbar hemorrhage, penetration of the globe, or injection of the anesthetic agent into an artery. The retrobulbar injection is usually given before the surgical preparation is done. A peribulbar block provides similar anesthesia. However, it is administered in the more anterior portion of the orbit.

Sequence of Events in the Operating Room

1. Suite cleaned with disinfecting solutions.
2. Supplies and instruments are selected by the circulator and/or scrub technician.
3. The circulator or the scrub technician checks all electrical equipment and machinery to ensure performance and safety.
4. Items are left opened on the sterile back table, according to aseptic technique.
5. The scrub technician scrubs.
6. Patient enters operating room and is positioned and prepared by the circulator and anesthetist.
7. Scrub technician puts on own gown and gloves and begins to arrange sterile supplies and instruments.
8. All sharps (needles and blades) are counted by the circulator and scrub technician.
9. Anesthesia is administered, if not previously administered in the holding area.
10. Surgeon or assistant gloves and prepares surgical area.
11. Scrub technician helps surgeon and assistant put on gowns and gloves. All gowns are turned and tied, and talc is removed from gloves.
12. Head-drape (or turban) is placed around patient's head, covering the hair.
13. Sterile drape is placed over the patient's body.
14. Towel, plastic drape, or "unidrape" is placed to surround surgical site.
15. If one is used, a bridle suture is placed next.
16. Microscopes, head lamps, and other visual aids are positioned by the circulator.
17. Case proceeds until wound is closed.
18. Appropriate drops, ointments, and injections are administered.
19. Re-count of all sharps is made by the scrub technician and circulator.
20. Surgical area is cleaned and prepared for dressing.
21. Dressing is applied to surgical area.
22. All drapes and towels are removed from table and disposed of.
23. Instruments are washed, rinsed, dried, and replaced in cases.
24. Soiled linens are placed in laundry hamper.
25. Patient leaves room.
26. All disposable items are discarded.
27. Items to be sterilized for next case are placed in wire mesh basket, then in autoclave.
28. Items to be resterilized with gas are wrapped and then taken to sterile supply.
29. Room is cleaned with disinfecting solution and mopped as required, to make ready for next case.

• ASEPTIC TECHNIQUE

Aseptic technique is the method of preventing infection, and of assuring maximum cleanliness and sterile conditions in and about the operating room. Strict adherence to its principles provides protection for the patient and health care staff.

Aseptic technique divides items and areas into sterile and nonsterile.

Sterile. This term covers all instruments, supplies, clothing, and skin that are free from living micro-organisms, including spores, after completion of a mechanical or chemical sterilization process.

Nonsterile. The term describes the condition wherein objects are not free of all living micro-organisms.

Surgically Clean. Objects that contain a reduced number of micro-organisms from mechanical, chemical, or physical methods, but still are not considered sterile come under this heading.

The main sources of contamination are

• Environment from air, floor, and furniture
• Equipment from supplies, instruments, linens, and clothing
• Operating room personnel, caused by exhaled breath, and uncovered skin
• Patient.

Principles of Aseptic Technique

Do not touch anything that is not sterile! Only sterile items may touch other sterile items. Even so, sterile items are handled as little as possible. After a sterile item touches a nonsterile item, it is contaminated. Remove it from the sterile field immediately and replace with a sterile item. If in doubt about the sterility of any item, consider it as not sterile. Resterilize before use.

After they are scrubbed, do not fold your arms across your chest against your gown. Hands in sterile gloves must stay in sight above the waist, away from your body and face, and away from nonsterile items. *Do not drop your hands below table level.* Even when scrubbed, only the uplifted arms just above the elbow, the face, and front of the gown from the waist up are considered sterile. Because you cannot see behind you to know if anything nonsterile has touched the back of your sterile gown, consider the back of your gown as nonsterile. Scrubbed personnel pass one another either face-to-face or back-to-back. The circulator passes behind scrubbed personnel. Sterile and nonsterile personnel always face the sterile field. In eye surgery, the microscope handles must be covered with a sterile plastic bag when the surgeon or the assistant touches the operating room microscope. Neither the microscope

Technique for Both Long and Short Scrubs

1. Open two prepacked sponges and place them on top of scrub sink for the first scrub of the day.

2. Turn water on and adjust it to a comfortable temperature.

3. Wash hands and arms thoroughly to remove gross dirt.

4. Clean beneath the fingernails with a nail cleaner (Fig. 25–2A).

5. Rinse one hand and arm to 2 inches above elbow.

6. Using the brush side of a sponge, begin scrubbing left hand (Fig. 25–2B)

    30 strokes to nails

    20 strokes to surface of fingers and nails, including areas between fingers. Bend knuckles.

    10 strokes to surface of arms. Divide arm into two area, hand to forearm, and forearm to 3 inches above elbow. Wet sponge and wash with a circular

motion to 3 inches above elbow (Fig. 25–2C). Wet sponge as needed to maintain good lather.

7. Transfer sponge to left hand.

8. Do right hand and arm in similar manner.

9. Rinse and discard sponge in trash receptacle.

10. Rinse finger tips first, then hand, arm, and elbow.

11. Keep hands above the level of the elbow so that the water drips off the elbow into the sink, not back down over hands or fingers.

12. Repeat steps 6 through 11 with a second sponge for the first scrub of the day.

13. Hold hands up with arms well away from body and proceed to operating room where hands will be dried (Fig. 25–2D).

Do not scrub if you have infection anywhere, or any broken skin on hands or forearms.

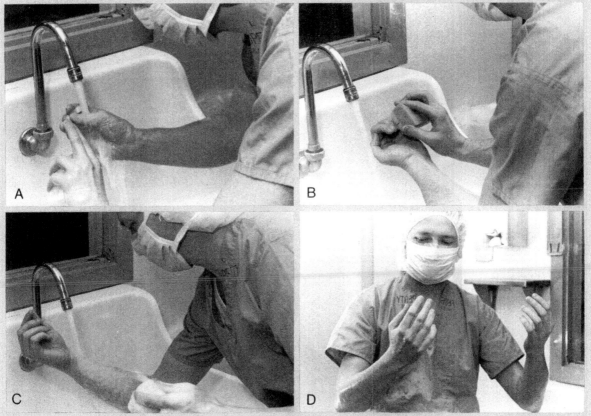

FIGURE 25–2. Technique for both long and short surgical scrubs. *A,* Clean beneath the fingernails with a nail cleaner with hand under running water. *B,* Scrub the fingernail surface with the brush side of a sponge. *C,* Use circular motions to scrub the arms, beginning with the fingers, then proceed up the arm to 2″ above the elbow. *D,* Hands are held above the elbows so that water runs off the elbows rather than over the clean arms and hands. Maintain this position during and after the rinse until arms are dried with a sterile towel.

Technique for Opening Sterile Items

Cloth or Paper-Wrapped Sterile Items.

1. Pull back the corner of the wrapping that unfolds away from the body. Grasp the item with one hand and the corner, now considered unsterile, with the other hand to prevent it from springing back (Fig. 25–3A).

2. Use the same technique to pull back the corner unfolding to one side (Fig. 25–3B).

3. Use the same technique to pull back the corner unfolding to the other side (Fig. 25–3C).

4. Pull the remaining corner back toward the body to expose the sterile contents. Toss the contents onto the sterile field or allow it to be removed by scrubbed personnel (Fig. 25–3D).

Sterile Items in Plastic Peel Packs

1. Grasp the ends of the plastic package so that the ends can be peeled back away from one another, exposing the sterile contents (Fig. 25–3E).

2. Toss the contents onto the sterile field or allow it to be removed by scrubbed personnel.

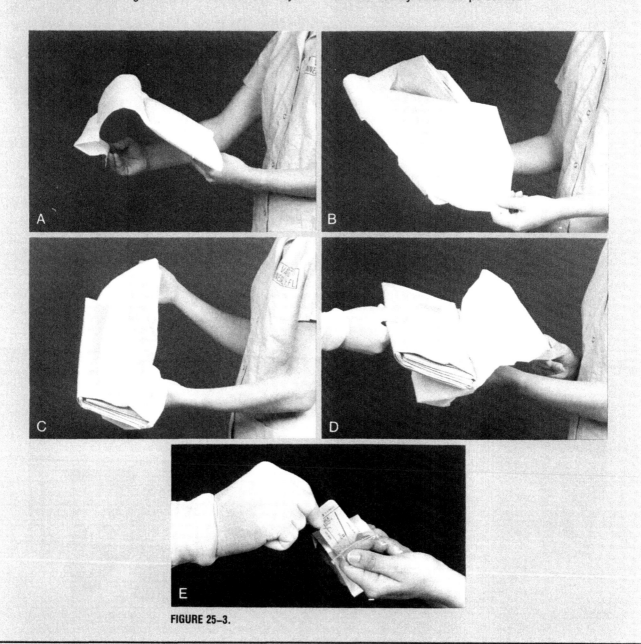

FIGURE 25–3.

nor the indirect ophthalmoscope are considered sterile.

Consider the patient as nonsterile. Avoid reaching across the sterile field with uncovered hands, arms, or nonsterile items. *Do not reach for anything that falls off the table.* It *is* contaminated. Only the tops of sterile drapes on tables are considered sterile.

Keep sterile cloth and paper items dry. Moisture allows micro-organisms from the nonsterile surface below to permeate and contaminate the drape.

Think of the skin, because it harbors micro-organisms as ''dirty.'' Avoid skin contact, especially if the skin is sweaty. Discard any needle or instrument that touches skin. Avoid coughing or sneezing, because the expired droplets carry bacteria. If you must sneeze or cough, turn away from the sterile field, then change your mask. If a scrubbed member of the surgical team touches any nonsterile item, that member is contaminated and cannot return to the sterile field until after re-gowning and re-gloving. Start each case with fresh solutions and sterile instruments. After each case, all items that come into contact with the patient or sterile field, whether used or not, are to be considered contaminated and to be removed from the operating room before the next patient arrives.

Members of the surgical team are obligated to mention, and attend to, any violation of sterile conditions. The patient's welfare is the most important concern in the operating room. Admit your mistakes.

Surgical Scrub

The surgical scrub is an orderly process that should result in clean hands and arms, with as little bacteria as possible. Because the skin harbors bacteria on its surface, a mechanical cleasing with an antimicrobial solution, known as the surgical scrub, is necessary before covering with sterile garments. This rids the hands and arms of dirt, oil, and microbes. An antimicrobial solution kills as many micro-organisms as possible. Scrub policy varies from one facility to another, but the process is based on either the *timed* anatomical scrub or the *counted* anatomical scrub. Each has a long and a short version. The counted anatomical scrub counts the number of brush strokes per area, e.g., 30 strokes to each hand, including all four surfaces. Many facilities require the long scrub as the first scrub of the day, or after a particularly infective case. The short scrub is done between cases, assuming the gown and gloves have not been removed. The timed anatomical scrub has a 10-minute (long) and a 5-minute (short) version. Because frequency of brush strokes is considered more important than the length of time spent scrubbing, by most surgeons, the counted scrub is more common.

Preoperative Preparations for the Surgical Team

Before entering the operating room, a scrub suit, foot and head coverings, and a mask are put on. Masks are changed after each case. Talking is kept to a minimum to prevent micro-organisms from being blown through the mask. The circulator and scrub technician prepare for the case before the patient enters the room, selecting the necessary instruments and supplies and ensuring that all electrical and mechanical equipment is working. They open all sterile supplies and count the sharps. All solutions, chemicals, and drugs are kept clearly labelled at all times.

The scrub technician prepares the Mayo stand, back table, and equipment necessary for the surgical case. Surgical instruments are placed on the draped Mayo tray and stand, where they are organized in the sequence preferred by the scrub technician to enhance comfort and efficiency. Additional or larger supplies and instruments are placed on the back table, which is also draped with a sterile covering. As the scrub technician prepares the surgical instruments and supplies, the patient is prepared for surgery (Fig. 25–4).

Preoperative Patient Preparation

Sixty to 90 minutes before intraocular surgery, the pupil of the operative eye is dilated or constricted as required by the type of anticipated procedure, e.g., the pupil is dilated before cataract surgery but is constricted before corneal transplant surgery. Explain to the patient what you are doing and why. Double-check to verify the correct medication in the correct strength at the correct interval for the correct number of times in the correct eye. Instillations of eye medications designated by the surgeon are administered approximately three times at 2- to 5-minute intervals.

The patient is wheeled into the operating room. A patient having surgery under local anesthesia is made as comfortable as possible in the supine position before the procedure because movement must be minimized after surgery begins. For this reason, patients are not allowed to fall asleep during the intraocular surgery because sudden awakening often produces equally sudden head movements that can prove disastrous. Oxygen or air is piped in through a nasal cannula or tube taped to the patient's chin to assure adequate oxygen under the drapes. The patient's arms are loosely restrained with a towel, sheet, or tape to prevent the patient's reaching up to the sterile field.

Once positioned on the operating table, the patient is attached to an electrocardiogram (ECG) with EGG electrodes placed on the chest to provide continuous readings; to an automatic blood pressure machine pro-

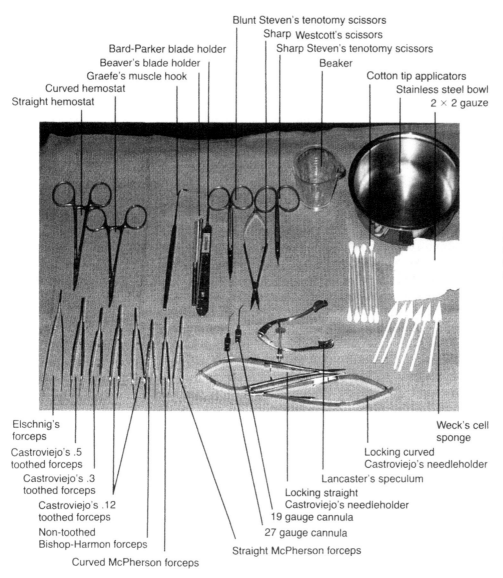

Straight hemostat
Curved hemostat
Graefe's muscle hook
Beaver's blade holder
Bard-Parker blade holder
Blunt Steven's tenotomy scissors
Sharp Westcott's scissors
Sharp Steven's tenotomy scissors
Beaker
Cotton tip applicators
Stainless steel bowl
2 × 2 gauze

Elschnig's forceps
Castroviejo's .5 toothed forceps
Castroviejo's .3 toothed forceps
Castroviejo's .12 toothed forceps
Non-toothed Bishop-Harmon forceps
Curved McPherson forceps
Straight McPherson forceps
27 gauge cannula
19 gauge cannula
Locking straight Castroviejo's needleholder
Lancaster's speculum
Locking curved Castroviejo's needleholder
Weck's cell sponge

FIGURE 25–4. Representative basic eye tray. The instruments included will vary considerably in different facilities.

grammed to record the patient's blood pressure every 5 to 10 minutes; and to a pulse oximeter. Routine monitoring continues throughout all local and general cases. The patient's head is steadied by resting on a doughnut-shaped cushion. General anesthesia is then administered or a regional block (retrobulbar/peribulbar), if not administered previously.

Facial Preparation

Now the surgical site is cleansed; the surgical preparation is done either by the scrubbed first assistant or by the circulator, while the ophthalmic surgeon scrubs his or her own hands and forearms. Care is taken to avoid getting the solution on the eye itself, as this could reduce visibility of the surgical site. The eye is rinsed with sterile saline from a bulb to reduce the toxic effects of the scrub solution (e.g., povidone-iodine [Betadine]) on the cornea.

Some surgeons require application of povidone-iodine paint to the area before blotting dry. This leaves a residual antimicrobial agent on the skin throughout the surgical procedure.

Surgical Drape

Sterile drapes are stacked on the back table for easy use in order to reduce handling. When draping, hold by the corners, cuffing the drape over your fingers to protect against possible contamination. Avoid flapping drapes because the created air currents may cause bacteria to rise up from the floor. Once in place, do not move them. Do not let drapes touch the floor.

The patient is draped, beginning with a sterile head and hair drape. A sterile body sheet is draped to extend from the patient's chin to the feet, covering the OR table and hanging over the sides. A plastic eye drape is placed over the operative eye area.

Facial Prep

1. All items and solutions for the preparation are arranged on a separate draped table (Fig. 25–5A).

2. The eyelids and lashes of the operative eye are mechanically cleansed with a cotton-tipped applicator soaked in an antimicrobial solution, e.g., an iodine-based soap such as povidone-iodine (Betadine) detergent, or hexachlorophene (pHisoHex) if the patient is allergic to Betadine (Fig. 25–5B).

3. The eyelids and surrounding area are cleansed in a circular fashion with a 4 × 4 gauze soaked in an antimicrobial agent, extending from the center out in all directions including the eyebrows, eye lids, bridge of the nose, forehead, and cheek (Fig. 25–5C). This is repeated three times using a clean 4 × 4 each time. Never return to a previously prepared area with the same 4 × 4.

4. Once thoroughly scrubbed, the preparation site may be rinsed off with a sterile saline solution, then blotted dry with a clean 4 × 4 (Fig. 25–5D).

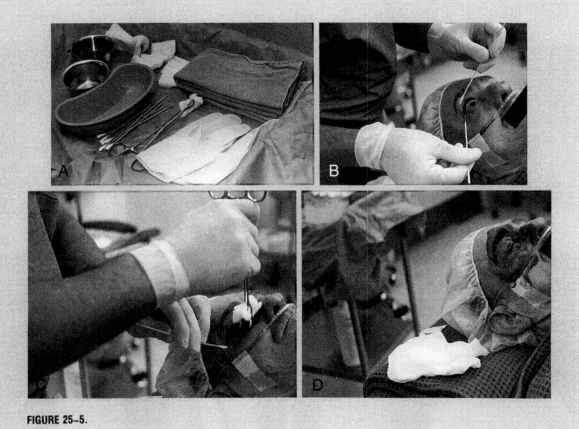

FIGURE 25–5.

Gowning and Gloving

After the surgical scrub is completed, a sterile gown and gloves are donned with a self-glove technique called *closed gloving.*

After anesthesia is administered, the surgeon and the surgical assistant begin their surgical scrub. The scrub technician assists the surgeon and the assistants with gowning and gloving.

When all members of the surgical team are in sterile attire, the gown is tied at the waist by having one scrubbed person hold the waist tie end as the other person turns around, so that the two ends can be tied. The first person then assists the scrub technician with the same turning procedure. After all members are turned and tied, excess talc is removed from the gloves with a damp cloth to prevent the talc from entering the surgical site.

Closed Glove Technique

1. The towel is grasped and lifted directly up without touching any article (Fig. 25–6A).

2. Unfold the towel while standing back away from any articles. Use one end of the towel to dry one arm, starting with the fingers and proceeding to the elbow (Fig. 25–6B). Use the opposite end of the towel for the other arm. Discard the towel as now contaminated.

3. Grasp the gown at the center and lift directly up (Fig. 25–6C). Move away to a clear area to avoid contamination during gowning.

4. Allow the gown to unfold while slipping the hands into the arm holes (Fig. 25–6D). A nonsterile member of the team will pull the gown over the shoulders and secure it at the neckline. *Only handle the inside of the gown while gowning.*

5. Do not allow fingers and hands to go through the gown's cuff at this time (Fig. 25–6E).

6. Open the glove package, exposing the gloves. Grasp the right glove with your left hand, with fingers still inside the cuff (Fig. 25–6F).

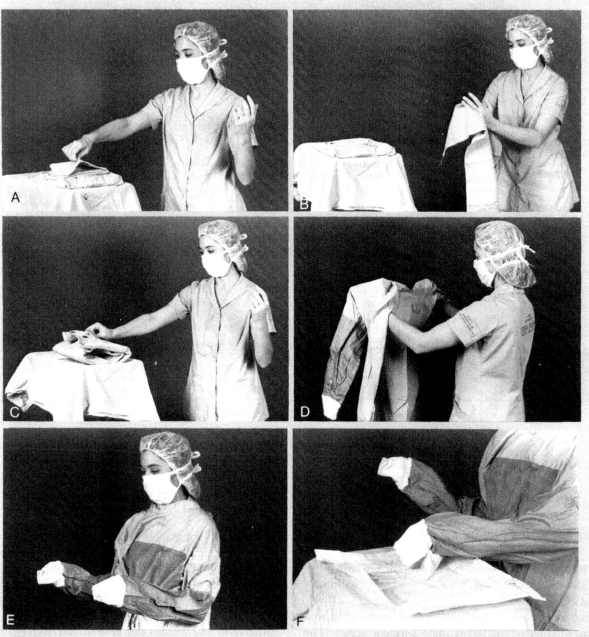

FIGURE 25–6.

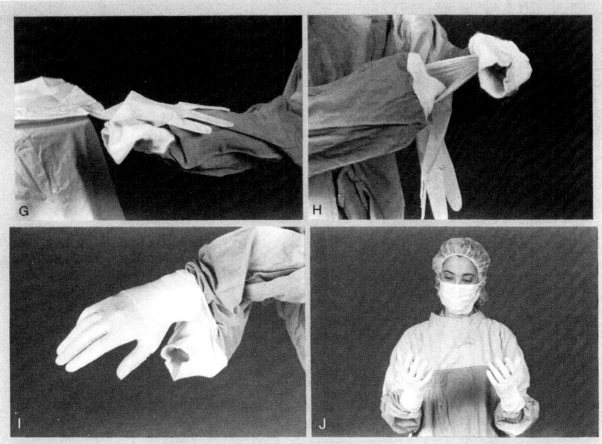

FIGURE 25-6. *Continued*

7. Lay the glove over the palm of your right hand (still inside *its* cuff) with the fingers of the glove facing your body (Fig. 26–6G). The thumb of the glove is on the same (right) side as your right thumb.

8. Grasp the edge of the glove's cuff with your right thumb (still inside the gown's cuff). Pull the opposite edge of the glove's cuff with the left hand (still in the gown's cuff) over the right hand, so that the right cuff of the gown is completely inside the glove (Fig. 25–6H).

9. Slip the right hand completely into the glove (Fig. 25–6I).

10. Repeat steps 6 through 9 for the left hand.

11. Now that gown and gloves are on, hands and arms must be kept away from the face and above waist level (Fig. 25–6J). The arms, hands, and front area of the gown from waist to chest are considered sterile at this time.

When removing gloves, the cuffs are pulled down. One gloved hand grasps the cuff of the other glove and pulls it off. The ungloved hand grasps the inside cuff of the first glove and pulls it off. In this way, neither hand touches the outside of either glove, which is now considered contaminated as it is removed.

Surgical Procedure

After the patient is prepared and steps are taken to make the surgical team and site sterile, an area in the operating room is designated as the sterile field. The eye, the surgical site, lies in the center. The Mayo

Assisting the Surgeon to Gown and Glove

1. The scrub technician hands the surgeon one end of an unfolded sterile towel (Fig. 25–7A). The technician dries the surgeon's hands employing the same technique described in 25–6B.

2. The scrub technician unfolds a gown, exposing the inside to the surgeon, who slips the hands into the arm holes (Fig. 25–7B). A nonsterile member of the team pulls the gown over the shoulders and secures it at the neck.

3. The scrub technician expands the edge of the right glove's cuff so that the surgeon can slip a hand into the glove (Fig. 25–7C).

4. Repeat for the left glove. The surgeon may assist in expanding the glove cuff for easier entry (Fig. 25–7D).

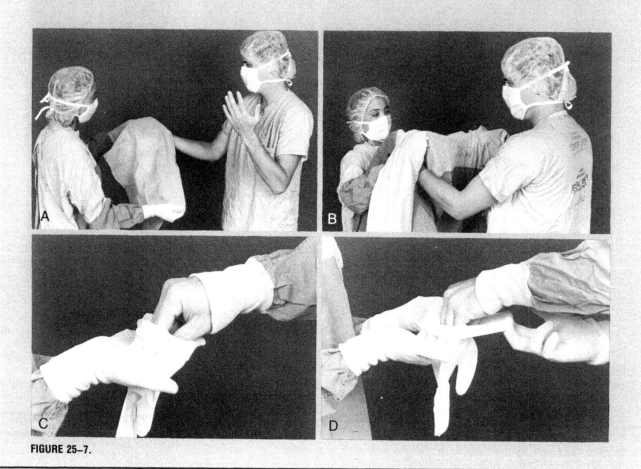

FIGURE 25–7.

stand, with the surgical instruments, and the back tables are moved into position. Attention is now directed to the surgical procedure. The surgical assistant and the scrub technician must remain alert, *anticipating* the surgeon's needs, by passing instruments, needles, blades, and sponges in sequence in the manner the surgeon prefers (Fig. 25–8). All operating room personnel work together for a smooth and problem-free procedure that ensures the best postoperative results for the most important person in the operating room—the patient.

Eye Patch

Following eye surgery, the eye is patched for comfort and protection. A patch does increase the temperature around the eye, however, enhancing bacterial growth. Therefore, a patch is to be discontinued as soon as possible. The patch must be firm enough to keep the eye lid closed under it, in order to prevent a corneal abrasion from the eye pad, as well as to provide pressure to avoid further swelling of tissues after surgery, such as an enucleation. The first pad may be folded in

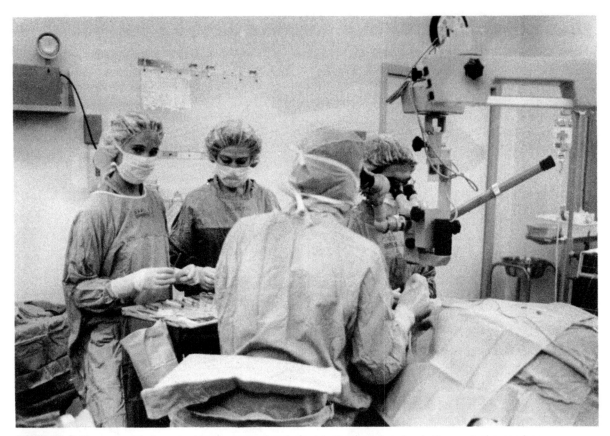

FIGURE 25–8. The assembled surgical team, gowned and gloved, stand ready to begin the surgical procedure.

half with a second pad placed flat on top of it to create a pressure patch. Oblique placement of strips of tape allows the mouth to open and close without disturbing the tape. A Fox shield guards against accidental trauma during this vulnerable postoperative period. It is applied after all intraocular surgery, e.g., cataract extraction, corneal transplant, and vitrectomy; in short, whenever the eye is surgically opened.

The eye patch is usually applied by the ophthalmologist. At the end of the case, the surgical assistant, or sometimes the scrub technician, is often too preoccupied in ridding the operating room of contaminated instruments to prepare for the next case. Postoperative orders are written in the chart by the surgeon. Written and verbal instructions are given to the patient by the Surgeon or Nurse, before discharge.

All sharps are counted as required by the facility before closure of any and all body cavities. At the end of each operation, after the patient is out of the room, contaminated supplies are either disposed of, or collected for cleaning and sterilizing. All items that came in contact with the patient or the sterile field are considered contaminated. All linens, gowns, gloves, masks, and instruments are removed as the OR table is stripped. Universal precautions are in effect on all cases to avoid cross-contamination. Before the next

case begins, the floor and all horizontal surfaces are disinfected with an antimicrobial agent, usually by a cleaning crew. The scrub assistant and circulator now prepare the room for the next case. The scrub technician, surgeon, and surgeon's assistant do not change their scrub suits unless they leave the operating room area, but they do change their head, beard, and foot coverings, as well as their masks.

Wound Closure

Surgical wound closure requires some form of tie, whether a suture, staple, clip, or other adhesive material. Ophthalmic sutures may be absorbable or nonabsorbable and are made of various materials, e.g., silk, nylon, Vicryl, each with intrinsic characteristics with regard to wound healing, ease of handling, and so forth. The suture may be composed of a single fiber (monofilament) or a group of fibers (multifilament). The material may be natural, e.g., silk, or synthetic, e.g., Vicryl. Silk is easy to handle, but like all natural sutures, it causes moderate tissue irritation and patient discomfort, which promotes faster healing. Monofilament nylon is less irritating but more difficult to tie. Vicryl is absorbable, strong, and has excellent knot security.

Patching the Eye

1. After removing the drapes, the eyelids and surrounding area are wiped clean with a damp 4 × 4 gauze (Fig. 25–9A).

2. The area is dried with a dry 4 × 4 and necessary drops or ointment instilled (Fig. 25–9B).

3. Two sterile oval eye pads are placed over the closed operative eye (Fig. 25–9C).

4. Surgical tape is applied diagonally with pressure from the forehead to the cheekbone (Fig. 25–9D).

5. A Fox eye shield is placed over the patch and secured with surgical tape (Fig. 25–9E).

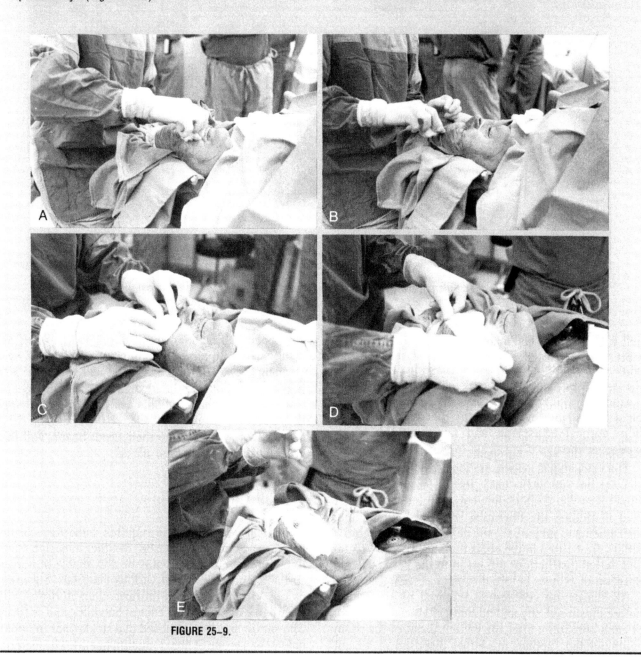

FIGURE 25–9.

The diameter of the suture is the width of the thread or fiber, designated by the number of the suture package. The lower the number, the larger the suture width; for example, a 10.0 suture is much finer than a 4.0 suture.

The tensile strength of a suture material is the amount of pull it can withstand before breaking. Suture material may have a relatively constant tensile strength or an initially high tensile strength, with a gradual reduction. For many types of intraocular ophthalmic surgical procedures, a circular, or semicircular, wound closure is required just outside the limbus. Two methods of suturing can be employed, *running* and *interrupted,* depending on the procedure and the surgeon's preference (Fig. 25–10).

Once placed inside the body, the suture is a foreign substance. Normal tissue reaction releases enzymes that try to degrade it. This rate of degradation, or absorption, is dependent on the material. Certain suture materials are especially formulated to prolong absorption. Absorbable sutures need not be removed. Nonabsorbable (nonbiodegradable) sutures are either removed or buried under tissue for an indefinite period. Improvement in wound closure and other surgical techniques have greatly reduced the necessity of restricting postoperative patient activity. Most patients are up and out of bed either the same day or the day after surgery.

Suture Needles

The needle has three components—the *eye,* the *body,* and the *point.*

The *eye* is where the suture fibers are attached to the needle. The eye is similar to the elongated opening of a sewing needle. Most sutures are prepackaged attached, i.e., swaged, to the needle, however. Most ophthalmic wounds are closed with a swaged needle (Fig. 25–11).

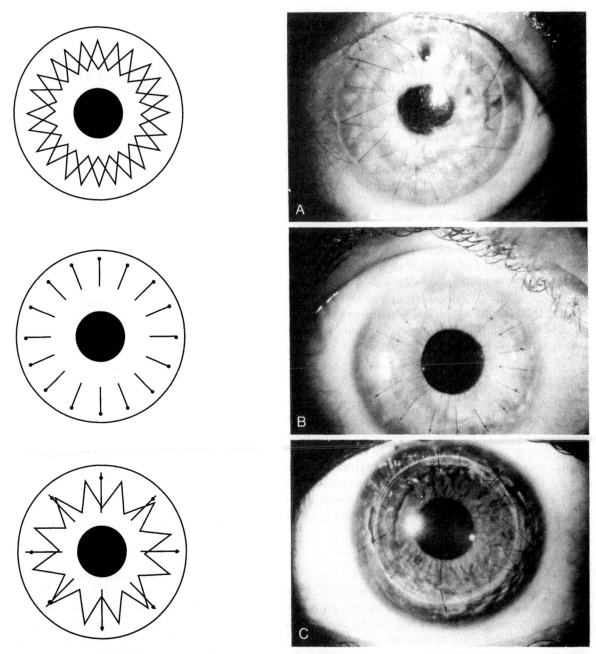

FIGURE 25–10. Ophthalmic suturing techniques. *A,* Running. *B,* Interrupted. *C,* Combination interrupted and running.

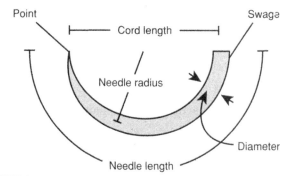

FIGURE 25–11. Surgical needle parameters.

The *body* of the needle extends from the eye to the point and is often referred to as the grasping area. The shape of the body may be round, oval, rectangular, triangular, or trapezoidal. The length of the body may be straight or curved to 90°, 145°, 180°, or 225°. Compound curved needles of fine gauge wire are often utilized in ophthalmic procedures.

The *point* of the needle is most important in suture placement. Cutting points have at least two sharp edges. The point may be triangular, with the apex inside the curve of the needle (conventional cutting) or with the apex outside the curve of the needle (reverse cutting). A side cutting point is trapezoidal, with the cutting edges on the side of the point. A taper point is a single, sharp point at the tip of the needle. Blunt point needles have no sharp edge. Taper and blunt points are rarely employed in ophthalmic surgery.

These delicate needles must be handled very carefully to avoid blunting the sharp tips and edges. Many types of tips, cutting edges, and curvatures exist. Each surgeon has preferences, which are usually recorded on a special card.

Applicators

Cotton-tipped and cellulose sponge applicators are common in ophthalmic surgery. Cotton-tipped swabs are available in 3- or 6-inch sizes, packaged by the manufacturer or purchased in bulk to be sterilized in smaller lots by the central supply department of the facility. Cellulose sponge applicators, also available in several sizes or shapes, are preferred in ophthalmology, because they are more absorbent and have no fibers or lint to shed.

Sponges

Sterile gauze or cloth pads, called sponges, especially 2 × 2 and 4 × 4, are used for various purposes. Some sponges have a dyed band woven through, to make them visible on a radiograph. In many institutions, no sponge or applicator count is performed, be-

cause they are so large compared with the eye and its orbit that the risk of one's accidentally being left in the ophthalmic surgical site is minimal. Cottonoids are counted.

Occasionally, delicate instruments are additionally cleaned and treated. Several methods may be employed.

Mechanical Hand Scrubbing. Cleaning with gentle abrasives may loosen clots and rust, especially in hard-to-reach areas. A soft toothbrush or nail brush works well with proper cleaning solutions. Rinse thoroughly with water.

Instrument Milk. This milky solution coats the cleaned instruments and prevents rust. It should be applied on a regular basis for instruments steam-sterilized frequently. Rinse instrument and wipe it off before using treated instrument in the eye.

• WRAPPING INSTRUMENTS FOR STERILIZATION

After cleaning, instruments must be wrapped to allow full exposure to either steam or gas sterilization. Inspect instruments for meshing of teeth, jaw alignment, and cutting ability before wrapping. Dissassemble detachable parts.

Wrap instruments in their open position, uncrowded in their case or wrap. Do not mix instruments of different materials, e.g., stainless steel, titanium, chrome-plated, together in the same wrap, because this may cause pitting. Place protective tips on sharp edges and place them securely in cases or in other packages. Wrap individual items in plastic packages; include chemical indicator strips. Do not use staples or clips to seal packages. Wrap cases in double cloth or paper and tape them securely with chemical sensor tape. Place heavier instruments near the bottom.

Label and date cases and packages clearly. Write expiration date on package (1 month for cloth or paper; 6 months for plastic). Any instrument with an unknown expiration date is considered nonsterile. Such "expired" items must be rewrapped before resterilizing. Do not reuse single use items. Preheat instruments in autoclave for 3 to 5 minutes before closing door.

• STERILIZATION

All instruments and supplies in a surgical procedure are cleansed of blood and bits of tissue in either mild detergent or an enzyme solution. After rinsing, they are placed in an ultrasonic unit before being brought to the room in the operating suite designated for sterilization. Instruments are placed in the ultrasonic unit disassembled and separated to avoid contact with other

Guidelines for the Care of Surgical Instruments

Because of the fragility and expense of ophthalmic surgical instruments, special, meticulous, "tender loving care" is required. The following list offers tips on cleaning, handling, and storing procedures.

1. During the case, gently wipe each instrument as you receive it from the surgeon with a sponge wet with sterile distilled water and place it back in the tray for possible reuse. Alternatively, soak the instrument in a 5 ml sterile beaker filled with sterile water (Fig. 25–12).

2. Rinse instruments with sterile water as soon as possible after use to remove blood, clots, serum, bits of tissue, and so forth. A sponge basin filled with sterile water may be made available to soak any instruments no longer needed in the procedure.

3. Flush all cannulas, reuseable needles, and infusion equipment with sterile water to remove all saline and tissue.

4. Use only mild, noncaustic detergent or enzyme solutions specified for cleaning surgical instruments. Clean with a soft toothbrush, never with steel wool, scouring powder, or high pH detergents.

5. Carefully wash instruments, then rinse them thoroughly with distilled water.

6. Disassemble detachable parts. Open hinged instruments.

7. Test function of instruments at end of each day, setting aside all those not in excellent working order.

8. Ultrasonic cleaning with proper solution is next. Place opened instruments in an ultrasound basket and immerse in appropriate cleaning solution. All instruments should be processed for 5 to 15 minutes in ultrasonic cycle. All lubrication must be removed. Rinse well with distilled water.

9. Dry with forced hot air.

10. Place rubber tips on sharp ends of instruments to protect their delicate edges.

11. Lubricate moving parts with instrument milk.

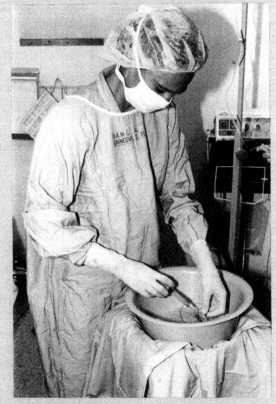

FIGURE 25–12. Instruments soaking in sponge basin.

12. Leave distilled water inside the lumen of the tubing or instruments because it will turn to steam as the temperature rises. Do not let tubing kink.

13. Place instruments in case, tray, or packaging for storage.

14. Prepare for sterilization—either in a wire mesh basket to "flash" or wrapped in cloth or plastic for steam or gas.

15. Include indicator strips or tape that darken when exposed to steam.

---

pieces. The ultrasonic unit cleans but does not sterilize. It utilizes high frequency sound energy to break up and remove debris from the serrations, box locks, and crevices of the instruments. In the designated work room, instruments are either organized into specialty sets or packaged individually. Instrument sets are placed on perforated trays, wrapped in paper or cloth, and secured with heat sensitive indicator tape. When the heat requirement for that tape is met, the tape color changes. Individual instruments are also wrapped in paper, cloth, or, more commonly, in transparent plastic pouches. Now they are ready for sterilization.

Sterilization kills micro-organisms by several means.

Steam Sterilization. This is the most common method. Pressurized steam kills micro-organisms including spores, the most resistant, by denaturing and coagulating proteins within each cell. Most metal instruments and supplies are placed in a mesh basket in an autoclave, which uses steam (moist heat) at 270°C under 30 pounds of pressure for 3 to 10 minutes to sterilize. The higher the temperature setting is, the shorter the cycle needed. Crowding of packs is inappropriate, because the moist heat must be able to penetrate. Because of its speed, this method is called "flashing." After the minimum 3 minutes of actual sterilization time, 6 to 7 minutes more is needed before opening the door. Some instruments cannot be sterilized by this method because of the moisture involved, or the high heat. The autoclave door is "cracked" open to allow drying and gradual temperature reduction before being fully opened. A sterilization indicator is used. Flashed items are considered sterile only for that particular case.

Required sterilization times for items flashed at 270°C:

Unwrapped loose instruments (5 or fewer)—3 minutes

Wrapped instrument set—15 minutes

Unwrapped tubing—10 minutes

Wrapped tubing—15 minutes

Linen packs—30 minutes

If steamed for 15 to 30 minutes, cloth- or paper-wrapped packages will remain sterile for 1 month and plastic-wrapped for 6 months. This method of sterilization is the most effective and least costly. The constant exposure to high temperature and moisture can damage delicate ophthalmic instruments, however. If the instrument was not cleaned properly before flashing, stains and discolorations will be seen.

Gas Sterilization. Micro-organisms, including spores, are killed by the gas's interfering with normal cell metabolism and reproduction. Instruments that are heat or moisture sensitive, like plastic spheres, are cleaned, dried, then wrapped in double muslin or paper or plastic. They are then exposed to ethylene oxide gas, one part per billion (ppb), for 3 to 6 hours. The package is aerated with heat (this keeps packing dense) and air (this removes gas particles) for an additional 6 hours to 7 days. Unlike steam sterilization, lumens of tubing and instruments must be dry before wrapping. Sensitive tape is included in the wrapping as a sterilization indicator. Sterility is maintained for 1 month with cloth or paper wrap, 6 months for plastic wrap.

Chemical Sterilization. Instruments and supplies are bathed with a potent chemical solution, an activated glutaraldehyde, such as Cidex (for 12 hours) or Glutarex (for 10 to 15 minutes; 25 if contaminated). These are then thoroughly rinsed *twice* with sterile water. This method, called "cold" sterilization (because no heat is involved), is rarely done in ophthalmology because of potential chemical reactions in the eye.

Ionizing Radiation. This is employed by many manufacturers of surgical supplies. Sutures, blades, applicators, and other equipment are sterilized by the manufacturer. Some have a sterility expiration date. As noted, supplies sterilized in the hospital have only limited sterility. Those exposed to ethylene oxide have the longest.

Bibliography

Atkison LJ, Kohn ML: Berry and Kohn's Introduction to Operating Room Technique, 7th ed. New York, McGraw-Hill, 1991.

Brightbill FS: Corneal Surgery, 2nd ed. St. Louis, CV Mosby, 1992.

Brooks SM: Fundamentals of Operating Room Nursing, 2nd ed. St. Louis, CV Mosby, 1979.

Casey TA, Mayer DJ: Corneal Grafting—Principles and Practice, 2nd ed. Philadelphia, WB Saunders, 1984.

Charles S: Vitreous Microsurgery, 2nd ed. Baltimore, Williams & Wilkins, 1987.

Emery JM, McIntyre DJ: Extracapsular Cataract Surgery, 2nd ed. St. Louis, CV Mosby, 1990.

Fuller JR: Surgical Technology, Principles and Practice, 3rd ed. Philadelphia, WB Saunders, 1993.

Instrument Care Book. Denville, NJ, Katena Instruments.

Meeker MH: Alexander's Care of the Patient in Surgery, 10th ed. St. Louis, CV Mosby, 1984.

Spaeth GL, et al: Ophthalmic Surgery—Principles and Practice, 2nd ed. Philadelphia, WB Saunders, 1989.

● CHAPTER 25 SURGICAL ASSISTING

1. Which of the following cranial nerves is *not* temporarily paralyzed by a retrobulbar injection?
    a. CN VI
    b. CN II
    c. CN IV
    d. CN V
    e. CN III

2. Which of the following is *not* a principle of aseptic technique?
    a. only touch sterile items
    b. handle sterile items as little as possible
    c. if in doubt, consider an item to be nonsterile
    d. hands in sterile gloves stay above waist level away from face and body
    e. once scrubbed and gowned, the front and back of the gown are sterile

3. Which of the following sequences for gowning and gloving is *incorrect*?
    a. Keep both hands inside the cuff of the gown's sleeves. With one cuffed hand pull first glove over the cuff of the other sleeve. Push other hand through cuff of other sleeve into first glove.
    b. With one cuffed hand pull first glove over the cuff of the other sleeve. Push other hand through cuff of other sleeve into first glove. Use this first gloved hand to pull second glove over cuff.
    c. Push other hand through cuff of other sleeve into first glove. Use this first gloved hand to pull second glove over this first cuff of first sleeve. Push ungloved hand through cuff into second glove.
    d. Keep one hand inside the cuff of the gown's sleeves. Use that hand to pull first glove over the hand and cuff of the other sleeve. Use first gloved hand to pull second glove over cuff of first sleeve.
    e. Slip scrubbed and dried hands into sterile gown. Keep both hands inside the cuff of the gown's sleeves. With one cuffed hand pull first glove over the cuff of the other sleeve. Push other hand through cuff of other sleeve into the first glove.

4. Which of the following guidelines for care of ophthalmic surgical instruments is *incorrect*?
   a. Rinse with sterile water as soon as possible.
   b. Keep detachable parts assembled.
   c. Place rubber tips on sharp ends.
   d. Flush all cannulas, reusable needles, and infusion equipment with sterile water.
   e. Lubricate moving parts with instrument milk.

5. What is the most common method for sterilizing ophthalmic surgical instruments?
   a. Autoclave (180° under 20 pounds pressure for 3 to 10 minutes)
   b. ethylene oxide gas (1 part/billion for 3 to 6 hours)
   c. ultrasonic unit
   d. activated glutaraldehyde
   e. flashing (270° under 30 pounds pressure for 3 to 10 minutes)

Alison Guber

Examination Strategy

LEARNING OBJECTIVE

● Devise a typical basic format for examination of the eyes depending on the type of problem presented

Ophthalmic technical personnel should approach any examination with two basic intentions. The first is to *document* all pertinent information. By *anticipating* what your ophthalmologist needs, you decide what information it is necessary to obtain. From hundreds of possible tests, you select the fewest necessary to obtain the information your ophthalmologist requires to diagnose the condition and advise the patient. Second, you perform the examination quickly and efficiently, approaching each as though expecting to find an eye dysfunction.

The patient assumes you are under the direction of the ophthalmologist and will know what to do. If an examination has ten parts, do not explain all ten parts initially. Explain each test to the patient as it is to be performed. A long, detailed explanation wastes time. A short one- or two-sentence explanation of the next phase is all that is required. Give additional instruction as each phase of each test is about to begin. Do not diagnose or explain what the results might mean to the ophthalmologist. There is a fine line between explaining what you are doing and telling the patient what the test has shown. The first can be done, but the second is not the function of technical personnel. If there is time after all testing is finished, while the patient is waiting and if he or she asks for clarification, details may be given. During testing, there are times when the patient may be pushed to produce additional responses. Sometimes this follows a 10- or 15-minute rest, but should never occur when the patient is too ill or too tired.

● *For example.* If a patient easily reads the 20/50 line without mistakes or hesitation, but then claims to

be able to see no farther, do not assume this is true. Smaller letters are not as clear and the patient may wish to avoid making a mistake. The patient needs to be encouraged with statements such as "Try this next line anyway," or "Tell me what you think you see." Only after the patient fails to recognize more than half the symbols can you record the best visual acuity.

Children and the elderly probably need the gentlest, most subtle encouragement the examiner can muster.

● FALSE-POSITIVE AND FALSE-NEGATIVE RESULTS

A false-positive result occurs when you record a test response indicating a nonexistent abnormality. A false-negative result occurs when you record a test as normal although there is an abnormality you missed. Missing a visual field defect is a false-negative result. Finding an enlarged blind spot caused by poor fixation is a false-positive. Try to avoid both situations. Attempt to document not only what is pertinent but also what is valid. False-positive and negative results are easier to avoid on objective than subjective testing. If in doubt, trust the objective test. You must nevertheless record what the patient tells you. Your ophthalmologist decides what is valid.

● MANIFEST REFRACTOMETRY

As part of your evaluation, many patients have a manifest refraction. This includes all new patients, and return patients with various signs and symptoms, such as

Headaches

Blurred or changed vision

More than 12 months since the last manifest refraction

Postoperative cataract return, after approximately two weeks

Postoperative glaucoma return, after 1 month

Postoperative retina return, after 1 month

Desire for a duplicate prescription more than a year old.

A manifest refraction is performed on these patients even without improvement with a pinhole (NI c ph, i.e., no improvement with pinhole). When the manifest refraction offers no improvement over the old lenses or the pinhole vision, do not write only no improve-

ment, but the day's manifest refraction with the visual acuity after it.

● *For example.*

> *VOD cc 20/60 c ph NI*
> *VOS cc 20/70 c ph NI*
> *MR +2.25 +2.00 × 90 = 20/60*
> *MR +2.50 +2.25 × 90 = 20/70*

Be sure to document whether the reflex or the patient's subjective responses are poor. If a copy of a prescription less than 1 year old is given without manifest refractometry, record this in the chart. If a difference from the last examination is encountered with retinoscopy of the right eye and you are unsure of the patient's

---

New Patient Work-up

1. Visual acuity is always tested first except for cases of emergency chemical burns and childhood strabismus. Whenever possible, vision is evaluated on Snellen letter or number charts with the patient's current refractive correction worn, either as eyeglasses or contact lenses. If vision is less than 20/200, or if the patient is over age 50, near vision is also tested. If vision is less than 20/20, vision is retested through a multiple pinhole. Vision is always evaluated separately for each eye by occluding the eye not being tested. A whole line of vision may be blocked off at a time, but isolating each letter is not advised, because amblyopia will be incompletely detected.

2. Applanation tonometry is performed, usually at the slit lamp. A Tono-pen may be substituted.

3. Motility is assessed by
   a. Evaluating stereopsis with the Titmus test. If the patient correctly identifies which circle "stands out" on the last three sets, it best indicates normal binocular vision. The patient may have a phoria or intermittent tropia but not a constant misalignment.
   b. Noting the equality or inequality of the position of the corneal light reflexes, and determining whether there is an eso-, exo-, or hyper-deviation.
   c. Proving the deviation with a cover test. If there is none, evaluate whether a phoria is present.
   d. Testing the six cardinal positions of gaze for any abnormalities of extraocular muscle versions.

4. Confrontation test for gross estimate of visual field loss. Using yourself as the control, test the patient's ability to correctly count the fingers you hold up in each of four quadrants, up and right, down and right, up and left, and down and left. Hold your fingers in the middle of the quadrant, midway between yourself and the patient.

Because the central field is most important, test this with an Amsler grid. If abnormal, you may want to repeat the test with the patient's near correction.

5. Test pupil function in dim illumination with distance fixation. Note pupil size, shape, reactivity to light, and whether or not any difference in pupillary response is seen in the two eyes.

6. View the fundus with a direct ophthalmoscope, noting the disc, vessels, macula, and background. Estimate the cup-to-disc ratio. Estimate the height of any lesion seen extending into the vitreous by remembering that for every diopter of change to keep the lesion in focus, there is 0.3-mm size variation.

7. Refer the following to your ophthalmologist without any work-up:
   a. Any penetrating injury
   b. Chemical burns *after* copious irrigation
   c. Red, painful eye
   d. Sudden painless loss of vision
   e. Flashing lights, curtain, scotoma
   f. Microscopic or deep foreign body; if superficial, irrigate and use wet swab under the lids to remove; if microscopic or deep, refer.

8. With approval from your ophthalmologist, instill dilating drops (e.g., cyclopentolate [Cyclogyl 1%], one drop each eye every 5 min 3×). The dropper bottle tip must never touch the eye or eyelid. Punctal occlusion for 30 sec, by holding one finger against the side of the nose next to the inner canthus of the eye being dropped, should be done whenever possible.

Evaluation of New Patient for Cataracts

1. History needs special questions. Why does the patient desire removal? What can he or she not do that he or she wants to do? Other questions concern

Glare
Decreased night vision
Foggy and hazy vision
Ghosting (monocular diplopia)
Haloes.

2. Check for visual acuity, pinhole vision, manifest refraction, and best corrected vision.
3. Perform keratometry for corneal curvatures.

4. Conduct glare test, slit lamp examination, and applanation tonometry. Record the red reflex seen in retinoscopy, or the reflex seen on slit lamp exam by retroillumination. Remember to describe lens changes, such as nuclear sclerotic, cortical, and posterior subcapsular changes, but do not attempt to diagnose the type of cataract.
5. Obtain approval to dilate the patient's pupils.
6. While the patient's pupils are dilating, and if visual acuity is sufficiently decreased to warrant consideration of cataract surgery, perform tests for the acuity potential of the retina (e.g., laser interferometry or the Potential Acuity Meter [PAM]).

---

cooperation, test the left eye. If no difference from the last examination is found, you conclude there was a problem with the right eye, not with patient cooperation.

Manifest refractometry is not necessary when return patients have

No visual complaint

No change in visual acuity

Manifest refractometry performed within the last 12 months, or not incorporated into the patient's prescription.

Place the results of that recent manifest refraction into a trial frame, however, and check and record the visual acuity. It may be necessary to use it for the best corrected vision that day.

Except for ocular motility dysfunction, all patients have vision tested first, then a manifest refraction if needed, then a slit lamp examination, and finally a measurement of intraocular pressure. Following that point, much depends on the reason for the visit. The eyes of new patients are always dilated after testing pupil function. As with all drops, avoid contacting the eye with the tip of the dropper bottle. Technical personnel may do the cycloplegic refraction, but the ophthalmologist evaluates the fundus and determines additional tests for that visit. If the patient has either glaucoma or ocular hypertension, *anticipate* and perform repeat visual fields, depending on when they were last recorded.

Every ophthalmologic practice is different. Expect variations of the following schemes depending on your supervisor, but these strategies are typical.

Preoperative Evaluation of Patient for Cataract Surgery

1. Obtain the best corrected vision for the day.
2. Perform a slit lamp examination.
3. Measure intraocular pressure by applanation tonometry.
4. Obtain approval to dilate the patient's pupils.
5. Work up next patient while waiting for full dilation.
6. Examine the lens from a 1-m distance with an ophthalmoscope or slit lamp for residual clear areas that might

be penetrated by the PAM or laser beam for interferometry.
7. Record vision from the PAM or laser interferometry for potential vision expected after surgery.
8. Find corneal curvature measurements (Ks) by keratometry.
9. Measure axial lengths by A-scan ultrasound. Axial lengths and Ks are used in calculating the power of the intraocular lens implant.

Postoperative Cataract Evaluation

1. During history taking, record date of surgery and any complaints, especially about pain and foreign body sensation.

2. Does the patient subjectively see better or worse?

3. Ask about medications: which drugs e.g., dexamethasone (Maxitrol, Maxidex, Decadron, AK-Dex) or tobramycin (Tobradex), how often, when was last application?

4. Evaluate vision without correction (sc) in each eye on each visit. If there is no intraocular lens implant, utilize a +10.00 lens. Retest with a pinhole.

5. Perform keratometry and manifest refraction on the postoperative eye.

6. Examine each eye on each visit using slit lamp examination and applanation tonometry. Results in the unoperated eye will tell you what is normal for that patient.

    a. Note corneal edema or folds in Descemet's membrane.

    b. Count sutures.

    c. Notice whether any sutures are tight or loose. If loose, does the wound leak? Does the wound gape? Is the wound secure?

    d. Is the anterior chamber deep and quiet or does it have cell and flare?

    e. Is the peripheral iridectomy patent (open)?

7. Measure intraocular pressure by applanation tonometry and record the time it was taken.

8. Dilate the eye 6 weeks postoperatively. If it is less than 4 weeks postoperatively or if vision is less than 20/100, ask about dilating (e.g., 2.5% phenylephrine (Neo-Synephrine) and 1% Mydriacyl) for a fundus examination.

8. Dilate the patient's pupils at the postoperative visit when the final prescription will be given.

9. The ophthalmologist will determine by the amount of astigmatism found on manifest refractometry when and which additional sutures to cut.

Neurological Work-up

1. History: any recent illness, any headaches, any new medications?

2. Measure visual acuity with correction (cc). Attempt to improve it with a manifest refraction.

3. Evaluate binocular vision and ocular motility.

4. Observe pupil function.

	Light response	Concensual response
OD size in mm	0 to +4	0 to +4
OS size in mm	Light response 0 to +4	Consensual response 0 to +4

5. Test color vision.

6. Test visual fields, especially at the vertical meridian.

Glaucoma Work-up

1. History: How long since diagnosis, what medication, how often and how compliant, when did patient last take each medication? Any change in vision? Any surgery? Was it by laser or microsurgery?

    Commonest drops:

        Timolol (T) 1/4% or 1/2% BID (yellow)

        Propine (DPE) .1% BID (green)

        Pilocarpine (P) .5% up to 6% (green)

    Less likely pills:

        Acetazolamide (Diamox) 215 mg or 250 mg QID

        Methazolamide (Neptazane) 50 mg or 100 mg BID (ask about stomach upset)

    Family history of glaucoma?

2. Evaluate visual acuity with correction (cc). If poorer than last visit, attempt to improve with manifest refraction.

3. Slit lamp examination: Observe anterior chamber for depth, notice any filtering bleb. If there is one, is it functioning or flat? Is the angle deep or narrow? Is any previous peripheral iridectomy open (patent)?

4. Review chart for date of last visual field. If longer than 6 months ago, repeat visual fields with same targets or programs used for last field.

5. If less than 6 months previously, review chart for note by ophthalmologist to have visual fields repeated on this visit. *All new patients have Goldmann's visual fields (GVF), or automated Humphrey's fields (HVF).*

6. Measure intraocular pressure by applanation tonometry.

7. Patients are usually dilated on first visit, but not on return visits.

Retina Work-up

1. History: Is patient diabetic? Dosage of insulin? Does patient have high blood pressure? Is there any sudden loss of vision or a "curtain" down over one eye (symptom of retinal detachment)? Are any flashes of light (photopsia) present? Was there surgery, laser or other?

2. Test visual acuity with correction (cc). Repeat with pinhole unless vision is 20/20.

3. Begin manifest refraction (MR) with retinoscopy results, then refine, unless vision is 20/20.

4. Slit lamp examination: If patient is diabetic, look for blood vessels at the pupillary border (sign of rubeosis iridis).

5. Test pupillary function.

6. Measure intraocular pressure by applanation tonometry and record when taken.

7. Obtain permission to dilate the patient's pupils. If any signs of rubeosis iridis or relative afferent pupillary defect are present, ask the ophthalmologist for confirmation prior to dilating the patient's pupils.

Bibliography

Please see Chapter 28.

● CHAPTER 26 EXAMINATION STRATEGY

1. Which of the following statements is true?
   a. Patient is given full explanation of entire examination at the beginning.
   b. Ophthalmic technical personnel do not make diagnostic decisions.
   c. Ophthalmic technical personnel record what they think is correct, not necessarily what patient says.
   d. All testing is completed before allowing patient a rest period.
   e. Do *not* note appropriateness of patient responses.

2. When is manifest refractometry recommended?
   a. If patient returns in 2 months without complaints about vision
   b. If patient returns in 4 months with no change in vision
   c. If more than 1 year has elapsed since last manifest refractometry
   d. If postoperative cataract patient returns after one week
   e. If patient wants a copy of manifest refractometry performed 6 months ago

3. Which of the following series of tests is typical for a new patient workup?
   a. Vision, slit lamp, tonometry, motility, confrontation, pupil function, and dilation
   b. Vision, slit lamp, tonometry, motility, automated perimetry, pupil function, and dilation
   c. Vision, slit lamp, tonometry, motility, pupil function, axial lengths, and dilation
   d. Vision, slit lamp, tonometry, motility, keratometry, pupil function, and confrontation
   e. Vision, manifest refractometry, slit lamp, keratometry, confrontation, pupil function, and dilation

4. Refer to your ophthalmologist, without further working up the patient, when there is which of the following?
   a. sudden double vision
   b. superficial foreign body
   c. slow loss of vision over years
   d. glare from night headlights
   e. sudden painless loss of vision

5. Which of the following workups is most likely to require color vision testing?
   a. glaucoma
   b. retina
   c. cataract
   d. neurological
   e. new

Abnormalities of the Eye

Barbara Cassin
Donna McDavid
Diana Shamis

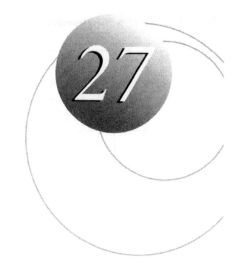

Eye Disorders

LEARNING OBJECTIVES

- List the primary causes of blindness in the United States
- Know what tests are used to detect age-related macular degeneration (ARMD)
- Describe the normal position of the upper eyelid margin
- Measure levator function
- Differentiate among normal, congenital, and acquired nystagmus
- Define a cataract
- Describe the difference among intracapsular cataract extraction, extracapsular cataract extraction, and phacoemulsification
- List tests used to evaluate patients with preoperative cataract for vision impairment and potential vision recovery

- Understand how cataract surgery can produce astigmatism
- Describe the difference between primary open angle glaucoma and closed angle glaucoma
- Understand the mechanisms by which intraocular pressure increases
- Understand how and why the optic nerve head and the anterior chamber angle are involved in glaucoma
- List the commonest sequence of visual field loss in glaucoma
- List at least six drugs regularly used to control glaucoma

● AGE-RELATED MACULAR DEGENERATION (ARMD)

The macula is the area of the retina responsible for the sharpest, clearest, central vision. ARMD is characterized by thinning and breaking down of the macular tissues. Bruch's membrane progressively thickens and drusen forms in the macula, causing atrophy and depigmentation of the retinal pigment epithelium. As the number of drusen increases, so does macular destruction. The macula shows areas of reduced pigmentation in the middle of streaks and specks of pigmentation. Sometimes small hemorrhages and exudates are found. The choriocapillaris bleeds, then develops abnormal new blood vessels (neovascular membranes) under the macula, along with fluid leaks (serous retinal detachment) which elevate the area. The fragile neovascular membranes rupture easily, developing subretinal hemorrhages which lead to scar formation. Vision decreases markedly. At the end stages of the process, the macula becomes a raised white elevated mass of subretinal scar tissue and exudate.

This gradual destruction of the macula is the leading cause of irreversible legal blindness (20/200 or less) in older white people. This causes the very center of view to become smudged, wavy, or distorted. One eye is often involved months or even years before the other. Patients over age 60 are at risk for this degenerative, incurable disease.

Initial symptoms often include distortion of straight lines and objects (metamorphopsia) and blurring. Testing with Amsler's grid is often useful (Fig. 27–1). Color vision may deteriorate. Symptoms are often not appreciated until the second eye becomes involved. Side (peripheral) vision stays intact. At an early stage of the disease, laser surgery can seal off abnormal areas, both reducing and retarding the spread of the disease. Fluorescein angiography is useful in detecting the extent of damage.

● PTOSIS

Ptosis (blepharoptosis) is the condition of the upper eyelid margin wherein it droops below its expected position as the eyeball looks straight ahead. Ptosis usually indicates deficient levator palpebrae superioris muscle function (Fig. 27–2).

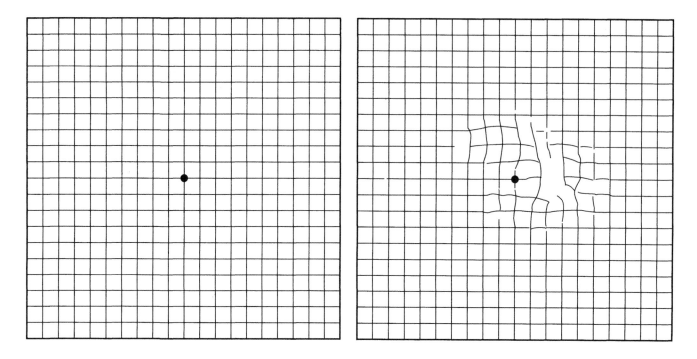

A   B

FIGURE 27–1. Amsler grid. *A,* Without metamorphopsia. *B,* With metamorphopsia.

The average palpebral fissure width, at midposition, is about 11 mm. The average palpebral fissure length is about 28 mm. The average corneal diameter is 12 mm horizontally, but 11 mm vertically. Assuming no vertical deviation, the corneal light reflection is 5.5 from either upper or lower limbus. The lower limbus is usually at the lower lid margin, or 0.5 mm below it. Using a clock face to describe lid position can be misleading for ptosis patients because the eyelid margins may slant lower on the nasal side than the temporal, or the reverse. Noting the midposition location in relation to the corneal reflex is more appropriate. The upper eyelid margin usually rides over the upper cornea about 1.5 mm, so that the upper eyelid margin midposition should be 4 mm above the corneal light reflection. If the upper eyelid margin is 1 to 2 mm below its normal

position, the ptosis is mild; at 3 mm below, it is moderate; and at 4 mm below, it is severe.

A lid fold that covers part of the tarsal portion is normally found in the upper eyelid (Fig. 27–3). The poorer the levator function, the less the fold. The less the fold, the more the tarsal portion of the lid shows. Poor levator function has no lid fold, only a lid crease. If even a minor lid crease is found in up gaze, some minimal levator function is indicated. Lack of a lid crease indicates no levator muscle function. Usually the lashes point down, and an everted lid cannot unflip itself. When levator function is poor, the upper eyelid is frequently 2 to 3 mm lower than normal when the eye is in primary position. If the ptosis is congenital, the palpebral fissure widens in down gaze because the levator malfunction prevents the upper lid from follow-

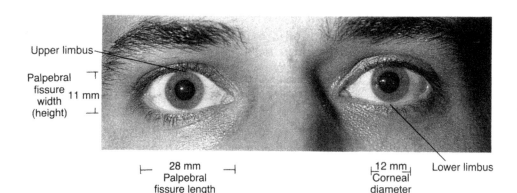

Upper limbus

Palpebral fissure width (height) 11 mm

├── 28 mm ──┤
Palpebral
fissure length

12 mm
Corneal
diameter

Lower limbus

FIGURE 27–2. Palpebral fissure terminology and measurement.

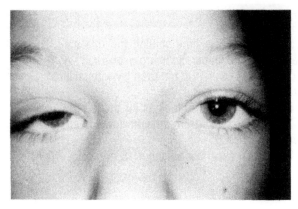

A

4 mm ptosis OD
lid crease

2 mm ptosis OS
lid fold

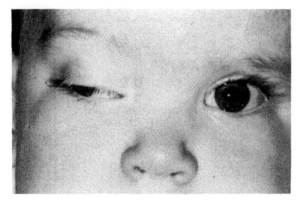

B

6 mm ptosis OD
no lid crease

no ptosis OS
lid fold

FIGURE 27–3. Blepharoptosis. *A,* Mild and moderate ptosis. Right eye; 5-mm tarsal portion of lid showing under lid crease. Left eye; 2-mm tarsal portion of lid showing under lid fold. *B,* Severe ptosis. Right eye; no lid fold, no lid crease. Left eye; no ptosis. Normal lid fold, 1-mm tarsal portion of lid showing under lid fold.

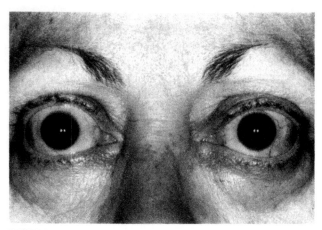

FIGURE 27–4. Proptosis from thyroid eye disease, Note sclera showing both above and below cornea, right eye more than left eye.

may be too low, also from proptosis, with sclera showing below the lower limbus. The resulting widened palpebral fissure gives the appearance of "stare," most often caused by thyroid ophthalmopathy (Fig. 27–4).

Sometimes the palpebral fissure opening appears too small. Enophthalmus may occur if the eye falls back into the orbit, because of less bulk, e.g., from loss of orbital fat with age. The eye and the orbital contents do not exert enough pressure to keep the eyelids apart as much as usual. Blepharophimosis is a condition of too little tissue in the eyelids. Less of the external eye peeps through, resulting in the upper eyelid's riding too low. For these mechanical reasons in eyeball position, the eyelids may be more open or more closed than usual.

● NYSTAGMUS

This disturbance of eye movement is characterized by involuntary, rhythmic, to-and-fro oscillations of one or both eyes. Most nystagmus is horizontal, but vertical, oblique, and rotary forms are encountered as well. Rotary nystagmus may be more circular or elliptical, as seen in patients with multiple sclerosis, but it can be torsional, as seen in patients with skew deviation from brain stem disease. Similar ocular oscillations that are not rhythmic are called nystagmoid movements. Vision is best when the eyes look in the direction where the movement is least. Patients with nystagmus adopt an abnormal head posture to take advantage of this, e.g., if the nystagmus dampens most in right gaze, a head turn to the left is adopted. There is no single

ing the eye down. The levator relaxes, as well as contracts, poorly.

Levator muscle function is tested by noting the difference in millimeters of how far down the upper eyelid is when looking in extreme down gaze, and then how far up it is in extreme up gaze. The brow must be manually blocked so that the frontalis muscle does not influence eyelid position. An arched eyebrow is an indication of use of the frontalis muscle to aid the levator.

If the upper eyelid is above the upper limbus with sclera showing, it is too high. This can be caused by the eyeball's being pushed forward, i.e., proptosis, because of extra bulk in the orbit. The lower eyelid margin

Levator Function Testing

1. Block both eyebrows by pushing down on them with your left thumb and forefinger. This prevents the use of the frontalis muscle to raise the upper eyelid.

2. Hold a millimeter rule vertically with your right hand just outside the center of the lid.

3. Tell the patient to look as far down as possible.

4. Note the centimeter mark position on the rule that is parallel to the upper lid margin position.

5. Do not waste time shifting the rule until the zero mark is at the upper lid margin position, unless it is accomplished easily. Do not even try with children. Settle for a centimeter mark.

6. Tell the patient to look as far up as possible.

7. The difference from straight down to straight up is levator function.

8. Normal excursion is about 15 mm (Fig. 27–5).

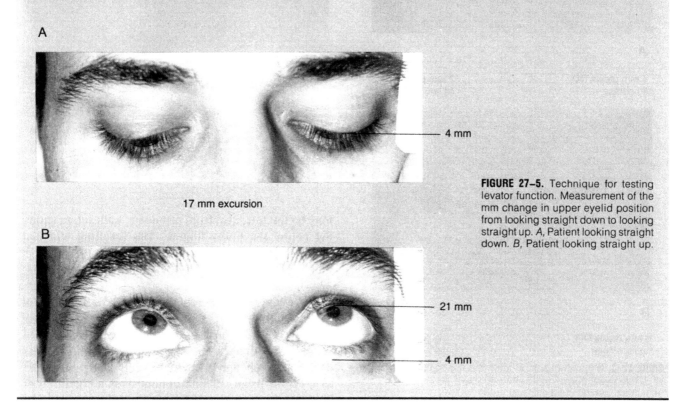

A

17 mm excursion

B

4 mm

21 mm

4 mm

FIGURE 27–5. Technique for testing levator function. Measurement of the mm change in upper eyelid position from looking straight down to looking straight up. *A*, Patient looking straight down. *B*, Patient looking straight up.

accepted classification, but the simple classification in Figure 27–6 includes the more common forms.

The underlying defect appears to be disturbed feedback to the gaze centers in the brain stem that interferes with control of the fixation mechanism. The result is a so-called motor defect from abnormal signals to the extraocular muscles for eye movement. The ability to fixate straight ahead may be defective or the vision may be too poor to provide sufficient visual stimulation for stable fixation. There may also be an imbalance of messages coming to the system from the two sides of the vestibular system. Nystagmus can be induced in normal patients by rotating the body, irrigating an ear with water, or moving the visual stimulus.

Patterns

There are two basic patterns. Jerk nystagmus occurs when the speed of the oscillations is more rapid in one direction than the other. The slow phase, which is caused by the underlying defect, is produced by the pursuit, vergence, vestibular, or fixation systems. The fast phase is the corrective repositioning produced by the saccadic system. Jerk nystagmus is named for the direction of the fast phase, e.g., right-beating and left-beating. The speed, amplitude, and even the direction may differ depending on the field of gaze. The other pattern, pendular nystagmus, occurs when the oscillations are horizontal with approximately the same speed in each direction.

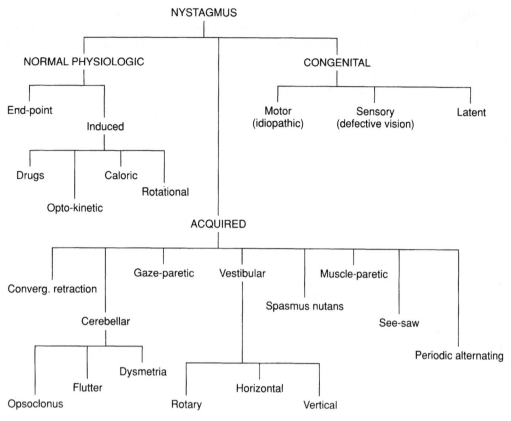

FIGURE 27-6. Classification of nystagmus.

Characteristics of Nystagmus

1. Usually decreases vision
2. May dampen with:
   a. Convergence. If so, near vision better than distance
   b. An abnormal head posture to take advantage of a null point
   c. Closing the eyes
   d. Sleep
   e. Slow tracking (pursuit) movements
3. Jerk or pendular in direction
4. Fast or slow speed
5. May have oscillopsia, i.e., visual environment appearing to move in the same direction as the fast phase (occurs with acquired nystagmus, not congenital)
6. Increases with:
   a. Fatigue
   b. Fast saccadic fixation
   c. Use of drugs or alcohol
7. Associated symptoms of acquired vestibular nystagmus:
   a. Spinning sensation (vertigo)
   b. Ringing in the ears (tinnitus)
   c. Nausea
8. Amplitude possibly fine (excursion $<3°$) $\rightarrow$, moderate (excursion of 5 to 15°), $\Rightarrow$ or coarse (excursion $>15°$). $\Rrightarrow$
9. Symbols often used: $\leftrightarrow$ pendular horizontal
   $\rightarrow$ left beating
   $\downarrow$ down beating
   $\cap$ pendular rotary
10. Possible change of speed, amplitude, and direction from one field of gaze to another, so-called laterality
11. Possible differences in form, speed, and amplitude in the two eyes, so-called dissociated
12. Acquired types follow Alexander's law, i.e., nystagmus increases when looking in the direction of the fast phase; examples include up beating nystagmus increasing in up gaze and right beating increasing in right gaze.

Normal Physiologic Nystagmus

This is a normal symmetrical response in both eyes to an induced imbalance in, or an excessive demand on, the feedback system from the vestibular system to the ocular motor system. An asymmetrical response in either eye is a sign of disease.

Induced nystagmus in normal patients provides evidence for normal labyrinthine function.

End-Point

If fixation is maintained for more than 30 sec in extreme limits of gaze, usually beyond the binocular field, a jerk nystagmoid movement is seen in 50% of normal patients. The fast phase is toward the limit of gaze. Although not a true nystagmus, it may be difficult to distinguish from gaze-paretic nystagmus associated with a defect of the gaze centers or muscle-paretic nystagmus associated with a defect in innervation to an extraocular muscle. In gaze-paretic, muscle-paretic, and normal end-point nystagmus, the eye drifts back toward primary position, followed by a jerk back to the extreme gaze.

Optokinetic Nystagmus (OKN)

Introducing and slowly moving a drum (or tape) with vertical stripes (or pictures) about a foot in front of a patient's eyes as the patient watches provokes a jerk nystagmus with the fast phase in the opposite direction of the tape movement (Fig. 27–7). The eyes fix and follow one stripe for a short distance, then quickly shift to fix and follow another stripe. Stripes moving to the right produce a normal physiological response with a slow pursuit to the right and a fast refixation saccade back to the left. If optokinetic nystagmus is symmetrical on testing both to the right and to the left, it verifies

that the sensory visual pathway, the saccadic system, the pursuit system, and the connections from the visual cortex to the ocular motor system are functioning as they should. This signifies that the ocular motor pathways are intact.

Asymmetrical or absent optokinetic nystagmus indicates that a pathological condition exists. For example, deep parietal lobe disease associated with hemianopsia disturbs the optokinetic response. The field defect results from damage to the optic radiations in the parietal area. The slow phase of optokinetic nystagmus is defective when the tape is moved toward the side of the lesion, e.g., moving the tape from left to right elicits a decreased response in the slow phase to the right when the disease is in the right parietal lobe. Interestingly, patients with a history of infantile esotropia have normal temporal to nasal optokinetic nystagmus, but decreased nasal to temporal optokinetic nystagmus under monocular viewing conditions.

Optokinetic nystagmus cannot be induced in blind patients. Alternatively, an optokinetic response is difficult for a patient to stop if there is vision. If optokinetic nystagmus is normal in a patient claiming blindness, it proves that the patient can see and may be malingering or may have a hysterical visual loss.

Drugs

Tranquilizers, barbiturates, anticonvulsants such as preoperative medications, alcohol, and so forth, will produce nystagmus that is up-beating in up gaze, left-beating in left gaze, and so forth.

Vestibular System

Head movement causes a flow of endolymph in the semicircular canals of the inner ear. Signals are transmitted to the brain stem gaze centers of the ocular motor system. This feedback mechanism stabilizes the movement of the eyes so that retinal images stay steady as the head and body move.

Testing the vestibular mechanism can be done by attempting to produce a doll's head maneuver. If the head is moved quickly to the right, the eyes move left, and vice versa. This vestibular ocular reflex (VOR) can be suppressed by fixating a target.

Under normal conditions, the labyrinths on both right and left sides are stimulated equally. No nystagmus is noted. If the amount of stimulation to one side is out of balance by either too much or too little stimulation, however, nystagmus results.

Labyrinthine nystagmus can be induced as a normal physiological response by spinning the body or by caloric stimulation. This verifies that the labyrinth and semicircular canals are transmitting these out-of-balance signals to the ocular motor system. The nystagmus induced can be horizontal, vertical, or rotary. In-

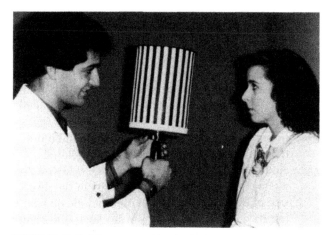

FIGURE 27–7. Twirling an optokinetic drum.

ducing nystagmus is not done by ophthalmic technical personnel but usually by a neuro-ophthalmologist or neurologist.

Rotational Testing. The patient's head is tilted 30° forward so that the horizontal semicircular canals are parallel to the floor. The eyes are closed. The patient is rotated rapidly in a chair for 20 sec, then abruptly halted. The eyes are opened, and the induced nystagmus is observed. After the rotation ends, the fast phase of the nystagmus should be in the direction opposite to the rotation, i.e., rotation to the right will result in left-beating nystagmus.

Calorics. The semicircular canals of the inner ears are stimulated with cold or warm water. Cold water blocks labyrinthine function, allowing the opposite labyrinth to work unopposed. When one ear is irrigated with cold water, nystagmus is produced with the fast phase toward the opposite ear. Warm water stimulates labyrinthine function. When one ear is irrigated with warm water, nystagmus is produced with the fast phase toward the same ear. In both instances the vestibular system drives the slow phase even though the resulting nystagmus is named for the fast phase. The mnemonic *COWS*, for Cold Opposite, Warm Same, is widely used to remember the expected results of this test.

Congenital Nystagmus

This type of nystagmus should more properly be labeled as infantile nystagmus because it is not found at birth. It occurs early in life, usually within a few months of birth. The term congenital has been, however, and continues to be the accepted term for this condition.

In congenital nystagmus the brain adapts by subtracting the eye movements from the environment. Patients do not have oscillopsia (the world does not jiggle along with the eyes). Head movements opposite to the nystagmus partly compensate, especially for visual tasks such as reading. The two types are sensory and motor.

Sensory Nystagmus. Poor vision precedes the nystagmus. Sensorily-induced nystagmus results from an anterior visual pathway problem, always with an associated afferent visual system disease. Once present, the nystagmus persists for life. The incoming visual information from the retina is too poor for normal development of steady foveal fixation.

If vision is decreased in only one eye, even if that eye deviates, no nystagmus develops. After the fixation reflex develops by about three months of age, subsequent bilateral visual loss never results in nystagmus. Vision must be decreased in both eyes early in life for sensory nystagmus to occur.

Sensory nystagmus may result from:

Macular hypoplasia (albinism, aniridia)

Congenital cataracts

Congenital optic nerve hypoplasia

Leber's congenital amaurosis

Achromatopsia

Retinopathy of prematurity

Congenital optic atrophy

High uncorrected refractive errors

Glaucoma

When the ocular defect is obvious, the cause is clear. When the defect is not obvious, congenital sensory nystagmus is 10 times commoner than congenital motor nystagmus. Often, the electroretinogram (ERG) will detect early changes undetected by fundus exam.

Motor Nystagmus. A defect in the fixation mechanism in one of the slow eye movement systems causes motor-induced nystagmus. The diagnosis tends to be one of exclusion if no sensory defect is found after the appearance of the nystagmus.

Although classically thought of as pendular, it may be jerk nystagmus. It is usually horizontal, but complex combinations often occur. When it is inherited, it is usually autosomally dominant. Motor nystagmus presents within the first few weeks of life and is bilateral and symmetrical both in amplitude and frequency. The infant may be otherwise healthy.

Congenital motor nystagmus often has a null point, i.e., that position where the nystagmus is least and vision is best. The null is a gaze position where both the amplitude and the frequency of the oscillations is at its minimum. The patient prefers to look into the field of gaze where the null point is located. To do so, the head turns away from the null. This abnormal head posture aims the null point straight ahead taking advantage of the improved vision found at the null. The level of vision depends on the amount of residual nystagmus. Vision often improves from 20/200 in the straight ahead position to the 20/40 range at the null. Vision is best tested by allowing the patient to employ the abnormal head posture. In the presence of horizontal nystagmus, normal vertical optokinetic nystagmus in an infant or a toddler is a sign of good vision.

These patients often see better when vision is tested with both eyes rather than each eye individually, because of superimposed latent nystagmus. This binocular vision replicates the patient's normal seeing conditions. The patient has better near vision than distant vision because convergence frequently dampens the oscillations. The oscillations may increase with attempted fixation, however.

When looking up or down, congenital motor nystagmus remains horizontal in direction, as do periodic alternating and peripheral vestibular nystagmus. Congenital nystagmus changes direction when the eyes pass the null point, always beating away from the null. When looking right or left, the nystagmus often changes to jerk nystagmus with the fast phase to the right in right gaze, and to the left in left gaze.

The null can also be moved to primary position by prisms, placing the apex toward the null point of both eyes. This replaces, however, the cosmetic blemish of the abnormal head posture with the cosmetic blemish of large prisms in eyeglasses (Fig. 27–8).

To eliminate the abnormal head posture, surgery (Kestenbaum's procedure) moves the null point to primary position. The *out* eye is moved in and the *in* eye is moved out. One pair of yoke muscles is recessed; the other is resected.

Latent Nystagmus. Only present when one eye is patched, this form is always congenital, usually bilateral, often asymmetrical, and often seen in patients with infantile esotropia. Vision assessment is difficult because the vision decreases with the onset of nystagmus when one eye is covered. To avoid this dilemma, visual acuity is tested in each eye separately but while keeping both eyes open by:

1. Blurring the eye not being tested with a + 10.00 lens
2. Using the distance A-O vectograph with polarized glasses
3. Using remote occlusion (holding the occluder in front of, but away from, the eye to allow peripheral vision)
4. Using a neutral density filter

Visual acuity is often better when both eyes are tested simultaneously. When either eye is patched, the fast phase is toward the uncovered eye.

Acquired Pathological Nystagmus

All acquired nystagmus is a sign of neurological disease. Acquired nystagmus is usually accompanied by oscillopsia. The jiggling image of the world often produces nausea.

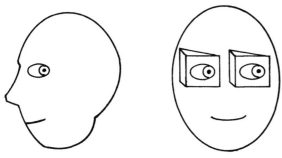

FIGURE 27–8. Eliminating marked head turn with prisms to shift null point to the straightahead head position.

Defects in the Fixation Mechanism

Seesaw Nystagmus. Alternate elevation and depression of the eye in opposite directions are characteristics of this form of nystagmus. As one eye goes up, the other goes down. The rising eye intorts, the descending eye extorts. Most commonly caused by parasellar tumors such as chiasmal gliomas producing bitemporal hemianopsia, it can also be caused by head trauma. One form is congenital.

Acquired Jerk Nystagmus. This disorder can be caused by drug abuse, tranquilizers, antiepileptic drugs, sedatives, antibiotics, or alcohol abuse, but it may indicate vestibular system disease. As with all jerk nystagmus, this is described by the fast phase, e.g., left beating nystagmus indicates that the fast phase oscillates to the left. Usually the amplitude and frequency increase when the patient looks in the direction of the fast phase, e.g., left-beating nystagmus becomes worse when looking to the left.

Spasmus Nutans. This asymmetrical, fine, very fast, quivering nystagmus is usually pendular and associated with head nodding and head tilting. Although the cause is unknown, the condition is usually benign. It appears in children about six months of age. It usually disappears spontaneously by age three, but always by kindergarten age. The child is otherwise healthy. A similar nystagmus entity is associated with chiasmal gliomas.

Defects in the Gaze Mechanism

Muscle-paretic Nystagmus. This disorder is similar to end-point nystagmus in normal patients. If an extraocular muscle is paretic, nystagmus may be seen when the muscle is moved into its field of action. The fast phase is toward the field of action. The nystagmus is usually only seen in the paretic eye.

Gaze-paretic Nystagmus. This disorder is similar to end-point nystagmus in normal patients, but is exaggerated, with more than six beats noted. In these cases, the defect is of the conjugate gaze mechanism on one side. The patient cannot maintain conjugate gaze in extreme positions. Gaze-paretic nystagmus is usually seen before extreme gaze is reached. Any area involved with gaze (frontal lobe, brain stem, and especially the cerebellum) is suspect. It is almost always drug induced, however.

Dissociated Nystagmus. This asymmetrical acquired jerk or pendular nsytagmus is often associated with a history of head trauma, neurosurgical intervention, demyelinating disease, or seizures.

● *For Example. Internuclear ophthalmoplegia (INO)— nystagmus in lateral gaze, primarily in the abducted eye with weakness of adduction in the opposite eye. Observed after strokes in older patients and with multiple sclerosis in younger patients.*

Vestibular Nystagmus

Jerk nystagmus is seen in primary position and is associated with brain stem, cerebellar, and labyrinthine defects. It may also have a rotary component. Symptoms include dizziness, balance problems, nausea, and ringing in the ears. Peripheral vestibular nystagmus from a labyrinthine defect or the inner vestibular nerve occurs abruptly but tends to disappear in a few weeks. Central vestibular nystagmus from the brain stem or cerebellum lasts much longer (Fig. 27–9).

Conditions causing vestibular nystagmus:

1. Multiple sclerosis (MS)
2. Vascular disease, e.g., stroke
3. Inner ear infection
4. Encephalitis
5. Lesions of vestibular nuclei, e.g., tumors from cerebellopontine angle or brain stem.

Special Related Forms

Voluntary Nystagmus. This disorder is characterized by small amplitude, high frequency, back-to-back saccades rather than nystagmus, which some patients are capable of producing voluntarily. Fatigue occurs within seconds. It has no clinical significance.

Wandering Eye Movements. Total or almost total blindness in both eyes before age two results in slow, irregular, large amplitude, wandering movements. Because they are not rhythmic and have no pattern, they do not qualify as nystagmus.

Cerebellar Disease. In addition to its association with various forms of true nystagmus (e.g., upbeat nystagmus), cerebellar disease may produce nystagmoid movements such as ocular dysmetria, ocular flutter, and opsoclonus (saccadomania). In evaluation of dysmetria, the patient is asked to look in the primary position. He or she overshoots, then refixates. Flutter produces bursts of back-to-back saccades that increase, then decrease, in amplitude. In opsoclonus, the oscillations are random, constant, chaotic, and unpredictable, but both eyes move in the same direction.

Up-beating and Down-beating Nystagmus. Vertical nystagmus that is present in primary position indicates possible underlying neurological dysfunction. In contrast, drug-induced nystagmus is usually not present in primary position but resembles an exaggerated form of end-point nystagmus. The most common form of vertical nystagmus is drug induced up-beat. When not drug induced, down-beating is associated with dysfunction in the area near the bottom of the brain stem at the cervical-medullary junction. This is seen in older patients after a brain stem stroke and in younger patients with Arnold-Chiari malformation. This form worsens in side gazes. Up-beating can occur from a defect at any brain stem level but is most commonly associated with the cerebellum. Usually, up-beating nystagmus increases in up gaze and down-beating nystagmus increases in down gaze, thus obeying Alexander's law. When up-beating increases in down gaze instead of decreasing, the medulla is probably involved.

Periodic Alternating Nystagmus (PAN). This is acquired horizontal jerk nystagmus without dizziness that changes direction periodically, usually approximately every minute and a half. Usually there are 10 or 15 sec of no nystagmus before the change. The nsytagmus still beats horizontally in vertical gaze, as do congenital

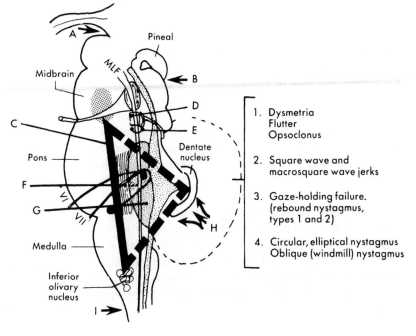

FIGURE 27–9. Schematic midsagittal section of brain stem pathology designating areas that produce acquired nystagmus. (Redrawn and adapted with permission from Burde RM, Savino PJ, Trobe JD: Clinical Decisions in Neuro-ophthalmology, 2nd ed. St. Louis, CV Mosby, 1992.)

motor and peripheral vestibular forms. This can be congenital but is usually associated with a cervical-medullary junction abnormality such as the Arnold-Chiari malformation, head trauma, or blood vessel insufficiency. Syphilis or multiple sclerosis (MS) is often found.

Superior Oblique Myokymia. This disorder causes brief, recurrent episodes of unilateral, benign, rapid microtremor with oscillopsia and torsional diplopia. These episodes usually afflict patients between 30 and 50 years of age. Spontaneous bursts of twitching last a few seconds and usually worsen in the reading position or field of action of the involved superior oblique. Superior oblique myokymia is thought to be a supranuclear response to a CN IV injury producing tetanic pulses from damaged motor neurons. The episodes may gradually subside or may persist for many years. This disorder appears and disappears spontaneously in otherwise healthy adults.

Convergence Retraction Nystagmus. The eyes appear to retract intermittently inward into the orbit, then slowly return. Convergence retraction nystagmus is seen with attempted convergence or up gaze in patients with dorsal midbrain syndrome. Voluntary up gaze is lost first, then pursuit. Moving an optokinetic nystagmus (OKN) tape down, which requires up-beating saccades, induces this nystagmus in affected individuals.

Ocular Bobbing. Vertical oscillations are noted with a fast downward phase followed by a slow staggered drift back up to the primary position. Seen with brain stem dysfunction, the patient also lacks horizontal eye movements. The patient is usually comatose from massive pontine lesions.

• CATARACT

The eye's natural, crystal clear lens has a central nucleus, covered by layered lens fibers making up a surrounding cortex with a flexible outer membrane, the capsule, that acts as an envelope. (Fig. 27–10).

Changes in the metabolism of the lens lead to its hardening and loss of transparency. A cataract is the gradual clouding of the lens until it becomes opaque. Opaque areas appear as gray or white spots. Just as a foggy camera lens blurs the picture taken, a cataract degrades the quality of the image produced on the retina, almost as if looking through frosted glass. Vision gradually and painlessly worsens as the cataract progresses (Fig 27–11).

An immature cataract is both opaque and clear in parts. No matter where in the lens these opacities and changes arise, the cataractous process ultimately may involve the entire lens. When the lens cortex is partially cloudy, the pupil appears gray rather than black, because some of the light is reflected back from the opacities.

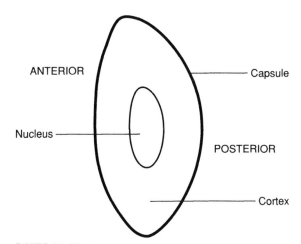

FIGURE 27–10. Structure of the lens.

A cataract is mature when all the lens fibers are opaque and somewhat swollen up to the capsule, which remains smooth. Now all light rays striking the lens surface are reflected. The pupil is white. At this stage the retina behind the lens can no longer be visualized. If left untreated, the lens becomes hypermature with a wrinkled outer capsule that is more permeable, and with a shrunken lens inside which has liquefied particles that can leak out into the anterior chamber. A morgagnian lens is a hypermature lens with liquefied lens cortex swelling the lens and an opaque nucleus floating inside.

Cataracts progress at various rates. The fastest changes follow a penetrating injury that breaks the lens capsule. The lens becomes totally opaque within hours. Cataracts can be caused early in life by eye injury or

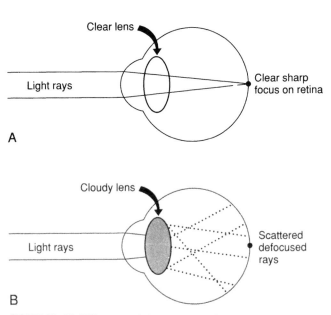

FIGURE 27–11. Differences in image clarity from clear and cataractous lenses. *A,* Clear lens refracts light rays to a clear, sharp image on the retina. *B,* Cataractous lens refracts light rays poorly to a blurred, defocused image on the retina.

chronic eye disease, or as a side effect of drugs, such as corticosteroids. Many cataracts in older patients take years to progress enough to cause a visual handicap (Fig. 27–12).

Cataract removal is usually not adivsed until visual acuity decreases to a level that significantly interferes with the patient's daily activities. Although cataracts can occur at any age, they are most common in the elderly. In the United States, 1.25 million people per year lose their vision from cataracts.

Types

The three major cataract types are based on location: cortical, nuclear, and posterior subcapsular. Both nuclear and cortical change occur with aging. In the nuclear type, the central part of the lens becomes harder and optically denser, taking on a yellow-brown color. These cataracts develop slowly and are usually associated with increasing nearsightedness caused by the lens changes.

Cortical cataracts affect the outer layers of the lens. Irregular spoke-like opacities appear from the periphery toward the center of the lens. Opacities develop that may affect both near and far vision. Frequently vacuoles (holes) are seen with cortical changes. Vacuoles are zones of reduced protein concentration and cellular remnants surrounded by fluid-filled spaces (Fig. 27–13).

Posterior subcapsular cataracts (PSCC) progress more rapidly. Characterized by clumping of abnormal epithelial cells at the posterior pole of the lens just inside the capsule, they initially look similar to cookie crumbs, rapidly forming an opaque plaque in the center of the visual axis. Visual acuity is often worse in bright sunlight when the pupil is smaller. Patients are incapacitated by severe problems with glare sensitivity as well as decreased vision. This type of lens opacity (8%) accounts for 40% of cataract extractions.

Congenital cataracts may develop from a genetic or prenatal injury or infection. Many congenital cataracts

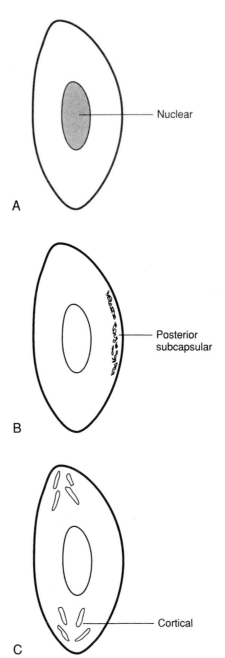

FIGURE 27–13. Three types of cataract.

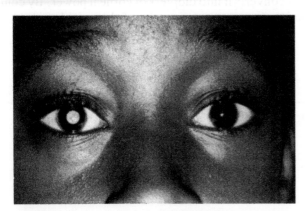

FIGURE 27–12. Traumatic cataract, right eye.

are incompletely opaque. If the cause is of short duration, clear lens fibers may encase opaque ones. If so, only one zone may be involved.

Cataracts are 10 times more common in diabetics than in the general population. They appear earlier in life and tend to progress more rapidly. These cataracts are caused by the same aging process. The true diabetic cataract, known as a sugar cataract, occurs in much younger patients. It appears suddenly, usually in juvenile-onset insulin-dependent diabetes (IDDM), from abnormally high levels of blood glucose (sugar). Osmosis occurs, and the cortical sugar cataract forms secondary to lens hydration. A snowflake cataract, characterized by white opacities in the cortex, results from poorly controlled juvenile-onset IDDM.

Occupational cataracts are seldom seen nowadays, because appropriate steps are taken to avoid lens changes. Certain occupations are at higher risk without protection: glassblowers, steelworkers, and radiographic technicians.

Symptoms

The most common early symptom is blurring of distant vision. As the cataract progresses, the lens nucleus hardens, increasing the lens optical power, shifting the eye's optical power toward nearsightedness. Reading vision tends to be affected much less than distance vision. In fact, near vision often improves. This counters the effect of presbyopia, resulting in so-called second sight. Distortion and glare are common complaints. The lens in an older patient is more dense, absorbing more of the short wavelengths of light at the blue end of the spectrum. This does not allow some shades of blue to be perceived, making what does appear slightly yellowish.

Discomfort, tearing, redness, or discharge are usually absent. Changes in diet, eye drops, or medication will neither prevent nor retard cataract formation. Excessive reading, sewing, watching television, or poor lighting will not cause or worsen cataract formation.

Preoperative Diagnostic Tests

A cataract no longer has to progress to maturity before removal. When the cataract decreases vision enough to interfere with the patient's lifestyle, removal is considered. It does no harm to delay surgery, but it needs periodic evaluation to avoid waiting so long that the cataract becomes *over-ripe* and leaks, with the possibility of developing secondary glaucoma. This is especially true for monocular cataracts. Patients do well with a single normal eye. Binocular depth perception markedly decreases, but otherwise, one-eyed patients do well visually. For example, most states require only 20/40 or better in one eye for a driver's license.

Visual acuity, best corrected vision, and retinoscopy are documented in immature cataracts. Ideally, postoperative vision should be as good as preoperative vision, i.e., before the cataract matured. The ability to predict visual potential of an eye with a mature cataract is not easy. It is often difficult to know whether retinal deterioration that cannot be viewed behind a dense cataract will make excellent vision impossible postoperatively. It is sometimes impossible to know the effect on postoperative visual acuity of corneal changes that *can* be seen.

If the patient is able to project light accurately, it usually means that there is not total retinal deterioration, and no absolute visual field defect. Patients with mature cataracts need a B-scan ultrasound to rule out partial retinal detachments, hemorrhages, tumors, and optic nerve (ON) abnormalities. B-scan ultrasound provides a two-dimensional view of the inside of the eye behind the cataract, like sonar scanning. Pupil function testing for a relative afferent defect can help. If pupil responses are normal, and the retina and optic nerve are normal, chances for the return of excellent vision improve.

Laser interferometry projects images of interference fringe patterns through the less dense areas of an incompletely cataractous lens onto the retina. This provides an estimate, by grating acuity, of the potential vision to be expected after surgery. Estimates of potential vision after surgery can also be obtained by using a potential acuity meter (PAM), which projects a brightly illuminated chart of Snellen's letters onto the retina through the less dense areas of the cataract.

Glare results from the separation of lens fibers by fluid. Visual acuity decreases with glare before visual acuity decreases in normal testing conditions. Glare testers help determine how disabled the patient has become in bright light conditions. They are the best device for documenting visual disability from immature cataracts.

To determine the appropriate power of an intraocular lens for implantation, A-scan ultrasound measures the axial length of the eyeball. The average axial length is 23.5 mm. Keratometry measures the corneal curvature and converts it into diopters of corneal power. By combining A-scan measurements of the axial length (AL)

● Cataract Symptoms

1. Fuzzy blurring of vision from induced myopia and astigmatism, especially at a distance
2. Distortion of images
3. Glare and dazzling effects, especially in bright sunlight
4. Ghosting of objects, usually described as monocular diplopia
5. Blue tones seen as yellowish
6. Vision helped by frequent changes in eyeglass correction in early stages (more nearsighted)

of the eye and keratometry measurements (K-readings), the numbers can be plugged into an SRK formula* to calculate the power of the intraocular lens (IOL) to be implanted. The average power of IOL implants is 20 to 25 diopters. SRK formula for IOL power

$$\text{IOL power} = 117 \text{ (a constant)} - 2.5 \text{ (AL)}$$
$$- .9 \text{ (average of K)}$$

Types of Surgery

The only cure for cataracts is surgical removal. Often surgery can be delayed until the vision in the better eye decreases. Microsurgical techniques using ceiling-mounted operating microscopes, precise instruments, and fine sutures have improved results so that most patients recover excellent vision. Before the natural lens is removed, the eye is phakic. Once the natural lens has been removed, the eye is aphakic. When an aphakic eye has a plastic intraocular lens surgically implanted, it becomes pseudophakic. Occasionally the remaining capsular bag also clouds, necessitating laser surgery to create a clear zone.

Following surgery, all patients require additional plus power correction to focus at near compared with their correction for distance viewing. Accommodation is lost with the lens removal. The lost power in the eye's optical system must be replaced by thick, aphakic spectacles, thin contact lenses, or implantation of a plastic lens (IOL) inside the eye (Fig. 27–14).

Although cataracts are the most common cause of blindness in the United States, vision can be markedly improved in most cases by removing the lens, either with its capsule (intracapsular extraction), or without it (extracapsular extraction). Cataract extraction is the most commonly performed surgical procedure in the United States. Even so, 1 of 5000 eyes are lost owing to infection. About 5% have significant postoperative complications.

Vision restoration is closest to natural with an IOL of an optical power selected to replace the power lost by removal of the eye's natural lens. An IOL is a clear, flexible plastic device fixated into the eye in or near the position of the natural lens following an extracapsular cataract extraction. The IOL is held in place by two haptics, or loops. If the implant is placed in the posterior chamber behind the iris in the capsular bag that is left empty by removal of the lens nucleus and cortex, it is a posterior chamber intraocular lens (PC IOL). If in the anterior chamber in front of the iris, it is an anterior chamber intraocular lens (AC IOL). An IOL produces minimal magnification and distortion with little loss of depth perception or peripheral vision (Fig. 27–15).

* S = Sanders, R = Retzlaff, K = Kraff.

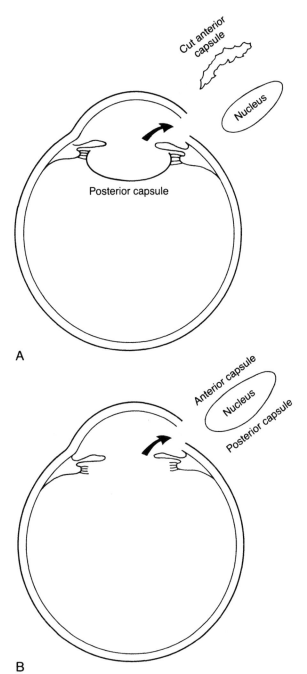

FIGURE 27–14. Two methods of cataract extraction. *A,* Extracapsular cataract extraction (ECCE). Anterior capsule and lens nucleus removed, leaving posterior capsule intact. *B,* Intracapsular cataract extraction (ICCE). Lens nucleus and entire capsule removed.

IOLs are permanent, require no maintenance or handling, and are not felt by the patient or noticed by other people. With an IOL, eyeglasses for reading and for near work are usually required and thinner eyeglasses at most may be needed for distant vision. For patients who have had cataract surgery without IOL implants, secondary procedures to insert a lens implant in the anterior chamber are possible. Rapid advances in IOL technology are continuing.

Both intracapsular cataract extraction (ICCE) and

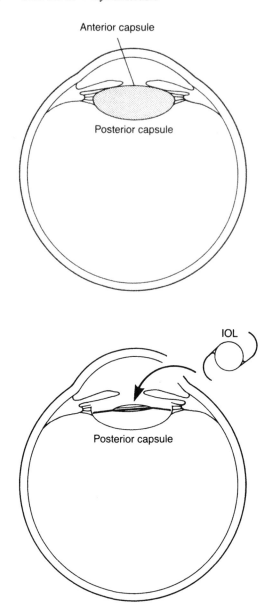

Anterior capsule

Posterior capsule

IOL

Posterior capsule

FIGURE 27-15. Intraocular lens implantation. *A,* Eye before cataract extraction. *B,* Eye with anterior capsule and lens removed and posterior chamber intraocular lens (IOL) implanted through corneal incision.

extracapsular cataract extraction (ECCE) do have disadvantages. An extracapsular cataract extraction is technically more difficult. Often the posterior capsule opacifies, requiring a secondary capsulotomy, frequently using a YAG laser. There is increased risk of vitreous loss, vitreous herniation into the anterior chamber, and retinal detachment and cystoid macular edema with an ICCE. Common complications include corneal edema, glaucoma, uveitis, and refractive problems.

After intracapsular cataract extraction without an intraocular implant, no improvement in vision is evident without optical correction. A contact lens can be used with a thin pair of eyeglass lenses for near, or

alternatively thick, magnifying, + power aphakic eyeglasses with bifocals for near vision. Often thick + 10.00 temporary eyeglasses are used until the final prescription, usually between + 10.00 to + 15.00 power, can be prescribed about two months after surgery.

Surgical Considerations

Cataract surgery is commonly performed on an outpatient basis, usually with local anesthesia even in patients in poor physical condition. If the condition of the patient's health demands hospital admission for the procedure, hospital stays range from two to four days. Cataract surgery is usually performed one eye at a time, in the eye with worse vision first. A cataract is removed when the level of vision is insufficient for the patient's daily needs. For Medicare coverage, Snellen acuity and glare acuity must be 20/50 or poorer. The goal of cataract extraction is a happy patient with relief from symptoms, improved vision, and avoidance of complications. Sources of dissatisfaction include lack of visual improvement, poorer results than expected, and complications.

After extracapsular cataract extraction with an intraocular implant, vision usually improves markedly—the next day in most patients. Other patients may require months before final improvement. Surgery may induce astigmatism caused by tight stitches (sutures). Postoperative astigmatism from the stitches has its axis in plus cylinder where the stitches are placed. Wound compression shortens the vertical meridian. With ECCE needing about seven to nine stitches in the vicinity of the vertical meridian (90°), the plus axis cylinder will be with the rule (see Chapters 13 and 14). Months later, the stitches may be cut to lengthen the vertical meridian and thereby reduce the final amount of astigmatism (Fig. 27–16).

Patients return for frequent examinations until the final eyeglasses are prescribed—within eight weeks after surgery. Patients may need a prescription for near vision because the intraocular lens does not have the variable power of the eye's natural lens. Although most patients will see better with some distance correction, usually of low power, many can perform daily activities without them.

● GLAUCOMA

Glaucoma, cataracts, and age-related macular degeneration are the three major causes of blindness in the United States. Glaucoma is the second commonest form of blindness, estimated to affect 1.6 million in the United States, damaging the eyeball by abnormally

Disadvantages of Aphakic Eyeglasses Following ICCE

1. These eyeglasses are extremely thick, heavy, and unattractive.
2. Although central vision is excellent, peripheral (side) vision is reduced and distorted. To best view an object seen out of the corner of the eye, the patient must move the head more than the eye.
3. These eyeglasses must be worn at a precise distance from the eye.

4. Until the second eye has cataract surgery, the increased image size (about 30%) resulting from the aphakic eyeglasses for the operated eye is not compatible with the normal image size from the unoperated eye, thus producing double vision.

---

high pressure. Some eyes can tolerate higher intraocular pressure (IOP) than others before destruction of optic nerve tissue.

This chronic disease affects both eyes. The insidious onset is gradual and asymptomatic. Slowly, relentlessly, nerve fiber destruction progresses. Slow, painless, progressive loss of vision occurs unless the intraocular pressure is sufficiently lowered. Routine glaucoma screening is a preventive measure that allows diagnosis to be made early before nerve fiber destruction occurs.

Most damage to nerve fibers probably occurs at the optic nerve head (ONH). The manner in which the increased IOP damages optic nerve fibers is disputed. One theory is that the fibers starve because of reduced blood supply. Another is that the mechanical compression of the nerve fibers as they bend and stretch into the ONH causes damage. Once destroyed, these cells and fibers cannot be restored. The increased IOP presses on the optic nerve at levels high enough to destroy neurons. Changes in optic nerve fibers at the ONH cause subsequent loss of peripheral visual field. As in age-related macular degeneration, glaucomatous changes are irreversible.

Because glaucoma is hereditary, siblings and children of glaucoma patients are at increased risk, as are patients whose IOPs are greater than 21 mm Hg or who have high myopia, blood vessel disease, or diabetes.

African-Americans appear to be more susceptible to damage from IOP and will not respond as well to drug therapy as whites. Glaucoma mostly develops in middle age or later; 2% of the population over age 40 have the disease. Over age 60, the incidence of both cataracts and glaucoma increases. Treatment of adults is mostly medical initially, with surgery performed when drugs can no longer control neuron destruction. Treatment of infants with congenital glaucoma is mostly surgical, because drugs usually are not effective.

Glaucoma is detected, and damage from the disease assesssed, using four criteria: increased IOP, the structure of the anterior chamber angle, the ratio of the optic cup size to optic disc size, and the effect of high IOP on the visual field. IOP is measured by tonometry, the anterior chamber angle by gonioscopy, the cup-to-disc ratio by the fundus examination, and the field loss by perimetry. The diagnosis cannot be made without documentation of visual field loss.

Pathophysiology

Aqueous humor is produced by the ciliary body; flows behind the iris in the posterior chamber through the pupil into the anterior chamber; bathes the anterior segment of the eye with oxygen and nutrients; and flows toward the anterior chamber angle with waste

---

Advantages of Contact Lenses Following ICCE

1. Contact lenses are attractive and lightweight.
2. Central and peripheral vision are good, without distortion.
3. The small magnification (about 5%) of the image size from the contact lens is well tolerated with the normal image from the unoperated eye. No double vision occurs.

4. Lens cleaning, insertion and removal, and lens fragility are well tolerated unless the patient is elderly with decreased dexterity, tremors, and other problems.

Advantages of IOL Following ECCE

1. Distance vision improves markedly almost immediately, although incompletely.
2. When eyeglasses or contact lenses are required for distance viewing, they are usually of low power.
3. The chance of postoperative complication from cystoid macular edema is decreased.
4. No image size difference is noted in operated and unoperated eyes.
5. No care is required for the IOL once implanted.

products, to percolate out through the sieve-like trabecular meshwork into Schlemm's canal (Fig. 27–17). From there, the aqueous enters collector channels and aqueous veins, finally exiting the eye through episcleral veins (Fig. 27–18). Resistance to flow through the trabecular meshwork creates internal pressure in the eye, reflecting a balance between the production of aqueous humor and its outflow through the trabecular meshwork. When the outflow is insufficient to prevent fluid accumulation within the eye, the nondistensible eye has an increase in pressure.

The optic nerve has over 1.2 million axons of ganglion cells. The nerve fiber layer of the retina runs in a specific arrangement of bundles to the optic disc, exiting through the disc as the optic nerve. The disc is located at the weakest part of the sclera, the lamina cribrosa. A small, pale depression in the middle of the disc is the optic cup. The physiological cup is reddish white, much lighter than the surrounding disc. The size of the cup is expressed as a ratio of its diameter to that of the disc. Without glaucoma, the cup is not usually more than one third the size of the horizontal diameter of the disc, but normal variations do occur. Any change in size or shape of the cup is a sign of optic nerve injury.

Early disc changes include thinning of the temporal disc margin and widening and deepening of the optic cup. The superior and inferior temporal nerve fibers of the optic disc are most vulnerable to increased pressure, and disc changes occur there first. Enlargement of the cup usually precedes visual field loss. The cup usually elongates vertically first, indicating nerve damage to fibers in bundles serving the arcuate area. Blood

vessels are displaced nasally. The affected areas degenerate and lighten in color as the lamina cribrosa becomes exposed. If evidence of progressive cup enlargement and excavation is found, the IOP is too high for that patient, no matter its level.

Most normal eyes maintain pressures between 10 and 21 mm Hg. A few eyes cannot tolerate even these normal pressures without damage. To prevent progressive visual field loss, these eyes must maintain pressure under 12 mm Hg. These patients have low tension glaucoma. Some patients can maintain pressures considerably above 21 mm Hg without evidence of optic disc changes or visual field loss. These cases, called ocular hypertensive, are followed closely. The patients are not treated with glaucoma medications until demonstration of disc changes or field loss meets the criteria for the diagnosis of glaucoma. Patients with ocular hypertension (OHT) are at increased risk to develop glaucoma, but treatment before evidence of glaucomatous changes is not preventive. Most ocular hypertensive individuals remain as measured 15 years later.

Because IOP usually increases slowly, glaucoma is insidious owing to a lack of symptoms. Early detection, and effective control of the IOP, either pharmaceutically or surgically, is vital to preserving vision. Because peripheral (side) vision is lost first, it is not noticed. Because field loss occurs in the periphery or around the optic disc first, visual acuity is not affected until much later in the disease process. Late in the progression, sharp, central vision is lost, with a disastrous decrease in vision. The end result in untreated glaucoma is a hard eye (from the high IOP) without light perception.

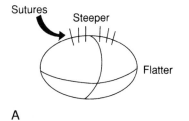

A

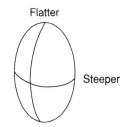

B

FIGURE 27–16. Astigmatic error induced by sutures and spectacle method of correcting. *A,* Tight stitches steepen cornea at 90°, giving eye too much plus at 90° (axis 180°). *B,* Correcting cylinder must be steeper 90° from corneal steepness. Need plus at 180 (axis 90°).

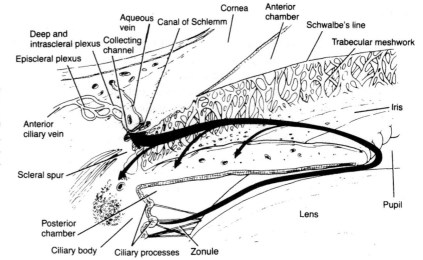

FIGURE 27–17. Aqueous flow produced by ciliary body leaves posterior chamber through the pupil into the anterior chamber and out of the eye through the trabecular meshwork into the canal of Schlemm. (From Snell RS, Lemp MA: Clinical Anatomy of the Eye. Boston, Blackwell Scientific Publications, 1989. Reprinted by permission of Blackwell Scientific Publications, Inc.)

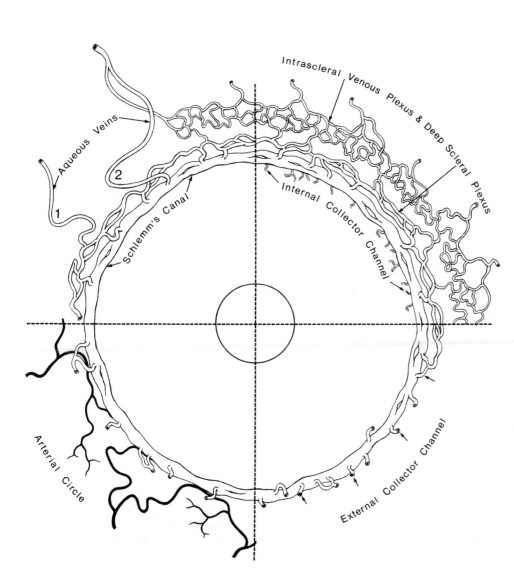

FIGURE 27–18. Schematic diagram of outflow channels and veins from Schlemm's canal. 1 and 2 = aqueous veins. (Redrawn and adapted from Hogan MJ, Alvarado JA: Histology of the Human Eye. Philadelphia, WB Saunders, 1971.)

Types

Although glaucoma has many causes and types, we concern ourselves with only three: primary open angle (POAG), closed angle (CAG), and infantile.

The overwhelming majority of glaucoma patients have POAG, as opposed to CAG. Open angle refers to the normally wide angle in the anterior chamber between the iris and the corneal-scleral junction where the aqueous humor drains into the trabecular meshwork. The sieve-like meshwork is defective and does not allow sufficient filtering of aqueous fluid. The drain is flawed, not the access to it.

An acute attack of CAG strikes suddenly, blurring vision and causing a perception of haloes around lights from corneal edema, often with severe pain and redness in and around the eye. The intraocular pressure usually exceeds 50 mm Hg. Nausea and vomiting often occur. The cause is a shallow anterior chamber with an accompanying narrow or closed angle. Because of the shallow chamber, especially when the pupil is mid dilated, the pupillary margin increases its contact with the lens surface and sticks to it. Aqueous flow through the pupil slows. Relative pupillary block has occurred. This increases the pressure in the posterior chamber, which bows the iris forward (Fig. 27–19). The peripheral iris near the angle pushes up against the trabecular meshwork, closing the angle. The iris extends its arc of contact with the trabecular meshwork, sticking to the posterior corneal surface, forming peripheral anterior synechiae (PAS), and blocking outflow of aqueous humor. When too much of the filtration angle is blocked for too long, the PAS become permanent. The effect of permanent closure of areas of the angle is similar to closing a zipper. Intermittent minor episodes often precede an acute attack. The drain can function, but access to it is cut off, like putting a stopper in the sink.

An acute attack of CAG is a medical emergency. The eye cannot tolerate such high pressure for long. The IOP must be lowered as soon as possible, within hours of the attack, to prevent irreversible loss of vision. Drugs to break the attack are employed, then surgery is used to prevent further attacks. Hyperosmotics such as glycerol or mannitol create an osmotic gradient between the plasma and ocular fluids, thus drawing water out of the eye quickly.

If the IOP stays elevated because the angle cannot be opened or the pupillary block broken, surgery, such as laser iridotomy, is indicated. Often surgery is also performed on the other eye to prevent a later acute attack.

Infantile glaucoma is rarer than either of the adult types. Malformation of the anterior chamber angle is the cause. The infant's eyes can stretch from the IOP, unlike an adult eye. *Big* eyes with enlarged corneas result. Other signs and symptoms are hazy, "steamy" corneas; intense photophobia; and tearing. Because of the malformation, drugs usually do not control the elevated pressure. Surgery, such as a goniotomy or trabeculotomy, to open or create drainage channels, is the treatment of choice.

Evaluation

Abnormal angle structures can be identified and the depth of the anterior chamber at the junction of the iris and the cornea estimated by gonioscopy with a

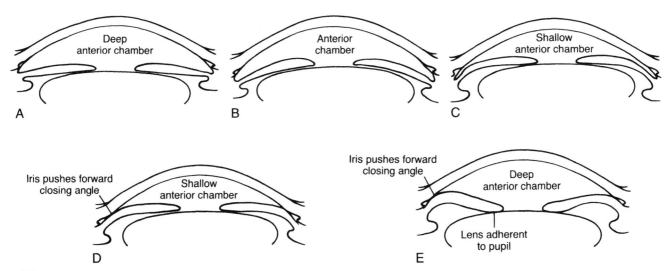

FIGURE 27–19. Impedance to aqueous outflow as the anterior chamber angle diminishes. *A,* Normal, wide open anterior chamber angle (40°). No impedance to aqueous outflow. *B,* Moderate anterior chamber angle (20°). Slight impedance to aqueous outflow. *C,* Narrow anterior chamber angle (10°). Some impedance to outflow. *D,* Narrow angle closed. Aqueous flow cannot reach trabecular meshwork. Intraocular pressure rises precipitously. *E,* Pupillary block, normal anterior chamber angle. If the iris adheres to the lens at the pupillary border, pressure builds up behind iris, bowing it forward, pushing the iris against the trabecular meshwork, closing the anterior chamber angle. Intraocular pressure rises precipitously.

contact lens with angled mirrors. Examination of the fundus with a direct ophthalmoscope or a goniolens with a slit lamp allows visualization of the optic nerve head to evaluate changes in the disc compatible with progression of the disease. Ophthalmic technical personnel are not usually required to perform these tests. They do, however, measure the intraocular pressure by tonometric means and record visual fields for documentation of progressive loss.

Tonometry

The pressure inside the eye is measured with tonometers. Two of the basic types of this instrument measure by the strength necessary to indent or to flatten (applanate) a small segment of cornea. Commonly used instruments include Schiotz tonometers, Goldmann applanation tonometers, and Tono-pens. Measurements are accurate unless the patient attempts to squeeze the eyelid shut.

Visual Fields

Perimetry detects and quantifies early glaucoma field defects because it is a sensitive method of documenting injury to axons of the optic nerve head. Destruction of nerve fibers is such that specific bundles are affected. Nerve fiber bundle defects are characteristic of damage to the visual pathway from the nerve fiber layer in the retina to the chiasm.

Glaucomatous field changes stop along the horizontal meridian on the nasal side. This contrasts with chiasmal and postchiasmal field defects that stop along the vertical meridian. The horizontal raphe temporal to the macula in the retina is the dividing line responsible for the nasal horizontal meridian of the visual field. It demarcates nerve fiber pathways above the raphe that arc above the macula to the disc from nerve fiber pathways that arc below the macula to the disc. These types of defects are typical of glaucoma but can occur from other causes, such as ischemic optic neuropathy.

Vertical enlargement of the blind spot or oval paracentral scotomas 10 to 25° from fixation not connected to the blind spot are the earliest visual field defects

found. Nasal steps are the other early common field defect. Paracentral scotomas enlarge and coalesce as forerunners of partial and then full arcuate (Bjerrum) scotomas. Vertical extensions of the blind spot (Seidel scotomas) into the Bjerrum area are not uncommon. The papillomacular bundle is more resistant to high pressure and is usually not affected until late in the disease. This preserves sharp central vision until this bundle gives way. The nasal retina, represented by the temporal field, appears to be most resistant. Temporal islands of field are the last to be lost (Fig. 27–20).

Repeat field testing on subsequent visits allows evaluation of the progress of the disease as well as the effectiveness of the treatment in preventing progression. If progressive field loss is documented, the level of IOP remains too high for that eye to tolerate.

Treatment

Without treatment, progression to failure to perceive light eventually occurs. Treatment does not cure glaucoma—it does slow its progress. The goal is to keep the intraocular pressure under control. Even with treatment, progression often occurs, but at a much delayed rate. Think of treatment as keeping a leaky ship afloat longer. Glaucoma in adults responds well to drugs. Patients must comply with the treatment regimen, but unfortunately, this does not always occur.

The current first choice is timolol, a beta-adrenergic blocker that works by decreasing aqueous production. It slows heart rate, reduces blood pressure, and causes bronchospasm, side effects of particular concern in patients with lung and heart disease. Timolol has few ocular side effects. Other beta-blockers are levobunolol and betaxolol.

Cholinergic miotic drugs, such as pilocarpine and carbachol, increase the efficiency of the outflow channels. The mechanism is probably mechanical traction. As the ciliary muscle contracts, it pulls the scleral spur and trabecular meshwork open. Brow ache, pseudomyopia, and decreased night vision are common side effects. Miotics are effective and inexpensive.

Long-acting anticholinesterases, such as phospholine iodide, have more significant side effects and are

---

● Most Common Order of Glaucomatous Field Defects

1. Enlarged blind spot
2. Paracentral scotoma
3. Nasal step
4. Seidel scotoma
5. Arcuate defects
6. Central 10° lost
7. Lost temporal island

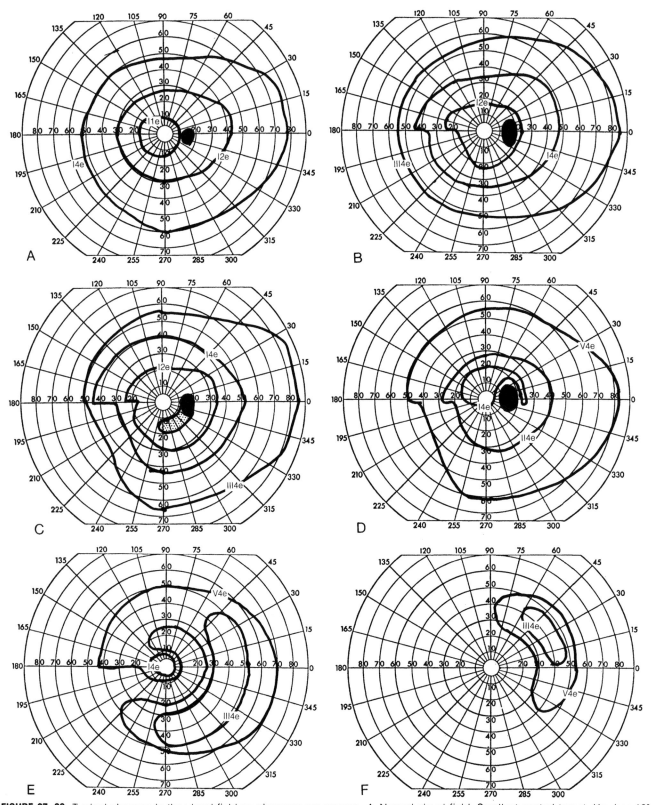

FIGURE 27–20. Typical changes in the visual field as glaucoma progresses. *A,* Normal visual field. Smallest central target, I1e, has 10° isopter; I2e central threshold target, has 30° nasal limit, 40° temporal limit to isopter; I4e peripheral target, has 50° nasal limit and 80° temporal limit to isopter; vision 20/20. *B,* elongated blind spot, loss of I1e field, nasal step to I2e and I4e; I2e and I4e isopters have lost at least 10° in all quadrants; III4e isopter same as I4e previously. *C,* Blindspot now has partial arcuate scotoma below with the I4e target; vision still 20/20. *D,* Loss of I2e isopter; baring of blind spot to the I4e with marked loss of the I4e isopter; V4e isopter almost the same as III4e isopter in last visual field. *E,* Small central 5° remaining to I4e and III4e; temporal island to III4e also; V4e has full arcuate scotoma broken through to periphery below, and partial arcuate scotoma above, vision still 20/40. *F,* Small temporal island to III4e. Larger temporal island to V4e; vision now 20/400.

Drugs that Increase Outflow

Cholinergic miotics
   Pilocarpine
   Carbachol
Anticholinesterases
   Demecarium (Humorsol)
   Phospholine iodide
Beta-adrenergic agonists
   Epinephrine

Drugs that Decrease Production

Carbonic anhydrase inhibitors
   Methazolamide (Neptazane)
   Acetazolamide (Diamox)
Beta-adrenergic blockers
   Timolol (Timoptic)
   Levobunolol (Betagan)
   Betaxolol

usually reserved for patients who are not candidates for surgery.

Sympathetic agonists, such as epinephrine, decrease aqueous production and increase outflow. Continued use causes redness and allergy to the eye. Propine is a synthetic agent that converts to epinephrine inside the eye and has fewer systemic side effects because it has better corneal penetration at lower concentrations.

Carbonic anhydrase inhibitors, such as methazolamide, decrease aqueous production markedly, but these drugs have side effects such as lethargy, malaise, and gastrointestinal upsets, which limit tolerance of them by patients.

Maximum medical therapy combines a beta-blocker, a miotic, a sympathetic agonist, and a carbonic anhydrase inhibitor. In the typical elderly patient with OAG, the potential side effects may be significant.

Surgery

Surgery is usually indicated if field loss is continuing despite maximum medical therapy. Several possible surgical procedures attempt to increase the flow of aqueous humor from the eye. When maximal medical therapy does not decrease IOP sufficiently to retard visual field loss and progressive cupping, surgery is advised. Laser surgery blasts a hole in the iris (iridotomy) for CAG, or blasts holes through the trabecular meshwork just in front of the scleral spur (trabeculoplasty) for POAG. A peripheral iridectomy cuts out iris tissue near the angle, creating a small hole between the posterior chamber and the anterior chamber, allowing aqueous flow to bypass a blocked pupil. With a filtering trabeculectomy, tissue is cut out under a scleral flap which is subsequently closed. This provides a filtering bleb (blister) under the conjunctiva.

Bibliography

Aaberg TM: Fluorescein angiography. In Peyman GA, Sanders DR, Goldberg MF (eds): Principles and Practice of Ophthalmology, vol II. Philadelphia, WB Saunders, 1980.

Anderson DR: The optic nerve in glaucoma. In Duane TD, Jaeger EA (eds): Clinical Ophthalmology, vol 3. Hagerstown, MD, Harper & Row, 1986.

Beard C: Ptosis, 3rd ed. St Louis, CV Mosby, 1981.

Brown B: Preoperative evaluation of cataract patient. J Ophthal Nurs Tech 7:204, 1988.

Burde RM, Savino PJ, Trobe JD. Nystagmus. In Clinical Decisions in Neuro-ophthalmology, 2nd ed. St Louis, Mosby Year Book, 1992.

Elman MJ, Fine SL: Exudative age-related macular degeneration. In Ryan SJ (ed): Retina, vol II. St Louis, CV Mosby, 1989.

Gay AJ, Newman NW, Keltrer JL, et al.: Nystagmus. In Eye Movement Disorders. St Louis, CV Mosby, 1974.

Jaffe NS, Jaffe MS, Jaffe GF: Cataract Surgery and Its Complications, 5th ed. St Louis, CV Mosby, 1990.

Kolker AE, Hetherington J: Becker-Shaffer's Diagnosis and Therapy of the Glaucomas, 4th ed. St Louis, CV Mosby, 1987.

Luntz MH: Clinical types of cataracts. In Duane TD (ed): Clinical Ophthalmology, vol 1. Hagerstown, MD, Harper & Row, 1985.

Miller N: Nystagmus and related ocular motility disorders. In Walsh and Hoyt's Neuro-ophthalmology, 4th ed, vol 2. Baltimore, Williams & Wilkins, 1985.

Nelson LB, Ullman S: Congenital and developmental cataracts. In Duane TD (ed): Clinical Ophthalmology, vol 1. Hagerstown, MD, Harper & Row, 1985.

Neumann A, McCarty G: The Relationship between indoor and outdoor Snellen visual acuity in cataract patients. J Cataract Refract Surg 14:35, 1988.

Paton D, Craig J: Glaucomas: Diagnosis and Management. Summit, NJ, Ciba Pharmaceutical, 1976.

Phelps CD: Examination and functional evaluation of the crystalline lens. In Duane TD (ed): Clinical Ophthalmology, vol 1. Hagerstown, MD, Harper & Row, 1985.

Phelps CD: Glaucoma: general concepts. In Duane TD, Jaeger EA (eds): Clinical Ophthalmology, vol 3. Hagerstown, MD, Harper & Row, 1986.

Sarks SH, Sarks JP: Age-related macular degeneration: atrophic form. In Ryan SJ (ed): Retina, vol II. St Louis, CV Mosby, 1989.

Shields MB: Textbook of Glaucoma, 3rd ed. Baltimore, William & Wilkins, 1991.

• CHAPTER 27 EYE DISORDERS

1. Which of the following is the leading cause of irreversible blindness in the United States?
   a. cataracts
   b. peripheral anterior synechiae
   c. glaucoma
   d. age-related macular degeneration
   e. central retinal artery occlusion.

2. What is the average height (mm) of the palpebral fissure in midposition?
   a. 11

b. 8
c. 10
d. 13
e. 6

3. Which one of the following is an example of Alexander's law?
   a. acquired nystagmus produces oscillopsia
   b. nystagmus decreases with drug or alcohol use
   c. right beating nystagmus increases in right gaze
   d. right beating nystagmus in right gaze changes to left beating nystagmus in left gaze
   e. nystagmus decreases with convergence.

4. Which of the following is an example of induced nystagmus?

   a. sensory
   b. optokinetic
   c. latent
   d. seesaw
   e. vestibular

5. In order to diagnose glaucoma, you must have evidence of which one of the following?
   a. visual field loss
   b. abnormal anterior chamber angle
   c. less than 0.3 cup to disc ratio
   d. more than 35 mm intraocular pressure
   e. increased aqueous production

Eye Diseases

LEARNING OBJECTIVES

- Discuss the signs and symptoms of Graves' disease
- Understand the systemic effects of hypothyroidism and hyperthyroidism
- Explain the abnormalities at the myoneural junction that cause myasthenia gravis
- Know the two characteristic findings in ocular myasthenia

- Define thrombus, embolus, clot, aneurysm, ischemia, infarct, arteriosclerosis, myocardial infarct, cerebrovascular accident, and neovascularization
- List three chronic systemic disorders caused by diabetes
- List four ocular disorders caused by diabetes

● GRAVES' DISEASE

The thyroid gland is involved in the regulation of the body's metabolic rate. When we eat foods containing iodine, it is taken in by the gut, absorbed, and combined chemically, so as to attach to an iodine-bound protein, thyroglobulin (TBG). This is synthesized and stored by the thyroid gland near the larynx. Thyroglobulin can be secreted from this storage reservoir to the bloodstream as hormones in the form of thyroxine (T_4) and, to a lesser extent, triiodothyronine (T_3), where it binds to TBG. T_3 and T_4 regulate the basal metabolic rate in each cell, tissue growth and development, and activity in the nervous system. Because T_3 is more potent than T_4, enzymes in the liver and kidney convert T_4 to T_3 when required by the body.

The hypothalamus releases thyroid releasing hormone (TRH). This stimulates the pituitary gland to release thyroid stimulating hormone (TSH), which is carried by the blood to the thyroid gland. The thyroid is stimulated to release T_3 and T_4. As thyroid hormone production increases, it has an inhibitory effect on the hypothalamus and pituitary gland, slowing their release of hormones. Otherwise, too much TRH would be released. This would, in turn, produce too much TSH and the thyroid would release more T_3 and T_4 than the body needs. In this closed-loop, self-regulating control system, each gland detects the blood levels of the other glands' hormones and regulates secretions appropriately. When this feedback mechanism is not controlled,

either too little or too much thyroid activity occurs (Fig. 28–1).

With *hyperthyroidism* thyroid activity is increased, accelerating both the body's uptake of iodine and the basal metabolic rate. The patient may be nervous, excitable, restless, anxious, irritable, sweaty, and hungry, but despite eating more, loses weight. The heart rate increases, the lower part of the legs swells, and the patient becomes intolerant of heat. This occurs when TSH and TRH escape regulation, such as from a tumor in young adults, or when the thyroid itself escapes regulation, as occurs with toxic thyroiditis or Graves' disease when excess T_3 and T_4 are released. Medical treatment with drugs such as propylthiouracil (PTU) or methimazole (Tapazole) targets the thyroid by interfering with hormone synthesis. Surgery to remove the thyroid can help, as can radioactive iodine therapy. Plasma concentrations for T_3 and T_4 levels and TRH stimulation are taken to verify thyroid gland malfunction.

Decreased thyroid production, or *hypothyroidism,* reduces the basal metabolic rate. The patient may be lethargic, constipated, depressed, weak, and may have dry skin. The patient is not hungry, but even eating less results in weight gain. The heart rate decreases and the patient is intolerant of cold because he or she feels cold already. This clinical presentation occurs when the thyroid is destroyed by tumors or destructive thyroiditis or when drugs for hyperthyroidism work too well. When thyroid function is impaired for a long time, an enlarged thyroid gland, *goiter,* develops.

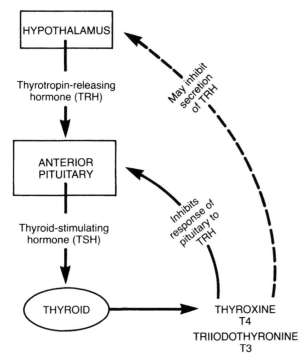

FIGURE 28–1. Self-regulation of thyroid activity by the hypothalamus-pituitary-thyroid axis. TRH increases the secretion of TSH. T4 and T3 suppress the secretion of TSH.

• THYROID EYE DISEASE

Graves' is a common disease of the thyroid gland. The body's immune system attacks the thyroid and the extraocular muscles. The relationship between thyroid gland function and the eye findings is not clear, however. There may be more than one mechanism, but an abnormal autoimmune process is suspected because abnormal antibodies that stimulate the thyroid are often found circulating in the blood of patients with Graves' disease. The cellular immune system (T cells) has also been implicated. About 25% of those patients with Graves' disease also develop myasthenia gravis, another autoimmune disease. As with most autoimmune disease, Graves' disease has a high predilection for females, especially those over age 40. It often occurs during or after an episode of a hyperthyroid dysfunction, but laboratory tests may show normal thyroid function (euthyroid). The effect is often asymmetric, i.e., one eye is more involved than the other.

Eye changes are described by the mnemonic **"NO SPECS"** from most mild to most severe ocular involvement.

N No eye signs or symptoms

O Only signs (upper lid retraction and stare, no symptoms, possible lid lag and mild proptosis [< 22mm])

S Soft tissue swelling (lids, conjunctiva) with signs and symptoms

P Proptosis > 3 mm

E Extraocular muscle involvement, usually with diplopia

C Corneal exposure with drying of eyes secondary to lid lag

S Sight loss from optic nerve compression

Mild symptoms are excessive tearing, gritty sensation, discomfort behind the eyeball, and photophobia. Mild signs are conjunctival and lid swelling, conjunctival injection, orbital fat extrusion, lid lag, lid retraction, and staring. Along with proptosis and restricted eye movements, these signs are hallmarks of Graves' disease. The proptosis and upper lid retraction (Dalrymple's sign) produce the typical appearance of stare, with exposure of sclera above the cornea: you see too much eyeball and too little eye lid. Upper lid lag (von Graefe's sign) occurs when the eye moves from primary to down gaze, but the upper eye lid fails to move as far down as it should (Fig 28–2).

Thyroid eye disease is the most common cause of proptosis in adults. Although the average proptosis from Graves' is 3 mm greater than the usual 18 to 20 mm, it ranges from a minimum of 22 mm to a more marked 28 mm. The proptosis prevents the eye lids from closing completely, thus producing corneal irritation with the symptoms of a gritty sensation and photophobia. Chronic corneal exposure leads to corneal dehydration, which, in turn, leads to corneal epithelial stippling, ulceration, clouding, and finally, if not controlled, perforation. Often the eye lids are swollen because venous drainage from the orbit is impaired. When the proptosis is marked, the extraocular muscles are so stretched that eye movement is markedly restricted. If symptoms are also severe, optic neuropathy is possible from the optic nerve's being compressed at the

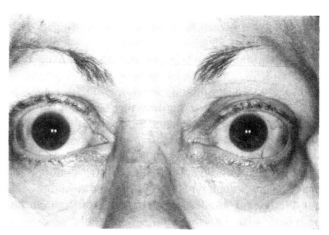

FIGURE 28–2. Patient with thyroid eye disease. Note the upper eyelid retraction giving the appearance of "stare." Also note sclera showing under lower limbus.

apex of the orbit, because all the tissues at the orbital apex become crowded.

Signs and symptoms generally progress for 1 to 2 years, then subside. As the inflammation subsides, collagen and mucopolysaccharides are deposited in the normally elastic muscles, causing fibrosis and shortening, which restrict eye movement. The involved muscle can contract to pull the eye for its normal function, but the fibrosis does not allow the involved muscle to relax when innervated to do so in order for its direct antagonist to contract. The eye is restricted in its range of excursion in the opposite direction from the one where the fibrosed muscle functions.

Thyroid eye disease often produces inflammation of all the extraocular muscles, particularly the rectus muscles. The muscle tendons that insert onto the eyeball are spared. The inferior rectus muscle appears to be involved preferentially, followed closely by the medial rectus. Involvement of these two muscles affects the eye's ability to look up (inferior rectus is unable to relax) and to look out (medial rectus is unable to relax). Superior rectus involvement is less common, and the lateral rectus still less. The "thyroid spiral" is a method of recalling the order in which the extraocular muscles are involved (Fig 28–3). The misalignment produced is incomitant, measuring different amounts in different positions of gaze. Usually extraocular muscles in both eyes are involved, but the amount of enlargement is usually markedly asymmetric.

This tethering effect on the extraocular muscles produces diplopia in the field opposite the restriction (Fig 28–4).

- *For example. The left inferior rectus is a depressor, moving the eye down. When the inferior rectus is fibrosed and shortened by thyroid eye disease, the left eye can still move down, but it cannot move*

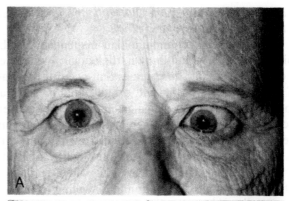
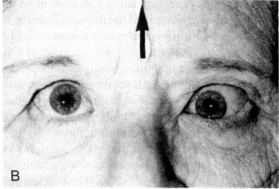
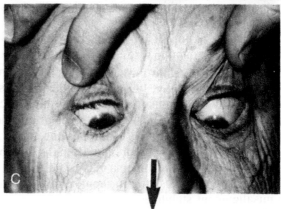

FIGURE 28–4. Restriction of eye movement from thyroid eye disease. *A,* Restriction of left medial rectus (LMR) and left inferior rectus (LIR) causing left eye to be pulled in and down. *B,* On attempted up gaze neither eye elevates well. Left eye cannot rise to midline. LIR is more restricted than right inferior rectus (RIR). *C,* On attempted down gaze both eyes depress well. Inferior recti can contract to pull eyes down.

THYROID SPIRAL

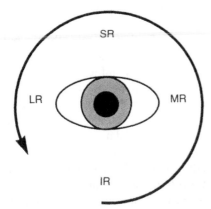

FIGURE 28–3. Thyroid spiral. Similar to Tillaux's spiral for EOM insertions. This spiral reverses the first two muscles and the direction of the spiral.

up because the inferior rectus cannot relax "on the stretch" when the superior rectus contracts to pull the eye up. The left inferior rectus is bound down, the left eye is pulled down, producing a left hypotropia, and the patient has vertical diplopia when attempting to look up. By adopting a chin-up head position, the diplopia is avoided. From examining the eye's movements, it appears as though the left superior rectus is weakened, but it is not. Likewise, when the left medial rectus is fibrotic, the left eye is pulled in, producing horizontal diplopia worse when looking to the left from what appears to be a weak left lateral rectus, but it is not.

Although the exact immunologic mechanism for thyroid eye disease is not known, the ocular involvement is clearly secondary to changes that occur at the back of the orbit. Orbital fat and orbital blood vessels are not affected, but the lacrimal gland is. There is a predilection for injurious changes in the extraocular muscles, but not in the tendons. Rather slowly, connective tissue spaces within the muscles are lightly infiltrated by mononuclear lymphocytes and water to cause a diffuse inflammatory reaction and swelling. The muscles swell and become distended. Because most of the swelling occurs in the belly of the muscles near the back of the orbit, patients develop exophthalmos (proptosis) because the enlarged muscles take up most of the orbital space, thus pushing the eyeball out. This accounts for the massive increase (three to eight times normal size) in extraocular muscle size that overflows the orbit, resulting in increased orbital pressure. As the eye pushes out, it may stretch the optic nerve. As the orbital pressure pushes against the optic canal, the optic nerve may be squeezed. The increased pressure does not allow normal removal of fluids collecting in connective tissue spaces within the muscles, i.e., venous outflow is impaired.

Fibrotic restriction of extraocular muscles is confirmed by forced duction testing. Orbital ultrasound or CT scans demonstrate the muscle swelling, helping rule out an orbital tumor as the cause of the proptosis. Improved high resolution orbital CT scans allow excellent visualization of the enlarged extraocular muscles, especially coronal views. Prisms over the more restricted eye often allow partial relief from the diplopia. Surgery to eliminate the diplopia may be performed on the extraocular muscles after the acute phase ends and the misalignment stabilizes.

Lubricating medications are given for relief of the gritty sensation accompanying corneal dehydration. Sewing the eye lids together on the temporal side (partial tarsorrhaphy) may prevent corneal dehydration with its resulting loss of corneal sensation from epithelial decompensation. Once the inflammatory process "burns out," proptosis may be relieved by surgical orbital decompression of the inferior, nasal, or lateral walls of the orbit, thus creating more space into which the orbital contents can fit.

Those patients most severely affected suffer vision loss from chronic corneal exposure or optic nerve compression at the orbital apex. As with other optic neuropathies, optic nerve involvement is evaluated by color vision testing, pupil function testing, ophthalmoscopy looking for disc pallor, and visual field testing looking for central scotomas, often with inferior field loss. Patients with optic nerve involvement are often treated with corticosteroids, such as prednisone, to reduce the inflammation.

• MYASTHENIA GRAVIS

This chronic autoimmune disorder is characterized by weakness and progressive fatiguability of striated muscles from defective transmission of impulses at the nerve-muscle junction. One theory is that gamma G immunoglobulin (IgG) antibodies circulating in the blood bind to the muscle end plate receptors and compete with acetylcholine for attachment sites. Another theory is that circulating antibodies damage the acetylcholine receptor sites. In either case, the autoimmune system attacks the neuromuscular junction, decreasing the availability and sensitivity of the acetylcholine receptors. Because acetylcholine is unable to bind normally to the postsynaptic membrane, the nerve impulse is unable to excite the muscle effectively.

Myasthenia gravis can be restricted to the extraocular muscles as ocular myasthenia, but it often affects the entire body as generalized myasthenia. Half of all patients presenting with ptosis and diplopia have myasthenia gravis. Most myasthenic patients have symptoms of ptosis and diplopia. Most ocular myasthenia patients develop systemic involvement within 18 months of the ocular signs. Pupillary and accommodative muscle fibers are not involved. If they are, suspect another disorder. Another autoimmune disorder, thyroid eye disease, sometimes occurs in myasthenic patients.

Weakness without other signs of neurologic deficit (no tendon reflex changes, sensory loss, or muscle atrophy), and *variability* of muscle functions within minutes, hours, or weeks, with remissions and exacerbations, is typical. Other signs are difficulty in swallowing, talking, or breathing, weakness of the jaws or limbs; all these signs become more pronounced with fatigue. Fatigue increases toward the end of the day. The most feared complication is respiratory weakness, which may combine with paralysis of swallowing. Because symptoms become progressively more severe with fatigue or infection, a myasthenic patient may develop acute respiratory failure leading to death following any respiratory infection. Diplopia may be caused by involvement of any one, or several, of the extraocular muscles, but upward movement is usually affected first. The extraocular muscle involvement is such, however, that ocular myasthenia can mimic an internuclear ophthalmoplegia, a gaze palsy, a muscle palsy, or a thyroid eye disease and may be unilateral or bilateral. *Variability* of levator and extraocular muscle involvement is the characteristic that offers the clue to myasthenia gravis.

Ptosis shifts from one eye to the other. It may be asymmetric, unilateral, or bilateral. Ptosis is usually absent on awakening but worsens throughout the day. Often the affected upper eye lid twitches when the eye moves from down gaze to straight ahead. On asking the patient to keep the eyes in up gaze, the affected upper eye lid begins to droop from fatigue after 30 seconds. Repeated closure of the eye lids also worsens the ptosis. If unilateral, the unaffected eye lid may retract because it receives extra innervation required by the affected eyelid. Occluding the eye with the ptosis eliminates the retraction.

The onset of myasthenia gravis is most common in the second or third decade of life, but it may occur at any age. It is diagnosed by intravenously injecting a rapid, short acting, anticholinesterase agent such as edrophonium chloride (Tensilon). This acts rapidly, but only for a short period. Severe slowing of the heart rate, bradycardia, is a possible side effect of this drug. Atropine should be available as an antidote. Because edrophonium inhibits the action of cholinesterase, acetylcholine concentration increases. More binding of receptor sites occurs at the nerve-muscle junction. Extraocular muscle action and ptosis improve within 1 minute of injection. Slurred speech may improve, rounded shoulders may lift up, and the droopy look of the face may disappear. Objective diplopia measurements before and after edrophonium injection can be documented on a Lancaster red-green screen. Approximately 5 minutes after injection, the diplopia returns to the preinjection amount.

Treatment depends on the severity of the disease. The eye muscles are the least responsive. Usually long-acting anticholinesterase agents such as pyridostigmine bromide (Mestinon) or neostigmine (Prostigmin) reduce symptoms with little risk. Steroids such as prednisone may be employed, sometimes with dramatic improvement, but side effects are a problem with long-term use. Thymectomy, or removal of the thymus gland, suppresses the production of the IgG antibodies. This form of treatment is reserved for patients who do not respond to anticholinesterase drugs and have medical contraindications to steroids. Patients should be managed by an ophthalmologist-internist-neurologist team.

● BLOOD VESSEL DISEASE

A thrombus is a blood clot attached to a blood vessel wall. An embolus is a thrombus that breaks off and travels through the bloodstream. A clot, embolus, or thrombus can obstruct a blood vessel, thus markedly decreasing the blood flow through it. The reduced blood supply causes ischemia, a lack of nutrients and oxygen to those tissues normally supplied by the blood. With ischemia the tissues become starved for oxygen and may die. The resulting area of tissue death is an infarct.

Sometimes closed capillaries open and form an anastomosis. This provides an alternate route for blood, a collateral circulation. The collateral circulation comes from another artery that reaches that area by a nearby but different route. If a blood vessel becomes blocked, this allows blood to circulate around that area.

Hypertension is the most common blood vessel disease, occurring when the cardiovascular system escapes regulation by at least one of its many control systems. Blood pressure higher than 140/90 mm Hg is considered hypertensive, too high for the continued health of the cardiovascular system. Most patients with hypertension have no particular underlying cause and no symptoms. It is a leading cause of death in the United States.

When blood pressure is high, the heart uses more energy to pump and gradually enlarges. When the heart's pumping ability becomes damaged, the result is congestive heart failure. Fluid fills the lungs, causing shortness of breath. Beta blockers, such as timolol, are contraindicated in patients with congestive heart failure. These blockers decrease the heart rate and contractility and thereby decrease the amount of blood pumped out by a heart already in trouble.

Arteriosclerosis, a straightening, hardening, and narrowing of arterioles, is part of the aging process. From being stretched over long periods, the elastic arteries harden and scar. The heart, kidneys, and brain are the organs most affected.

Atherosclerosis is an important type of arteriosclerosis. Atherosclerosis is an infiltration in the walls of large arteries by fatty deposits, such as cholesterol, that partially block blood flow. This damages the lining in the walls, by thickening and deforming it and decreasing the elasticity. Other bits of tissue in the blood stick to the fatty deposits, further narrowing the blood vessel diameter. As flow slows, clots form. If the clot breaks off, the embolus may block a smaller blood vessel in another part of the body. Atherosclerosis is the most common cause of myocardial infarctions (heart attacks) and strokes or cerebrovascular accidents (CVA). As with hypertension, retinal changes can be followed by direct visualization with ophthalmoscopy and intravenous fluorescein angiography. Hypertensive patients often develop atherosclerosis and kidney disease. When kidney function decreases because of the arteriosclerotic changes, chronic renal failure develops as well as hypertension.

The risk of developing blood vessel disease can be decreased by regular exercise, by controlling cholesterol and high blood pressure levels by diet and drugs, and by not smoking. The incidence of blood vessel disease increases with age, with predisposing heredity, with diabetes, and possibly with stress. It is more common in men than in women, and it is more common in African-Americans than in whites.

● CEREBRAL BLOOD VESSEL DISEASE

Cerebral blood vessel disease in adulthood is the most common cause of acquired neurologic disorders. Either a blood vessel becomes blocked by a clot or increased blood pressure puts a severe strain on the cerebral arteries, which rupture and hemorrhage. Either mechanism produces a CVA, which is a sudden disruption of the blood supply to part of the brain and interferes with the body functions controlled by that part of the brain. The most common type of stroke, thrombotic, is caused by a partial closing of arteries in the brain by atherosclerosis, slowing the flow of blood in that area. Thrombi form and lodge on the fatty deposits, totally blocking the artery and cutting off the blood supply to that area of the brain. Embolic strokes occur when such blood clots clog a cerebral artery.

An aneurysm is a weakening of a blood vessel with formation of a bubble that forms in the blood vessel wall. As the aneurysm enlarges, the blood vessel walls weaken and sometimes rupture, often with disastrous results. Hemorrhagic strokes occur when an aneurysm weakens enough to burst, causing loss of blood to that area. The body supplies collateral circulation whenever possible following the loss of blood supply. Aspirin helps to ward off stroke by preventing the clotting of blood.

Internal carotid artery insufficiency, usually from atherosclerosis, often results in a monocular visual loss on the affected side. Carotid artery insufficiency is the cause of a *transient ischemic attack (TIA)*, a brief spasm of a cerebral blood vessel diminishing the flow of oxygen to the brain on a temporary basis, causing discomfort but no lasting damage. This type of ministroke lasts from a few minutes to a few hours. The signs include fainting; double vision; blurred vision; field loss; temporary blindness; sudden headache; forgetfulness; weak or numb muscles on one side; deafness; ringing in the ears; irritability; and problems with swallowing, speaking, or understanding speech. Transient ischemic attack warns of an impending stroke. Any transient visual loss is called amaurosis fugax.

Vertebrobasilar insufficiency usually results in a binocular visual loss, such as a congruous homonymous bilateral visual field loss from an affected occipital lobe. Because the vertebrobasilar system also supplies the 3rd, 4th, and 6th nerve nuclei in the brain stem, insufficiency can cause double vision. Vertebrobasilar TIAs cause clumsiness, dizziness, bilateral blurring, and vision dimming.

● RETINOPATHY

Hypertensive Retinopathy

Retinal blood vessels are final branches of the ophthalmic artery, itself a branch off the internal carotid artery. Whenever disease affects the blood vessels of the body, it also affects the retinal blood vessels. Because retinal blood vessels can be directly observed by ophthalmoscopy, any changes in blood vessel disease can be monitored. Hypertensive retinopathy alters the blood vessels over the retina. Choroidal blood vessels are often more severely affected than retinal blood vessels. Fluorescein angiography is a method of photographing the damage to the retinal blood vessels.

These pathologic changes in blood vessels begin in the arterioles with irregular areas of narrowing and straightening. The next phase, after the blood-retinal barrier is disrupted, causes the blood vessels to act like leaky pipes. Findings include "cotton-wool" spots, flame-shaped bleeds, fat deposits (hard exudates), arteriosclerotic changes, small branch arteriole and vein occlusions, disc swelling, both micro- and macroaneurysms, central retinal artery and vein occlusions, and epiretinal membrane formations. The bleeding and cotton-wool spots indicate lack of oxygen and nutrients from capillaries.

Drugs can reverse all changes, especially if these are taken in the early stages. Hypertensive retinopathy is an excellent indicator of how well the body responds to the control of hypertension by drugs. If patients with severe hypertensive retinopathy do not have any evidence by ophthalmoscopy or fluorescein angiography of the changes being reversed with powerful antihypertensive drugs, they have a poor chance of survival. Retinal hemorrhages, exudates, and disc swellings may take months to resolve after blood pressure has been lowered to normal levels. Fluorescein leakage and disc swelling often improve markedly.

Central Retinal Artery Occlusion (CRAO)

This is an ophthalmic emergency wherein the ophthalmic artery or internal carotid artery is blocked and blood flow to the central retinal artery is stopped. An acute blockage leads to immediate catastrophic loss of vision in the involved eye. The disc appears pale with very narrow arterioles and enlarged, tortuous veins. This is often caused by an embolus; an attempt is made to dislodge the embolus into a smaller blood vessel that supplies a smaller portion of the retina, because the area supplied by the blocked blood vessel dies. Decreasing the intraocular pressure by withdrawing some anterior chamber fluid or massaging the eye may unblock the artery. If accomplished within an hour of the block, some vision may return. After that point, no further recovery is possible. The macula acutely develops a cherry red spot, and the optic nerve eventually atrophies.

Central Retinal Vein Occlusion (CRVO)

Vision loss from CRVO is neither as quick nor as severe as that from CRAO. The patient may notice a contraction of the visual field or that objects appear red. Classic findings are retina and disc swelling, and enlarged tortuous veins with huge nerve fiber layer blot hemorrhages, especially near the macula. About half these patients eventually develop neovascularization (rubeosis) of the iris and anterior chamber angle. Gradually over months, the fundus returns to a more normal appearance. Another form without the retinal ischemia occurs with little change in vision and gradual improvement over several years. There is usually no pain, but there is no proven therapy, either.

Ischemic Optic Neuropathy (ION)

Sudden painless vision loss, which may continue to deteriorate over a few days, and may not recover is known as ischemic optic neuropathy. Part or all of the optic disc has a milky swelling. Arcuate and altitudinal, especially inferior, visual field defects are common. When the cause can be found, it is often temporal arteritis, but it may be hypertension or diabetes.

• DIABETES MELLITUS

Sugar (glucose) found in blood is the major source of energy for the body. The blood glucose level is mostly maintained by insulin and glucagon, two hormones with opposing actions secreted by the pancreas. After eating, nutrient sugars are transported by the blood to the liver where they are changed to glycogen and stored until released to the blood as glucose for transport to the cells. Insulin lowers the blood glucose level by increasing the amount of glucose taken into the cells, which increases the amount of glucose stored in the liver and muscles. When the blood glucose level drops long after eating, glucagon releases glucose by the liver

and muscles, elevating the blood glucose level to normal. The concentration of glucose is kept in balance by the insulin level.

Diabetes mellitus is an abnormality of glucose metabolism caused by an insufficient supply of insulin produced by the pancreas when its beta cells are destroyed. Beta cells release insulin, which drives glucose from the blood into the inside of the cells. With too little insulin, the increased blood glucose concentration makes the patient hyperglycemic. The elevated blood glucose level is too high for the kidneys to reabsorb. The excess spills over into the urine, attracts large amounts of water, and dehydrates the patient.

Making matters worse, glucagon increases the formation of acids called ketones. With a decreased insulin supply, the body's energy requirements are met by fat, using up the body's reserve, also producing ketones. When the ketone concentration builds up in the blood, the excess also spills over into the urine, dragging along sodium and potassium ions that the body requires. As the fat is transported by the blood, some is deposited on blood vessel walls, leading to atherosclerosis.

Diabetes is characterized by increased urine production, increased thirst, increased hunger (especially for sweets), and weight loss. Because it leads to arteriosclerosis, diabetes is also considered a blood vessel, especially small blood vessel, disease. Diabetes leads to other chronic disorders, especially in the blood vessels of the kidneys, nerves, and eyes. If a diabetic takes insulin, but does not eat shortly after, the blood glucose level will drop too low, causing hypoglycemia. The diabetic patient needs sugar or fruit juice. Otherwise, he or she shakes, sweats, feels tired, and becomes mentally confused. The heart may race and cause fainting.

Ocular Manifestations

Despite advances in delivery of insulin to diabetics, the disease still decreases life expectancy, although not as severely as previously. Diabetics are more prone to glaucoma and cataracts than nondiabetics. When diabetics develop extraocular muscle palsies from cranial nerve involvement, recovery is frequently spontaneous within 2 to 3 months. The third (oculomotor) cranial nerve (CN III) and the sixth (abducens) cranial nerve (CN VI) are affected more commonly than the fourth (trochlear) cranial nerve (CN IV), usually with pupil sparing when CN III is involved. Diabetic patients have difficulty with refraction, because their retinoscopy fluctuates with their blood glucose levels. An elevated blood glucose level increases the index of refraction of the lens as the glucose enters it. Diabetics develop intermittent episodes of blurry vision from induced nearsightedness.

Diabetic Retinopathy

Diabetic background retinopathy begins with an increased blood flow. In the deterioration of retinal capillary walls, which leak blood when they should not, small dot and blot hemorrhages, hard exudates, cotton-wool spots, and swelling, mostly in the posterior pole, are found. As capillaries are destroyed, the retina is supplied with less blood and, thus, less oxygen and nutrients. The retinal veins dilate in an attempt to receive more blood and oxygen, producing nerve fiber layer infarcts (i.e., cotton-wool spots). The lowered oxygen supply from the lowered blood supply, or ischemia, causes all these changes.

Gradually this leads to the sprouting of small, abnormal, new blood vessels (neovascularization). Neovascularization forms on the venous side of the blood vessel system on the retinal surface. These new blood vessels are larger but weaker than normal and thus bleed easily and profusely. Neovascularization is the major sign of proliferative diabetic retinopathy. Fortunately, most diabetics have only the background retinopathy described previously, which is less severe than proliferative retinopathy.

If neovascularization is untreated, these areas can bleed massively into the vitreous or exert traction on the retina, which may result in a retinal detachment. Traction bands can be cut and peeled away. A vitrectomy may be required to clear a path through blood or cloudy areas. If the iris develops new blood vessel growth, rubeosis iridis, the angle may "zip shut" and may produce secondary glaucoma.

The progress of diabetic retinopathy is often followed by repeat fluorescein angiography. Microaneurysms in the capillaries show areas of hyperfluorescence from leakage of dye, whereas loss of capillaries shows areas of hypofluorescence because no dye is seen. Panretinal photocoagulation by a laser cauterizes the neovascular areas, seals off the affected retina, and prevents catastrophic visual loss.

Bibliography

Graves' Disease

Cassin B: The thyroid spiral. Am Orthoptic J 36: 87, 1986.
Miller NR: Walsh & Hoyt's Clinical Neuro-ophthalmology, 4th ed, vol 2. Baltimore, Williams & Wilkins, 1985.
Sergott RC, Glaser JS: Graves' ophthalmopathy: a clinical and immunological review. Surv Ophthalmol 26: 1, 1981.
Sisler HA, Jakobiec FA, Trokel SL: Ocular abnormalities and orbital changes of Graves' disease. In Duane TD, Jaeger EA (eds): Clinical Ophthalmology, vol 2. Philadelphia, Harper & Row, 1986.
Smith BR, Hall R: Thyroid stimulating immunoglobulins in Graves' disease. Lancet 2: 42, 1974.

Trokel SL, Jakobiec, FA: Correlation of CT scanning and pathologic features of ophthalmic Graves' disease. Ophthalmology 88: 553, 1981.
Werner SC: Classification of the eye changes of Graves' disease. J Clin Endocrinol Metab 29: 982, 1969.
Werner SC: Modification of the classification of the eye changes of Graves' disease. Am J Ophthalmol 83: 725, 1977.

Myasthenia Gravis

Drachman DB: Myasthenia gravis. N Engl J Med 298: 136, 1978.
Miller NR: Myasthenia gravis. Ophthalmology 86: 2165, 1979.
Miller NR: Walsh and Hoyt's Clinical Neuro-ophthalmology, 4th ed, vol 2. Baltimore, Williams & Wilkins, 1985.

Blood Vessel Disease

Andreoli TE, Carpenter CCJ, Plum F, et al: Cecil's Essentials of Medicine. Philadelphia, WB Saunders, 1986.
Berne RM, Levy MN: Physiology, 2nd ed. St Louis, Mosby-Year Book, 1988.
Fishman MC, Hoffman AR, Klausner RD, et al: Chapter 10 Hypertension. In Medicine, 2nd ed. Philadelphia, JB Lippincott, 1985.
Jampol L: Ocular manifestations of selected systemic diseases. In Peyman GA, Sanders DR, Goldberg M (eds): Principles and Practice of Ophthalmology. Philadelphia, WB Saunders, 1980.
Tso M, Jampol L: Pathophysiology of hypertensive retinopathy. Ophthalmology 89: 1132, 1982.
Walsh J: Hypertensive retinopathy: description, classification, and prognosis. Ophthalmology 89: 1127, 1982.

Diabetes Mellitus

Andreoli TE, Carpenter CCJ, Plum F, et al: Cecil's Essentials of Medicine. Philadelphia, WB Saunders, 1986.
Hoffman AR, Klausner RD, Fishman MC, et al: Medicine, 2nd ed. Philadelphia, Lippincott, 1985.

● CHAPTER 28 EYE DISEASES

1. Which two extraocular muscles are most commonly restricted in Graves' disease?
   a. IR and SR
   b. SR and MR
   c. IR and MR
   d. SR and LR
   e. IR and LR

2. Weakness and variability of muscle function are typical of which disorder?
   a. myasthenia gravis
   b. diabetes
   c. orbital tumor
   d. Graves' disease
   e. ischemic optic neuropathy.

3. What is a sudden disruption of the blood supply to part of the brain called?
   a. cerebrovascular accident
   b. aneurysm
   c. amaurosis fugax
   d. myocardial infarction
   e. transient ischemic attack.

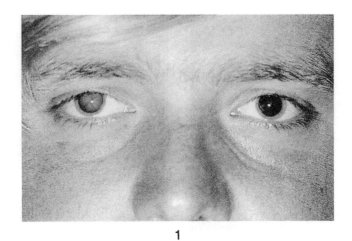

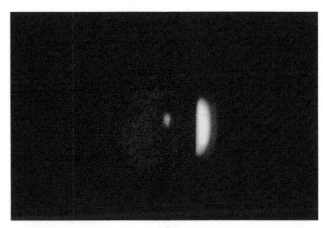

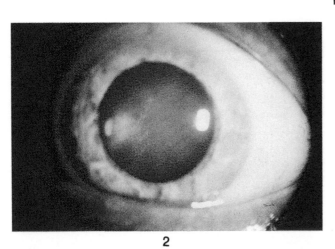

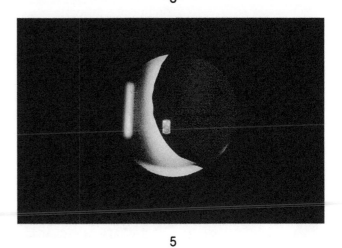

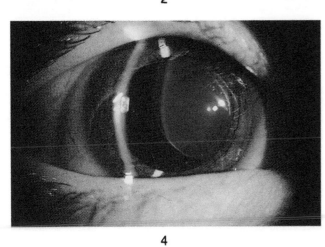

COLOR PLATE 1. Patient with cataract in right eye.
COLOR PLATE 2. Posterior subcapsular cataract, shown using diffuse illumination as seen on slit lamp.
COLOR PLATE 3. Same posterior subcapsular cataract, shown using retroillumination as seen on slit lamp.
COLOR PLATE 4. Subluxated (partially dislocated) lens, as seen with thin beam on slit lamp.
COLOR PLATE 5. Same subluxated lens, with retroillumination on slit lamp.

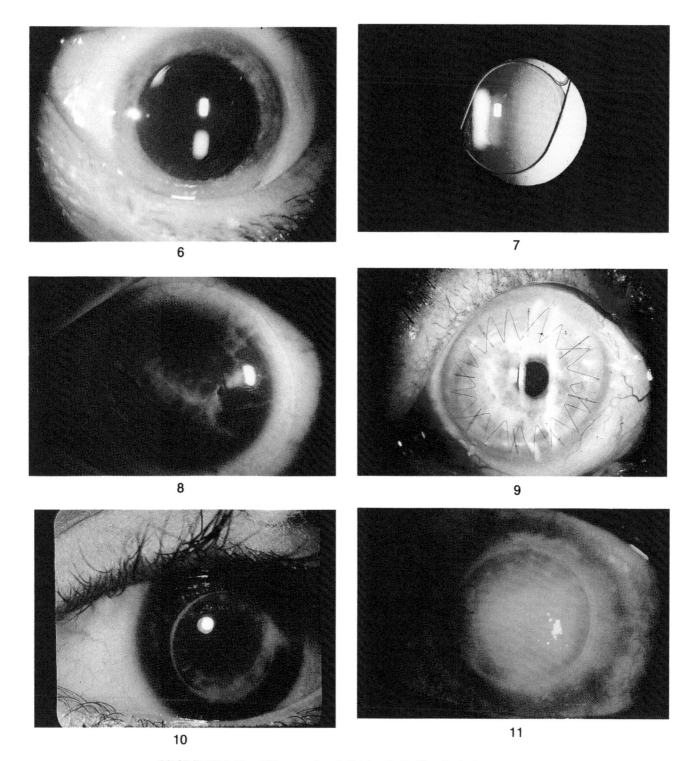

COLOR PLATE 6. Edge of IOL as seen through dilated pupil with diffuse illumination on slit lamp.
COLOR PLATE 7. Same edge of IOL as seen with retroillumination on slit lamp.
COLOR PLATE 8. Corneal scar after traumatic corneal laceration.
COLOR PLATE 9. Post-penetrating keratoplasty (corneal transplant) with running sutures.
COLOR PLATE 10. Post-penetrating keratoplasty after sutures removed.
COLOR PLATE 11. Post-penetrating keratoplasty with graft failure.

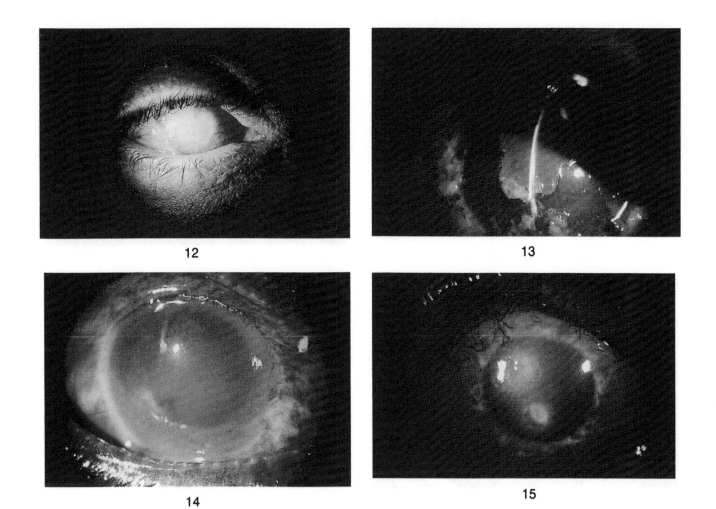

COLOR PLATE 12. Severe alkaline (lye) burn.
COLOR PLATE 13. Acid burn, several hours after occurrence, with sloughed corneal epithelium.
COLOR PLATE 14. Same acid burn, after 3 weeks, showing healed epithelium but residual corneal haze.
COLOR PLATE 15. Corneal ulcer due to an infective organism.

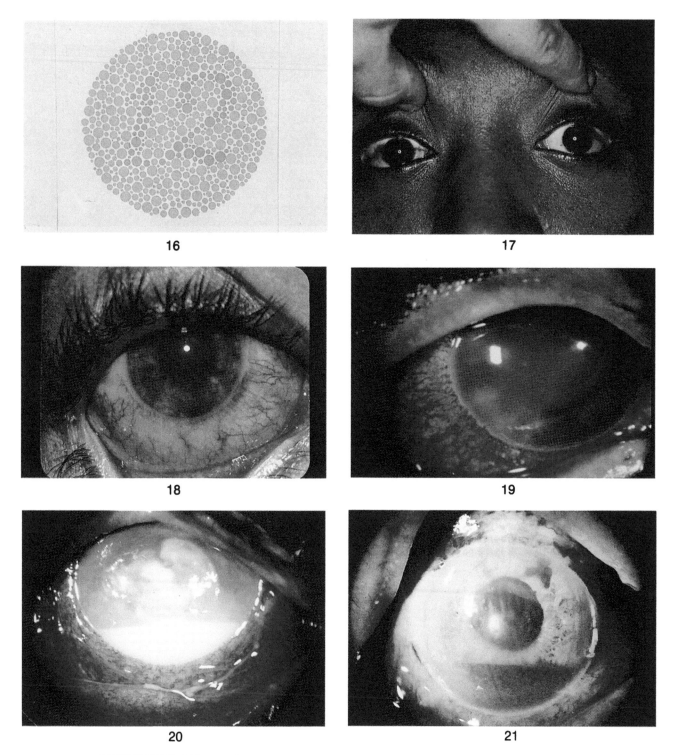

16

17

18

19

20

21

COLOR PLATE 16. Ishihara test plate.
COLOR PLATE 17. Subconjunctival hemorrhage.
COLOR PLATE 18. Viral conjunctivitis (pink eye).
COLOR PLATE 19. Acanthamoeba corneal infection, associated with contact lens wear and contaminated contact lens solution.
COLOR PLATE 20. Hypopyon. White line demarcates layered collection of pus in bottom of anterior chamber.
COLOR PLATE 21. Hyphema. Red line denotes layered collection of blood in bottom of anterior chamber.

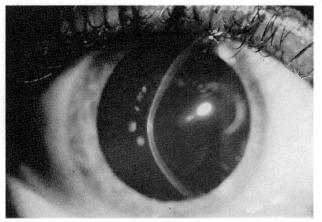

22

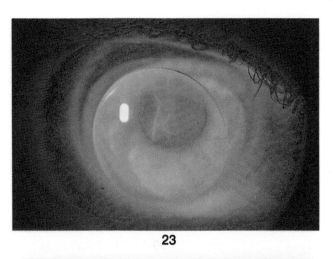

23

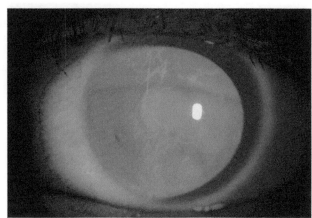

24

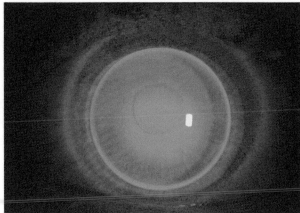

25

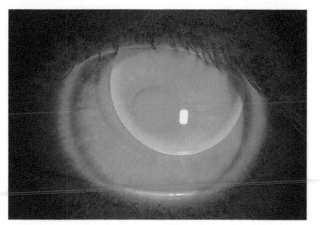

26

COLOR PLATE 22. Desçemet's folds in patient with keratoconus.
COLOR PLATE 23. Corneal abrasion under contact lens seen with fluorescein dye.
COLOR PLATE 24. Foreign body under a rigid gas permeable contact lens seen with fluorescein dye.
COLOR PLATE 25. Appearance with steep fit of a rigid gas permeable contact lens seen with fluorescein dye.
COLOR PLATE 26. Appearance with flat fit of a rigid gas permeable contact lens seen with fluorescein dye.

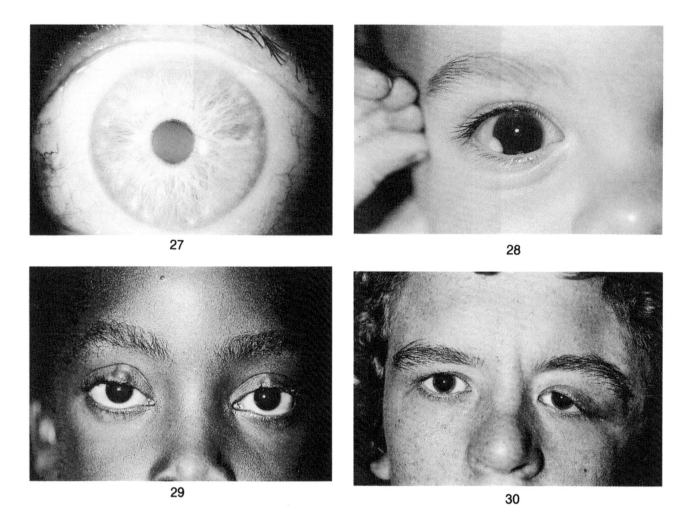

27

28

29

30

COLOR PLATE 27. Iris nevus at 4 o'clock position.
COLOR PLATE 28. Epibulbar dermoid cyst in a patient with Goldenhar's syndrome.
COLOR PLATE 29. Multiple chalazia of the eyelids.
COLOR PLATE 30. Characteristic S-shaped deformity of the upper left eyelid, as seen with neurofibromatosis.

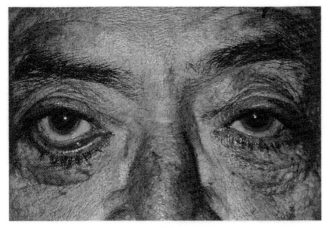

31

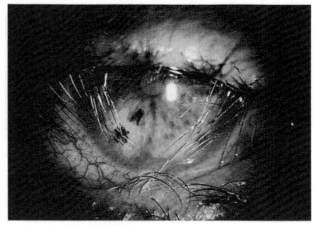

32

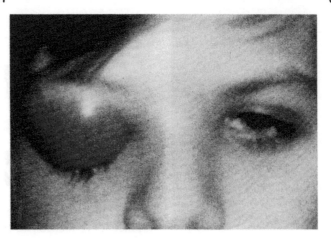

33

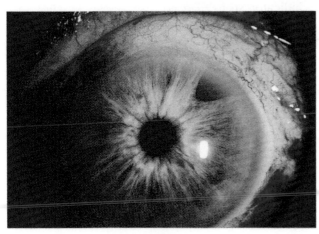

34

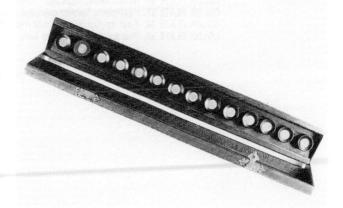

35

COLOR PLATE 31. Ectropion. Lower right eyelid margin falls away from eyeball.
COLOR PLATE 32. Entropion. Lower eyelid margin turns inward toward eyeball, with lashes touching cornea (trichiasis).
COLOR PLATE 33. Orbital cellulitis, right eye
COLOR PLATE 34. Peripheral iridectomy at one o'clock.
COLOR PLATE 35. Farnsworth D-15 test for color vision.

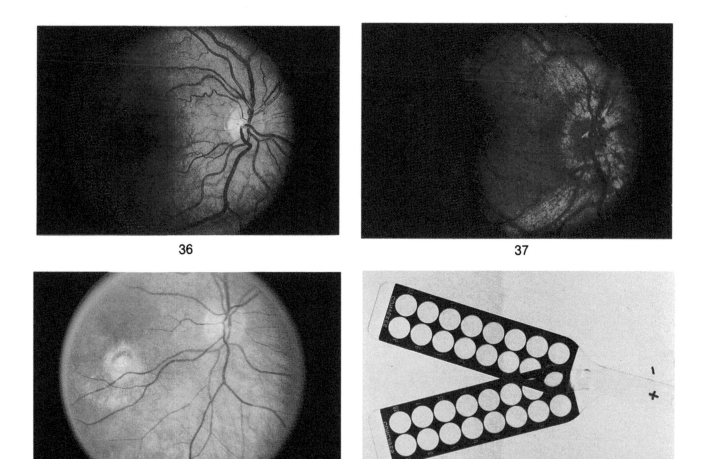

COLOR PLATE 36. Normal fundus, right eye.
COLOR PLATE 37. Papilledema. Swollen optic disc with obscuration of vessels at disc margin and engorged veins.
COLOR PLATE 38. Focal macular scar that may result from a variety of disorders.
COLOR PLATE 39. Plus and minus skiascopy bars.

4. What is an immediate catastrophic vision loss in one eye most likely caused by?
   a. central retinal vein occlusion
   b. ischemic optic neuropathy
   c. myasthenia gravis
   d. Graves' disease
   e. central retinal artery occlusion.

5. What do diabetics have problems with?
   a. too much insulin
   b. hyperglycemia
   c. induced farsightedness
   d. decreased urine production
   e. hypoglycemia.

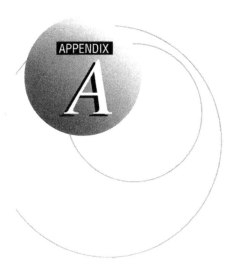

Appendix

MATHEMATICS REFERENCE

Geometric and physiological optics use basic math and algebra to solve lens problems, convert diopters to meters, and transpose spherocylinders. As a reference, this appendix reviews elementary mathematics concepts for technical personnel.

● TRANSFORMATION OF AN EQUATION

Equations often need to be rearranged to solve them. We can add, subtract, multiply, or divide both sides of an equation by the same number without changing the validity of the equation, but whatever you do to *one* side you *must* do to the other.

Adding and Subtracting

- *Example.* $-4 + P = +7$
- *To solve for P we need to rid the left side of the equation by -4. To do this, we add $+4$ to both sides.*
$$-4 + P + 4 = +7 + 4$$
$$P = +7 + 4$$
$$P = 11$$
- *Simplify this maneuver by moving a letter or number across the equal sign but changing its sign.*

- *For Example. To eliminate -4 from the left side of the foregoing equation, you move it across the equal sign to the right side of the equation but change its sign to $+4$. You just saved one step.*
$$-4 + P = +7$$
$$P = +7 + 4$$
$$P = 11$$

Multiplication and Division

To eliminate a denominator, both sides are multiplied by that denominator.

- *Example.* $AC/A = +5 + \dfrac{(+10) - (+4)}{3}$
$$AC/A = +5 + \frac{6}{3}$$
$$(3)AC/A = (+5)(3) + \frac{(+6)(3)}{3}$$
$$(3)AC/A = +15 + (+6)$$
$$(3)AC/A = +21$$
- *What we did was move the denominator 3 across the equal sign but reverse its function; i.e., we multiplied 3 into what was on the other side.*
- *Now we need to eliminate the 3 on the left side of the equation to solve for AC/A, so we divide both sides by 3.*
$$\frac{(3)(AC/A)}{3} = \frac{(+21)}{3}$$
$$AC/A = +7$$

● ADDITION AND SUBTRACTION OF POSITIVE AND NEGATIVE NUMBERS

Positive and negative numbers are used in transposing spherocylinders from minus to plus form, and plus to minus, and when finding the spherical equivalent, and measuring lens strength on a lensometer. Plus and minus numbers are continuous on a numberline but begin counting in opposite directions.

Relate this to reading a thermometer. To get from 10° below zero to 15° above zero is a plus change of 25° (Fig. App.–1).

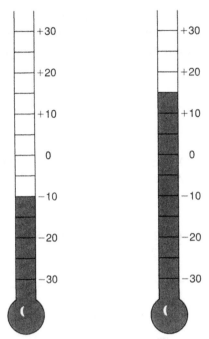

FIGURE App.–1. Relating a numberline to a thermometer.

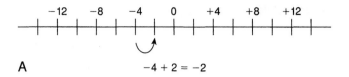

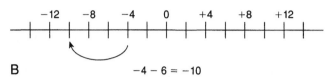

FIGURE App.–2. *A,* Adding a positive number to a negative number on a numberline. *B,* Adding two negative numbers on a numberline.

● ***For Example.*** *If we have a −4 D lens and add +2D to it, the new lens strength becomes −4 +2, or −2D (Fig. App.–2).*

To add two negative numbers, add the numbers but keep the minus sign. If we have a −4 D lens and add −6 D to it, we get −4 −6, or −10 D lens.

To subtract a negative number, you add it, because two minus signs make one plus.

● ***For Example.*** *In the formula A = F − N below, we need to subtract −5.*
● *The two minus signs become a plus sign:*
$$+15 = F - (-5)$$
$$+15 = F + 5$$
$$F + 5 = +15$$
● *Now we subtract +5 from both sides by moving the +5 from the left side of the equation to the right side and change its sign:*
$$F + 5 = +15$$
$$F = +15 - 5$$
$$F = +10$$

● OPTICAL CROSSES

The optical cross below has a value of −1.00 + 4.00 × 180. To go from a negative to a positive meridian, you move along the numberline to zero first.

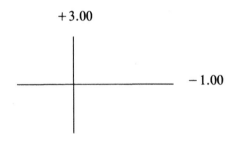

A +4.00 added to a −1.00 produces +3.00. If this spherocylindrical lens were measured on a lensometer, the thin sphere lines would come into focus at −1.00 with the axis dial at a 180° setting, and the thick lines would come into focus at +3.00 with the axis dial at the 180° setting.

The same change occurs when measuring ocular misalignments. If the distance and near measurements are

10^Δ X and 8^Δ X′, you have a positive (+) change of 2.

10^Δ X and 12^Δ X′, you have a negative (−) change of 2.

10^Δ X and 0′, you have a positive (+) change of 10.

10^Δ X and 8^Δ E′, you have a positive (+) change of 18.

To add a positive and a negative number, you do what the signs say (Fig. App.–2).

● ACCOMMODATIVE CONVERGENCE/ ACCOMMODATION RATIOS

When calculating AC/A ratios, we use + for esodeviations and − for exodeviations. If we have a patient with 20^Δ XT + 35^Δ XT′ with a 6-cm pupillary distance, we have:

$$AC/A = PD + \frac{N - D}{3}$$
$$= 6 + \frac{(-35) - (-20)}{3}$$
$$= 6 + \frac{-35 + 20}{3}$$
$$= 6 + \frac{-15}{3}$$
$$= 6 - 5$$
$$= 1$$

• DIVIDING BY A FRACTION

Sometimes we need to divide a whole number by a fraction, such as

$$\frac{2}{1/3}$$

The part of the fraction doing the dividing is the denominator (1/3). We invert it (change 1/3 to 3/1) and multiply the numerator and denominator by its inversion.

• *For Example.*

$$\frac{2}{1/3} =$$
$$\frac{2 \times 3/1}{1/3 \times 3/1} =$$
$$\frac{6}{1} =$$
$$6$$

• RATIOS AND PROPORTIONS

A ratio is a fraction that compares two quantities. The AC/A ratio compares how much accommodative convergence is produced by a given level of accommodation.

• *For Example. If 18 prism diopters of accommodative convergence is produced by 6 D of accommodation, the ratio is:*

$$18^\Delta/6 \text{ D (or } 3^\Delta/1 \text{ D)}.$$

Visual acuity is a ratio of the testing distance as the numerator, compared with the size print seen as the denominator.

• *For Example. 20/80 vision occurs when someone sees at 20 ft the size print they ought to see 80 ft away.*

Sometimes visual acuity is measured metrically, sometimes with English notation. To change from one system to the other, we compare two equal ratios; a type of equation called a proportion. As one numerator (or denominator) increases, so does the other, by the same proportion. As one decreases, so does the other, by the same proportion. They are directly proportional. The numerator, denoting distance, is 20 ft (English

notation) or 6 m (metric notation). If we have 6/24 visual acuity in metric notation and want to know its English notation equivalent, we set up the direct proportion like this:

$$\frac{6}{24} = \frac{20}{X}$$

To solve for X, both sides need to eliminate their denominators. We multiply both sides by both denominators.

$$\frac{(6)(24)(X)}{24} = \frac{(20)(24)(X)}{X}$$
$$\frac{144X}{24} = \frac{480X}{X}$$
$$6X = 480$$
$$X = 80$$
$$\text{Thus, } \frac{6}{24} = \frac{20}{80}$$

This can be simplified in one step by cross multiplying. We multiply the numerator of the first fraction (6) by the denominator (X) of the second fraction, and the denominator of the first fraction (24) is multiplied by the numerator (20) of the second fraction. Cross multiply:

$$\frac{6}{24} = \frac{20}{X}$$
$$6 \times X = 20 \times 24$$
$$6X = 480$$
$$X = \frac{480}{6}$$
$$X = 80$$

Alternatively, you can divide the denominator by the numerator to determine the multiple (ratio). Then use that ratio to obtain the converted denominator.

• *For Example.*
• *In the English notation 20/40, the ratio is 2 : 1 because 20 is half 40. To convert to the metric system, begin with the numerator 6. To find the denominator, you multiply the numerator by the same ratio 2. In this case: 6 × 2 = 12.*
Therefore, $\frac{20}{40} = \frac{6}{12}$

To convert from metric to English notation, the same procedure is followed.

- *For Example.*
- *The metric 6/18 (ratio is 3 : 1) uses a multiple of three to get from the numerator 6 to the denominator 18. To convert to the English system, you use the same multiple of 3 to get from the numerator 20 to the denominator 60.*

  Therefore, $\dfrac{6}{18} = \dfrac{20}{60}$

● MAGNIFICATION

Magnification of image and object size is proportional to image and object distance. Cross multiplying is used for solving magnification problems.

$$\frac{\text{image size (Is)}}{\text{object size (Os)}} = \frac{\text{image distance (Id)}}{\text{object distance (Od)}}$$

- *For Example.*
- *If the Is is 2 cm, the image distance Id is 1 m, and the Od is 3 m;*

$$\frac{2\,cm}{X} = \frac{1\,m}{3\,m}$$
$$2 \times 3 = 1 \times X$$
$$6 = X$$
$$\therefore 6\,cm = Os$$

Note that both numerator and denominator on the left side of the equation are in cm, and both numerator and denominator on the right side of the equation are in m. Both quantities of size are expressed by the same unit of measurment, and both quantities of distance are expressed by the same unit of measurement.

Because of the direct proportion we can alternatively solve by noting that Od is 3 times more than the Id. Therefore, the Os will be 3 times the Is of 2 cm.

● DIOPTERS TO METERS

In optics, focal length is usually measured in mm, cm, or m. It can be converted to dioptric power by the formula:

$$D = 1/f$$

Where D = dioptric power, measured in diopters (D) and f = focal length, measured in meters (m).

Now we are not comparing equal ratios. Focal length and dioptric power are inversely proportional. As one increases, the other decreases. The higher the dioptric power, the shorter the focal length, and vice versa. A 6 D lens has a focal length of 1/6 m, or 16 cm. A 2 D lens has a focal length of 1/2 m, or 50 cm.

Distances from lenses are usually measured in cm or m and converted to dioptric power by this means.

If a patient's near point of accommodation is 25 cm from his or her nose while wearing glasses,

$$25\,cm = .25\,m = \frac{25}{100}\,m = \frac{1}{4}\,m$$
$$D = 1/f = \frac{1}{1/4} = 4$$

so the near point dioptric equivalent of 25 cm equals 4 D of accommodation power.

When comparing the power of lenses, or the vergence of light rays, focal lengths and their dioptric equivalents are used in almost equal amounts. Vergence power must be all in diopters or all in m to compare. Beware of comparing diopters with m.

We obtain the *reciprocal* of a number by dividing it into 1; e.g., the reciprocal of 5 is 1/5. The reciprocal of 1/3 is

$$\frac{1}{1/3}, \text{ or } 3.$$

● METERS TO FEET

Ophthalmic medical personnel use the metric system as well as the English system. The patient's near point of accommodation, interpupillary distance, distance from the fixation target, and the size of the target are measured using the metric system, with meters (m), centimeters (cm), and millimeters (mm). To correlate metric measurements with the English system, remember that a meter is slightly more than a yard.

$$1\,m = 3.28\,ft = 39\,3/8\,in. = 39.375\,in.$$

To help keep your perspective, because 1 m is almost 40 in., 1/2 meter is about 20 in., 1/4 meter about 10 in.

The conversion formula is 1 in. = 2.54 cm. If 1 in. = 2.54 cm, then 12 in. = 30.5 cm (approximately 1/3 m).

The metric system uses multiples of 10 or 100.

$$10\,mm = 1\,cm$$
$$100\,cm = 1\,m$$

Just as there are 100 cents in a dollar, there are 100 cm in a meter. Just as 1 cent can be expressed as $.01, 1 cm can be expressed as .01 m. You shift from one to another by just moving the decimal point.

- *For Example.*
- *25 cm = .25 m = 1/4 m*
  25 cents = $.25 = a quarter

Occasionally, with wavelengths of light, you will need to deal with nanometers (nm), which equal millimicrons (term being phased out); 1000 nm equals a micrometer (μm), 1000 μm equals a millimeter. Laser speeds are expressed in picoseconds (psec).

$1 \text{ cm} = .01 \text{ m} = 10^{-2} \text{ m}$

$1 \text{ mm} = .001 \text{ m} = 10^{-3} \text{ m}$

$1 \text{ } \mu\text{m} = .000001 \text{ m} = 10^{-6} \text{ m}$

$1 \text{ nm} = .000000001 \text{ m} = 10^{-9} \text{ m}$

$1 \text{ psec} = .000000000001 = 10^{-12} \text{ m}$

One meter equals

100 cm

1000 mm

1,000,000 μm

1,000,000,000 nm

1,000,000,000,000 psec

When we convert from a larger unit (such as meters) to a smaller, (such as centimeters), we multiply. If one wishes to convert from meters to centimeters, one multiplies by 100.

- *For Example.*
- *a. 3m = 3 × 100 cm = 300 cm*
  b. $\frac{1}{6}$ m = $\frac{1}{6}$ × 100 cm = $\frac{100\,cm}{6}$ = 16 cm = .16 m

---

To convert from meters to millimeters, one multiplies by a thousand:

- *a. 3m = 3 × 1000 mm = 3000 mm*
  b. $\frac{1}{6}$ m = $\frac{1}{6}$ × 1000 mm = $\frac{1000\,mm}{6}$ = 160 mm

---

To convert from a small unit to a larger unit, we divide. To convert from centimeters to meters, the decimal point is moved two numbers to the left, or divided by 100.

- *For Example.*
- *16 cm = $\frac{16}{100}$ m*

  $\frac{16}{100}$ m = .16 m
- *Or you may prefer a fraction.*

- *For Example.*
- *16 cm = $\frac{16}{100}$ m*

  = $\frac{16/16}{100/16}$ m

  = 1/6m

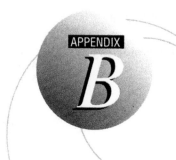

APPENDIX

B

Answers to Review Questions

Chapter One

1. c
2. d
3. d
4. a
5. e

Chapter Two

1. e
2. c
3. d
4. a
5. d

Chapter Three

1. d
2. a
3. d
4. c
5. b

Chapter Four

1. b
2. c
3. a
4. a
5. c

Chapter Five

1. b
2. e
3. a
4. c
5. d

Chapter Six

1. d
2. b
3. c
4. c
5. a

Chapter Seven

1. d
2. e
3. e
4. a
5. a

Chapter Eight

1. c
2. c
3. a
4. e
5. e

Chapter Nine

1. a
2. d
3. e
4. a
5. b

Chapter Ten

1. b
2. a
3. d
4. b
5. d

Chapter Eleven

1. d
2. e
3. b
4. b
5. e

Chapter Twelve

1. a
2. e
3. c
4. b
5. d

Chapter Thirteen

1. c
2. a
3. b
4. c
5. d

Chapter Fourteen

1. d
2. a
3. b
4. b
5. e

Chapter Fifteen

Visual Assessment

1. d
2. d
3. c
4. e
5. a

Pupil Function

1. b
2. c
3. a
4. e
5. b

Biomicroscopy

1. b
2. a
3. c
4. d
5. a

Tonometry

1. b
2. d

Refractometry

1. a
2. c
3. c
4. e
5. b

Lensometry

1. c
2. a

Keratometry

1. d
2. a
3. c

Interpupillary Distance

1. b
2. e

Exophthalmometry

1. c

Biometry

1. e
2. b

Chapter Sixteen

1. d
2. b
3. b
4. e
5. b

Chapter Seventeen

1. c
2. a
3. c
4. d
5. e

Chapter Eighteen

1. e
2. c

3. b
4. a
5. e

Chapter Nineteen

1. d
2. b
3. c
4. e
5. b

Chapter Twenty

1. e
2. d
3. b
4. a
5. c

Chapter Twenty-One

1. b
2. a
3. c
4. e
5. d

Chapter Twenty-Two

1. a
2. c
3. e
4. a
5. d

Chapter Twenty-Three

1. a
2. d
3. b
4. e
5. b

Chapter Twenty-Four

1. d
2. a
3. b
4. e
5. c

Chapter Twenty-Five

1. c
2. e

3. d
4. b
5. e

Chapter Twenty-Six

1. b
2. c
3. a
4. e
5. d

Chapter Twenty-Seven

1. d
2. a
3. c
4. b
5. a

Chapter Twenty-Eight

1. c
2. a
3. a
4. e
5. b

Index

Note: Page numbers in *italics* refer to illustrations; page numbers followed by (t) refer to tables.

Printed and bound by CPI Group (UK) Ltd, Croydon, CR0 4YY

03/10/2024

01040367-0020